Surgical Management of Eld

Antonio Crucitti
Editor

Surgical Management of Elderly Patients

sicg
società italiana
chirurgia geriatrica

Springer

Editor
Antonio Crucitti
Department of General and Mininvasive Surgery
Cristo Re Hospital
Rome, Italy

ISBN 978-3-030-09656-4 ISBN 978-3-319-60861-7 (eBook)
https://doi.org/10.1007/978-3-319-60861-7

Softcover re-print of the Hardcover 1st edition 2018

Printed on acid-free paper

This Springer imprint is published by the registered company Springer International Publishing AG part of Springer Nature
The registered company address is: Gewerbestrasse 11, 6330 Cham, Switzerland

To my wife Fiorella, driving force, sense, and sensibility of my life

Foreword

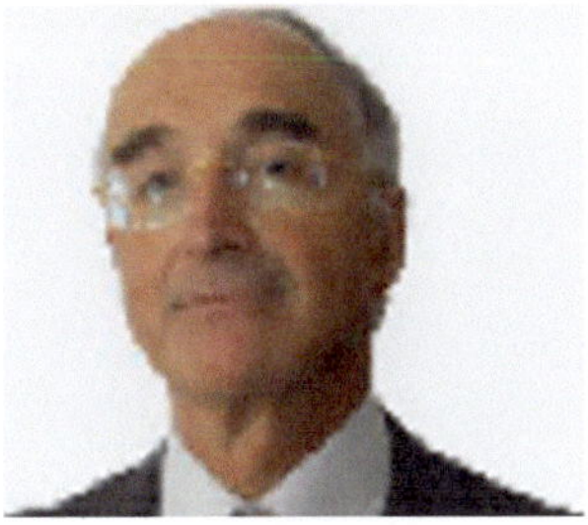

It's with great pleasure that I present this book *Surgical Management of Elderly Patients* by Antonio Crucitti, President of the Italian Society of Geriatric Surgery.

I think the editor and all the other distinguished contributors have to be commended for their efforts to put together a complete and exhaustive list of topics covering the entire spectrum of surgical diseases in the elderly patient.

Geriatric surgery is not to be intended as a new surgical specialty, since most surgeons already act as "geriatric surgeons," due to the constant increase of elderly population and the need to face surgical problems even in the very old patients.

So it's timely and very useful to assemble a comprehensive book that will allow the entire surgical community and other healthcare providers to understand the issues involved in choosing surgery as a treatment option for their patients.

I'm quite sure that this text will find its definite place in the bookshelf of all surgeons.

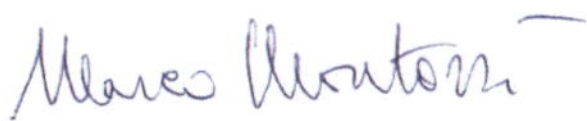

Marco Montorsi
President of the ITALIAN SOCIETY of Surgery
Rozzano, Italy

Preface

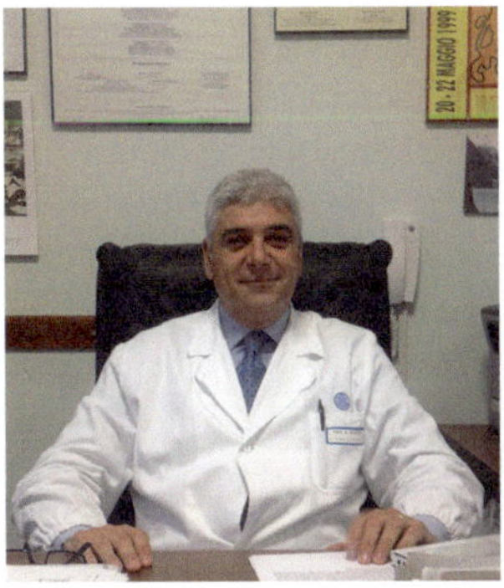

The geriatric population is incredibly increasing worldwide.

Europe and many other countries in the world are currently facing increasingly complex and systemic societal challenges. Due to healthcare advances, increased wealth, improved well-being, and living standards, life expectancy has dramatically increased during these past decades. The world will have more people who live to see their 80s or 90s than ever before, even because we are attending the baby boomer generation growing and becoming older.

It is projected that between 2010 and 2060, the number of Europeans aged over 65 will double, from 88 to 153 million (about 30% of the EU population will be aged 65 + [14]). The rise of the "oldest old" is the fastest-growing part of the total population, since those over 80 will nearly triple, from 24 to 62 million.

What happens in Europe is the counterpart of a global situation: the world's population aged 65 and over is projected to grow from 524 million to nearly 1.5 billion between the years 2010 and 2050. The number of people aged 65 or older will outnumber children under age 5, and this population aging is not only going to continue but also accelerate.

This impressive growing prompted us, as health operators, to propose continuous and adaptable clinical routes, especially related to geriatric patients. It's time for us all to focus on approved protocols, shared clinical course, and referring centers dedicated to geriatric evaluation, with closed relations with public or academic hospitals or territorial centers, to better select surgical candidates.

We all must also be ready to recognize that multiparametric evaluation has to be related to surgical procedures; we need to create a trans-institutional relationship and multidisciplinary models that have to consider old-aged criticisms during their route, not only gaining their health status or social value but also preserving their quality of life.

Only through these modalities could we reach real advantages, considering the growing "health needs" and the more specific surgical issues, approaching these "frailty" and "demanding" patients, with new comprehensive eyes and not only from an exclusively surgical point of view.

The purpose of this book is to provide an updated, synthetic guide on the most important surgical pathologies of the elderly. Here is also supplied an essential contribution from geriatrician and anesthesiologists, and a particular focus is also present on hemostasis and thrombosis and vascular and emergency surgery.

I sincerely thank the Board of the Italian Society of Geriatric Surgeons, for its support in writing this book.

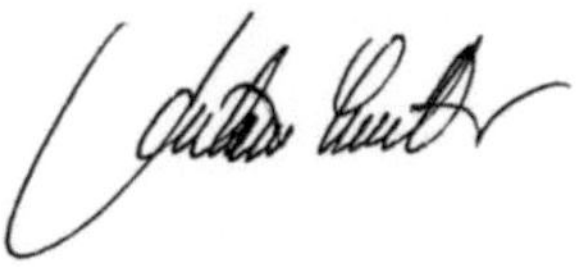

Rome, Italy
October 6, 2017

Antonio Crucitti
President of the Italian Society of Geriatric Surgeons
Rome, Italy

Contents

Part III Gastrointestinal System

Part IV Vascular Disorders

Contributors

Sergio Alfieri Department of Digestive Surgery, Catholic University, "A. Gemelli" Hospital, Rome, Italy

Bruno Amato Dipartimento Medicina Clinica e Chirurgia, Università degli studi di Napoli Federico II, Naples, Italy

Binda Gian Andrea Department of Surgery, Galliera Hospital, Genoa, Italy

Giulio Angelini E.O. Ospedali Galliera, Genova, Italy

Luca Ansaloni Unit of General and Emergency Surgery, Papa Giovanni XXIII Hospital, Bergamo, Italy

Nicola Avenia General and Endocrine Surgery Unit, S. Maria University Hospital, University of Perugia, Terni, Italy

Gianandrea Baldazzi Department of General Minimally-invasive and Robotic Surgery, Policlinic of Abano Terme, Padua, Italy

Maddalena Baraghini Department of Surgical Sciences, "Sapienza"—University of Rome, Rome, Italy

Andrea Barberis E.O. Ospedali Galliera, Genova, Italy

Francesco Basile Department of Surgery and Medical-Surgical Specialties, Surgical Clinic, Vittorio-Emanuele University Hospital of Catania, Catania, Italy

Guido Basile Department of Surgery and Medical-Surgical Specialties, Emergency Abdominal Surgery Unit, University Hospital of Catania, University of Catania, Catania, Italy

Domenico Benevento Department of Medicine, Surgery and Neurosciences, Vascular and Endovascular Unit, Siena University, Siena, Italy

Carlo Bergamini General, Emergency and Minimally Invasive Surgery Unit, Careggi University Hospital, Florence, Italy

Camilla Bing General Surgery Department, San Giuseppe Hospital, Empoli, Italy

Antonio Biondi Department of Surgery and Medical-Surgical Specialties, Surgical Clinic, Vittorio-Emanuele University Hospital of Catania, Catania, Italy

Silvestro Canonico Department of Medical, Surgical, Neurological, Metabolic and Geriatric Sciences, University of Campania Region "Luigi Vanvitelli", Caserta, Italy

Laura Capoccia Vascular and Endovascular Surgery, Department of Surgery "Paride Stefanini", "Policlinico Umberto I", "Sapienza" Università di Roma, Rome, Italy

Fausto Catena Department of Emergency Surgery, Maggiore Hospital, Parma, Italy

Roberto Cirocchi General Surgical and Surgical Oncology Unit, University of Perugia, Perugia, Italy

Federico Coccolini Unit of General and Emergency Surgery, Papa Giovanni XXIII Hospital, Bergamo, Italy

Anna Claudia Colangelo General Surgery Residency Program of the University of Padua, Padua, Italy

Francesco Colombo General Surgery, Department of Medical Sciences L. Sacco, University of Milan, Milan, Italy

Graziamaria Corbi Department of Medicine and Health Sciences, University of Molise, Campobasso, Italy

Antonio Corcione Dipartimento Area Critica A.O.R.N. dei Colli, Monaldi - Cotugno – CTO, Naples, Italy

UOC Anestesia e TIPO, Ospedale Monaldi, Naples, Italy

Antonio Crucitti Department of General and Mini-invasive Surgery, Cristo Re Hospital, Rome, Italy

Simone Cuozzo Vascular and Endovascular Surgery, Department of Surgery "Paride Stefanini", "Policlinico Umberto I", "Sapienza" Università di Roma, Rome, Italy

Alessandro d'Adamo Vascular and Endovascular Surgery, Department of Surgery "Paride Stefanini", "Policlinico Umberto I", "Sapienza" Università di Roma, Rome, Italy

Cassini Diletta Department of General Minimally-invasive and Robotic Surgery, Policlinic of Abano Terme, Padua, Italy

Giovanni Battista Doglietto Department of Digestive Surgery, Catholic University, "A. Gemelli" Hospital, Rome, Italy

Marcello Donati Department of Surgery and Medical-Surgical Specialties, Surgical Clinic, Vittorio-Emanuele University Hospital of Catania, Catania, Italy

Giuseppe de Donato Department of Medicine, Surgery and Neurosciences, Vascular and Endovascular Unit, Siena University, Siena, Italy

Anna Falanga Division of Immunohematology and Transfusion Medicine, Thrombosis and Hemostasis Center, Hospital Papa Giovanni XXIII, Bergamo, Italy

Massimo De Falco Department of Medical, Surgical, Neurological, Metabolic and Geriatric Sciences, University of Campania Region "Luigi Vanvitelli", Caserta, Italy

Federico Fazio E.O. Ospedali Galliera, Genova, Italy

Nicola Ferrara Department of Translational Medical Sciences, Federico II University of Naples, Naples, Italy

Marco Filauro E.O. Ospedali Galliera, Genova, Italy

Martina Formiconi Vascular and Endovascular Surgery, Department of Surgery "Paride Stefanini", "Policlinico Umberto I", "Sapienza" Università di Roma, Rome, Italy

Diego Foschi General Surgery, Department of Medical Sciences L. Sacco, University of Milan, Milan, Italy

Stefano de Franciscis Department of Medical and Surgical Sciences, Interuniversity Center of Phlebolymphology (CIFL), International Research and Educational, Program in Clinical and Experimental Biotechnology, University Magna Graecia of Catanzaro, Catanzaro, Italy

Marsilio Francucci General Surgery and Day Surgery Unit, Hospital of Terni, Terni, Italy

Paola Fugazzola General, Emergency and Trauma Surgery Department, Papa Giovanni XXIII Hospital, Bergamo, Italy

Francesco Gabrielli Department of General Surgery, University of Milan Bicocca, Zucchi Hospital, Monza, Italy

Erico Gallitto Vascular Surgery - Bologna University, Bologna, Italy

Giuseppe Galzerano Department of Medicine, Surgery and Neurosciences, Vascular and Endovascular Unit, Siena University, Siena, Italy

Antonio Gasbarrini Internal Medicine, Gastroenterology and Hepatology, Agostino Gemelli Hospital, Rome, Italy

Giulia Gibiino Internal Medicine, Gastroenterology and Hepatology, Agostino Gemelli Hospital, Rome, Italy

Massimiliano Walter Guerrieri Department of Medicine, Surgery and Neurosciences, Vascular and Endovascular Unit, Siena University, Siena, Italy

Angelo Guttadauro Department of General Surgery, University of Milan Bicocca, Zucchi Hospital, Monza, Italy

Louis Banka Johnson Department of Colorectal Surgery, University Hospital of Malmoe-Lund, SUS, Lund, Sweden

Maria Agnese Kelly Department of Colorectal Diseases, St. Vincent's University Hospital, Dublin, Ireland

Klara Komici Department of Translational Medical Sciences, Federico II University of Naples, Naples, Italy

Domenico Landi General and Day Surgery Unit, AOU San Giovanni di Dio e Ruggi d'Aragona, Department of Medicine Surgery and Dentistry, University of Salerno, Salerno, Italy

Renata Lorenzetti Geriatric Surgery Unit, University of Padua, Padua, Italy

Monaco Luigi General and Laparoscopic Surgery, Nursing Home Villa Esther Avellino, Avellino, Italy

Ileana Maria Luppino Gastroenterology and Endoscopy Unit, AO Annunziata, Cosenza, Italy

Wassim Mansour Vascular and Endovascular Surgery, Department of Surgery "Paride Stefanini", "Policlinico Umberto I", "Sapienza" Università di Roma, Rome, Italy

Cristina Marmorale Formazione in Chirurgia Generale—Ospedali Riuniti di Ancona, Ancona, Italy

Direttrice della Scuola di Specialità in Chirurgia Generale—Università Politecnica delle Marche, Ancona, Italy

Bruno Martella Geriatric Surgery Unit, University of Padua, Padua, Italy

Chiara Mascoli Vascular Surgery - Bologna University, Bologna, Italy

Matteo Maternini Department of General Surgery, University of Milan Bicocca, Zucchi Hospital, Monza, Italy

Franco Mazzalai General Surgery, Treviso Hospital, Treviso, Italy

Andrea Mazzari Department of General and Mini-invasive Surgery, Cristo Re Hospital, Rome, Italy

Maria Agnese Mele Department of Medicine, Surgery and Neurosciences, Vascular and Endovascular Unit, Siena University, Siena, Italy

Cecilia Merli Unit of Emergency Medicine, Papa Giovanni XXIII Hospital, Bergamo, Italy

Dario Di Miceli Department of Digestive Surgery, Catholic University, "A. Gemelli" Hospital, RomeItaly

Viola Milesi Division of Immunohematology and Transfusion Medicine, Thrombosis and Hemostasis Center, Hospital Papa Giovanni XXIII, Bergamo, Italy

Carmelo Militello Geriatric Surgery Unit, University of Padua, Padua, Italy

Giulia Montori General, Emergency and Trauma Surgery Department, Papa Giovanni XXIII Hospital, Bergamo, Italy

Mario Nano University of Turin—Honorary President of the Italian Society of Geriatric Surgery, Orbassano, Turin, Italy

Di Martino Natale Division of General and Gastroenterologic surgery, University of Campania "Luigi Vanvitelli", Naples, Italy

Giulio Orlando University Magna Graecia of Catanzaro, Catanzaro, Italy

Giulia Pacella General and Day Surgery Unit, AOU San Giovanni di Dio e Ruggi d'Aragona, Department of Medicine Surgery and Dentistry, University of Salerno, Salerno, Italy

Piergaspare Palumbo Department of Surgical Sciences, "Sapienza"—University of Rome, Rome, Italy

Baggi Paolo Unit of General and Emergency Surgery, Papa Giovanni XXIII Hospital, Bergamo, Italy

Nicoletta Pecora Department of General Surgery, University of Milan Bicocca, Zucchi Hospital, Monza, Italy

Gianluca Pellino Unit of General and Geriatric Surgery, I Policlinico, Università degli Studi della Campania "Luigi Vanvitelli", Naples, Italy

Federico Perrone Department of General and Mini-invasive Surgery, Cristo Re Hospital, Rome, Italy

Gennaro Perrone Department of Emergency Surgery, Maggiore Hospital, Parma, Italy

Dario Piazzalunga Unit of General and Emergency Surgery, Papa Giovanni XXIII Hospital, Bergamo, Italy

Rodolfo Pini Vascular Surgery - Bologna University, Bologna, Italy

Vanessa Polenta Clinica Chirurgica—Ospedali Riuniti di Ancona, Ancona, Italy

Andrea Polistena General and Endocrine Surgery Unit, S. Maria University Hospital, University of Perugia, Terni, Italy

Andrea Polistena Unit of Endocrine Surgery, Department of Surgical Sciences, School of Medicine University of Perugia, Terni, Italy

Francesca Romana Ponziani Internal Medicine, Gastroenterology and Hepatology, Agostino Gemelli Hospital, Rome, Italy

Chiara Pranteda Vascular and Endovascular Surgery, Department of Surgery "Paride Stefanini", "Policlinico Umberto I", "Sapienza" Università di Roma, Rome, Italy

Giorgia Prestigiacomo Department of Surgical Sciences, "Sapienza"—University of Rome, Rome, Italy

Alessandro Puzziello General and Day Surgery Unit, AOU San Giovanni di Dio e Ruggi d'Aragona, Department of Medicine Surgery and Dentistry, University of Salerno, Salerno, Italy

Emanuele Rausa Unit of General and Emergency Surgery, Papa Giovanni XXIII Hospital, Bergamo, Italy

Giuseppe Rengo Department of Translational Medical Sciences, Federico II University of Naples, Naples, Italy

Nascimbeni Riccardo Department of Molecular and Translational Medicine, University of Brescia, Brescia, Italy

Fausto Rosa Department of Digestive Surgery, Catholic University, "A. Gemelli" Hospital, Rome, Italy

Gianluca Sampietro General Surgery, Department of Medical Sciences L. Sacco, University of Milan, Milan, Italy

Sergio Sandrucci Sarcoma Unit, Città Della Salute e della Scienza, S. Giovanni Battista Hospital, University of Turin, Turin, Italy

Alessandro Sanguinetti Unit of Endocrine Surgery, Department of Surgical Sciences, School of Medicine University of Perugia, Terni, Italy

Giuseppe Santangelo Department of Medical, Surgical, Neurological, Metabolic and Geriatric Sciences, University of Campania Region "Luigi Vanvitelli", Caserta, Italy

Massimo Sartelli Department of Surgery, Macerata Hospital, Macerata, Italy

General and Emergency Surgery, Macerata Hospital, Macerata, Italy

Salomone Di Saverio Department of Surgery, Maggiore Hospital, Bologna, Italy

Marco Scatizzi Chief Surgical Dept. Usl 4 - Prato, Florence, Italy

Via Alessandro Serpieri, 13, 00197, Rome, Italy

Francesco Selvaggi Unit of General and Geriatric Surgery, I Policlinico, Università degli Studi della Campania "Luigi Vanvitelli", Naples, Italy

Raffaele Serra Department of Medical and Surgical Sciences, Interuniversity Center of Phlebolymphology (CIFL), International Research and Educational, Program in Clinical and Experimental Biotechnology, University Magna Graecia of Catanzaro, Catanzaro, Italy

Carlo Setacci Department of Medicine, Surgery and Neurosciences, Vascular and Endovascular Unit, Siena University, Siena, Italy

Francesco Setacci Department of Medicine, Surgery and Neurosciences, Vascular and Endovascular Unit, Siena University, Siena, Italy

Federico Sicoli Department of General and Mini-invasive Surgery, Cristo Re Hospital, Rome, Italy

Pasqualino Sirignano Vascular and Endovascular Surgery, Department of Surgery "Paride Stefanini", "Policlinico Umberto I", "Sapienza" Università di Roma, Rome, Italy

Mario Solej University of Turin, San Luigi Gonzaga University Hospital, Turin, Italy

Alessia Sonetto Vascular Surgery - Bologna University, Bologna, Italy

Francesco Speziale Vascular and Endovascular Surgery, Department of Surgery "Paride Stefanini", "Policlinico Umberto I", "Sapienza" Università di Roma, Rome, Italy

Andrea Stella Vascular Surgery - Bologna University University, Bologna, Italy

Pasquina Tomaiuolo Department of General and Mini-invasive Surgery, Cristo Re Hospital, Rome, Italy

Concezione Tommasino Department of Biomedical, Surgical and Odontoiatric Sciences, University of Milano, Milan, Italy

ASST Santi Paolo e Carlo University Hospital, Milan, Italy

Andrea Valeri General, Emergency and Minimally Invasive Surgery Unit

Careggi University Hospital, Florence, Italy

Roberto Vergari Clinica Chirurgica—Ospedali Riuniti di Ancona, Ancona, Italy

Fernando Vicinanza General and Day Surgery Unit, AOU San Giovanni di Dio e Ruggi d'Aragona, Department of Medicine Surgery and Dentistry, University of Salerno, Salerno, Italy

Marina Vinciguerra General Surgery and Day Surgery Unit, Hospital of Terni, Terni, Italy

Part I

General Principles and Epidemiology

Aging: from Demography to Epidemiology

1

Nicola Ferrara, Klara Komici, Giuseppe Rengo, and Graziamaria Corbi

1.1 Demographic Aspects of Aging

Aging of the worldwide population is progressively increasing, in relation to augmented life expectancy (LE), which in 2016 was around 71.4 years according to the World Health Organization (WHO), with a greater expectation in women than men all over the world [1]. Today, for the first time in history, even in less developed countries, most people can expect to live for more than 60 years, especially because of the reduction in childhood mortality [2], while in high-income countries, it is mainly due to the increase in life expectancy of over 60-year-old individuals [3, 4]. Currently, it has been estimated that life expectancy of 60-year-old people rose from 18.7 years in 2000 to 20.4 years in 2015, with different regional rates. In particular, 12 European countries, including Italy, in 2015 showed a life expectancy that exceeded 82 years of age, with women living longer than men in every part of the world [1]. In 2016, WHO data underlined that LE was 73.8 years for women and 69.1 years for men, quite similar to 2015 data [1].

In Europe, Eurostat data demonstrated that in 2015 over 65-year-old persons represented 18.9% of the total population [5], with an expected increase to a peak of 525.5 million around 2050 followed by a gradual decline to 520 million in 2080 [6]. The comparison of 2015 and 2080 data projection shows that Europe's population will continue to age, especially because of the "baby boomer" progressive aging [6]. Importantly, the progressive aging of the older population itself should be considered, given the increase at a faster rate of the over 80-year-old population, which is expected to double between 2015 and 2080, rising from 5.3 to 12.3%. As a result of these population changes between different age groups, the old-age dependency

N. Ferrara (✉) • K. Komici • G. Rengo
Department of Translational Medical Sciences, Federico II University of Naples, Naples, Italy
e-mail: nicola.ferrara@sigg.it

G. Corbi
Department of Medicine and Health Sciences, University of Molise, Campobasso, Italy

A. Crucitti (ed.), *Surgical Management of Elderly Patients*,
https://doi.org/10.1007/978-3-319-60861-7_1

ratio (the ratio between the elderly population and the working age population (15–64)) is projected to change from 28.8% in 2015 to 51.0% by 2080 [6]. The Italian Institute of Statistics (IIS) showed that in 2016, Italy was at third place in Europe for longevity, with a LE of 84.7 years for women and 80.1 years for men, and the prediction for 2065 reached 91.5 years for women and 86.6 years for men [7].

Beyond LE if we consider health life expectancy (HLE), it is clear that between the two parameters there is a gap. HLE provides a comprehensive indicator of health in a population, representing the average number of years in full health that a newborn could expect to live considering the specific mortality rates by age and average age-specific levels of health status for a given period [8]. Globally it is estimated that in 2015 the global HLE was 63.1 years for both women and men. The gap between LE and HLE is the equivalent of the years spent in comorbidity and disability [8]. The main factors contributing to these conditions are represented by chronic diseases (particularly depression, neurological disorders, loss of vision and hearing, cardiovascular disease, and diabetes) [1]. The majority of these conditions increase with age, and for many of them, the prevalence, even after correction for age, does not tend to decline. Therefore, the proportion of years spent in illness increases, with a consequent slower increase of HLE compared to LE [1]. In 2016, the WHO has calculated that the HLE was 61.5 years for men and 64.6 years for women with substantial gender differences in all regions of the world [1]. In Italy, beyond the longevity, the quality of survival is also improved, particularly among young seniors (65–74 years) [9], with 65-year-old subjects expected to experience a LE without functional limitations of 12.7 years for men and 14.2 for women in 1994, compared to the 15.5 years for men and 16.2 for women reached in 2013 [9].

1.2 Epidemiological Aspects of Aging

According to WHO data in 2016, noncommunicable chronic diseases were the main cause of health loss in more than half of cases [10]. Eurostat data shows that the elderly (≥65 years old) represented more than 2/5 (42.2%) of all disabled persons in the European Union in 2012 [11], with a probability of 4.2 times higher for the presence of disability in subjects ≥65 years compared to those aged between 15 and 44 years [11]. In Italy, in 2013 the first generation of "baby boomers" arrived at the old-age threshold in better health condition than previous generations: functional limitation is lower and also the self-reporting of "feeling bad or very bad" [9]. Aging itself determines an overall increasing level of chronic diseases in the elderly, although analysis of generation reports that particularly among young seniors (65–74 years) [9], the presence of serious chronic diseases is diminishing over the years, primarily as a result of preventive measures implemented in recent years. In 2015, IIS data showed that 24.8% of over 75-year-old persons enjoy good health, while 85.2 and 65.4% are, respectively, affected by at least one or two chronic diseases. Among over 75-year-old subjects with chronic diseases, 20.4% appear to be in good health [12], although 88.1% of them report at least one drug use in the last 2 days [13]. From 2011 to 2015, we find an increase in the use of drugs: in over 65-year-old subjects from 79.6% in 2011 to 82.1% in 2015 [14], with an increase in consumption also in relationship to age (75.8% in subjects 65–74 years against 88.1% of those over 75) [14]. As a result, drug-related adverse events in general practice are an important cause of morbidity and are thought to be responsible for 10–30% of all hospital admissions in older patients [15]. Importantly different studies have shown that 52.3% of elderly patients use an inappropriate drug therapy [16]. The 2015 OSMED report shows that 44.8% of reported adverse drug reactions (excluding vaccines) relate to subjects of ≥65 years [17].

With regard to hospitalization frequency, although the total number of hospital admissions has been reduced (by over 12.8 million in 2001 to 9.4 million in 2014) (−26.7%), affecting only the component of acute care hospitalization (−29.2%), which is the main reason for admission (91.1% in 2014), in the geriatric population, 45.1% of men ≥65 years (24.7% in those ≥75 years) and 40.8% of women of the same age (23.9% in those ≥75 years) appeared to have been hospitalized in 2014 [18]. Furthermore, in contrary to what occurs in the general population, by comparison with 2001, in 2014 admissions of persons ≥75 years had an increased cost: equal to 7.3% in men and stable in women, because of disease severity [18].

With regard to "frailty," its definition has been debated for a long time in the context of geriatrics [19–23]. According to Fried, frailty can be defined as a condition characterized by a reduction in the functional reserve with an age-dependent increase of vulnerability (so-called preclinical frailty) [21]. Acute events, which in non-vulnerable subjects are easily managed, may precipitate the clinical conditions of patients with preclinical frailty. A typical example of an acute event, which can achieve a critical framework in a fragile subject, is represented by the glyco-metabolic decompensation of both hyper- and hypoglycemic types. For these reasons these subjects need a more careful monitoring of the glyco-metabolic compensation.

The preclinical frailty framework is further aggravated in presence of particular characteristics of clinical frailty including comorbidity, polypharmacy with the relative high risk of iatrogenic damage, social and economic problems, and characteristics that lead inexorably toward a severe disability framework. Such a clinical phenotype has been proposed by Rockwood et al. [24] that focuses on the disease at the center of frailty.

In this framework diabetes and its complications play a central role in determining frailty.

The indices of Fried [19] and Rockwood [22] certainly represent the most used indexes in the definition of frailty, but they have also had more confirmations from the point of view of prognostic value in the literature.

Fried's index (Table 1.1) is used to define the fragile phenotype in preclinical phase. Recently Op et al. [25] reported that in 8684 elderly patients, this tool effectively discriminated the social, psychological, and functional treatment of vulnerable subjects, allowing a better definition and treatment. In addition, several studies confirm its prognostic value in falls, disability, fractures, and death [26].

Frailty in the clinical index of Rockwood was constructed by counting the number of deficits accumulated over time, within a very extensive list of 70 clinical deficits (Table 1.2).

Table 1.1 Definition of preclinical frailty phenotype (*modified*) [24]

(A) Characteristics of frailty
Weight loss (unintentional)
Sarcopenia (muscle mass loss)
Weakness
Poor endurance
Low activity
(B) Cardiovascular health study measures
>4.5 kg (10 lbs) in the year before the current evaluation or unintentional weight loss of at least 5% of the previous year's body weight
Grip strength of the dominant hand lower than 20% (for sex, body mass index)
Self-reported exhaustion
Reduced energy consumption
Kcal/week: lower than 20%
M: <383 kcal/week
F: <270 kcal/week
(C) Presence of frailty
Frail phenotype: ≥3 positive criteria

Table 1.2 Frailty hypothesis of Rockwood (*modified*) [27]

1. Very fit. People who are robust, active, energetic, well motivated, and fit; these people commonly exercise regularly and are the fittest for the age
2. Well. People without active disease symptoms, but less fit than category 1. Often, they exercise or are very active occasionally, e.g., seasonally
3. Managing well. People whose medical problems are well controlled, but are not regularly active beyond routine walking
4. Vulnerable. While not dependent on others for daily help, often symptoms limit activities. A common complaint is being "slowed up" and/or being tired during the day
5. Mildly frail. These people often have more evident slowing and need help in high-order IADLs (finances, transportation, medications, heavy housework). Typically, mildly frail progressively impairs shopping and walking outside alone, meal preparation, and housework
6. Moderately frail. People need help with all outside activities and with keeping house. Inside they have problems with stairs and need help with bathing and might need minimal assistance (cuing, standby) with dressing
7. Severely frail. Completely dependent for personal care from whatever cause (physical or cognitive). Even so they seem stable and not at risk of dying (within 6 months)
8. Very severely frail. Completely dependent, approaching the end of life. Typically, they could not recover even from a minor illness
9. Terminally ill. Approaching the end of life. This category applies to people with a life expectancy <6 months, who are not otherwise evidently frail

It was developed based on a comprehensive geriatric assessment by counting the number of accumulated deficits, including diseases, physical and cognitive impairments, the psychosocial risk factors, and geriatric syndromes other than weakness [27, 28]. To consider a different variable as a deficit, it must be acquired, associated with age, and with a negative outcome. The total number of deficits that can be used is considered to be equal to 80, with 30–70 elements typically evaluated [29].

In comparison with Fried's index, Rockwood seems to be a more sensitive predictor for adverse health outcomes, due to its more finely graduated scale of risk and the inclusion of deficits that probably have causal relationships with adverse clinical outcomes [30].

Conclusions

To meet the challenges that demography and epidemiology are bringing to our societies, even those with a high standard of living, several care and health strategies that have been followed until now should be reviewed. In particular, the care interventions for the elderly, considered as frail and complex subjects, must be planned and implemented to be effective as part of a network of geriatric continuing care. Then interventions should respond to a multidisciplinary and multiprofessional logic and take place in organized and specialized structures, where the criterion for admission must not be related to age, but should be reserved mainly for the frail elderly, after a careful assessment performed using validated multidimensional tools.

References

1. WHO. World Health Statistics. Monitoring health for the SDGS (Sustainable Development Goals); 2016: http://www.who.int/gho/publications/world_health_statistics/2016/en/ (Accessed on 04 Jan 2017).
2. Bloom DE. 7 billion and counting. Science. 2011;333:562–9.
3. Olshansky SJ, Antonucci T, Berkman L, et al. Differences in life expectancy due to race and educational differences are widening, and many may not catch up. Health Aff. 2012;31:1803–13.
4. Beard JR, Officer A, de Carvalho IA, Sadana R, Pot AM, Michel JP, Lloyd-Sherlock P, Epping-Jordan JE, Peeters GM, Mahanani WR, Thiyagarajan JA, Chatterji S. The world report on ageing and health: a policy framework for healthy ageing. Lancet. 2016;387(10033):2145–54. https://doi.org/10.1016/S0140-6736(15)00516-4.
5. Eurostat. Dati 2016. http://ec.europa.eu/eurostat/tgm/refreshTableAction.do?tab=table&plugin=1&pcode=tps00010&language=en (Accessed on 04 Jan 2017).
6. Eurostat. Eurostat yearbook. statistics explained. http://ec.europa.eu/eurostat/statistics-explained/index.php/Population_structure_and_ageing (Accessed on 04 Jan 2017).
7. ISTAT. Popolazione. Italia in cifre edizione 2016. http://www.istat.it/it/archivio/popolazione-e-famiglie (Accessed on 04 Jan 2017).
8. WHO. An overarching health indicator for the post-2015 development agenda. Brief summary of some proposed candidate indicators. Background paper for expert consultation, 11–12 December 2014, Geneva: World Health Organization; 2014 (http://www.who.int/healthinfo/indicators/hsi_indicators_SDG_TechnicalMeeting_December2015_BackgroundPaper.pdf?ua=1).
9. ISTAT. Rapporto annuale 2016. La situazione del paese. http://www.istat.it/it/files/2016/05/Ra2016.pdf.
10. Benziger CP, Roth GA, Moran AE. The global burden of disease study and the preventable burden of NCD. Glob Heart. 2016;11(4):393–7. https://doi.org/10.1016/j.gheart.2016.10.024.
11. EUROSTAT. Disability statistics - prevalence and demographics; 2015. http://ec.europa.eu/eurostat/statistics-explained/index.php/Disability_statistics_-_prevalence_and_demographics#How_prevalent_are_activity_difficulties_and_disabilities.3F (Accessed on 06 Jan 2017).

12. ISTAT. Stato di salute: Classi di età. Salute e sanità I.Stat. http://dati.istat.it (Accessed on 03 Jan 2017).
13. ISTAT. Consumo di farmaci: Classi di età. Salute e sanità I.Stat. http://dati.istat.it (Accessed on 05 Jan 2017).
14. ISTAT. Italia in cifre 2016. http://www.istat.it/it/files/2016/12/ItaliaCifre2016.pdf Accessed on 07 Jan 2017).
15. Thomas R, Huntley AL, Mann M, et al. Pharmacist-led interventions to reduce unplanned admissions for older people: a systematic review and meta-analysis of randomised controlled trials. Age Ageing. 2014;43(2):174–87.
16. Corbi G, Gambassi G, Pagano G, Russomanno G, Conti V, Rengo G, Leosco D, Bernabei R, Filippelli A, Ferrara N. Impact of an innovative educational strategy on medication appropriate use and length of stay in elderly patients. Medicine (Baltimore). 2015;94(24):e918. https://doi.org/10.1097/MD.0000000000000918.
17. Osservatorio Nazionale sull'impiego dei farmaci -AIFA. L'uso dei farmaci in Italia. Rapporto Nazionale Anno 2015. http://www.agenziafarmaco.gov.it/sites/default/files/Rapporto_OsMed_2015.pdf.
18. WHO. Global report on diabetes. Executive summary, World Health Organization; 2016. www.who.int/diabetes/global-report (Accessed on 05 Jan 2017).
19. Brody KK, Johnson RE, Douglas RL. Evaluation of a self-report screening instrument to predict frailty outcomes in aging populations. Gerontologist. 1997;37:182–91.
20. Carlson JE, Zocchi KA, Bettencourt DM, Gambrel ML, Freeman JL, Zhang D, et al. Measuring frailty in the hospitalized elderly: concept of functional homeostasis. Am J Phys Med Rehabil. 1998;77:252–7.
21. Fried LP. Conference on the physiologic basis of frailty. April 28, 1992, Baltimore, Maryland, U.S.A. introduction. Aging Clin Exp Res. 1992;4:251–2.
22. Rockwood K, Fox RA, Stolee P, Robertson D, Beattie BL. Frailty in elderly people: an evolving concept. CMAJ. 1994;150:489–95.
23. Rockwood K, Hogan DB, MacKnight C. Conceptualization and measurement of frailty in elderly people. Drugs Aging. 2000;17:295–302.
24. Fried LP, Tangen CM, Walston J, Newman AB, Hirsh C, Gottdiener J, et al. Cardiovascular health study collaborative research group: frailty in older adults: evidence for a phenotype. J Gerontol A Biol Sci Med Sci. 2001;56A:M146–56.
25. Op het Veld LP, van Rossum E, Kempen GI, de Vet HC, Hajema K, Beurskens AJ. Fried phenotype of frailty: cross-sectional comparison of three frailty stages on various health domains. BMC Geriatr. 2015;15:77. https://doi.org/10.1186/s12877-015-0078-0.
26. Ensrud KE, Ewing SK, Taylor BC, Fink HA, Cawthon PM, Stone KL, Hillier TA, Cauley JA, Hochberg MC, Rodondi N, Tracy JK, Cummings SR. Comparison of 2 frailty indexes for prediction of falls, disability, fractures, and death in older women. Arch Intern Med. 2008;168(4):382–9. https://doi.org/10.1001/archinternmed.2007.113.
27. Rockwood K, Song X, MacKnight C, Bergman H, Hogan DB, McDowell I, Mitnitski A. A global clinical measure of fitness and frailty in elderly people. CMAJ. 2005;173(5):489–95.
28. Jones DM, Song X, Rockwood K. Operationalizing a frailty index from a standardized comprehensive geriatric assessment. J Am Geriatr Soc. 2004;52(11):1929–33.
29. Searle SD, Mitnitski A, Gahbauer EA, Gill TM, Rockwood K. A standard procedure for creating a frailty index. BMC Geriatr. 2008;8:24. https://doi.org/10.1186/1471-2318-8-24.
30. Rockwood K, Mitnitski A. Frailty defined by deficit accumulation and geriatric medicine defined by frailty. Clin Geriatr Med. 2011;27:17–26.

Anesthesia for the Elderly Patient

2

Concezione Tommasino and Antonio Corcione

2.1 Introduction

In Europe, the elderly population (≥65 years of age) will account for 30% of the population by 2060 [1]. Advances and improvement in medical science have increased life expectancy for most people, and according to the latest World Health Organization (WHO) data, life expectancy in Italy is very high, being 82.7 years (male 80.5, female 84.8 years). Although the mechanisms that control the aging process and life span remain unknown, we can speculate that a very important factor contributing to the Italian longevity is the healthcare system, which is ranked second according to WHO and which has the third best medical performance worldwide.

In parallel with the increasing longevity of the population, the volume of surgery is growing rapidly, and anesthesia in the elderly patient has become an extremely important issue, mostly because this segment of the population is the most vulnerable and is likely to have the highest number of comorbidities, to suffer from frailty, and to have diminishing physiological reserve.

C. Tommasino
Department of Biomedical, Surgical and Odontoiatric Sciences, University of Milano, Milan, Italy

Anesthesia and Intensive Care, ASST Santi Paolo e Carlo University Hospital, Via di Rudinì 8, 20142 Milan, Italy
e-mail: concezione.tommasino@unimi.it

A. Corcione (✉)
Dipartimento Area Critica A.O.R.N. dei Colli, Monaldi - Cotugno – CTO, Naples, Italy

UOC Anestesia e TIPO, Ospedale Monaldi, Via L. Bianchi 1, 80131 Naples, Italy
e-mail: antonio.corcione@libero.it

A. Crucitti (ed.), *Surgical Management of Elderly Patients*,
https://doi.org/10.1007/978-3-319-60861-7_2

In order to minimize the perioperative adverse events, anesthesiologists need to focus on the risks related to the operative procedure, the anesthetic and analgesic techniques, and the patient's underlying medical, physical, and functional condition.

2.2 Physiology Considerations in the Geriatric Patient

Aging is a universal physiological phenomenon, associated with a progressive loss of functional reserve in all organs and systems; however, the extent and onset of these changes vary significantly from patient to patient. Understanding of the physiological consequences of aging represents one of the prerequisites to administer good anesthetic care to elderly patients.

Every major organ system experiences physiological changes, which result mostly in cognitive impairments (nervous system), higher blood pressures and lower cardiac output (cardiovascular system), reduction of arterial oxyhemoglobin (respiratory system), delayed gastric emptying and reduction of hepatic metabolism (gastrointestinal system and liver), and reduced glomerular filtration rate (renal system) (Fig. 2.1). These physiological changes, mostly when combined with coexisting diseases, create a very complex condition [2].

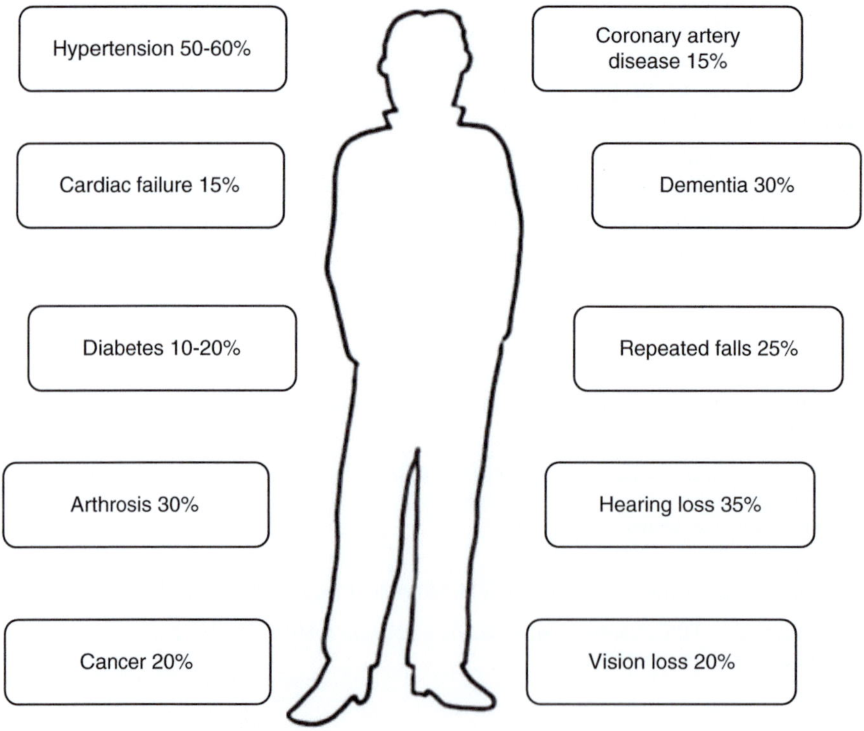

Fig. 2.1 Frequency of main comorbidities in elderly patients

2.3 Central Nervous System (CNS)

The CNS is the target organ for almost every anesthetic drug, and age-related alterations in CNS have unquestionable implications for anesthesia care. Aging universally produces a reduction in neuronal density, and the volume of the brain declines by almost 5% per decade, after age 40. There is a greater loss of white matter, and neuronal cell death is believed to be the main reason for the reduction of gray matter. Coupling of cerebral electrical activity, cerebral metabolic rate, and cerebral blood flow remains intact in older individuals in the absence of disease, as well as autoregulation and cerebrovascular response to CO_2 and hypoxemia. However, there is a depletion of brain neurotransmitters (acetylcholine, dopamine, serotonin, brain-derived neurotrophic factor) that could explain the reduced synaptic plasticity regulation and neurogenesis. These changes may partly be responsible for depression, loss of memory, and motor dysfunction in elderly patients. Increasing age is associated with increasing blood-brain barrier permeability (likely because of endothelial glycocalyx alterations), allowing inappropriate passage of mediators from the plasma into the CNS. This may result in an increased inflammatory response and structural damage in the brain, as well as altered patterns of neuronal activity, by modulating synthesis of neurotransmitters and changing expression of neurotransmitter receptors [3]. Cognitive decline does not always accompany aging but it is common. Slowed reaction time and cognitive processing and impaired short-term memory are very frequent in elderly patients.

2.4 Peripheral Nervous System (PNS)

Aging deeply influences several morphologic and functional features of the PNS. In older individuals, there is a reduction in the number of neurons within the spinal cord, and the diameter and number of myelinated fibers in the dorsal and ventral nerve roots are decreased. In peripheral nerves, inter-Schwann cell distance is decreased, as is afferent and efferent conduction velocity [4]. These changes tend to make older individuals more sensitive to neuraxial and peripheral nerve blocks.

2.5 Cardiovascular and Autonomic Nervous System

Aging is one of the largest risk factors for the development of cardiovascular disease. The physiological alterations in structure and function of the autonomic nervous system, heart and blood vessels, affect cardiovascular performance and explain why hypertension and increased pulse pressure, ischemic heart disease, conduction abnormalities, and congestive heart failure are frequent in older patients. The most relevant age-related changes are the increased myocardium and vasculature stiffness, decreased beta-adrenergic responsiveness, and impaired autonomic reflex control of heart rate, all of which may have considerable consequences during cardiovascular stress [5] (Table 2.1). Arterial stiffening leads to systolic hypertension,

Table 2.1 Age-related cardiovascular changes and possible clinical impairments

Cardiovascular change	Pathophysiology	Clinical impairment
Cardiac		
• Increased myocardial stiffness • Altered conduction • Increased LA size	• Decrease LV compliance • Irregular conduction • Increased LA pressure/distension	• Dyspnea • Arrhytmias • Atrial fibrillation
Vascular		
• Increased vascular stiffness	• Increased aortic impedance	• Systolic hypertension, LV hypertrophy
Cardiovascular		
• Increased stiffness (myocardial and vascular)	• Decreased cardiovascular reserve	• Reduced excercise tolerance • Heart failure
+ Autonomic dysfunction + Decreased beta-adrenoreceptor responsiveness	• Decreased baroreceptor reflex activity	• Postural hypotension • Syncope

LA left atrium, *LV* left ventriculum. Modified from [5]

impaired impedance matching, and myocardial hypertrophy. Aortic valve sclerosis is common in older individuals and is associated with an increase in the risk for adverse cardiovascular and coronary events. Venous stiffening decreases the ability to buffer changes in blood volume and blood distribution and will impair the ability to keep preload constant. Impairment of diastolic relaxation leads to diastolic dysfunction, and diastolic heart failure (prevalent in females) is now recognized as heart failure with preserved ejection fraction [6]. Clinical diagnosis of diastolic dysfunction is difficult, since the clinical picture resembles left ventricular systolic failure, and echocardiography is the diagnostic modality of choice. Cardiac performance in the elderly depends on the preload; as a consequence of myocardium and vasculature stiffness, decreased beta-adrenergic responsiveness, and autonomic dysfunction, low preload can lead to fall in cardiac output and induce marked hypotension. On the other hand, an inappropriate high preload can precipitate left ventricular insufficiency, with pulmonary edema, dyspnea, and impaired oxygenation [5].

2.6 Respiratory System

The maximal functional status of the lungs is achieved in the third decade of life, after which lung function gradually declines [7]. Environmental factors and smoking are mostly responsible for the deterioration of lung function. Chronic obstructive pulmonary disease (COPD), pneumonia, and obstructive sleep apnea syndrome (OSAS) are very frequent in the elderly. Age-related generalized loss of the lung elastic recoil, increased chest wall rigidity, and decreased functional alveolar surface area lead to a decrease in vital capacity (about 30 mL/year), increase in residual volume, decrease in expiratory flows, and increase in ventilation-perfusion mismatch. Respiratory muscle strength declines, and the work of breathing increases. Arterial oxygen tension decreases progressively with age-induced ventilation-perfusion

Table 2.2 Normal values for arterial partial pressure of oxygen (PaO_2) according to age

Age (years)	PaO_2 mmHg (mean and range)
20–29	94 (84–104)
30–39	91 (81–101)
40–49	88 (78–98)
50–59	84 (74–94)
60–69	81 (71–91)
>70	80–85

mismatch and anatomical shunt [8] (Table 2.2). Gas exchange may be well preserved at rest; however, pulmonary reserve is diminished, and there is a decreased response to hypoxemia and hypercapnia. Increased sensitivity to respiratory depressants (narcotics) and muscle weakness pose additional risks for perioperative pulmonary complications in elderly patients, as well as under conditions of positive fluid balance, positioning for surgery, and increased metabolic demand.

2.7 Hepatic Function

Increased age is associated with a reduction in liver size (almost 50% by the age of 80 years) and blood flow (10% per decade) [9]. The production of albumin (binding for acidic drugs) by the liver is decreased, whereas alpha-1-acid glycoprotein (binding for basic drugs) level is increased, affecting plasma protein binding of specific drugs, and hepatic synthesis of cholinesterase is reduced, mostly in males. The reduced perfusion of the hepatic tissue may delay drug clearance, especially rapidly metabolized drugs.

2.8 Renal and Volume Regulation

Aging alters renal function affecting the renal vasculature, and the decline is more pronounced in males [10]. The number of functioning glomeruli declines, as well as the renal blood flow (by 10% per decade after 40 years), with reduction in responsiveness and autoregulation of volume status [10]. Because of the decreased muscle mass, serum creatinine is within normal limits, and it is a poor predictor of renal function. Glomerular filtration rate declines by 6–8% per decade (almost 50% by the age of 80 years). Consequently, drugs (or metabolites) that are primarily eliminated via the renal system have a longer half-life and reach higher peak levels, likely leading to toxicity. Medications that are renally cleared should have dosages adjusted, based on the patient's estimated glomerular filtration rate (eGFR):

$$\text{eGFR} = \left[(140 - \text{age}) \times \text{body weight}\,(\text{kg}) \times (0.85\text{ if female})\right] / \left[72 \times \text{serum creatinine}\,(\text{mg/dL})\right].$$

The renal/pituitary response to dehydration is compromised in elderly subjects, with reduced ability to concentrate the urine and to excrete an acid load. Decreased ability of the kidney to control electrolyte homeostasis, especially under stress, makes fluid and electrolyte balance challenging [10].

2.9 Gastrointestinal System

Geriatric individuals may have prolonged gastric emptying, which predisposes to higher risk for aspiration during anesthetic induction or in the postoperative period.

2.10 Pharmacokinetic and Pharmacodynamic Differences in the Elderly

Aging influences the pharmacologic responses to drugs, because of alterations in the absorption, distribution, metabolism, and excretion. Anesthetic agents, to some extent, are bound to plasma proteins; since in the elderly protein binding is less efficient, this will result in an exaggerated pharmacologic effect. Body composition changes with age, and there will be a progressive decrease in lean body mass, an increase in body fat (greater volume of distribution of lipophilic drugs), and a decrease in total body water (smaller central compartment and increased serum concentrations of hydrophilic drugs). As discussed previously, drug metabolism and clearance are reduced because of the effects of aging on the liver and kidney. All these factors will affect the drugs' pharmacokinetic and pharmacodynamic, and the anesthetic drug dosage needs to be adjusted accordingly [11] (Table 2.3).

2.11 Anesthetic Requirement

2.11.1 Inhaled Anesthetics

Older patients will generally require lower absolute doses of inhalational anesthetics to obtain equivalent anesthetic effects. The minimum alveolar concentration (MAC) decreases 6.7% per decade for most volatile agents [12] (Table 2.3), likely because of neurophysiological changes in the brain (ion channels, synaptic activity, or receptor sensitivity modifications). In the clinical setting, however, anesthesiologists tend to deliver higher age-adjusted doses of volatile anesthetics during maintenance of anesthesia in elderly patients, 3.8% less volatile anesthetics per decade rather than the recommended 6.7% [13], and this should not be the case since emerging, although controversial, evidence suggests that increased depth of anesthesia may be associated with postoperative cognitive dysfunction, delirium, and increased mortality [14]. The best strategy is to titrate volatile anesthetics with the assistance of depth of anesthesia monitoring [15].

Table 2.3 Suggested dose adjustments in geriatric patients for drugs frequently used in anesthesia

Drug	Adult dose	Geriatric dose
Propofol	• Bolus 2-2.5 mg/kg • Infusion 100-250 mcg/kg/min	• 1.2-1.7 mg/kg or 20% reduction in bolus dose • 30% reduction in infusion
Midazolam	0.2–0.3 mg/kg	• 0.05–0.15 mg/kg in premedicated patients • 20% reduction in patients aged >55 years • 75% reduction in patients aged > 90 years
Sevoflurane	MAC closest to age 40 = 2.1%	MAC is reduced by 6.7% per decade of increasing age • 60 years ≅ 1.6% • 70 years ≅ 1.5% • 80 years ≅ 1.4% • 90 years ≅ 1.3%
Desflurane	MAC closest to age 45 = 6.0%	MAC is reduced by 6.7% per decade of increasing age • 60 years ≅ 5.8% • 70 years ≅ 5.5% • 80 years ≅ 5.1% • 90 years ≅ 4.8%
Morphine	• 0.1–0.2 mg/kg intraoperatively • 1–2 mg boluses titrated to effect for acute postoperative analgesia	• 50% reduction in dose • No change
Fentanyl	1–2 mcg/kg for short-term analgesia	50% reduction in dose
Remifentanil	• Bolus 0.5–1 mcg/kg • Infusion 0.03–0.1 mcg/kg/min	• 50% reduction in bolus dose • 33% reduction in infusion dose

MAC minimum alveolar concentration, MAC values for geriatric patients from [12]

2.11.2 Intravenous Anesthetic Agents

Thiopental is not used in modern anesthesia and has been replaced by propofol, a rapid, short-acting alkylphenol. The brain becomes more sensitive to the effects of propofol with age [16], and for patients older than 60 years, the elimination clearance decreased linearly. Therefore, propofol dosing needs to be reduced (Table 2.3), mostly when administered with any other induction agent, narcotics or benzodiazepines, as anesthetic depth is synergistically increased. Induction dose with 1.0–1.5 mg/kg in the elderly produces a rapid onset of anesthesia (<1 min), lasting 5–10 min; the dose must be reduced to 0.5–1.0 mg/kg with opioids or when midazolam is given. The induction dose should be further reduced for patients over the age of 70–80 [17]. Propofol is a good choice because of rapid recovery time and few side effects. For example, patients older than 80 years exhibit less postanesthetic cognitive impairment as compared to other hypnotic agents.

Aging may influence sedation and cardiorespiratory functions in response to midazolam, a short-acting benzodiazepine, widely used as an anxiolytic, sedative, and anesthetic adjuvant. These effects are related to increased brain sensitivity and decreased drug clearance. A dosage of 0.02 mg/kg for preoperative sedation is effective in reducing anxiety, without compromising cardiorespiratory function [18]. Sedation with midazolam is safe and well tolerated in the elderly, provided that the dosage is reduced according to patient age (Table 2.3). Induction of general anesthesia with midazolam is feasible, and the dose should be 0.1–0.15 mg/kg, with further reduction to <0.1 mg/kg if synergistic drugs, such as opioids, are used.

2.11.3 Opioid Analgesics

Opioids suppress pain by their action in the brain, spinal cord, and peripheral nervous system and provide the analgesic component of anesthesia, especially during total intravenous anesthesia (TIVA). With age, the brain becomes more sensitive to opioids and older patients are more sensitive to the respiratory depressant effects of opioids.

Morphine is metabolized (>90%) mainly in the liver, with most of the conversion to morphine-3-glucuronide (M3G) and morphine-6-glucuronide (M6G, analgesic effects). Patients with renal insufficiency may have impaired elimination of morphine glucuronides, and this may account for some of the enhanced analgesia from a given dose of morphine in the older patient [19].

Sufentanil, alfentanil, and fentanyl are approximately twice as potent in older patients, and the dose requirements decrease by 50% over the age range 20–89 years [20] (Table 2.3). These findings are related to brain increased sensitivity to opioids with age, rather than alterations in pharmacokinetics [20].

Remifentanil, a relatively new synthetic opioid, is quickly hydrolyzed by nonspecific plasma and tissue esterases to essentially inactive compounds, which are excreted by the kidneys. Remifentanil has a context-sensitive half-time that is very short, is not influenced by hepatic or renal failure, and is also independent on the duration of infusion. In the older adults, remifentanil is approximately twice as potent. Minto et al., comparing 20- vs. 80-year-old patients, demonstrated an age-dependent reduction of both central compartment volume and clearance, and a much smaller remifentanil dose infusion is required in the elderly [21]. With the Minto model for target-controlled infusion of remifentanil, elderly patients receive less drug for a similar target concentration than younger patients of similar height and weight [22].

Although recommendations currently exist for intravenous dosing, recent studies have found that elderly patients are routinely given intravenous anesthetic drugs greater-than-recommended doses for their age, and this is associated with clinically significant hypotensive episodes (MAP < 60 mm Hg or reduction by >40% from baseline) [17, 23].

2.11.4 Neuromuscular Blocking Agents

Muscle relaxation is one of the components of balanced anesthesia. Aging can have significant effects on the pharmacokinetics of neuromuscular-blocking drugs, when the drug depends on liver or renal metabolism [24]. Intermediate-acting relaxants, vecuronium and rocuronium, which depend on end-organ elimination, may have a significantly prolonged duration of action in elderly patients, and appropriate changes must be made to drug dosage and dose intervals. Atracurium and cisatracurium, eliminated primarily by temperature-dependent, spontaneous Hoffman degradation, do not have prolonged duration. Recovery time is almost identical to young subjects, with no difference in dosage requirements in the elderly. Mivacurium action is prolonged, due to the decreased plasma acetylcholinesterase that accompanies aging. Short- to intermediate-acting muscle relaxants should be used in all elderly patients when extubation is planned at the end of the surgery. Pharmacological reversal of neuromuscular blockade must be a standard procedure in the geriatric population, since postoperative residual curarization may increase postoperative pulmonary complications, such as pneumonia and atelectasis [25].

2.11.5 Local Anesthetics

In the elderly, the response to local anesthetics is more intense [26]. With aging, there is a decline in the number of neurons within the spinal cord and slowing of conduction velocity in the peripheral nerves. A progressive sclerotic closure of the intervertebral foramina occurs with aging, and the epidural compliance increases, and a lower dose of epidural local anesthetic is required to block the same number of segments. After epidural administration, there is an increased spread of the local anesthetic, intensity of the motor blockade is enhanced, and the level of the block may be higher [27]. Both bupivacaine and ropivacaine enhance the intensity of motor blockade, and bupivacaine provides a fast onset time.

When local anesthetics are administered in the subarachnoidal space (spinal anesthesia), the spread of analgesia varies with the baricity of the solution. With hyperbaric bupivacaine, sensory analgesia develops more rapidly in patients older than 80 years, and the maximum level of analgesia is also higher (at least by one dermatome) [28]. Hemodynamic changes (bradycardia, hypotension) after neuraxial anesthesia are more frequent with advancing age [29], requiring continuous and careful hemodynamic monitoring.

The effects of local anesthetic agents, administered for obtaining peripheral nerve blocks, have longer duration in the elderly population. Ropivacaine (0.75%) induces sensory and motor blocks that last longer, likely as a consequence of alterations of nerve physiology and sensitivity to local anesthetics [30].

2.12 Preoperative Assessment

The preoperative assessment of the elderly patient must embrace not only physical status and comorbidities but also domains, such as cognition, functionality, frailty, polypharmacy, nutrition, and social support [31]. The patient should be evaluated several days before the surgery, possibly after medical information has been obtained from the surgeon or primary care physician. The assessment includes history, physical examination, and review of the medical chart. Due to the high frequency of postoperative neurologic, pulmonary, and cardiac complications in the elderly, the anesthesiologist should pay special attention to these specific organ systems.

With the aim of improving the quality of care, recent guidelines recommend precise preoperative assessments for every geriatric patient [32, 33]. The punctual assessment emphasized in the guidelines is intended to be as a multidisciplinary approach from the full team involved in the care of the patient: the physician (internist, geriatrician), the surgeon, and the anesthesiologist.

2.12.1 Performing Complete History and Physical Examination

Clinical history and physical examination allow the assessment of the physical status, the comorbidities, and the functional reserve of the patient. During the visit, the anesthesiologist should recognize the alterations that may require preoperative correction (dehydration, hypovolemia, anemia, electrolyte disturbances, arrhythmias).

2.12.2 Conducting Cognitive Assessment, Including the Patient's Ability to Understand the Purpose of the Planned Surgical Procedure

Assessment and documentation of the baseline cognitive status will facilitate recognition of postoperative cognitive dysfunctions. Simple-to-administer and reproducible tests can be useful, such as the Mini-Cog, a composite of three-item recall and clock drawing [34], or the Mini-Mental Status Examination, with scores from 0 to 30 (a score less than 17 indicates dementia) [35]. The patients must understand the anesthesia plan and give his/her consent to treatment. When the patient loses decision-making capacity, because of cognitive dysfunction, it will be necessary for a legal representative to grant informed consent, according to the laws of the country [36].

2.12.3 Screening for Depression

Depression has been associated with higher pain perception and increased postoperative analgesic use. To evaluate depression, the anesthesiologist may use very simple tools, such as the Patient Health Questionnaire-2 [37], or ask for advice from a psychiatrist.

2.12.4 Determining Risk Factors for Postoperative Delirium

Delirium is an acute decline in cognitive function with reduced awareness and disturbance of attention that tends to fluctuate throughout the day. The main predisposing risk factors for delirium are cognitive impairment (Mini-Mental State Examination score < 24) [35], dementia (main predisposing factor), depression, multimorbidity, reduced functional status (i.e., reduced levels of independence, abilities, and socialization) and/or frailty, malnutrition (low serum albumin), dehydration (blood urea nitrogen-to-creatinine ratio < 18), alcohol abuse, sensory impairment (hearing and visual), drug interactions (anticholinergics, benzodiazepines), pain, hypoxia, and metabolic disturbances [38].

2.12.5 Screening for Substance Abuse/Dependence, Including Alcohol

Alcohol abuse and dependence are associated with increased rates of postoperative mortality and complications, including pneumonia, sepsis, wound infection, and prolonged hospitalization [39]. Prophylaxis for withdrawal syndromes should be considered, and in the case of alcohol abuse, patients should receive, in the perioperative period, daily multivitamins (with folic acid) and high-dose oral or parenteral thiamine (100 mg).

2.12.6 Performing Cardiac Evaluation

Older patients are more vulnerable to perioperative cardiac adverse events [40]. Therefore, it is critical to evaluate the cardiac functional reserve of the patient and plan the appropriate perioperative screening (Fig. 2.2) and management. Functional capacity can be measured in metabolic equivalents (METs) and can be used as a predictor of future cardiac events. One MET equals the basal metabolic rate (oxygen consumption at rest = 3.5 mL O_2/kg bw/min), and exercise testing provides an objective assessment of functional capacity. Without testing, functional capacity can be estimated from the ability to perform daily living activities. Walking on level ground (about 6 km/h) or climbing two flights of stairs demands 4 METs, while strenuous sports, such as swimming, >10 METs. Generally, <4 METs indicates poor functional capacity, associated with increased incidence of postoperative cardiac events and worse short- and long-term outcome in patients undergoing noncardiac surgery. Cardiac risk estimation is based on patient characteristics and type of surgery (nature and duration of the surgical procedure), and laboratory measurements and noninvasive/invasive testing are required accordingly, following evidence-based algorithms (Fig. 2.2) [41].

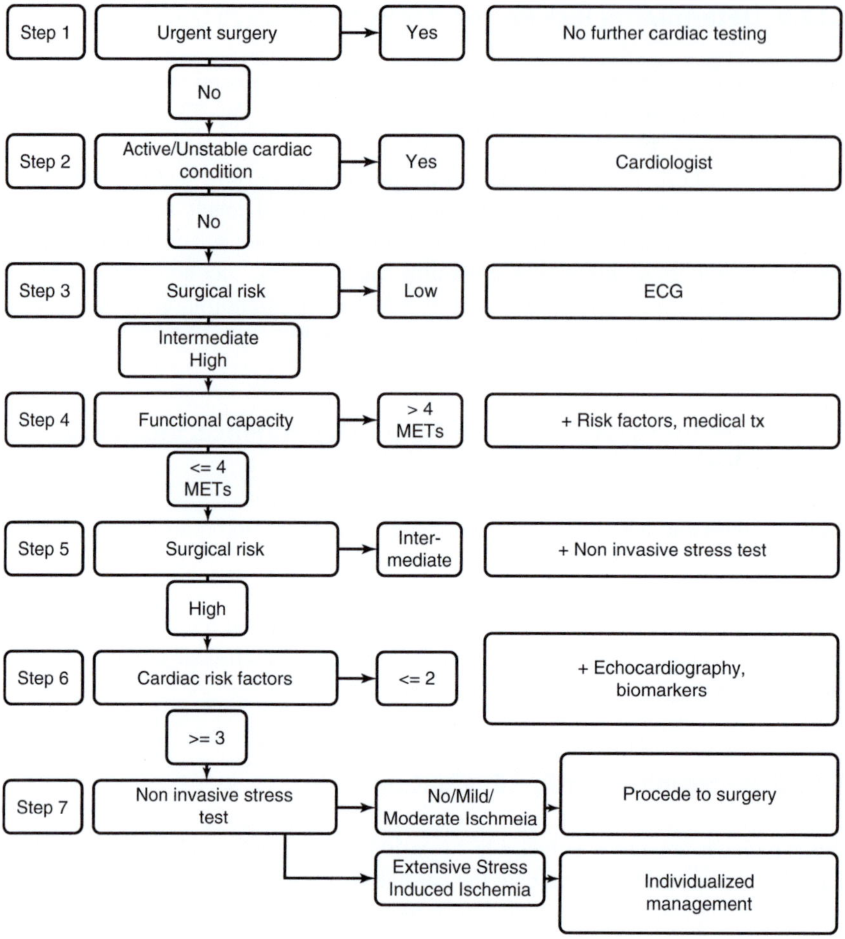

Fig. 2.2 Algorithm for patients undergoing noncardiac surgical procedure

2.12.7 Assessing Risk Factors for Postoperative Pulmonary Complications

Postoperative pulmonary complications have an incidence of 40% in the elderly and contribute to overall morbidity and mortality. Many independent variables are associated with respiratory failure, as the American Society of Anesthesiologists (ASA status) classification, emergency and/or complex surgery, preoperative sepsis, and elevated creatinine. Older age, male patients, smokers, and patients with a history of congestive heart failure or COPD, or both, are also predisposed [42].

2.12.8 Documenting Functional Status and Fall History

Reduced levels of independence, abilities, and socialization are common among the elderly, as a result of gait alteration, loss of coordination, reduced or nullified sphincter control, malnutrition, associated illnesses, and/or cognitive deterioration. Impaired functional status is associated with surgical site infection, increased mortality, and complication rate [43]. Functional status can be measured by activities of daily living (ADL, physical day-to-day self-care) and instrumental ADL (IADL, complex task activity) [44]. Patients who are not able to complete the Timed Up and Go test in less than 20 s are regarded as being at risk of falls [45].

2.12.9 Calculate Frailty Score at Baseline

Frailty, a condition of critically reduced functional reserves, involving multiple organ systems, is an age-associated decline in five domains: shrinking (weight loss), weakness (decreased grip strength), exhaustion, low physical activity, and slowed walking speed (measured by the speed at which the patient walks a fixed distance). These domains can be easily assessed using the frailty index [46]. Hypoalbuminemia, hypocholesterolemia, and high levels of inflammation, together with muscular atrophy, are specific markers. Frailty (6.9% in older patients) independently predicts postoperative complications, length of stay, and discharge to a skilled or assisted living facility [46].

2.12.10 Assessing Nutritional Status and Considering Implementation of Preoperative Interventions for High-Risk Patients

Suitable tools for evaluating the nutritional status are the body mass index and weight loss within the last 6 months. Among acutely hospitalized older patients, the prevalence of malnutrition is 52%, and the most widely used test to assess nutritional status and diagnose malnutrition is the Mini-Nutritional Assessment, which can be performed at the bedside using a questionnaire, with scores ranging from 0 to 30 (<17 indicates malnutrition) [47]. Malnutrition may be secondary to somatic, psychic, or social problems, is associated with a worse prognosis, and is an independent risk factor for morbidity and mortality. Reversing established preoperative nutritional deficit, especially in short periods of time, is challenging. In high-risk patients, improvement in the nutritional status can be achieved over time by adequate diet, hand feeding, additional sip feeding, or enteral nutrition [48]. A multimodal rehabilitation program, consisting of exercise training and nutritional and psychological support, seems to improve the ability to undergo the stress of surgery and provides faster recovery [49]. Every effort should be made to prevent the development of malnutrition during hospitalization.

2.12.11 Taking a Complete Medication History, Making Needed Perioperative Adjustments, and Monitoring for Polypharmacy

Older patients take multiple medications, which can be appropriate, but increase the risk of adverse drug reactions (ADRs), impaired physical and cognitive function, and hospital admission. To minimize the risk for ADRs, the anesthesiologist needs to identify potential interactions between medications and anesthetic drugs and medications that should be discontinued or avoided before surgery, according to the Beers criteria, which must be used as a guide of good practice [50]. Polypharmacy is defined as taking more than five regular prescribed medicines. Deprescribing (reducing specific classes of medicines) may decrease ADRs and improve quality of life. This process, however, should be the aim of the full team taking care of the patient, because it can be a difficult task for the anesthesiologist when the preoperative visit is very close to the surgery or in case of emergency.

2.13 Perioperative Anesthetic Procedure

2.13.1 Preoperative Testing

Screening in the elderly patient should always include hemoglobin, renal function tests (blood urea nitrogen, creatinine), and albumin evaluation. Further diagnostic tests may be required on an individual basis, according to preoperative clinical assessment and surgical plan, to confirm the presence or absence of diseases (e.g., Fig. 2.2).

2.13.2 Preoperative Fasting

Clear fluids (water, tea, black coffee, fruit juices without pulp) can be given up to 2 h before anesthesia (general anesthesia, regional anesthesia, or sedation/analgesia), and the minimum fasting period for a light solid meal should be 6 h [51]. A carbohydrate-rich beverage before elective surgery improves subjective well-being, reduces thirst and hunger, and reduces postoperative insulin resistance. Recent evidence suggests that the carbohydrate-rich beverage attenuates fasting-induced stress in the elderly, without known risks of pulmonary aspiration [52].

2.13.3 Choice of Anesthetic Technique

Scientific evidence is insufficient to recommend the "most appropriate" anesthetic approach for elderly patients. General and regional anesthetic techniques have advantages and disadvantages, and the baseline functional status of the patient (as well as the type of surgery) needs to be considered when selecting anesthetic drugs

Table 2.4 Geriatric physiology and anesthetic implication

System	Geriatric physiology	Anesthetic implications
Cardiovascular	Decresed sympathetic tone	Labile blood pressure
	Decreased venous compliance and preload	Sensitivity to hypotension and volume overload
	Impaired baroreceptor response Cardiac diastolic dysfunction	Cardiac function decline with inadequate cardiac filling
Pulmonary	Increased pulmonary arterial pressure	Raised PAO_2-PaO_2 gradient
	Decreased responce to hypoxia and hypercarbia	Sensitivity to hypoxia and hypercarbia
	Decreased muscle mass and lung elasticity	Increased dead space ventilation and work of breathing
	Decreased cough reflex and esophageal motility	Sensitivity to residual anesthetic effects
		Aspiration risk
Nervous system	Decreased neurotransmitters	Increased risk of postoperative cognitive dysfunction
Endocrine system	Impaired glucose tolerance	Increased intraoperative hyperglycemia
Hepatic/renal system	Altered drug metabolism	Decreased drug clearance
Thermoregulation	Decreased muscle mass and vascular reactivity	Increased risk of hypothermia

and technique (Tables 2.3 and 2.4). Intensity of monitoring, during and following anesthesia, is determined on an individual basis, considering the patient's physical status and the surgical procedure. Monitoring depth of anesthesia (with processed EEG signal, e.g., Bispectral Index monitoring) may be a useful guide for effective titration of hypnotic drugs administration and avoids deep level of anesthesia, detrimental for elderly patients [15, 53].

Anesthesia-related complications are rare, and postoperative complications in the elderly are mostly related to the entire perioperative procedure [54]. General and locoregional techniques are both appropriate for older patients [55]. Neuraxial anesthesia, however, is increasingly viewed as a reasonable alternative to general anesthesia, and some surgical procedures, especially hip fracture surgery, seem to benefit from locoregional approaches [56]. Various beneficial effects from neuraxial blocks (epidural, spinal, or combined spinal-epidural techniques) have been reported, such as reduced 30-day mortality, decreased risk of pneumonia, opiate-sparing effects, and postoperative inhibition of fibrinolysis [57]. General anesthesia has a lower incidence of systemic hypotension and cerebrovascular accidents compared to neuraxial anesthesia [56], and the occurrence of hypotension is a strong and highly significant predictor for worse outcome in the elderly [53, 58]. Future studies will indicate whether the anesthesia choice will affect outcome in elderly patients. The recently started REGAIN trial is a multicenter randomized trial that will compare several outcomes, including recovery of functional independence, in patients undergoing spinal or general anesthesia for hip fracture surgery in the USA and Canada [59].

2.13.4 Intraoperative Fluid Management

The use of fixed-volume (mL/kg/h) fluid strategy should be avoided in elderly patients, because fluid in excess may have deleterious effects on cardiac and pulmonary functions, recovery of gastrointestinal motility (postoperative ileus), tissue oxygenation, wound healing, and coagulation [60]. A goal-directed fluid strategy should be preferred [61], and accurate intraoperative fluid balance should always be pursued.

2.13.5 Postoperative Nausea and Vomiting

Postoperative nausea and vomiting (PONV) constitutes a major unpleasant symptom after anesthesia and surgery, and risk stratification is essential in preventing and managing PONV [62]. Older adults at moderate or high risk for PONV should receive prophylactic interventions avoiding medications (anticholinergics) that can precipitate confusion and postoperative delirium [50].

2.13.6 Acute Postoperative Pain Treatment

Pain evaluation should be integrated into perioperative care, and verbal pain scales produce better pain assessment compared to nonverbal scales. In older patients, the use of tools appropriate to cognitive abilities [63] facilitates the regular evaluation and documentation of pain intensity, efficacy, and side effects of pain therapy. An individual multimodal analgesic plan should be developed for every older patient, according to baseline functional status, pain history, and type of surgery. Inappropriate pain medications should be avoided [50]. Opioid-based acute pain management may be used, with age-adjusted dose to avoid adverse side effects (somnolence, respiratory depression, constipation), and this is especially important in frail patients who poorly tolerate systemic opioids. Meperidinc has been always associated with an increased risk of delirium in elderly surgical patients and should be avoided [64]. Opioid-sparing techniques, such as perioperative paracetamol, and/or regional techniques (neuraxial blockade or peripheral nerve blocks) are good choices for treating acute postoperative pain, and in collaborative patients, patient-controlled analgesia (PCA) should be considered.

2.14 Postoperative Cognitive Impairment

After surgery, older adults are at high risk of cognitive impairments, and the most common disorders are postoperative delirium and postoperative cognitive dysfunction. When feasible, hospitalization of older patients should be avoided or reduced to a minimum, since postoperative cognitive dysfunction occurs less frequently after outpatient surgery [65].

2.14.1 Postoperative Delirium

Delirium (acute and fluctuating changes of cognitive function) is diagnosed according to the *Diagnostic and Statistical Manual of Mental Disorders* [66]. In older adults, even a single episode of postoperative delirium (POD) has been related to prolonged hospitalization, loss of functional independence, declined cognitive ability, and death [67].

The exact mechanism of POD is not fully understood. POD is a reversible condition and is mainly influenced by risks related to the patient, and not by the anesthesia mode, general or locoregional, although drugs such as anticholinergics and benzodiazepines should be avoided in patients at risk for delirium [38]. Screening for POD should start in the recovery room and continue during the complete hospitalization period. Delirium can be diagnosed with several tools. The Confusion Assessment Method (CAM), which considers onset and course of POD, attention, thinking, and level of consciousness, is the most used tool. CAM is a bedside rating scale developed to assist clinicians, not trained in psychiatry. Delirium can manifest as hyperactive (combative or agitated), hypoactive (lack of awareness and decreased motor activity), and mixed (hypo-/hyperactive) form, with an incidence, respectively, of 1.4, 67.6, and 31.1% in older adults [68]. To prevent or attenuate POD, it is recommended to implement proactive nonpharmacological measures, consisting mostly of orientation (clock, communication, etc.), visual/hearing aids, noise reduction and maintenance of a day/night rhythm, avoidance of unnecessary indwelling catheters, early mobilization, and early nutrition [69]. Prevention of any precipitating medical cause is the best therapy. It is of utmost importance to anticipate and treat pain and to correct any metabolic and electrolyte disturbances; pharmacologic therapy for neuropsychiatric disorders should be continued in the perioperative period, and drugs known to trigger delirium should be used with caution. In case pharmacologic intervention is advisable, low-dose haloperidol (0.25 mg stepwise titrated up to maximum of 3.5 mg, maximum dose/day < 6 mg) can be given [38, 70].

2.14.2 Postoperative Cognitive Dysfunction

Postoperative cognitive dysfunction (POCD) is a reversible decline in cognitive functions, especially memory, which lasts weeks or months after surgery. Unlike delirium, POCD cannot be recognized according to DSM criteria [66]. The risk of POCD increases with age, is frequent in older patients, and implies impairment in several cognitive domains (attention, memory, and psychomotor ability) [71]. Because of its intricate nature, a battery of neuropsychological tests is required to detect POCD, and the diagnosis can be made only by comparing pre- and postoperative neuropsychological tests.

2.14.3 Persistent Cognitive Dysfunction

Reversible postoperative decline in cognitive functions, which lasts from days to few months, must not be confused with *persistent* cognitive dysfunction. Surgery and anesthesia are unlikely to produce persistent cognitive decline. In a study of more than 8500 middle-aged and elderly Danish twins, recently published in *Anesthesiology*, researchers found no clinically significant association between surgery and general anesthesia with long-term cognitive decline [72]. Persistent deterioration in cognitive function reflects a cognitive impairment that was already present before surgery. Cognitive function is not currently assessed in the preoperative period, and when elderly individuals experience persistent cognitive decline after a surgical procedure, the surgery is usually a coincidence pretending to be the cause.

Conclusions

The knowledge of the physiological changes associated with aging and a careful preoperative evaluation of the patient are essential to plan and optimize the anesthetic care of older adults. The comprehensive care of elderly patients, however, needs to rely on a multidisciplinary dedicated team, including at the very least the physician, the surgeon, and the anesthesiologist, and this approach may significantly improve periprocedural results and both short- and long-term outcomes in senior patients requiring surgical procedures.

References

1. Grifasi C, Calogero A, Esposito A, Dodaro C. Perioperative care of elderly outpatients. A review. Ann Ital Chir. 2015;86(2):100–5.
2. Alvis BD, Hughes CG. Physiology considerations in geriatric patients. Anesthesiol Clin. 2015;33(3):447–56.
3. Brown EN, Purdon PL. The aging brain and anesthesia. Curr Opin Anaesthesiol. 2013;26(4):414–9.
4. Tsui BC, Wagner A, Finucane B. Regional anaesthesia in the elderly: a clinical guide. Drugs Aging. 2004;21(14):895–910.
5. Priebe HJ. The aged cardiovascular risk patient. Br J Anaesth. 2000;85(5):763–78.
6. Scantlebury DC, Borlaug BA. Why are women more likely than men to develop heart failure with preserved ejection fraction? Curr Opin Cardiol. 2011;26(6):562–8.
7. Sprung J, Gajic O, Warner DO. Review article: age related alterations in respiratory function - anesthetic considerations. Can J Anaesth. 2006;53(12):1244–57.
8. Sorbini CA, Grassi V, Solinas E, Muiesan G. Arterial oxygen tension in relation to age in healthy subjects. Respiration. 1968;25(1):3–13.
9. Schmucker DL. Age-related changes in liver structure and function: implications for disease ? Exp Gerontol. 2005;40(8–9):650–9.
10. Martin JE, Sheaff MT. Renal ageing. J Pathol. 2007;211(2):198–205.
11. Kruijt Spanjer MR, Bakker NA, Absalom AR. Pharmacology in the elderly and newer anaesthesia drugs. Best Pract Res Clin Anaesthesiol. 2011;25(3):355–65.

12. Nickalls RWD, Mapleson WW. Age-related iso-MAC charts for isoflurane, sevoflurane and desflurane in man. Br J Anaesth. 2003;91(2):170–4.
13. Van Cleve WC, Nair BG, Rooke GA. Associations between age and dosing of volatile Anesthetics in 2 academic hospitals. Anesth Analg. 2015;121(3):645–51.
14. Monk TG, Saini V, Weldon BC, Sigl JC. Anesthetic management and one-year mortality after noncardiac surgery. Anesth Analg. 2005;100(2):4–10.
15. Matsuura T, Oda Y, Tanaka K, Mori T, Nishikawa K, Asada A. Advance of age decreases the minimum alveolar concentrations of isoflurane and sevoflurane for maintaining bispectral index below 50. Br J Anaesth. 2009;102(3):331–5.
16. Schnider TW, Minto CF, Shafer SL, Gambus PL, Andresen C, Goodale DB, et al. The influence of age on propofol pharmacodynamics. Anesthesiology. 1999;90(6):1502–16.
17. Phillips AT, Deiner S, Lin HM, Andreopoulos E, Silverstein J, Levin MA. Propofol use in the elderly population: prevalence of overdose and association with 30-day mortality. Clin Ther. 2015;37(12):2676–85.
18. Sun GC, Hsu MC, Chia YY, Chen PY, Shaw FZ. Effects of age and gender on intravenous midazolam premedication: a randomized double-blind study. Br J Anaesth. 2008;101(5):632–9.
19. Wolff J, Bigler D, Christensen CB, Rasmussen SN, Andersen HB, Tønnesen KH. Influence of renal function on the elimination of morphine and morphine glucuronides. Eur J Clin Pharmacol. 1988;34(4):353–7.
20. Shafer SL. The pharmacology of anesthetic drugs in elderly patients. Anesthesiol Clin North Am. 2000;18(1):1–29.
21. Minto CF, Schnider TW, Egan TD, Youngs E, Lemmens HJ, Gambus PL, et al. Influence of age and gender on the pharmacokinetics and pharmacodynamics of remifentanil I. Model development. Anesthesiology. 1997;86(1):10–23.
22. Minto CF, Schnider TW, Shafer SL. Pharmacokinetics and pharmacodynamics of remifentanil. II. Model application. Anesthesiology. 1997;86(1):24–33.
23. Akhtar S, Liu J, Heng J, Dai F, Schonberger RB, Burg MM. Does intravenous induction dosing among patients undergoing gastrointestinal surgical procedures follow current recommendations: a study of contemporary practice. J Clin Anesth. 2016;33(9):208–15.
24. Cope TM, Hunter JM. Selecting neuromuscular-blocking drugs for elderly patients. Drugs Aging. 2003;20(2):125–40.
25. Berg H, Roed J, Viby-Mogensen J, Mortensen CR, Engbaek J, Skovgaard LT, et al. Residual neuromuscular block is a risk factor for postoperative pulmonary complications. A prospective, randomised, and blinded study of postoperative pulmonary complications after atracurium, vecuronium and pancuronium. Acta Anaesthesiol Scand. 1997;41(9):1095–103.
26. Veering BT. Pharmacological aspects of local anesthetics in the elderly. Acta Anaesthesiol Belg. 1998;49(2):117–22.
27. Simon MJG, Veering BT. Factors affecting the pharmacokinetics and neural block characteristics after epidural administration of local anaesthetics. Eur J Pain Suppl. 2010;4(S4):209–18.
28. Racle JP, Benkhadra A, Poy JY, Gteizal B. Spinal analgesia with hyperbaric bupivacaine: influence of age. Br J Anaesth. 1988;60(5):508–14.
29. Simon MJC, Veering BT, Stienstra R, van Kleef JW, Burm AGL. The effects of age on neural blockade and hemodynamic changes after epidural anesthesia with ropivacaine. Anesth Analg. 2002;94:1325–30.
30. Paqueron X, Boccara G, Bendahou M, Coriat P, Riou B. Brachial plexus nerve block exhibits prolonged duration in the elderly. Anesthesiology. 2002;97(5):1245–9.
31. Bettelli G. Preoperative evaluation in geriatric surgery: comorbidity, functional status and pharmacological history. Minerva Anestesiol. 2011;77(6):637–46.
32. Chow WB, Rosenthal RA, Merkow RP, Ko CY, Esnaola NF, American College of Surgeons National Surgical Quality Improvement Program; American Geriatrics Society. Optimal preoperative assessment of the geriatric surgical patient: a best practices guideline from the American College of Surgeons National Surgical Quality Improvement Program and the American Geriatrics Society. J Am Coll Surg. 2012;215(4):453–66.

33. Mohanty S, Rosenthal RA, Russell MM, Neuman MD, Ko CY, Esnaola NF. Optimal perioperative management of the geriatric patient: a best practices guideline from the American College of Surgeons NSQIP and the American Geriatrics Society. Am Coll Surg. 2016;222(5):930–47.
34. Borson S, Scanlan J, Brush M, Vitaliano P, Dokmak A. The mini-cog: a cognitive 'vital signs' measure for dementia screening in multi-lingual elderly. Int J Geriatr Psychiatry. 2000;15(11):1021–7.
35. Folstein MF, Folstein SE, McHugh PR. Mini-mental state. A practical method for grading the cognitive state of patients for the clinician. J Psychiatr Res. 1975;12(3):189–98.
36. Lautrette A, Peigne V, Watts J, Souweine B, Azoulay E. Surrogate decision makers for incompetent ICU patients: a European perspective. Curr Opin Crit Care. 2008;14(6):714–9.
37. Li C, Friedman B, Conwell Y, Fiscella K. Validity of the patient health questionnaire 2 (PHQ-2) in identifying major depression in older people. J Am Geriatr Soc. 2007;55(4):596–602.
38. Aldecoa C, Bettelli G, Bilotta F, Sanders RD, Audisio R, Borozdina A, Cherubini A, et al. European Society of Anaesthesiology evidence-based and consensus-based guideline on post-operative delirium. Eur J Anaesthesiol. 2017;34(4):192–214.
39. Nath B, Li Y, Carroll JE, Szabo G, Tseng JF, Shah SA. Alcohol exposure as a risk factor for adverse outcomes in elective surgery. J Gastrointest Surg. 2010;14(11):1732–41.
40. Davenport DL, Ferraris VA, Hosokawa P, Henderson WG, Khuri SF, Mentzer RM Jr. Multivariable predictors of postoperative cardiac adverse events after general and vascular surgery: results from the patient safety in surgery study. J Am Coll Surg. 2007;204(6):1199–210.
41. Poldermans D, Bax JJ, Boersma E, De Hert S, Eeckhout E, Fowkes G, et al. Guidelines for pre-operative cardiac risk assessment and perioperative cardiac Management in non-Cardiac Surgery: the task force for preoperative cardiac risk assessment and perioperative cardiac management in non-cardiac surgery of the European Society of Cardiology (ESC) and endorsed by the European Society of Anaesthesiology (ESA). Eur J Anaesthesiol. 2010;27(2):92–137.
42. Johnson RG, Arozullah AM, Neumayer L, Henderson WG, Hosokawa P, Khuri SF. Multivariable predictors of postoperative respiratory failure after general and vascular surgery: results from the patient safety in surgery study. J Am Coll Surg. 2007;204(6):1188–98.
43. Inouye SK, Peduzzi PN, Robison JT, Hughes JS, Horwitz RI, Concato J. Importance of functional measures in predicting mortality among older hospitalized patients. JAMA. 1998;279(15):1187–93.
44. Mahoney FI, Barthel DW. Functional evaluation: the Barthel index. Md State Med J. 1965;14(2):61–5.
45. Podsiadlo D, Richardson S. The timed 'up & go': a test of basic functional mobility for frail elderly persons. J Am Geriatr Soc. 1991;39(2):142–8.
46. Makary MA, Segev DL, Pronovost PJ, Syin D, Bandeen-Roche K, Patel P, et al. Frailty as a predictor of surgical outcomes in older patients. J Am Coll Surg. 2010;210(6):901–8.
47. Guigoz Y, Lauque S, Vellas BJ. Identifying the elderly at risk for malnutrition. The mini nutritional assessment. Clin Geriatr Med. 2002;18(4):737–57.
48. Jie B, Jiang ZM, Nolan MT, Zhu SN, Yu K, Kondrup J. Impact of preoperative nutritional support on clinical outcome in abdominal surgical patients at nutritional risk. Nutrition. 2012;28(10):1022–7.
49. Carli F, Scheede-Bergdahl C. Prehabilitation to enhance perioperative care. Anesthesiol Clin. 2015;33(1):17–33.
50. The American Geriatrics Society 2012 Beers Criteria Update Expert Panel 1. American Geriatrics Society updated beers criteria for potentially inappropriate medication use in older adults. J Am Geriatr Soc. 2012;60(4):616–31.
51. Smith I, Kranke P, Murat I, Smith A, O'Sullivan G, Søreide E, et al. Perioperative fasting in adults and children: guidelines from the European Society of Anaesthesiology. Eur J Anaesthesiol. 2011;28(8):556–69.
52. Hellström PM, Samuelsson B, Al-Ani AN, Hedström M. Normal gastric emptying time of a carbohydrate-rich drink in elderly patients with acute hip fracture: a pilot study. BMC Anesthesiol. 2017;17(1):23.

53. Sessler DI, Sigl JC, Kelley SD, Chamoun NG, Manberg PJ, Saager L, et al. Hospital stay and mortality are increased in patients having a "triple low" of low blood pressure, low bispectral index, and low minimum alveolar concentration of volatile anesthesia. Anesthesiology. 2012;116(6):1195–203.
54. Luger TJ, Kammerlander C, Luger MF, Kammerlander-Knauer U, Gosch M. Mode of anesthesia, mortality and outcome in geriatric patients. Z Gerontol Geriatr. 2014;47(2):110–24.
55. GALA Trial Collaborative Group, Lewis SC, Warlow CP, Bodenham AR, Colam B, Rothwell PM, et al. General anaesthesia versus local anaesthesia for carotid surgery (GALA): a multicentre, randomised controlled trial. Lancet. 2008;372(9656):2132–42.
56. Luger TJ, Kammerlander C, Gosch M, Luger MF, Kammerlander-Knauer U, Roth T, et al. Neuroaxial versus general anaesthesia in geriatric patients for hip fracture surgery: does it matter? Osteoporos Int. 2010;21(Suppl 4):S555–72.
57. Guay J, Choi P, Suresh S, Albert N, Kopp S, Pace NL. Neuraxial blockade for the prevention of postoperative mortality and major morbidity: an overview of Cochrane systematic reviews. Cochrane Database Syst Rev. 2014;1:CD010108.
58. Bijker JB, van Klei WA, Vergouwe Y, Eleveld DJ, van Wolfswinkel L, Moons KGM, et al. Intraoperative hypotension and 1-year mortality after noncardiac surgery. Anesthesiology. 2009;111(6):1217–26.
59. Neuman MD, Ellenberg SS, Magaziner JS, Feng R, Carson JL, the REGAIN Investigators. Regional versus general anesthesia for promoting independence after hip fracture (REGAIN): protocol for a pragmatic, international multicentre trial. BMJ Open. 2016;6(11):e013473.
60. Holte K, Sharrock NE, Kehlet H. Pathophysiology and clinical implications of perioperative fluid excess. Br J Anaesth. 2002;89(4):622–32.
61. Cecconi M, Fasano N, Langiano N, Divella M, Costa MG, Rhodes A, et al. Goal-directed haemodynamic therapy during elective total hip arthroplasty under regional anaesthesia. Crit Care. 2011;15(3):R132.
62. Tommasino C. Management of postoperative nausea and vomiting. In: Brambrink AM, Kirsch JR, editors. Essential of neurosurgical anesthesia & critical care. Springer, New York; 2012. p. 709–18.
63. Hadjistavropoulos T, Herr K, Prkachin KM, Craig KD, Gibson SJ, Lukas A, et al. Pain assessment in elderly adults with dementia. Lancet Neurol. 2014;13(12):1216–27.
64. Fong HK, Sands LP, Leung JM. The role of postoperative analgesia in delirium and cognitive decline in elderly patients: a systematic review. Anesth Analg. 2006;102(4):1255–66.
65. Canet J, Raeder J, Rasmussen LS, Enlund M, Kuipers HM, Hanning CD, et al. Cognitive dysfunction after minor surgery in the elderly. Acta Anaesthesiol Scand. 2003;47(10):1204–10.
66. American Psychiatric Association. Diagnostic and statistical manual of mental disorders (DSM-V). 5th ed. Washington: Amer Psychiatric Pub Inc; 2013.
67. Saczynski JS, Marcantonio ER, Quach L, Fong TG, Gross A, Inouye SK, et al. Cognitive trajectories after postoperative delirium. N Engl J Med. 2012;367(1):30–9.
68. Robinson TN, Raeburn CD, Tran ZV, Brenner LA, Moss M. Motor subtypes of postoperative delirium in older adults. Arch Surg. 2011;146(3):295–300.
69. Björkelund KB, Hommel A, Thorngren KG, Gustafson L, Larsson S, Lundberg D. Reducing delirium in elderly patients with hip fracture: a multi-factorial intervention study. Acta Anaesthesiol Scand. 2010;54(6):678–88.
70. Pisani MA, Araujo KL, Murphy TE. Association of cumulative dose of haloperidol with next-day delirium in older medical ICU patients. Crit Care Med. 2015;43(5):996–1002.
71. Rasmussen LS. Postoperative cognitive dysfunction: incidence and prevention. Best Pract Res Clin Anaesthesiol. 2006;20(2):315–30.
72. Dokkedal U, Hansen TG, Rasmussen LS, Mengel-From J, Christensen K. Cognitive functioning after surgery in middle-aged and elderly Danish twins. Anesthesiology. 2016;124(2):312–21.

Principles of Geriatric Surgery

3

Mario Nano and Mario Solej

3.1 Introduction

Geriatric surgery is the branch of medicine concerned with the surgical care of older adults. To meet the special needs of these patients and restore the highest possible level of practical functioning, it applies the principles of general surgery coupled with the formal assessment of potential risks and benefits, treatment options, and outcomes. Because preservation of functional independence is considered a more meaningful patient-reported end point than disease-free survival, determining the factors that can predict the maintenance of functional status is of critical importance in health-care delivery to the elderly [1–4].

Broadly defined, aging is a complex, differentiated process. Age-related biological parameters diverge as people grow older, whereas they tend to converge toward a narrower range of mean values in the young. Moreover, the trajectory of functional decline is malleable and can be reversed in many organs and systems. In living organisms, aging is a physiological, genetically programmed, universal, and heterochronic process. The term "heterochronic" describes the phenomenon that organs and systems senesce at different rates in the same organism. Heterochronic senescence is of central importance to geriatric medicine and surgery for distinguishing between diseases (curable or treatable) and incurable heterochronic conditions. For example, a 70-year-old with diabetes has a condition that a physician can treat. Conversely, a 70-year-old afflicted with panvasculopathy has a heterochronic

M. Nano (✉)
Full Professor of General Surgery—Honorary President of the Italian Society of Geriatric Surgery, Orbassano, Turin, Italy

M. Solej
University of Turin, Aggregate Professor San Luigi Gonzaga University Hospital, Orbassano, Turin, Italy
e-mail: mario.solej@unito.it

A. Crucitti (ed.), *Surgical Management of Elderly Patients*,
https://doi.org/10.1007/978-3-319-60861-7_3

condition in which the cardiovascular system shows clinical signs of premature aging that would normally be expected to be seen in a centenarian and about which the physician can do nothing.

Another aspect of aging is the difference between normality and normal: normality refers to physiological function in relation to biological age; normal is a statistical concept that refers to levels of functioning according to age class. To illustrate, arthrosis in an 80-year-old can be regarded as "normal" because it occurs statistically in many patients; however, it is not the normality since joint aging does not lead to severe cartilage deterioration. In fact, not all older adults suffer from arthrosis. Whereas normality refers to a physiological-functional and, hence, is an objective fact, normal refers to a subjective evaluation of functioning along a spectrum of cultural norms and social compliance. A 90-year-old woman with urinary incontinence, but otherwise self-sufficient and cognitively oriented, would be regarded by her family as being "normal" but not by nursing home administrators since her condition would mean extra work for the facility staff.

A third distinction to be made in aging concerns the difference between physiological condition and pathological condition. While the boundary between the two is usually clear in younger patients, it is blurred in the elderly and is more of a qualitative than a quantitative nature. This leads to a discussion of the differences between chronologic age and biological age.

Aging is characterized by homeostasis: a functional older adult may maintain good health into old age but will become increasingly vulnerable to stress and illness as physiologic reserve decreases [5, 6]. The difference between chronologic age and biological age derives from the difference between the functional reserve statistically expected for a given age group and the physiological reserve an individual patient actually has. Over the past century, the average life expectancy has increased, and with it, a life span beyond age 80 is now more common in Europe and the United States. At this stage of older age, an elderly person's sociofunctional status can be classified from robust to frail conditions (fit, pre-frail, frail).

In older adults, the surgical management of diseases is often complicated by age-related physiological changes and altered response to treatment. Besides prolonged hospitalization and bed rest, other factors including immobilization, reduced plasma volume, sensory deprivation, and reduced dietary intake can deplete the patient's physiologic reserve, precipitating further functional decline or irreversible dependence. Biological age, which is the cumulative result of pathophysiological aging, comorbidity, and genetic factors, seems to be a better predictor of the degree of fitness and performance status of a patient during an illness [5].

For this reason, geriatrics (medical and surgical) embraces a holistic approach rather than the disease-based model of conventional medicine. Consistent with this holistic view is the notion that there are no "elderly diseases" (like there are childhood diseases) but that certain diseases occur more often in older age. Central to geriatrics is the assessment of how an older adult's organism reacts to a disease, which will differ from that of a younger adult. In geriatric surgery, successful patient outcome is not the result of surgical technique but rather of a deep understanding of the geriatric patient.

In the surgical care of older patients, several factors increase susceptibility to perioperative stress:

- Low physiological reserve
- Slow recovery rate
- Difficult adaptation
- Increased susceptibility to bleeding, hypotension, hypovolemia, and anoxia
- Increased susceptibility to constipation and meteorism
- Lower resistance to infections
- Increased susceptibility to intravasal coagulation
- More catabolic metabolism
- Hypoventilation due to rigid rib cage and weak diaphragm

These factors categorize the older adult as a high-risk surgical patient. Based on personal experience [7], 25% of risk is attributable to age and surgical disease, while the general condition of body systems needed to respond to surgical stress accounts for the remaining 75%. To illustrate this point, we can take as an example a risk calculation model for a patient with diabetes [8]. The model uses a simple equation for calculating biological age: anagraphic age plus duration of diabetes in years. For instance, a 65-year-old with a 10-year history of diabetes presents the same clinical problems as those statistically expected for a 75-year-old. Surgical treatment of a diabetic patient involves not only glycemic control but also management of the risks associated with the systemic complications of diabetes. Because of the age-related decline in organ and system function, older age constitutes a surgical risk factor per se: the older the patient, the lower the functional reserve and the higher the surgical risk irrespective of associated pathologies.

"The traditional view in surgical and clinical care is that age does not matter when survival outcomes involve the oldest-old patients." This notion has been challenged by strong evidence to the contrary. Because the aging process diminishes the physiological functional reserve of vital organs, chronologic age in itself constitutes an established risk factor [3, 9]. This is, in fact, substantiated by the observation of a decline in renal function (slower glomerular filtration rate, decreased ability to concentrate, and dilute urine), cardiocirculatory function (lower maximal heart rate, decreased myocardial and vascular adrenergic response), and respiratory function (reduced elastic lung recoil and closing volume, altered ventilation/perfusion ratio with increased intrapulmonary shunt). Since these changes can affect the entire geriatric population, advanced age represents a surgical risk and poses both the patient and the surgical care team with difficult decisions about major surgery.

In geriatric surgery, risk assessment is of fundamental importance. The origin of modern geriatric surgery can be traced back to a presentation by William Parsons (The Elderly Patient as a Surgical Risk, presented at the 56th Annual Meeting of the Western Surgical Association, St. Louis, MI, 4 December 1948). Several models for the assessment of surgical risk in the elderly have been developed, some of which involving complex mathematical calculations [10]. Despite its limitations, the American Society of Anesthesiologists (ASA) Physical Status classification system, initially created in

1941 and revised several times since then, is the simplest and most practical grading system currently available to evaluate a patient's preoperative physical state and surgical risk also in geriatric patients. When coupled with the comprehensive geriatric assessment (CGA) scheme, it can be used to assess various physical, social, and psychosocial dimensions in the elderly. Other classification systems, such as the Reiss Index [11, 12], also investigate these variables. A simple arithmetic calculation is insufficient to predict surgical risk in such complex patients, however. Treatment options need to be personalized and based on a deep understanding of geriatrics. "An expert opinion would be required at the bedside. Scoring will never replace clinical judgment" [13]. Two common risk factors in the elderly are the immobilization syndrome and malnutrition, both of which are more often present in institutionalized patients.

3.2 Immobilization Syndrome

Immobilization refers to the physical restriction or limitation of the body and limbs, as may result from altered physiological function following prolonged bed rest (more than 3 days), with inability to move in bed, get into or out of bed, or walk. Decreased activity and gradual deconditioning lead to the function-limiting complications commonly seen in the immobilization syndrome [14]. The immobilization syndrome is a multisystem degenerative process that affects the body's major systems and structures. Initially reversible, it may progress, severely compromising function and result in irreversible organ damage. It is also one of the leading causes of morbidity and mortality in the elderly. Prolonged immobilization, which is rarely justifiable, ultimately affects all body systems and structures.

Loss of orientation to person and mental deterioration may occur, manifesting with abulia and psychomotor agitation. Abulia is characterized by the loss or impairment of the ability to perform voluntary actions or to make decisions, whereas psychomotor agitation is characterized by restless activity inappropriate to context that tends to increase at night due to the reduction in orientation stimuli.

The most conspicuous effect of prolonged immobilization is loss of muscle strength and endurance. Muscle atrophy sets in early, already after a few days of bed rest. A muscle at complete rest loses 10–15% of its strength each week, and nearly half of normal strength is lost within 3–5 weeks of immobilization [15]. With prolonged bed rest, contractures (or, more accurately, pseudocontractures) may occur due to progressive shortening of muscle fibers. Ankylosis, particularly of the lower limbs, is a common complication of immobilization. Ankylosis and pseudocontractures make it increasingly difficult to mobilize the patient or achieve and maintain upright posture. Bones can develop disuse osteoporosis, leading to increased risk of bone fracture, loss of bone mass, hypercalcemia, and negative calcium balance.

One of the most common complications of immobilization is the development of pressure sores, which tend to occur more often and earlier (within 2 weeks of bed rest) with advancing age. The incidence of pressure sores is estimated to be more than 70% in patients aged over 70 years and to increase nursing costs by up to 50% [16]. Common sites at higher risk for the development of pressure sores are the areas with little fat and muscle over bony prominences: the sacrum, lower back, heels, greater trochanters, ankles, and ischial tuberosities. Pressure sores can become infected, leading to secondary sepsis and death.

Cardiovascular deconditioning with prolonged bed rest includes increased resting heart rate and decreased ejection fraction and stroke volume. The shorter diastolic filling period reduces coronary blood flow and oxygen delivery to cardiac muscle, leading to a decline in cardiovascular function that appears to stabilize over time. A typical complication is orthostatic hypotension, which increases the risk of syncopal episodes and cerebral hypoperfusion on assumption of upright posture. This occurs within 2–3 weeks of bed rest due to an excessive pooling of blood in the lower extremities and a decrease in circulating blood volume [15]. Another potential complication is venous thrombosis. Venous thromboembolism is due primarily to venous stasis and to a lesser degree to increased blood coagulability. Stasis occurs in the legs owing to decreased contraction of the gastrocnemius and soleus muscles. Most deep venous thrombi occur in the calf muscles and originate mainly in the soleus sinus. Length of bed rest is directly related to the frequency of deep venous thrombosis. Patients with venous thrombosis have a 50% higher likelihood of developing pulmonary emboli; the mortality rate is about 20–35%.

Reduction of rib cage expansion and displacement of the diaphragm cephalad due to the pressure from the bed are predisposing factors to hypoventilation of the dependent areas of the lungs. Failure to fully expand the chest wall results in a 25–50% decrease in respiratory capacity [16]. In the horizontal position, lung perfusion is altered, leading to changes in the ventilation/perfusion ratio, and results in respiratory insufficiency and hypoxemia. In addition, the mucociliary clearance and the cough reflex are impaired, increasing the risk of infection of the lung parenchyma.

Irrespective of the patient's emotional state, anorexia and constipation are common complications of immobilization. Uncomfortable bed position and feelings of embarrassment can inhibit the defecation reflex, resulting in the buildup of stool in the colon and dehydration. Stool retention and impaction stretch the rectum and colon. Over time, the stretch receptors in the rectum are inhibited, with loss of the urge to defecate. In paradoxical diarrhea, liquid stool flows around a hard, impacted fecal mass inside the rectum. The continued presence of the fecal mass irritates the rectal mucosa, leading to the overproduction of mucus and the formation and leakage of watery stool. Fecal impaction can also put pressure on the bladder neck, creating an obstacle to urination already impaired by prostate hypertrophy in older men.

The best method to manage the immobilization syndrome is to prevent it by not immobilizing the patient in the first place. Very few situations require complete bed rest beyond a couple of days. Patients should be kept in a sitting or semi-sitting position to facilitate respiratory and cardiovascular function. Patients should also be encouraged to get up and walk at least two to three times over the course of a day to use the bathroom or around mealtimes, for example. In this way, intestinal and urinary problems and orthostatic hypotension can be avoided. For patients who must not or cannot get out of bed, mobilization exercises of the lower extremities can enhance cardiovascular function and prevent deterioration of musculoskeletal function. Patients should also be taught how to perform breathing exercises. For patients unable to do active exercises in bed, passive mobilization exercises with frequent position changes should be performed to prevent contracture, ankylosis, and pressure sores.

3.3 Malnutrition

Malnutrition is one of the leading causes of postoperative complications and mortality in elderly surgical patients, particularly among the institutionalized elderly. Malnutrition places the older patient at higher risk for delayed surgical wound healing, development of surgical wound complications, and onset and worsening of pressure sores. These problems stem from social issues (extrinsic factors) and from age-related changes in the gastrointestinal tract (intrinsic factors). The combination of both sets of factors makes malnutrition in the elderly often difficult and complex to correct.

Extrinsic factors associated with malnutrition include decreased physical ability, social isolation (widowers are at increased risk of dietary deficiency) [17], poor nutritional knowledge, economic hardship, alcoholism, monotonous diet, lack of exposure to sunlight, refusal to change eating habits, indiscriminate use of medications, and preference for foods that hold a symbolic meaning or for gratifying foods to compensate for frustration.

Though age-related changes in the gastrointestinal tract vary considerably from person to person, they typically lead to altered function of affected areas. For example, inadequate mastication may result from masticatory muscle fatigue and poor dentition (often due to financial constraints that preclude oral restoration). The senses of smell and of taste, in particular due to loss of gustatory papillae, are diminished. The taste sensation most often affected is salty, followed by bitter, whereas the threshold perception of sweet is usually preserved [18]. This, along with economic and psychological factors, explains the predilection for sweet foods among the elderly despite reduced glucose tolerance. Muscle incoordination, even when cerebrovascular disease is absent, results in altered deglutition [19]. Changes in muscular structure and function within the esophagus of adults over 80 years of age, as described under the term "presbyesophagus" [20], include reduced speed of propagation of the peristaltic wave, particularly to the upper third and the lower third segments and incoordination between opening and closing of the lower esophageal sphincter and propagation of the peristaltic wave. In addition, the production of hydrochloric acid, pepsin, and intrinsic factor is decreased, with malabsorption of iron and vitamin B_{12}. In the liver, the production of hepatic enzymes and albumin is diminished, and drug metabolism is altered. While the overall morphology of the small intestinal mucosa remains largely unchanged, the relatively poorly differentiated, immature enterocytes present are functionally incapable of normal absorption [21]. Active transport mechanisms are impaired, and lactase production is decreased (resulting in lactose malabsorption). Also correlated with advanced age are zinc malabsorption (an essential element for numerous metabolic, enzymatic, and immune functions) and deficiency of vitamins A, D, E, and K (typically associated with laxative overuse).

Small intestinal bacterial overgrowth syndrome (SIBO) is the most common cause of malabsorption in older adults. It is caused by the presence of excessive bacteria in the small intestine and is implicated as the cause of megaloblastic anemia. SIBO is caused by the decreased production of gastric juices and local secretion of immunoglobulins by the gastrointestinal tract. The colon is characterized by a marked reduction in peristalsis and thinning of the colon wall due to loss of muscle fibers. In patients who use excessive amounts of laxatives, the mucosa appears brown to black in color (melanosis), the rectal wall gradually loses elasticity, and the mucosa becomes less sensitive.

Extrinsic and intrinsic factors can combine to put the older patient at risk for nutritional deficiencies that complicate the postoperative course. Often, however, nutritional deficiencies are not related to age but rather to reduced food intake. History taking should investigate for social factors that can potentially affect dietary habits. Involuntary weight loss of 4–5% over the past year is associated with a significant increase in morbidity and mortality. Beyond social and psychological factors, weight loss may be a sign of undiagnosed illness (neoplasia, hyperthyroidism, malabsorption, and, more rarely, cardiorespiratory and renal diseases) [22].

Correction of nutritional status should be achieved with enteral nutrition therapy to promote epithelial maintenance and function, as well as mucosal immune function. Enteral nutrition therapy should be supplemented with dietary integrators to correct specific deficiencies [17]. Parenteral nutrition therapy administered via a peripheral line or central access should be reserved for patients who cannot or must not or do not want oral administration or in situations in which the time for renutrition is short (preoperative period). It should be remembered, however, that parenteral nutrition is not devoid of complications (patient positioning and management of infections). During the postoperative period (but also during the preoperative period if there is sufficient time), the return to oral intake should not coincide with complete discontinuation of parenteral nutrition therapy. Both types of nutrition therapy should be continued for several days to ensure adequate caloric intake. Continuation of parenteral hydration may be indicated, as often occurs in patients who do not have adequate oral fluid intake.[1]

Where geriatric medicine and surgery differ from other branches of medicine, the extent to which a patient's medical history, epidemiology of diseases, presence of coexisting conditions, need for functional assessment, decompensation cascade, drug therapy, and real-life circumstances all come into play in the delivery of care. One of the principal challenges of clinical geriatrics is early diagnosis owing to the difficulty in obtaining a history and the problems with interpreting symptoms [23].

[1] The authors wish to thank Dr. Marco Tinivella, Head of Dietary and Clinical Nutrition Service, San Luigi Gonzaga Hospital, for critical review of this section.

History taking in the elderly takes extra effort: they are not in a hurry, they have their own pace for telling their story, and they need time to tell it. Since reaction times are slower, quick answers should not be expected. The patient's age is often far older than that of the physician, creating a generational divide in life rhythm. Questions may not always be correctly or completely understood. An ill older adult is particularly vulnerable to the burden of illness, distressed by anxiety and physical pain, and distracted by these complicating factors. Often, hearing is impaired, a condition the patient may be reluctant to disclose. Symptoms may go unmentioned because it is thought to be merely typical of growing old. Moreover, associating certain diseases with age-related changes is deeply ingrained in medical culture. Members of the care team need to distinguish previous physiological alterations from specific diseases: aging of the arterial wall is not the same as arteriosclerosis, nor is cerebral aging indicative of dementia or joint senescence a sure sign of osteosclerosis. Also important in this context is the difference between normality and normal.

Interpreting symptoms is challenging, particularly so in older adults. A helpful mnemonic is the triad: altered signs and symptoms, masked signs and symptoms, and variable signs and symptoms.

- *Altered signs and symptoms*. Pain symptoms may be attenuated or absent (silent suffering of organ systems). Because signs of peritonism may be vague, and hyperthermia and leukocytosis limited to the acute event (e.g., diverticular perforation), the event may go unrecognized, resulting in delayed diagnosis and hospitalization for an advanced stage of generalized peritonitis. There are other associated diseases which, if complicated, can mimic a surgical disease. For example, metabolic acidosis in a diabetic patient can resemble acute surgical abdomen manifesting with abdominal pain, rebound tenderness (positive Blumberg sign), vomiting, fever, cutaneous hyperesthesia, and leukocytosis. Establishing the differential diagnosis between diabetic ketoacidosis-induced false acute abdomen and true acute surgical abdomen is complicated by ketoacidosis. A useful clue in the diagnosis of the former is that pain is preceded by nausea, vomiting, and polydipsia.
- *Masked signs and symptoms*. The presence of coexisting conditions further complicates interpreting symptoms. In addition, an acute event may precipitate a coexisting illness, distracting attention away from the acute event and delaying diagnosis. For example, in a patient with heart disease, an initially oligosymptomatic peritonitis may be the cause of an episode of congestive heart failure, drawing clinical attention only to the acute event.
- *Variable signs and symptoms*. There are certain diseases that can manifest very differently from those typically seen in younger patients. Hyperthyroidism can manifest with the classic symptoms of hypothyroidism (apathetic hyperthyroidism), making it difficult to establish the clinical diagnosis in relation to senile involutional cerebropathy.

Collectively, these risk factors place the elderly in a precarious situation of distress. Distressing symptoms are associated with psychophysical and emotional decline and frailty, one of the hallmark characteristics of high-risk elderly surgical patients. Closely linked to frailty is delirium, usually but not always occurring during the postoperative period, which significantly diminishes the quality of life of older adults.

3.4 Frailty

The term "frailty" in reference to the elderly was coined in 1973 when the US Congress created the Federal Council on the Aging (FCA) with a mandate to inform policies and program interventions addressing the special needs of older Americans and armed forces veterans. In 1974, the FCA created the Task Force on the Frail Elderly, with the Reverend Monsignor Charles Fahey of the Roman Catholic Diocese of Syracuse, New York, appointed as chairman. Under his chairmanship, the Task Force was responsible for defining the concept of the frail elderly to describe a range of conditions in older people, including general debility, cognitive impairment, and living in a structurally and socially marginalized environment [24].

Frailty encompasses socioeconomic, psychological, health-care, and biological aspects, any one of which may predominate in an individual older person, though there is a common denominator. Well-being means not only the absence of disease. Indeed, an older person may feel unwell even when no organic illness is present. The geriatric patient represents a new concept of health composed of various different components, the principal ones being absence of disease, residual functioning, affective and cognitive capacities, and social resources. Largely ignored by conventional medicine, the frail elderly are considered scientifically uninteresting, ungratifying professionally, unhealable, troublesome to manage, costly, and difficult to discharge [25]. The prevention, identification, and treatment of frailty are the core concern and main challenge in modern geriatric medicine [26, 27].

The general profile of the frail elderly patient is characterized by advanced or very advanced age, multiple chronic illnesses, disability, socioeconomic problems, loneliness and poverty, and precarious homeostasis due to multisystem failure that trigger the so-called failure cascade associated with elevated mortality. Added to these conditions are biological and biochemical abnormalities of uncertain origin that are the hallmarks of frailty: elevated C-reactive protein (CRP), interleukin-6 (IL-6), tumor necrosis factor-α (TNF-α), D-dimer, osteopenia, sarcopenia, anemia, insulin resistance, and decreased iron, vitamin B12, folate, and albumin levels [28–30].

In 1976, Bernard Isaac described the four giants of geriatrics—incontinence, immobility, instability (falls), and intellectual impairment—from which five geriatric syndromes were subsequently derived: pressure ulcers, incontinence, falls, functional decline, and delirium [31–33]. The frail elderly patient is categorized as such when three of these five syndromes are present.

Frailty is a dynamic condition that can be measured. The two major models for the assessment of frailty are the frailty phenotype devised by Fried and coworkers [27] and the fragility index proposed by Rockwood and colleagues [34]. The frailty phenotype (FP) is based on the assessment of five parameters [29]:

1. Unintentional weight loss over the past year (10 lbs or 4.5 kg)
2. Self-reported exhaustion on at least 3 days/week
3. Reduced muscle strength as evaluated by handgrip (less than 13 lbs or 5.85 kg for men and 7.5 lbs or 3.37 kg for women)
4. Reduced physical activity as measured with the Physical Activity Scale for the Elderly (PASE)
5. Reduced gait speed over a known distance (more than 7 s to cover 4.57 m)

If three of these five features are present, the patient is deemed as frail; if one to two are present, the patient is categorized as pre-frail; if none are present, the patient is considered robust.

The frailty index (FI) conceptualizes frailty as a syndrome characterized by the loss of physiological reserve due to the accumulation of deficits, resulting in vulnerability to stress. The index is derived from the Canadian Study of Health and Aging (CSHA) and comprises 70 items. It is calculated by dividing the number of deficits in a patient by the number of deficits measured [35–38]. The index is composed of four scores: 0 (no positive items), 0.33 (1/4 positive items), 0.67 (3/4 positive items), and 1 (all positive items—indicating maximum severity of frailty).

However, neither of these assessment tools takes into account many of the other important factors that contribute to frailty, such as living alone, social engagement, empowerment/life control, and socioeconomic status. The best instrument for assessing frailty is the comprehensive geriatric assessment (CGA) defined as a multidimensional diagnostic process intended to determine an older person's medical, psychosocial, and functional limitations. Among the many assessment scales described in the literature, the most widely used are the Clinical Frailty Scale (CFS), the Growing Frailty Indicator (GFI), the Tilburg Frail Indicator (TFI), and the Edmonton Frailty Scale (EFS) [39].

Since more and more older patients with comorbidities undergo surgery [40], surgeons have begun to use frailty as a predictive tool to identify those at risk for poor outcomes [32, 33, 36]. In patients over age 75 years, frailty is associated with increased postoperative mortality, postoperative complications, prolonged hospital stay, discharge to residential care, unplanned 3-month readmission, increased 3-month mortality, and a three- to eightfold higher incidence of postoperative delirium in elective and emergency abdominal surgery [31, 41–43]. The CGA has been shown to predict postoperative complications in frail elderly patients better than chronological age predicts postoperative mortality [44]. Unfortunately, none of these three tools (CGA, FI, FP) has been adopted in routine preoperative assessment. The CGA is the most comprehensive, while the FP is the simplest. Although the FP measures only physical performance, it may provide a valid clinical tool and starting point for the assessment of frailty in surgical patients [45].

3.5 Delirium

Delirium is an acute, fluctuating disturbance characterized by a reduced ability to focus, maintain, or shift attention; it is accompanied by changes in cognition and perceptual disturbances secondary to a general medical condition. In the surgical setting, emergency admission for an acute condition may precipitate preoperative delirium. There are no prevalence data for preoperative delirium; however, depending on patient age and risk category, its occurrence is estimated to range between 9 and 87%, with older patients undergoing cardiac surgery at greater risk (80%) than those receiving an orthopedic procedure (up to 40%) [46].

Postoperative delirium is closely correlated with frailty. An episode of postoperative delirium in a previously non-frail elderly patient may herald the onset of frailty. It is associated with a variety of poor outcomes, including functional decline, prolonged hospital stay, higher heathcare costs, risk of falling, pressure ulcers, transfer to a nursing home (institutionalization), and an increase in postoperative mortality from 4 to 20% [47]. Moreover, it may be an early signal of postoperative complications such as atrial fibrillation, myocardial infarction, respiratory difficulty, urinary tract infection, and line infection [48]. Risk factors include preexisting dementia, older age, functional impairments, multiple comorbidities, poor vision or hearing, ongoing infections, self-reported alcohol abuse, and psychopathological symptoms.

The acronym VINDICATE was created as a mnemonic denoting the causes of postoperative delirium: vascular infections, nutrition, drugs, injury, cardiac, autoimmune, tumors, and endocrine) [49]. While autoimmune and endocrine causes are rarely encountered in elderly patients, preexisting dementia appears to be the strongest predictor for the development of postoperative delirium [50], and male sex is reportedly a significant predictor though its association with postoperative delirium is unclear [51]. Commonly used medications may also precipitate an episode. The Beers criteria, developed in 1997 and updated in 2003, for inappropriate medication use in the elderly list antihistamines, benzodiazepine, muscle relaxants, meperidine, cimetidine, corticosteroids, belladonna, warfarin, and antiparkinson agents [52].

Postoperative delirium does not manifest immediately after surgery when the patient is lucid; instead, it may develop in 1–3 days following the lucid interval [53]. In addition to preoperative risk factors, there are several postoperative factors that may predispose to the development of delirium, including incomplete pain control, electrolyte abnormalities, presence of a bladder catheter, immobility, and sleep deprivation. Postoperative delirium is also correlated with frailty, duration of the operation, and blood loss. Though less often and less severe, delirium can develop after administration of local and locoregional anesthesia.

Delirium is usually transient and self-limiting, though it can persist through hospital discharge in up to 50% of cases [54]. Its etiology is not yet fully understood and is probably multifactorial. Central cholinergic deficiency is the leading hypothesized mechanism. Three subtypes are distinguished: hyperactive delirium characterized by agitation and hallucination; hypoactive delirium with decreased activity, decreased speech, and reduced awareness, which may be overlooked in patients who are withdrawn or calm; and mixed hyper-hypoactive delirium. Hypoactive delirium is associated with higher mortality. Diagnosis is often challenging and goes unrecognized in nearly 50% of cases [50].

According to the *Diagnostic and Statistical Manual of Mental Disorders, Fourth Edition (DSM-IV)*, four of the following criteria are needed to establish a diagnosis of postoperative delirium [55]:

1. Disturbance of consciousness, i.e., reduced clarity of awareness of the environment, with reduced ability to focus, sustain, or shift attention.
2. A change in cognition (such as memory deficit, disorientation, language disturbance) or the development of a perceptual disturbance that is not better accounted for by a preexisting, established, or evolving dementia.
3. The disturbance develops over a short period of time (usually hours to days) and tends to fluctuate during the course of the day.
4. There is evidence from the history, physical examination, and laboratory findings that the disturbance is caused by the direct physiological consequences of a general medical condition, developed during substance intoxication or during or shortly after a withdrawal syndrome.

Inattention is the cardinal symptom in the aged patient [56]. There are no specific tests for the diagnosis. As seen in frailty, inflammation markers are often elevated, though it is unclear whether the alterations are the cause or the effect of delirium [53]. Imaging studies may be useful to exclude other causes. Chest radiography, magnetic resonance imaging of the head, or abdominal computed tomography should be ordered when there is clinical suspicion of specific pathologies such as infection or stroke.

Treatment is based on a multicomponent approach. Pharmacological treatment is not recommended as a first-line therapy. The American Geriatrics Society has developed a core set of strategies for the prevention and treatment of postoperative delirium [56].

Behavioral and Nonpharmacologic Strategies for Prevention/Treatment of Delirium

1. Sensory enhancement (ensuring glasses, hearing aids, or listening amplifiers)
2. Mobility enhancement (ambulating at least twice per day if possible)
3. Cognitive orientation and therapeutic activities (tailored to the individual)
4. Pain control with scheduled acetaminophen if appropriate
5. Cognitive stimulation (if possible, tailored to the individual's interests and mental status)
6. Simple communication standards and approaches to prevent the escalation of behaviors
7. Nutritional and fluid repletion enhancement
8. Sleep enhancement (daytime sleep hygiene, relaxation, nonpharmacologic sleep protocol, and nighttime routine)

9. Medication review and appropriate medication management
10. Daily rounding by an interdisciplinary team to reinforce the interventions

Strategies should usually include these core elements, but this list is not all inclusive.

The drug of choice is haloperidol, which may induce extrapyramidal side effects. Low-dose benzodiazepine should be reserved for patients with a previous or current history of alcohol abuse or have consumed alcohol during the preoperative period and are experiencing symptoms of alcohol or benzodiazepine withdrawal.

References

1. Ugolini G, Pasini F, Ghignone F, Zattoni D, Bacchi Reggiani ML, et al. How to select elderly colorectal cancer patients for surgery: a pilot study in an Italian academic medical center. Cancer Biol Med. 2015;12(4):302–7. https://doi.org/10.7497/j.issn.2095-3941.2015.0084.
2. PACE participants, Audisio RA, Pope D, Ramesh HS, Gennari R, van Leeuwen BL, et al. Shall we operate? Preoperative assessment in elderly cancer patients (PACE) can help. A SIOG surgical task force prospective study. Crit Rev Oncol Hematol. 2008;65(2):156–63.
3. Kim YW, Kim IY. Factors associated with postoperative complications and 1-year mortality after surgery for colorectal cancer in octogenarians and nonagenarians. Clin Interv Aging. 2016;11:689–97. https://doi.org/10.2147/CIA.S104783.
4. Hamel MB, Henderson WG, Khuri SF, Daley J. Surgical outcomes for patients aged 80 and older: morbidity and mortality from major noncardiac surgery. J Am Geriatr Soc. 2005;53(3):424–9.
5. Dewan SK, Zheng SB, Xia SJ. Preoperative geriatric assessment: comprehensive, multidisciplinary and proactive. Eur J Intern Med. 2012;23(6):487–94. https://doi.org/10.1016/j.ejim.2012.06.009.
6. Feng MA, McMillan DT, Crowell K, Muss H, Nielsen ME, Smith AB. Geriatric assessment in surgical oncology: a systematic review. J Surg Res. 2015;193(1):265–72. https://doi.org/10.1016/j.jss.2014.07.004.
7. Masera N. Principi e Fondamentali della Chirurgia Geriatrica. In: Masera N, Ferrara L, Nano M, editors. Chirurgia Geriatrica. Torino: Minerva Medica; 1990.
8. Fumelli P. Chirurgia e Diabete Senile. In: Masera N, Ferrara L, Nano M, editors. Chirurgia Geriatrica. Torino: Minerva Medica; 1990.
9. Chung JY, Chang WY, Lin TW, Lu JR, Yang MW, Lin CC, et al. An analysis of surgical outcomes in patients aged 80 years and older. Acta Anaesthesiol Taiwanica. 2014;52(4):153–8. https://doi.org/10.1016/j.aat.2014.09.003.
10. Nano M. Problemi Chirurgici. In: Tammaro AE, Casale G, Frustaglia A, editors. Manuale di Geriatria e Gerontologia. Milano: McGraw-Hill; 1996.
11. Leardi S, De Santis C, Ciuca B, Risetti A, Pietroletti R, Simi M. Risk indices in geriatric surgery: ASA index versus Reiss index. Minerva Chir. 1997;52(3):255–60. Italian.
12. Reiss R, Deutsch AA, Nudelman I, Gutman H. Multifactorial analysis of prognostic factors in emergency abdominal surgery in patients above 80 years. Analysis of 154 consecutive cases. Int Surg. 1989;74(2):93–6.
13. Marchionni N, Moschi G, Di Bari M, Burgisser C, Fumagalli S, Boncinelli L, et al. Acute and long-term effects of flosequinan in patients with chronic cardiac failure. Am Heart J. 1993;126(1):147–54.
14. Laksmi PW, Harimurti K, Setiati S, Soejono CH, Aries W, Roosheroe AG. Management of immobilization and its complication for elderly. Acta Med Indones. 2008;40(4):233–40.

15. Dittmer DK, Teasell R. Complications of immobilization and bed rest. Part 1:musculoskeletal and cardiovascular complications. Can Fam Physician. 1993;39:1428–32. 1435-7.
16. Teasell R, Dittmer DK. Complications of immobilization and bed rest. Part 2: other complications. Can Fam Physician. 1993;39:1440–2. 1445-6.
17. Bosello O, Montesanti F, Armellini F, Zamboni M. Aspetti terapeutici della supplementazione orale nel paziente anziano. G Gerontol. 1997;45:769–76. Italian.
18. Zamboni M, Perbellini C, Bellini R. Fisiopatologia della nutrizione nell'anziano. G Gerontol. 1999;47:563–7. Italian.
19. Holt PR. Effect of aging on the gastrointestinal tract. G Gerontol. 1996;44:445–9.
20. Fradà G, Mitra M, Riggio D, Mauceri ML. Effetti dell'invecchiamento sulla motilità esofagea. G Gerontol. 1992;40:207–11. Italian.
21. Corazza GR, Malservisi S, Taglieri G. L'intestino tenue nell'anziano: molte domande, poche risposte. G Gerontol. 1996;44:363–7. Italian.
22. Lagoo-Deenadayalan SA, Jacobs DD. Nutrition. In: Rosenthal RA, Zenilman ME, Katlic MR, editors. Principles and practice of geriatric surgery. 2nd ed. New York: Springer; 2011.
23. Katlic MR. Principles of geriatric surgery. In: Rosenthal RA, Zenilman ME, Katlic MR, editors. Principles and practice of geriatric surgery. 2nd ed. New York: Springer; 2011.
24. Ruggiero C, Cherubini A, Senin U. Alla scoperta delle origini dell'anziano fragile. G Gerontol. 2007;55:183–90.
25. Makary MA, Segev DL, Pronovost PJ, Syin D, Bandeen-Roche K, Patel P, et al. Frailty as a predictor of surgical outcomes in older patients. J Am Coll Surg. 2010;210(6):901–8. https://doi.org/10.1016/j.jamcollsurg.2010.01.028.
26. Pilotto A, Ferrucci L. Verso una definizione clinica della fragilità: utilità dell'approccio multidimensionale. G Gerontol. 2011;59:125–9.
27. Fried LP, Tangen CM, Walston J, Newman AB, Hirsch C, Gottdiener J, et al. Cardiovascular health study collaborative research group. Frailty in older adults: evidence for a phenotype. J Gerontol A Biol Sci Med Sci. 2001;56(3):M146–56.
28. Orandi BJ, Winter JM, Segev DL, Makary MA. Frailty and surgery in the elderly. In: Rosenthal RA, Zenilman ME, Katlic MR, editors. Principles and practice of geriatric surgery. 2nd ed. New York: Springer; 2011. p. 129–34.
29. Foroni M, Mussi C, Erzili E, Salvioli G. L'anziano fragile e il paziente anziano fragile: problema solo terminologico? G Gerontol. 2006;54:255–9.
30. Partridge JS, Harari D, Dhesi JK. Frailty in the older surgical patient: a review. Age Ageing. 2012;41(2):142–7. https://doi.org/10.1093/ageing/afr182.
31. Jones TS, Dunn CL, Wu DS, Cleveland JC Jr, Kile D, Robinson TN. Relationship between asking an older adult about falls and surgical outcomes. JAMA Surg. 2013;148(12):1132–8. https://doi.org/10.1001/jamasurg.2013.2741.
32. Robinson TN, Wu DS, Pointer L, Dunn CL, Cleveland JC Jr, Moss M. Simple frailty score predicts postoperative complications across surgical specialties. Am J Surg. 2013;206:544–50. https://doi.org/10.1016/j.amjsurg.2013.03.012.
33. Robinson TN, Eiseman B, Wallace JI, Church SD, McFann KK, Pfister SM, Sharp TJ, Moss M. Redefining geriatric preoperative assessment using frailty, disability and co-morbidity. Ann Surg. 2009;250(3):449–55. https://doi.org/10.1097/SLA.0b013e3181b45598.
34. Rockwood K, Song X, MacKnight C, Bergman H, Hogan DB, McDowell I, Mitnitski A. A global clinical measure of fitness and frailty in elderly people. CMAJ. 2005;173(5):489–95.
35. Fagard K, Leonard S, Deschodt M, Devriendt E, Wolthuis A, Prenen H, et al. The impact of frailty on postoperative outcomes in individuals aged 65 and over undergoing elective surgery for colorectal cancer: a systematic review. J Geriatr Oncol. 2016;7(6):479–91. https://doi.org/10.1016/j.jgo.2016.06.001.
36. Robinson TN, Walston JD, Brummel NE, Deiner S, Brown CH 4th, Kennedy M, et al. Frailty for surgeons: review of a National Institute on Aging conference on frailty for specialists. J Am Coll Surg. 2015;221(6):1083–92. https://doi.org/10.1016/j.jamcollsurg.2015.08.428.

37. Op het Veld LP, van Rossum E, Kempen GI, de Vet HC, Hajema K, Beurskens AJ. Fried phenotype of frailty: cross-sectional comparison of three frailty stages on various health domains. BMC Geriatr. 2015;15:77. https://doi.org/10.1186/s12877-015-0078-0.
38. Lin HS, Watts JN, Peel NM, Hubbard RE. Frailty and post-operative outcomes in older surgical patients: a systematic review. BMC Geriatr. 2016;16(1):157. https://doi.org/10.1186/s12877-016-0329-8
39. Stoicea N, Baddigam R, Wajahn J, Sipes AC, Arias-Morales CE, Gastaldo N, Bergese SD. The gap between clinical research and standard of care: a review of frailty assessment scales in perioperative surgical settings. Front Public Health. 2016;4:150.
40. Bettelli G. Preoperative evaluation in geriatric surgery: comorbidity, functional status and pharmacological history. Minerva Anestesiol. 2011;77(6):637–46.
41. Preston SD, Southall AR, Nel M, Das SK. Geriatric surgery is about disease, not age. J R Soc Med. 2008;101(8):409–15. https://doi.org/10.1258/jrsm.2008.080035.
42. Jung P, Pereira MA, Hiebert B, Song X, Rockwood K, Tangri N, et al. The impact of frailty on postoperative delirium in cardiac surgery patients. J Thorac Cardiovasc Surg. 2015;149(3):869–75.e1-2. https://doi.org/10.1016/j.jtcvs.2014.10.118.
43. Revenig LM, Canter DJ, Taylor MD, Tai C, Sweeney JF, Sarmiento JM, et al. Too frail for surgery? Initial results of a large multidisciplinary prospective study examining preoperative variables predictive of poor surgical outcomes. J Am Coll Surg. 2013;217(4):665–670.e1. https://doi.org/10.1016/j.jamcollsurg.2013.06.012.
44. Kristjansson SR, Nesbakken A, Jordhøy MS, Skovlund E, Audisio RA, Johannessen HO, et al. Comprehensive geriatric assessment can predict complications in elderly patients after elective surgery for colorectal cancer: a prospective observational cohort study. Crit Rev Oncol Hematol. 2010;76(3):20817. https://doi.org/10.1016/j.critrevonc.2009.11.002.
45. Berrut G, Andrieu S, Araujo de Carvalho I, Baeyens JP, Bergman H, et al. Promoting access to innovation for frail old persons. IAGG (International Association of Gerontology and Geriatrics), WHO (World Health Organization) and SFGG (Société Française de Gériatrie et de Gérontologie) workshop-Athens January 20-21, 2012. J Nutr Health Aging. 2013;17(8):688–93. https://doi.org/10.1007/s12603-013-0039-2.
46. Ritchie K, Polge C, de Roquefeuil G, Djakovic M, Ledesert B. Impact of anesthesia on the cognitive functioning of the elderly. Int Psychogeriatr. 1997;9(3):309–26.
47. Hempenius L, Slaets JP, van Asselt D, de Bock GH, Wiggers T, van Leeuwen BL. Outcomes of a geriatric liaison intervention to prevent the development of postoperative delirium in frail elderly cancer patients: report on a multicentre, randomized, controlled trial. PLoS One. 2013;8(6):e64834. https://doi.org/10.1371/journal.pone.0064834.
48. Parikh SS, Chung F. Postoperative delirium in the elderly. Anesth Analg. 1995;80(6): 1223–32.
49. McCabe M. From disease to delirium: managing the declining elderly patient. Geriatrics. 1990;45(12):28–31.
50. Robinson TN, Eiseman B. Postoperative delirium in the elderly: diagnosis and management. Clin Interv Aging. 2008;3(2):351–5.
51. Jeong YM, Lee E, Kim KI, Chung JE, In Park H, Lee BK, et al. Association of preoperative medication use with post-operative delirium in surgical oncology patients receiving comprehensive geriatric assessment. BMC Geriatr. 2016;16:134. https://doi.org/10.1186/s12877-016-0311-5.
52. Fick DM, Cooper JW, Wade WE, Waller JL, Maclean JR, Beers MH. Updating the beers criteria for potentially inappropriate medication use in older adults: results of a US consensus panel of experts. Arch Intern Med. 2003;163(22):2716–24. Erratum in: Arch Intern Med. 2004 Feb 9;164(3):298.
53. Deiner S, Silverstein JH. Postoperative delirium and cognitive dysfunction. Br J Anaesth. 2009;103(Suppl 1):i41–6. https://doi.org/10.1093/bja/aep291.

54. Whitlock EL, Vannucci A, Avidan MS. Postoperative delirium. Minerva Anestesiol. 2011;77(4):448–56.
55. American Psychiatric Association. Diagnostic and statistical manual of mental disorders. 4th ed. Washington: American Psychiatric Association; 1994.
56. American Geriatrics Society expert panel on postoperative delirium in older adults. Postoperative delirium in older adults: best practice statement from the American Geriatrics Society. J Am Coll Surg. 2015;220(2):136–48.e1. https://doi.org/10.1016/j.jamcollsurg.2014.10.019.

Perioperative Management

4

Piergaspare Palumbo, Marco Scatizzi, Giorgia Prestigiacomo, and Maddalena Baraghini

4.1 The Challenge of Aging in Elderly Patients

In all the industrialized countries of the world, the elderly population is constantly increasing, having reached about 13.4 million people overall and 22% in relative terms, according to OMS data. Therefore, it represents the fastest increasing group in the entire population, which is expected to double by 2050.

This aging population sets constant healthcare challenges that aim to ensure an extended life expectancy and an improved quality of life.

Elderly patients have specific and different characteristics but in varying degrees, thus constituting their typical fragility: they have multiple diseases (hematological, hepatic, renal, cardiac, hypertension, diabetes mellitus, atherosclerosis, and chronic obstructive pulmonary disease (COPD)), as well as cognitive-behavioral and psychological problems due to old age. These show atypical presentations of disease and unstable homeostasis, which are accompanied by a high risk of complications and trigger a cascade of vicious circles. Above all, as a result of an acute pathological event or a surgical treatment, elderly patients have a physiological reduction of the functional reserve, in particular if this involves a long hospital stay or a re-hospitalization. Consequently, there is a more pronounced risk of comorbidities and complications. It is like configuring a permanent situation of disability and loss of independence, which will inevitably affect the overall health.

P. Palumbo (✉) • G. Prestigiacomo • M. Baraghini
Department of Surgical Sciences, "Sapienza"—University of Rome,
Viale del Policlinico, 155, 00161 Rome, Italy

Via Alessandro Serpieri, 13, 00197 Rome, Italy
e-mail: piergaspare.palumbo@uniroma1.it

M. Scatizzi
Chief Surgical Department, Usl 4 - Prato, Florence, Italy

Via Alessandro Serpieri, 13, 00197 Rome, Italy

A. Crucitti (ed.), *Surgical Management of Elderly Patients*,
https://doi.org/10.1007/978-3-319-60861-7_4

The ERAS (Enhanced Recovery After Surgery) method, a multimodal protocol aimed at ensuring the most rapid possible postoperative recovery, keeps the degree of elderly patient autonomy as close as possible to the previous level, limiting stress and significantly reducing the length of hospital stay and discharge and the rate of complications and readmission. To provide optimal care while maintaining high-quality standards and at the same time cope with the complexity of multiple health conditions of the elderly patient, the obvious priority is to reconsider the perioperative process starting with a careful analysis of the existing literature and providing common guidelines for proper management of the surgical geriatric patient.

In fact, by combining the latest available scientific evidence in the various disciplines that operate around the patient requiring major surgery, this method aims to positively change the response in preserving the physiological functional reserve.

4.2 The Pathophysiology of Surgical Stress

4.2.1 The Metabolic Response to Surgery

Surgery, and especially major surgery, is an insult to the body comparable to the intensity of the metabolic response to trauma or an extended burn.

The determining events are the result of the triggering of physiological compensation mechanisms which all together constitute the metabolic stress response to surgery.

The essential purpose of this response is to make the functional reserves available, from which the substrates are required to adapt to the stressful situation, repair damaged tissue, and protect the vital organs.

Three main events are identified, which act as a switch to all the other effects: the activation of the hypothalamic-pituitary-adrenal axis, the action of the immune system, and the systemic inflammatory response. They constitute the set of triggers that massively mobilize hormones and second messenger molecules, causing a series of cellular and metabolic changes in target organs. The result is a profound imbalance with complete disruption of homeostasis.

The paraventricular nucleus (NPV) acts as a coordinating center for signals from different brain areas devoted to the stress response. Its activation results in the secretion of corticotropin-releasing factor (CRF), which regulates the production of adrenocorticotropic hormone (ACTH), required for the production and release of glucocorticoids from the adrenal cortex, the most important of which is cortisol. Glucocorticoid hormones, in turn, exert significant influence on the immune system, acting both against the humoral and cellular effector arms. In fact, they regulate the production of interleukins, such as IL-1 and IL-6, interferon γ (IFNγ), and tumor necrosis factor α (TNFα) by T helper cells 1 and 2.

The dialogue between the nervous and immune systems does not seem to be confined to the hypothalamic-pituitary-adrenal axis. It extends potentially to the entire central nervous system, particularly the frontal lobe and the limbic system (hippocampus and amygdala), and determines some related events in inflammatory states and intense stress, such as the reduction of attention and interaction with the environment. This connection represents a pathophysiological basis for understanding the etiology of delirium that is very frequent in elderly patients undergoing surgery.

4.2.2 Stress Hyperglycemia

The liver is a target organ of the stress response. In fact, the production of proinflammatory cytokines and chemokines, catecholamines, and cortisol guides its function in favor of a massive production of glucose.

Protein catabolism induced by cortisol also acts on muscle tissue, until "muscle wasting"; this response leads to amino acid availability and increase hepatic gluconeogenesis. Also, the feedback mechanism responsible for the silencing of this pathway is inhibited by the presence of large amounts of proinflammatory molecules.

The TNFα and the IL-1 are, in fact, engaged in various actions: to directly stimulate gluconeogenesis and liver glycogenolysis, to cause a downregulation of synthesis and exposure of the glucose transporter GLUT4 membrane, and to interfere with insulin tyrosine kinase receptor signaling, repressing and thus triggering a resistance to the insulin response itself.

The result is an increase in hepatic glucose production and the onset of a marked insulin resistance, clinically defined as "stress hyperglycemia."

Hyperglycemia supports the inflammatory response and oxidative stress, contributing to the emergence of a vicious cycle that feeds on itself.

It also establishes a switch in hepatic protein synthesis, which is diverted to produce acute phase proteins and immunoglobulins and albumin in disadvantage.

This mechanism is amplified in the elderly patient, who already has a pre-existing condition of a depletion in protein stores and often of malnutrition.

This condition causes a reduction in oncotic pressure and the passage of fluid from the intravascular compartment to the interstitial, promoting a side effect of edema, which in the geriatric patient involves the onset of respiratory, cardiovascular, infective, and immune complications and contributes to increased postoperative morbidity and mortality. Moreover, the loss of protein is responsible for the state of sarcopenia and of delay in healing the surgical wound.

In addition, a marked lipolysis occurs, with cleavage of the fat reserves in the triglyceride which will take part, by increasing their blood concentration, in the intensification of the inflammatory response and the vicious circle described above, adding to the deterioration of other signaling processes with a reduction of cellular resistance to apoptosis.

Several studies also show that hyperglycemia and other stress-related disorders are associated at a statistically significant rate with an increased risk of perioperative adverse events, particularly in elderly patients with significant pre-existing comorbidities, and could therefore be considered predictive of mortality.

In clinical practice, the increase in blood glucose concentration appears to be related to the intensity of the surgical trauma and in major surgery can also record postoperative levels equal to 10–12 mmol/L. A glucose concentration higher than 7 mmol/L, frequently found in patients undergoing abdominal surgery, appears to be a predictor of mortality and the development of complications, and the patients show an increase of 15 times in the incidence of associated infections and hospital mortality.

The sudden and repeated fluctuations are mainly associated with worse outcomes, due to the consequences induced in the endothelial and cellular level; oxidative stress, in fact, has less serious effects when exposure lasts longer than the sudden exposure to high concentrations.

The elements that contribute to the onset of the state of insulin resistance in the postoperative period were identified in preoperative fasting, postoperative pain, and prolonged bed rest.

4.3 Risk Assessment in the Elderly Patient

The "Elderly Multidimensional Assessment (EMA)" must be used in this specific methodological approach, although it is not generally considered in the preoperative stage. It aims to assess the patient's geriatric functionality and status through performance measures, clinical data, laboratory, and also psychological and social measures.

The EMA uses specific rating scales, which differ in relation to the investigated areas. Several are validated and used in the international arena, including the Mini Mental State Exam (MMSE), which investigates the cognitive functions exploring temporal orientation, spatial, memory, and computing power. The Geriatric Depression Scale (GDS) aims to detect specific aspects of depression in the elderly. Activities of the Day Living (ADL) and Instrumental Activities of Day Living (IADL) reflect the elderly person's needs in their daily life and thus provide an indirect estimate of functional autonomy and social measures. The Barthel Index (BI) and the Modified Rankin Scale (MRS) are also commonly used for the assessment of disability. Finally, the scale of Tinetti is used to evaluate balance, posture, and gait [1].

Risk assessment can also use tools such as the POSSUM (Physiological and Operative Severity Score for the Enumeration of Mortality and Morbidity) score, which is very useful in predicting the postoperative outcomes and is appropriate in objectively evaluating the performance status of patients [2].

Finally, we need to apply a high degree of attention to the multiple comorbidities present. Elderly patients with two or more comorbidities have a higher risk of perioperative mortality (4–16%) than those with a single pre-existing pathology, confirming fragility as a predictor of morbidity and mortality.

The progressive interweaving of these elements and their interaction results in greater differentiation between patients and makes it difficult to find a standard risk assessment tool.

Score	1	2	4	8
Age (years)	≤60	61-70	≥71	
Cardiac signs	Normal	Diuretic, digoxin antianginal or antihypertensive therapy	Peripheral edema, warfarin therapy	Raised jugular venous pressure
Chest radiograph	Normal	—	Borderline cardiomegaly	Cardiomegaly
Respiratory history	Normal	Dyspnea on exertion	Limiting dyspnea (one flight of stairs)	Dyspnea at rest
Chest radiograph	Normal	Mild chronic obstructive airway disease	Moderate COAD	Fibrosis or consolidation
Systolic blood pressure (mmHg)	110–130	131–170	≥171	<89
		100–109	90–99	
Pulse (beats/min)	50–80	81–100	101–120	≥121
		40–49		≤39
Glasgow coma scale	15	12–14	9–11	≤8
Hemoglobin (g/dl)	13–16	11.5–12.9	10–11.4	≤9.9
		16.1–17	17.1–18	≥18.1
White cell count ($\times 10^{12}$/l)	4–10	10.1–20	≥20.1	
		3.1–4	<3	
Blood urea (mmol/l)	≤7.5	7.6–10	10.1–15	≥15.1
Sodium (mmol/l)	≥136	131–135	126–130	≤125
Potassium (mmol/l)	3.5–5	3.2–3.4	2.9–3.1	≤2.8
		5.2–5.3	5.4–5.9	≥6
Electrocardiogram	Normal		Atrial fibrillation (rate 60–90)	Any other change

COAD: Chronic obstructive airway disease

The POSSUM score (Copeland et al. [2]).

4.4 Eras Method

4.4.1 Rationale of Application

In recent years new topics in surgery and anesthesia have allowed demonstration of improvements for postoperative recovery in medium-high complexity surgery candidates.

The traditional care approach determines a significant postoperative reduction in functional capacity which can last up to several weeks.

In addition, in assessing the actual need and effectiveness of several standard approaches such as mechanical intestinal preparation, excessive fluid administration, and the prolonged use of the nasogastric tube, several studies have documented the uselessness and the risks of delaying the reacquisition of normal feeding and walking.

The usefulness of the ERAS protocol lies in the multimodal advanced management philosophy and perioperative route optimization, with the goal of limiting surgical stress as a factor conditioning the duration of hospital stay and at the same time restoring and supporting all those functions that enable rapid recovery of normal life activities of the patient, reducing the risk of complications and the hospital readmission rate.

This method, therefore, aims to modify the physiological response to major surgery and has proven effective in reducing complications, demonstrating a decrease in postoperative dysfunction in the geriatric patient and consequently greater satisfaction.

However, despite encouraging data, such innovations in the management of the surgical patient struggle to fully enter clinical practice because of cultural resistance anchored to conventional procedures and organizational difficulties.

4.5 The ERAS Protocol

Currently a single standardized protocol in any surgical procedure has yet been defined; however, some key elements are recognized as part of a rehabilitation program advanced in most adopted protocols. In applying the ERAS method, however, three common phases are recognized: the preoperative phase, the intraoperative phase, and the postoperative phase.

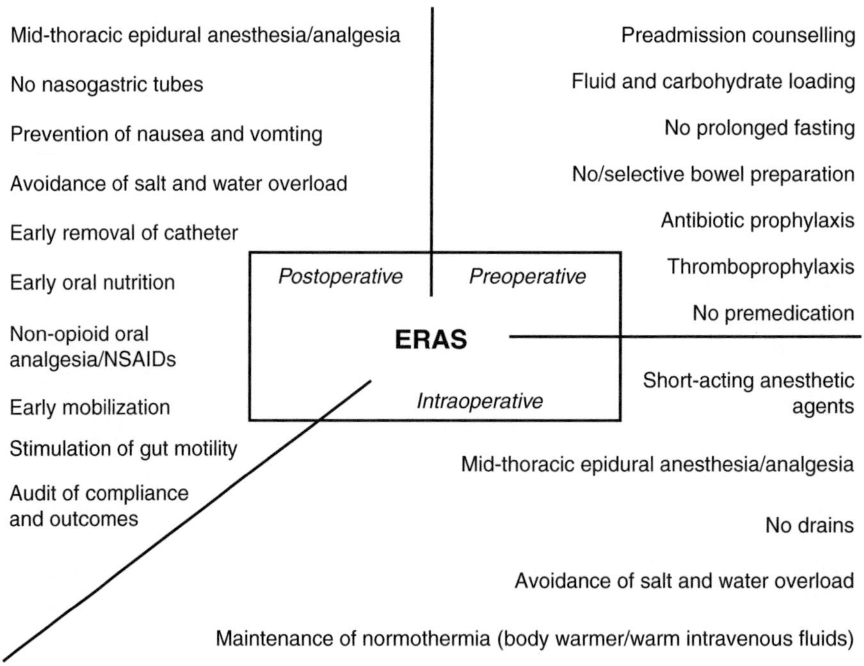

Fast-Track in Colorectal Surgery (Varadhan et al. [3]).

4.5.1 The Preoperative Phase

During the preoperative phase, counseling helps patients to better understand their overall health status, to become aware of the benefits and risks associated with the procedures, and to weigh up expectations based on these elements, especially with regard to pain treatment, the reacquisition of existing functionality, and other hurdles to be faced each postoperative day.

Therefore, the patient must have the opportunity to meet with all members of the multidisciplinary team to discuss details of various aspects of their treatment and to outline to the team members a complete picture of what they will face so that the team will be ready to put in place resources to help them cope.

Elderly patients who have had major surgery are often burdened with important comorbidities, which should be identified and treated to adequately limit their effects. This will significantly change the rate of occurrence of complications and affect the postoperative course.

Uncontrolled diabetic patients with elevated glycated hemoglobin levels show a more increased risk of major postoperative complications than patients with glucose intolerance or those without diabetes. Similarly, patients with cardiac comorbidity, COPD, and other homeostatic disorders have an increased risk of adverse events. Although anemia is a condition often found in the elderly, it needs to be identified and corrected before surgery. The anemic state in the preoperative period, in fact, is closely associated with increased morbidity and postoperative mortality, so it can be considered a predictor.

Malnutrition operates like other comorbidities to the establishment of an unfavorable condition to the body's response to surgical stress and impairs the patient's general condition. It is characterized by a negative impact on outcome and requires special attention to the correction of deficiencies of essential nutrients.

The European Society of Parenteral and Enteral Nutrition (ESPEN) defined severe nutritional risk patients as those who present with one or more of the following characteristics:

- Significant weight loss (from 10 to 16%) in 6 months
- BMI <18.5 kg/m^2
- Serum albumin <30 g/L

The ESPEN provides a screening questionnaire, the Nutritional Risk Screening, for the evaluation and stratification of patients, similar to the Malnutrition Universal Screening Tool (MUST); it identifies malnourished adults, with elevated risk of malnutrition or obesity based on a five-step process. Both are easy to use in the hospital setting.

Within the ERAS protocol, the achievement of a satisfactory nutritional state is carried out by administration of nutritional supplements to patients, generally by mouth or, if necessary, enterally. Scientific evidence supports preoperative nutrition as it has shown that administration of glucose solutions before surgery is safe and can have a positive effect on clinical outcomes, reducing the rate of complications and the length of stay [4].

Further addition of nutritional support is represented by immunonutrition, a term which defines the formula enriched with amino acids such as arginine and glutamine, unsaturated fatty acids, omega-3, vitamins, and minerals.

In conventional practice the preoperative fasting in its form "nihil per os" (NPO) from midnight of the day before surgery is considered standard. This recommendation is still very strong in clinical practice and is justified in the attempt to prevent aspiration pneumonia. Several studies have disproved the claim that fasting provides an "empty stomach," confirming that during fasting the stomach can secrete up to 50 mL/h of gastric juice and thus highlighting the limits of preoperative fasting and its potential harmfulness. The treatment provided by the ERAS protocol consists of the administration of a preoperative carbohydrate load (PCL) orally. The PCL causes a more rapid recovery of bowel function, reducing the length of stay without causing any side effects. Several randomized controlled trials (RCTs) show that the administration of the PCL will result in a faster metabolic response in the postoperative period, a reduction of insulin resistance, and contained protein loss, with greater preservation of muscle functional reserve. In fact, a Cochrane systematic review of 22 RCTs showed how fasting from midnight does not reduce gastric contents and also does not reduce the rate of complications of fasted patients compared to those who were allowed the ingestion of solid foods up to 6 h before the operation and clear liquids (water, fruit juices without pulp, carbonated drinks, tea, and coffee) up to 2 h before. The advantage of the pathophysiological preoperative glucose load lies in increasing the production of insulin which causes a cellular metabolism shift toward an anabolic state [5–7].

The traditional management of abdominal surgery candidate patients, in particular colorectal ones, provides for a complete mechanical cleaning of the colon with a duration of one or more days in combination with a diet low in slag and to an intestinal antibiotic prophylaxis.

Mechanical preparation allows a significant reduction in stool weight and, in synergy with the antiseptic preparation, results in a reduction of 80–90% of the colonic bacterial flora.

Recently, mechanical bowel preparation has been shown to be useless in multiple randomized clinical trials and in a Cochrane review, since it involves dehydration and electrolyte imbalances [8, 9].

Both lead to a significant reduction in muscle strength and exercise tolerance, as well as weight loss; also, they determine an increase in hematocrit and hemodynamic alterations, increased plasma osmolarity with rising concentrations of urea, and a falling of concentrations of calcium and potassium.

These results in elderly patients with several comorbidities lead to dangerous postural hypotension, which may cause syncope and increase the risk of falls and injuries.

Therefore, the utility of MBP is strongly challenged, and its avoidance does not cause an increased incidence of anastomotic leakage or the risk of infection.

Undergoing surgery is usually a strong emotional stress. In traditional perioperative management, patients receive the administration of atropine and benzodiazepines from 1 h to 30 min prior. A recent meta-analysis showed that the pre-anesthesia does not involve a substantial reduction of postoperative pain but leads to an extended phase of postoperative unconsciousness [10].

The use of anxiolytics with short action is preferred in ERAS protocol and can help anxious patients during insertion of the epidural catheter and generally in the postoperative period in controlling the pain and avoiding the excessive use of opioids. Long half-life sedatives should not be used for routine procedures and should be avoided 12 h prior to the surgery as they can hinder a rapid recovery of mobility and oral nutrition.

4.5.2 The Intraoperative Phase

Antibiotic prophylaxis, in the elderly as in younger patients, is effective in reducing infectious complications and therefore uniformly recommended for all major surgical operations. The single-dose ("ultra-short-term prophylaxis") and a multidose regimens ("short-term prophylaxis") have proven equally effective, although multiple doses are indicated for interventions exceeding 3 h, in accordance with the pharmacokinetics of the chosen antibiotic [11].

In traditional management opioids are often used for intraoperative analgesia. The choice of the anesthetic technique specified in the ERAS protocol must take two fundamental aspects into account: on the one hand the use of short-acting agents (such as Propofol®) that allow a more rapid onset of postoperative recovery and, on the other, an anesthetic procedure that minimizes surgical stress.

Epidural analgesia is an important anti-catabolic tool, used to prevent postoperative insulin resistance. The surgical trauma causes the stimulation of central and peripheral nerve pathways and leads to the catabolic response to surgery. In this light, the nociceptive segmental block at the spinal cord level guarantees not only adequate pain control but helps to limit catabolic effects, participating directly in a better outcome.

The anesthetic technique with neuraxial block and epidural analgesia is the only one able to alter the stress response. The benefits could result from different mechanisms, including an increase in blood flow, more effective breathing without pain, and, not least, by a reduction of multifactorial components of the response to surgical stress. The use of epidural catheters is also increasingly widespread in the management of postoperative pain: it provides for the systemic administration of different types of analgesics or for the application of systemic and regional analgesia together, making the control of pain and the reduction of side effects associated with the use of opioids possible in this way.

Epidural analgesia has also been shown to be superior to intravenous analgesia in postoperative pain control in both traditional surgery and in minimally invasive surgery, allowing a reduction in the paralytic ileus due to selective blockade of δ nociceptive fibers. Although there are few studies that have evaluated the impact of different anesthetic techniques on postoperative outcomes, there is no evidence that compares intravenous anesthetic to that of inhaled. It seems clear that the ERAS protocol makes a great effort to minimize the impact of anesthetic agents in order to promote rapid postoperative awakening and thus facilitate the recovery of the functions [12].

For this reason, the use of short-acting hypnotic inductor agents, such as propofol, is recommended, combined with a short half-life opioid such as fentanyl and remifentanil in bolus or continuous infusion. With regard to the maintenance phase, the ERAS method does not provide for the use of exclusive inhaler agents, in order to obtain the reduction in the incidence of PONV caused by nitric oxide, even if it is administered in the antiemetic prophylaxis.

The blockade of the neuraxial system prolonged to the postoperative phase involves additional benefits in many patients: a recent meta-analysis showed an overall reduction in mortality of 30% and significant reduction of other complications [13].

By virtue of these multiple benefits of epidural analgesia, this procedure is preferable in the ERAS protocol.

The trauma resulting from surgery involves two types of damage:

1. The primary injury determined by surgical incision, by tissue manipulation, and by the mobilization of the viscera
2. Secondary damage related to blood loss during surgery, the effects of the anesthetic technique, and the intraoperative administration of drugs

Reduction of these two types of damage can be obtained by exploiting the advantages offered by the use of minimally invasive surgical techniques.

Minimally invasive surgery allows the optimization of surgical damage through minimizing the incision extent and carefully carrying out dissection without compromising radicality and surgical accuracy.

In this way, the muscle fibers are moved away from each other instead of being etched (splitting vs. cutting); also, a better hemostatic control can be achieved, with easier identification of cleavage planes in a bloodless field. The magnification of images also proves beneficial in reducing the irritation of the serous, in limiting the formation of adhesions and incidence of hematoma or postoperative bleeding.

The minimally invasive approach seems to have significant short-term advantages over open surgery, such as the reduction of postoperative pain, early recovery of intestinal motility, improved lung function, reduced hospitalization, and a better quality of life in the first 30 days.

However, the use of minimally invasive techniques proved that it is not possible to completely change the effects of the endocrine-metabolic responses to surgical stress while limiting the immunodysfunction, the inflammatory response, pulmonary stress, and hypoxemia when compared with the laparotomic approach.

Moreover, some long-term outcome studies do not reveal the substantial difference expected, but report as equivalent the use of open and minimally invasive techniques [14].

By contrast, the multicenter study "LAFA Study 1" and other scientific research demonstrated a real benefit in the application of laparoscopic techniques in the multimodal strategy of rapid postoperative recovery [15, 16].

In recent years, the spread of new and alternative minimally invasive surgery techniques, including robotic surgery, laparoscopic techniques with single incision (SILS), and the "hand-assisted laparoscopic surgery" (HALS), has shown that it is possible to reduce invasiveness.

These techniques are mainly used in highly specialized centers, but their use is still not widespread, as there are not substantial data in favor of showing any real advantage to justify their becoming more widespread.

The metabolic response to surgical stress determines the alteration of the balance of fluids and electrolytes, as well as temperature and blood rheology. Through the AT1 receptor placed on the muscular coat of the vessels, angiotensin causes vasoconstriction and the production and release of several proinflammatory cytokines. The resulting water retention is accompanied by a reduced excretion of sodium and increased excretion of potassium.

In addition, the activation of inflammatory responses compromises the ability of the organism to achieve a proper metabolic balance and to maintain the volume and composition of the extracellular and intracellular fluid constant. The colloid osmotic pressure is altered in a negative sense, and this leads to an increased permeability of capillaries and a passage of fluids from the capillary bed interstitium.

The management of fluid therapy provided in the ERAS protocol is designed to counter these events: strong recommendations in this program suggest the adoption of a restrictive regime, as the excessive administration of fluids can affect the circulatory district and heart function.

Therefore, it must be recommended to limit the infusion of colloids and crystalloids, generally administered in order to avoid transfusions and the reduction in renal blood flow. In fact, excessive preload, particularly in the elderly, may depress cardiac function and lead to increased comorbidity such as cardiology and pulmonary ones, to the point of acute lung injury (ALI) and acute respiratory distress syndrome (ARDS).

The physiological electrolyte balance should therefore remain stable throughout the perioperative period, and in every single moment of the care path, this should be monitored to achieve the maintenance of the "steady state," which represents the state in which the volume and composition of the body fluids remain constant despite the quantitative and qualitative changes of water and solutes.

For this purpose, not more than 3 L of fluid per day is administered, and a bowel preparation is avoided; moreover, fluid intake control before treatment also allows the prevention of edema, associated with a prolongation postoperative ileus and reduced cell oxygenation.

"Goal-directed fluid therapy" involves the administration of intraoperative crystalloid at a rate of 2–3 mL/kg/h adequate to prevent an increase in weight of more than 2.5 kg, preferring isotonic and balanced solutions than the 0.9% saline solution.

Regarding colloidal solutions, their adoption has been deprecated by recent studies. In elderly patients, they significantly alter hemostasis and can lead to acute renal failure.

The ERAS protocol provides for the removal of the nasogastric tube even before the patient's awakening from anesthesia. There is no evidence to support its use in the postoperative period; a Cochrane meta-analysis of 37 studies, enlisting more than 5000 patients undergoing laparotomy for abdominal surgery, documented a slower functional recovery after surgery, a higher incidence of postoperative ileus, and an increased risk of complications in subjects in which the SNG is left in place [17].

Finally, intraoperative hypothermia prevention reduces the endocrine response and the sympathetic reflexes, allowing a limitation of the body's response to surgical stress caused by the intervention; in addition, it does not impair the coagulation tests, resulting in a reduction of bleeding.

Preventing hypothermia through the infusion of fluids at appropriate temperatures or the use of a thermal blanket reduces surgical site infections, cardiac complications, bleeding, and the need for blood transfusion.

In the immediate postoperative period, it also prevents the effects of desaturation and myocardial ischemic accidents due to the sudden increase in blood concentrations of norepinephrine caused by the drop in body temperature and prolongs the overall time for anesthesia.

4.5.3 The Postoperative Phase

Postoperative nausea and vomiting (PONV) are the most common complications in the immediate postoperative period, affecting 20–30% of patients undergoing abdominal surgery.

It appears within 24 h after surgery and contributes to postoperative morbidity, as possible causes of aspiration pneumonia, wound dehiscence, and hydroelectrolytic alterations.

Some endogenous molecules such as serotonin (5-HT), substance P, and other mediators capable of transmitting a signal to the afferent nerve fibers would assume relevant importance.

Various risk factors have been associated with the development of postoperative nausea and vomiting. Among them the strongest predictor appears to be gender, with women at double the risk compared to men. A system of stratification of the PONV risk is represented by the Apfel simplified score.

To avoid the unpleasant effects of PONV, it is necessary to focus attention on strategies that include the use of regional anesthesia, the use of short-acting anesthetic agents, the avoidance of nitric oxide, adequate hydration, and a restricted use of opioids.

In addition, administration of supplemental oxygen has been shown to have a clear benefit in reducing PONV. Goll et al. in a randomized study observed 240 patients and concluded that 2 h of oxygen at 80% is more effective and less costly than ondansetron in reducing PONV [18].

In high-risk patients, a combination therapy with the use of multiple drugs is recommended, increasing the probability of success over monotherapy, since the use of just one drug has only proved able to reduce the incidence by around 25%.

Delirium is perhaps the most significant age-related postoperative complication.

It is characterized by a sharp decline in cognitive function and attention and episodes of consciousness fluctuation and occurs in approximately 40% of patients undergoing surgery. It can occur in patients of any age but is most common in the elderly, especially those who have already shown cognitive impairment in the preoperative stage. Its etiology is multifactorial, depending on physiological imbalances caused by stress related to the intervention, the use of drugs in the intraoperative and postoperative period, or by a pre-existing condition of fragility and the susceptibility of the patient. The pathogenetic mechanism is not entirely clear, but several studies show a predominant role of the pathways of systemic inflammation and increased production of cytokines such as TNF. Delirium is associated with worse surgical outcomes, longer hospital stays, functional decline, higher institutionalization rates, mortality, and costs due to increased resource utilization.

To fully understand the pathophysiological basis of this phenomenon, consideration must be given to the risk factors and precipitating factors; for this purpose, different scores are considered to assist in recognizing patients at higher risk of postoperative delirium. The basic elements for risk stratification are age; pre-existing cognitive impairment; the use of antianxiety drugs such as benzodiazepines (BDZ); sleep disorders; alteration of laboratory values, particularly the function tests of the liver and kidney; and a history of alcohol abuse.

Hospital environments should favor proper hydration, the limited use of opioids and benzodiazepines, and an early empowerment.

Postoperative pain is one of the main variables in the recovery of patients and is one of the main factors that contributes to prolonging the postoperative hospital stay.

Traditionally, the control of postoperative pain is entrusted to plentiful intravenous administration of morphine. However, its use is burdened by side effects poorly tolerated by the patient especially if elderly, important among which are respiratory depression, inhibition of cough reflex, paralytic ileus, orthostatic hypotension, nausea, and vomiting. Moreover, the activation of opioid receptors for neuropeptides in the myenteric plexus inhibits the release of acetylcholine from the nerve endings, causing a decrease in the tonus of the smooth muscle cell and an impaired motility of the intestinal wall.

In the geriatric patient, multimodal pain control is more appropriate. The surgical incision and the manipulation of the intestinal bowel tissue cause the release of chemical mediators such as adenosine, bradykinin, cytokines, prostaglandins, TNF, and IL-1 that determines a sensitization of the peripheral sensory system, resulting in a lowering of the threshold of activation of nociceptors.

In particular, the prostaglandin 2 (PGE-2) at the spinal level leads to liberation of additional excitatory mediators, amplifying pain and allowing maintenance.

The thoracic epidural analgesia (TEA) involves the insertion of the catheter preferably at the mid-thoracic level (T6–T7, T7–T8) for both analgesia and the sympathetic block, avoiding the paralysis of the intestinal tract. This method is the gold standard for proper pain management in patients undergoing laparoscopic abdominal surgery [19].

If activated before the surgery, neuraxial blockade prevents hormonal release and attenuates postoperative insulin resistance, reducing the need for administering anesthetic agents.

Alternatives for the control of postoperative pain are represented by the use of opioids intravenously issued from a patient's device on demand (patient-controlled analgesia—PCA). An additional method is the "continuous wound infusion of local anesthetic"; in this technique, a "multiholed" catheter (multiperforated) is placed by the surgeon at the end of the intervention, increasing the duration of action of the drug and the tissue infiltration effectiveness. The incidence of failure of this technique is very low (1%) and its toxicity almost none. In addition, further multimodal analgesia strategies are to be considered. The block of the transverse abdominis plane (TAP) and the rectus fascia represents alternative solutions and may play an important role in the context of major abdominal surgery. Finally, another technique is represented by the infiltration of local anesthetic into the peritoneal cavity (IPLA) by elastomeric pump: it allows the blocking of nociceptive pathways of visceral pain.

The postoperative ileus is one of the main iatrogenic complications occurring in the postoperative period; its onset is part of the metabolic response to surgical stress.

Its etiology is multifactorial: factors favoring and triggering are represented by inflammation, changes in fluid and electrolytes, and the administration of drugs; the set of these triggers determines the contractility and altered bowel motility and edema of the wall.

It is one of the major factors that increases the morbidity of the patient, resulting in prolonged recovery time and hospital stay, but nevertheless is considered a normal and inevitable response to laparotomy and other surgical procedures.

The postoperative ileus involves a series of negative and unpleasant consequences, especially for the geriatric patient submitted to surgery: an increase of postoperative pain, an increased likelihood of pulmonary complications, and a postponement of the return to a normal oral feeding are observed. This latest issue is of crucial importance for the activation of the immune system and in the recovery of residual functionality.

In ERAS protocol, epidural analgesia is essential to prevent postoperative paralytic ileus and to stimulate intestinal motility. At the level of the abdominal area, it allows a reduction of the adrenergic tone and the pathway's transmission of the nociceptive signal activation. Furthermore, the use of restrictive infusion therapy prevents the accumulation of liquids in the intestine, thus preventing an overdistension of the fibers of the bowel wall. Also available to the ileum, prevention tools are the "opioid-sparing analgesia," the avoidance of the use of SNG in the postoperative phase, early removal of urinary catheter and drainage when positioned, the use of magnesium oxide per os, as well as early oral nutrition.

This should be initiated some hours after surgery, with at least the administration of clear liquids and, in the absence of PONV, continuing with solid foods from the first postoperative day. This supports the early resumption of intestinal motility.

The lure not only promotes the risk of venous thrombosis, insulin resistance, and muscle breakdown resulting in decreased strength and osteoporosis but also has a negative effect on lung function and oxygenation of tissues.

Patients should be encouraged to early mobilization as from the first postoperative day. A daily exercise program must be established, and the daily compilation, in patient care, of a diary helps achieve the objectives. From the day of surgery, patients should stay out of bed for 2 h, increasing to at least 6 h after the first postoperative day.

Various factors oppose early mobilization, poor compliance by patients, comorbidities, and the effects of any complications occurring after surgery; these all represent barriers to early ambulation and are the main causes of failure in the ERAS protocol.

The rationale behind early mobilization is in reducing the length of hospital stay, but, above all, it conveys a positive and important message of psychological empowerment for elderly patients, which in turn plays an active role in the healing and recovery process, essential to a speedy return to normal daily life.

Conclusions

Geriatric patients, always considered "unfit" for their poor performance status, are often excluded from the development of ERAS paths because they are considered high risk.

In several randomized controlled trials, the elderly represented only a small part of the recruited sample. A recent systematic review by Bagnall et al. [20] reports that the ERAS protocol is safe and can be applied in elderly patients, allowing a reduction in postoperative morbidity and a reduction in the length of stay (LOS) when compared with traditional care pathways. In addition, the data show that neither advanced age nor a high degree ASA has resulted in a higher rate of complications or postoperative mortality, in contrast to what is generally stated.

Patient compliance is considered, on the basis of the scientific evidence, as a predictor of success of the surgical procedure, as well as having a better postoperative outcome and a lower rate of complications; this is valid in the advanced age of the patient, in whom the overall health status components are closely connected to each other.

Few data have been reported regarding the compliance of the elderly patient, but recent studies show that optimal compliance can also be obtained in these subjects, with a positive impact on outcome in the short term, even in patients with a higher ASA grade and poorer performance status [21].

Evidence shows that the multidisciplinary team should always work toward a strong common goal and make a continuous effort to educate patients in order to involve them in all stages of the surgical pathway.

References

1. Sue Brown A, Brummel-Smith K, Burgess L, D'Agostino RB, Goldschmidt JW, Halter JB, Hazzard WR, Jahnigen DW, Phelps C, Raskind M, Schrier RW, Sox HC, Sankey VW. National Institutes of Health consensus development conference statement: geriatric assessment methods for clinical decision-making. J Am Geriatr Soc. 1988;36(4):342–7.

2. Copeland GP, Jones D, Walters M. POSSUM: a scoring system for surgical audit. Br J Surg. 1991;78(3):355–60.
3. Varadhan KK, Lobo DN, Ljungqvist O. Enhanced recovery after surgery: the future of improving surgical care. Crit Care Clin. 2010;26(3):527–47.
4. Noblett SE, Watson DS, Huong H, Davison B, Hainsworth PJ, Horgan AF. Pre-operative oral carbohydrate loading in colorectal surgery: a randomized controlled trial. Color Dis. 2006;8(7):563–9.
5. Green CR, Pandit SK, Schork MA. Preoperative fasting time: is the traditional policy changing? Results of a national survey. Anesth Analg. 1996;83:123–8.
6. Alexander NG, Smith G. Gastroesophageal reflux and aspiration of gastric contents in anesthetic practice. Anesth Analg. 2001;93:494–513.
7. Brady M, Kinn S, Stuart P. Preoperative fasting for adults to prevent perioperative complications. Cochrane Database Syst Rev. 2003;4:CD004423.
8. Guenaga KF, Matos D, Castro AA, Atallah AN, Wille-Jørgensen P. Mechanical bowel preparation for elective colorectal surgery [update of: Cochrane Database Syst Rev. 2003;(2):CD001544]. Cochrane Database Syst Rev. 2005;1:CD001544.
9. Ram E, Sherman Y, Weil R, Vishne T, Kravarusic D, Dreznik Z. Is mechanical bowel preparation mandatory for elective colon surgery? A prospective randomized study. Arch Surg. 2005;140(3):285–8.
10. Smith AF, Pittaway AJ. Premedication for anxiety in adult day surgery [update of: Cochrane Database Syst Rev. 2000;(3):CD002192]. Cochrane Database Syst Rev. 2003;1:CD002192.
11. Bratzler DW, Houck PM, Surgical Infection Prevention Guidelines Writers Workgroup; American Academy of Orthopaedic Surgeons; American Association of Critical Care Nurses; American Association of Nurse Anesthetists; American College of Surgeons; American College of Osteopathic Surgeons; American Geriatrics Society; American Society of Anesthesiologists; American Society of Colon and Rectal Surgeons; American Society of Health-System Pharmacists; American Society of Perianesthesia Nurses; Ascension Health; Association of Perioperative Registered Nurses; Association for Professionals in Infection Control and Epidemiology; Infectious Diseases Society of America; Medical Letter; Premier; Society for Healthcare Epidemiology of America; Society of Thoracic Surgeons; Surgical Infection Society. Antimicrobial prophylaxis for surgery: an advisory statement from the National Surgical Infection Prevention Project. Clin Infect Dis. 2004;38(12):1706–15.
12. Kehlet H, Wilmore DW. Evidence-based surgical care and the evolution of fast-track surgery. Ann Surg. 2008;248(2):189–98.
13. Madsen MV, Staehr-Rye AK, Gatke MR, Claudius C. Neuromuscular blockade for optimising surgical conditions during abdominal and gynaecological surgery: a systematic review. Acta Anaesthesiol Scand. 2015;59:1–16.
14. Khan S, Gatt M, MacFie J. Enhanced recovery programmes and colorectal surgery: does the laparoscope confer additional advantages? Color Dis. 2009;11(9):902–8.
15. Vlug MS, Wind J, Hollmann MW, Ubbink DT, Cense HA, Engel AF, Gerhards MF, van Wagensveld BA, van der Zaag ES, van Geloven AA, Sprangers MA, Cuesta MA, Bemelman WA, LAFA study group. Laparoscopy in combination with fast track multimodal management is the best perioperative strategy in patients undergoing colonic surgery: a randomized clinical trial (LAFA-study). Ann Surg. 2011;254(6):868–75.
16. Spanjersberg WR, van Sambeeck JD, Bremers A, Rosman C, van Laarhoven CJ. Systematic review and meta-analysis for laparoscopic versus open colon surgery with or without an ERAS programme. Surg Endosc. 2015;29(12):3443–53.
17. Nelson R, Edwards S, Tse B. Prophylactic nasogastric decompression after abdominal surgery. Cochrane Database Syst Rev. 2007;3:CD004929.
18. Goll V, Akca O, Greif R, et al. Ondansetron is no more effective than supplemental intraoperative oxygen for prevention of postoperative nausea and vomiting. Anesth Analg. 2001;92:112–7.

19. Young Jin Kim MD, Hyun Min Cho MD, Chee Soon Yoon MD, Chan Kyu Lee MD, Tae Yeon Lee MD, June Pill Seok MD. Thoracic epidural Anesthesia and analgesia (TEA) in patients with rib fractures. Korean J Thorac Cardiovasc Surg. 2011 Apr;44(2):178–82.
20. Bagnall NM, Malietzis G, Kennedy RH, Athanasiou T, Faiz O, Darzi A. A systematic review of enhanced recovery care after colorectal surgery in elderly patients. Color Dis. 2014;16:947–56.
21. Braga M, Pecorelli N, Scatizzi M, Borghi F, Missana G, Radrizzani D. Enhanced recovery program in high-risk patients undergoing colorectal surgery: results from the perioperative Italian society registry. World J Surg. 2017;41(3):860–7.

5 Risk of Venous Thromboembolism in Surgical Elderly Patients

Anna Falanga and Viola Milesi

5.1 Introduction

Venous thromboembolism (VTE), which includes deep vein thrombosis (DVT) and pulmonary embolism (PE), is recognized as a complex multifactorial disease, involving clinical and genetic risk factors as well as environmental interactions. The annual incidence varies from 1 to 3 events for every 1000 people in the world. In particular, the annual incidence of VTE in Europe varies from 104 to 180 per 100,000 persons per year [1]. Numerous factors, both transient (i.e., surgery, trauma, prolonged immobility, long trips, hormone therapy, pregnancy, and postpartum) and permanent (i.e., incurable tumors, antiphospholipid syndrome), favor its development. Therefore, when VTE occurs concomitantly or after any of these recognizable risk factors, it is classified as "secondary" VTE. Otherwise, when it occurs in the absence of any of these risk factors, it is classified as "idiopathic" VTE.

Survival after VTE is worse than expected, and survival after PE is even worse than after DVT alone; in fact the risk of early death among patients with symptomatic PE is 18-fold higher compared to patients with DVT alone [2]. PE is an independent predictor of reduced survival for up to 3 months after onset. For almost one-quarter of PE patients, the initial clinical presentation is sudden death. Independent predictors of reduced early survival after VTE include increasing age, male gender, lower body mass index, confinement to a hospital or nursing home, congestive heart failure, chronic lung disease, serious neurological disease, and active malignancy [3].

VTE also recurs frequently. About 30% of patients develop recurrences within the next 10 years. The hazard of recurrence varies with the time since the incident event and is highest within the first 6–12 months. However, even 10 years after an

A. Falanga, MD (✉) • V. Milesi
Division of Immunohematology and Transfusion Medicine, Thrombosis & Hemostasis Center, Hospital Papa Giovanni XXIII, Piazza OMS, 1, Bergamo 24127, Italy

A. Crucitti (ed.), *Surgical Management of Elderly Patients*,
https://doi.org/10.1007/978-3-319-60861-7_5

Table 5.1 Individual risk factors for VTE (Ref. [8])

Individual risk factors
• Advanced age
• Female gender
• Prior VTE or varicose veins
• Patient comorbidities (hypertension, infection, obesity, anemia, pulmonary, liver or renal disease)
• Prolonged immobilization
• Major surgery
• Trauma
• Inherited thrombophilic factors
• Active malignant neoplasm with or without concurrent chemotherapy
• Central vein catheterization or transvenous pacemaker
• Neurological disease with extremity paresis

incident DVT or PE, VTE patients are still at risk of recurrence [4]. Consistently across studies, the risk of recurrence is higher when risk factors are unknown (idiopathic VTE) or persistent as compared with risk factors that are transient. In general, the greater the transient nature of the risk factor, the lower the risk for recurrence after anticoagulant withdrawal. For example, Baglin and colleagues showed that in patients with a first episode of VTE, during a 2-year follow-up period, the incidence of recurrent VTE was 0% with surgery-related VTE, 19.4% with unprovoked VTE, and 8.8% with VTE associated with nonsurgical risk factors (fracture, illness, immobilization, travel, or estrogen) [5].

VTE is a common complication among hospitalized patients. In the absence of appropriate thromboprophylaxis, the reported incidence ranges from 10 to 40% in medicine and general surgery populations and from 40 to 60% in patients undergoing major orthopedic surgery [6]. PE may occur in up to 5–10% of high-risk hospitalized patients and represents one of the most common causes of preventable in-hospital death [7].

In order to improve survival, avoid recurrence, prevent complications, and reduce health-care costs, the occurrence of VTE must be reduced. To achieve this goal, it is very important that persons at risk for VTE are accurately identified. A number of known individual risk factors for VTE are summarized in Table 5.1 [8].

In this chapter, we will focus on the risk of VTE associated with surgery, especially in elderly patients, and on the available tools for stratifying patients undergoing surgery according to their risk level. Furthermore, we will provide information on the various forms of thromboprophylaxis and on the efficacy and safety of thromboprophylaxis in very high-risk type of surgery, i.e., orthopedic and oncological surgery.

5.2 Venous Thromboembolism in Elderly Patients

The incidence of VTE increases significantly with age for both idiopathic and secondary VTE, suggesting that the risk associated with advancing age may be due to the biology of aging rather than simply an increased exposure to VTE risk factors with advancing age. Incidence rates of VTE increase dramatically at about age 55 and by age 80 are nearly 1 in 100 per year, approximately 1000-fold higher than for subjects aged 45 or younger [9, 10]. Furthermore, rates of PE rise faster than DVT in the elderly so that the disease has a greater fatal impact.

Frequent VTE risk factors in older adults include recent hospitalization, recent surgery, cancer (occult or active), infection, immobility, chronic cardiopulmonary disease and exacerbation, and prior history of VTE. Frailty has also recently been found to be a risk factor for VTE. Other less common, but actual, VTE risk factors in older adults include nephrotic syndrome, myeloproliferative disorders, antiphospholipid antibody syndrome, and heparin-induced thrombocytopenia [11]. There are also age-specific factors that are almost exclusively present in the older population, such as reduced muscle strength, endothelial dysfunctions, and venous insufficiency. Overall muscle strength declines starting from the age of 50 years [12]. It is likely that this also affects the calf muscle pump. Although the role of muscle strength of the lower limbs and the concomitant deterioration in the venous hemodynamics is not yet clarified, diminished function or efficacy of the calf muscle pump could lead to reflux and stasis, which subsequently may predispose to thrombus formation. Also, the prevalence of chronic venous insufficiency increases with age. The pathophysiology of this functional disease consists of failure of valves through dilation of the venous wall or remodeling of the valve leaflets, which can then lead to stasis and elevation of distal venous blood pressure.

Other common findings with aging are important changes in the hemostatic balance, with appearance of a prothrombotic state, characterized by an increase in plasma levels of fibrinogen, Factor VII, Factor VIII, fibrinopeptide A, D-dimer, and PAI-1 and by an increased platelet activation in vivo with changes in platelet function related to variation in the membrane lipid composition [13]. For example, plasma fibrinogen levels increase with age, with an approximate 10 mg/dL incremental rise per decade in healthy subjects, and in some settings correlate with VTE risk in older adults. von Willebrand factor and FVIII levels also increase with aging and may be associated with increased risk of thrombosis. Components of the fibrinolytic pathway, such as fibrinolysis inhibitors, show a true age-related increase, which contributes to the overall thrombotic risk [11]. Finally, in elderly subjects, the occurrence of laboratory features of hypercoagulability, as shown by increased levels of circulating thrombotic markers, including D-dimer, underlies a prothrombotic background.

5.3 Risk Stratification in Surgery

In surgical patients, indication for VTE prophylaxis varies according to the individual risk of VTE (Table 5.1) and the type of surgical procedures. As shown in Table 5.2, two types of surgery are distinguished based on the length of intervention (i.e., greater or lower than 45 min).

The risk for VTE is increased in all patients undergoing general surgery, including elderly patients. However, the relative risk for postoperative

Table 5.2 Classification of surgical interventions

Minor surgery[a]	Major surgery
• Radical neck dissection • Inguinal hernia repair • Appendectomy • Laparoscopic cholecystectomy • Transurethral prostatectomy • Repair of a cystocele or rectocele • Cruciate ligament repair • Thyroid or parathyroid surgery	Abdominal or thoracic surgery that requires general anesthesia lasting ≥45 min

[a]In case of interventions with a greater duration of 30–45 min or associated with serious bleeding or extended dissections, the risk becomes comparable to that of major surgery

development of this complication varies among individual patients based on several factors, i.e., the length of immobilization following surgery, the type of surgery performed, and the presence of comorbid conditions. Immobilization for an extended period is a well-established risk factor for VTE, and early mobilization following surgery has been shown to lower the risk for postoperative VTE [14]. There is also strong evidence that the type of surgical procedure is predictive of the risk of postoperative VTE. Major general surgery (i.e., abdominal or thoracic operations that require general anesthesia lasting ≥45 min) is associated with a high risk of VTE. Orthopedic surgery is associated with an even higher risk [15]. Other procedures associated with a substantially increased risk include major vascular surgery, small or large bowel resection, gastric bypass, radical cystectomy, kidney transplantation, and below-the-knee amputation [16]. A lower risk of VTE was reported with radical neck dissection, inguinal hernia repair, appendectomy, laparoscopic cholecystectomy, transurethral prostatectomy, repair of a cystocele or rectocele, cruciate ligament repair, and thyroid or parathyroid surgery (Table 5.2).

In recent years, risk stratification has been suggested as a means of determining the risk for VTE in patients undergoing surgery and of guiding the selection of appropriate prophylactic measures. Several risk assessment models that stratify patients according to their risk of VTE have been published, the most notable being the Caprini score, that estimates VTE risk by adding points for various VTE risk factors (Table 5.3). The Caprini score was introduced in 2005 to improve compliance with VTE prophylaxis guidelines for surgical patients and uses a point-scoring system; the relative scores for individual risk factors are summed to produce a cumulative risk score that defines the patient's risk level (low, moderate, high, or highest risk) and the associated prophylaxis regimen [17]. An appropriate method of VTE prophylaxis can be chosen based on the patient's level of risk, taking into consideration any contraindications to prophylaxis that may be present.

Although this model was not developed using rigorous statistical methods, and includes some variables that were later found not to be associated with VTE risk, it is relatively easy to use and appears to discriminate reasonably well among patients

Table 5.3 Caprini risk assessment model (Ref. [17])

1 point	2 points	3 points	5 points
Age 41–60 years	Age 61–74 years	Age ≥ 75 years	Stroke (<1 month)
Minor surgery	Arthroscopic surgery	History of VTE	Elective arthroplasty
BMI >25 kg/m^2	Major open surgery (>45 min)	Family history of VTE	Hip, pelvis, or leg fracture
Swollen legs	Laparoscopic surgery (<45 min)	Factor V Leiden	Hip, pelvis, or leg fracture
Varicose veins	Malignancy	Prothrombin 20210A	Acute spinal cord injury (<1 month)
Pregnancy or postpartum	Confined to bed (>72 h)	Lupus anticoagulant	
History of unexplained or recurrent spontaneous abortion	Immobilizing plaster cast	Anticardiolipin antibodies	
Oral contraceptives or hormone replacement	Central venous access	Elevated serum homocysteine	
Sepsis (<1 month)		Heparin-induced thrombocytopenia	
Serious lung disease, including pneumonia (<1 month)		Other congenital or acquired thrombophilia	
Abnormal pulmonary function			
Medical patient at bed rest			
Congestive heart failure (<1 month)			
History of inflammatory bowel disease			
Acute myocardial infarction			

at low, moderate, and high risk for VTE. The incidence of VTE in patients in the low-risk category (1 risk factor) is so low (approximately 2%) that prophylactic measures would most likely not further reduce the risk. Thus, no measures above early ambulation are recommended in this patient population. The incidence of VTE ranges from 10 to 80% in the remaining groups; therefore, prophylactic measures are recommended in these groups. As opposed to an increasingly precise stratification and individual thrombotic risk, the definition of bleeding risk is instead limited to suggestions, even in the latest guidelines. Furthermore, there are differences between guidelines in the definitions of what are the contraindications to pharmacological anticoagulant prophylaxis. For example, concerning thrombocytopenia as a known bleeding risk factor, the National Institute for Health and Clinical Excellence (NICE) guideline [18] contraindicates the anticoagulant thromboprophylaxis in case of platelet count <20,000/μL, while in other guidelines the cutoff value is <50,000/μL. The decision to start or not pharmacological thromboprophylaxis must necessarily be based on an individual assessment of the thrombotic/bleeding risk balance.

5.4 Methods of Perioperative Thromboprophylaxis

Methods of thromboprophylaxis are typically divided into mechanical and pharmacological modalities. It is recommended that early and "aggressive" ambulation be a routine part of postoperative care in all patients unless there is an absolute contraindication. Although early mobilization following surgery has been shown to significantly lower the risk for postoperative VTE [14], it is recommended as a single method only for low-risk patients, those younger than 40 years without any additional risk factor for VTE, and who are undergoing minor surgery (outpatient surgery lasting less than 45 min). For surgical patients at moderate risk for VTE (major surgery with 2 additional risk factors), mechanical methods of prophylaxis have been safe and effective modalities.

Mechanical methods include:

- Graduated compression stocking
- Intermittent pneumatic compression
- Venous foot pump

These devices act by reducing venous stasis and increasing venous outflow in the lower extremities. Mechanical thromboprophylaxis is an attractive option for surgeons because it does not increase the risk for bleeding complications. However, although these devices have been demonstrated to decrease the incidence of DVT, they have not been shown to decrease the risk of PE or death [15]. For these reasons, the 8th ACCP guidelines recommend the use of mechanical tools as a single method of thromboprophylaxis exclusively in case of active bleeding or in presence of extremely high risk of bleeding; otherwise, they recommend the medical methods be used in association with pharmacological prophylaxis in patients at very high risk of VTE.

Commonly used pharmacologic agents for prevention of VTE in surgery include subcutaneous unfractionated heparin (UFH), low molecular weight heparins (LMWH), fondaparinux, and oral anticoagulants.

Low-dose subcutaneous UFH was the first pharmacologic agent to be widely investigated for prevention of VTE in patients undergoing general surgery. It is generally administered subcutaneously at a dose of 5000 I.U. every 8 or 12 h, beginning 2 h before the surgical procedure. Although UFH is effective for the prevention of DVT and PE, bleeding complications associated with this regimen present safety concerns. The short half-life of UFH (0.5–2 h) as compared to other anticoagulants is a limitation of UFH because it necessitates more frequent administrations; however, the short half-life can also be an advantage in case of bleeding complications or renal failure.

LMWHs appear to be at least as effective as UFH for the prevention of DVT in clinical trials of patients undergoing general surgery. It is produced by depolymerization of heparin into smaller molecules. These formulations have a more favorable pharmacokinetic profile, including improved bioavailability, longer half-life allowing for one time daily administration, and decreased interindividual variability in anticoagulant response, thus obviating the need for therapeutic monitoring in most patient populations. In summary, the advantages of LMWHs over UFH include a higher anti-Xa activity compared with antithrombin activity, better bioavailability at low doses, no monitoring required, and longer half-life (4–6 h vs. 0.5–2 h), once-daily fixed dosing. However, a long half-life can sometimes be a disadvantage in case of bleeding complications.

Fondaparinux is the first in a new class of antithrombotics known as factor Xa inhibitors, which are characterized by targeted inhibition of coagulation. It is administered subcutaneously at the dose of 2.5 mg once a day. Similar to LMWH, fondaparinux has the advantage of single-dose administration and seems not to be correlated to heparin-induced thrombocytopenia.

The oral antivitamin K anticoagulants at low doses (INR 1.5) have a limited use in surgery in Europe, whereas the new oral direct Factor X or Factor II inhibitors (DOAC), including dabigatran, rivaroxaban, and apixaban, are currently indicated for VTE prophylaxis in elective orthopedic surgery (i.e., replacements of prosthetic hip and knee). Indeed, in this setting, DOAC can be a viable alternative to parenteral anticoagulants, as shown by international randomized clinical trials of Phase II and III, documenting that DOAC are as effective and safe as LMWH in the prevention of VTE in orthopedic surgery.

5.5 Management of Thromboprophylaxis in Surgery

5.5.1 General Surgery

Based on the Caprini score, the 9th American College of Chest Physicians (ACCP) guidelines have developed recommendations for thromboprophylaxis in general surgery (Table 5.4) [19]. Indications for VTE prophylaxis vary according to the individual risk of VTE and the surgical procedure.

The 9th ACCP guidelines do not recommend specific thromboprophylaxis for low-risk surgery patients, such as ambulatory patients or those undergoing minor procedures and without additional VTE risk factors. For these patients, only an early mobilization is recommended. For patients at moderate or high risk of VTE who undergo major general surgery, prophylaxis with LMWH, UFH, or fondaparinux is recommended. The combination of either LMWH, UFH, or fondaparinux with mechanical prophylaxis with graduated compression stockings and/or intermittent pneumatic compression is recommended for general surgery patients with multiple risk factors for VTE. The 9th ACCP guidelines recommend continuing prophylaxis at least until patient discharge for patients undergoing major general surgical procedures. Extended prophylaxis for up to 28 days should be considered for selected high-risk patients, such as those undergoing oncological or orthopedic surgery.

For laparoscopic surgery, the routine use of thromboprophylaxis is not recommended, with the exception of patients with additional risk factors, for whom the use of one among UFH, LMWH, fondaparinux, compression elastic stockings, or intermittent pneumatic compression is recommended.

Table 5.4 Prevention of VTE in non-orthopedic surgical patients (modified from ACCP Guidelines 2012) (Ref. [19])

Category of risk	Recommendations
Very low risk (score 0)	No specific pharmacologic (Grade 1B) or mechanical (Grade 2C) prophylaxis be used
Low risk (score 1–2)	Mechanical prophylaxis, preferably with intermittent pneumatic compression (IPC), over no prophylaxis (Grade 2C)
Moderate risk (score 3–4)	LMWH (Grade 2B), low-dose UFH (Grade 2B), or mechanical prophylaxis, preferably with IPC (Grade 2C), over no prophylaxis
High risk (score ≥ 5)	LMWH (Grade 1B) or low-dose UFH (Grade 1B) over no prophylaxis. Mechanical prophylaxis with elastic stockings (ES) or IPC should be added to pharmacologic prophylaxis (Grade 2C)
High risk (score ≥ 5) in whom both LMWH and UFH are contraindicated or unavailable and who are not at high risk for major bleeding complications	Low-dose aspirin (Grade 2C), fondaparinux (Grade 2C), or mechanical prophylaxis, preferably with IPC (Grade 2C), over no prophylaxis
High-VTE-risk patients surgery for cancer	Extended duration of pharmacologic prophylaxis (4 weeks) with LMWH over limited-duration prophylaxis (Grade 1B)
High-VTE-risk patients who are at high risk for major bleeding complications	Use of mechanical prophylaxis, preferably with IPC, over no prophylaxis until the risk of bleeding diminishes and pharmacologic prophylaxis may be initiated (Grade 2C)
For all patients	Inferior vena cava (IVC) filter should not be used for primary VTE prevention (Grade 2C)

5.5.2 Oncological Surgery

There is a particularly strong association between cancer and VTE [20]. Clinically apparent VTE is present in as many as 15% of all cancer patients, with much higher incidences reported in postmortem studies. In addition, among patients with DVT, those with cancer have a more than twofold increased risk for VTE recurrence than those without cancer. The likelihood for the development of VTE in cancer patients varies by tumor types and is increased among patients with more advanced disease [21, 22]. Malignancies stemming from the uterus, brain, ovary, pancreas, stomach, kidneys, and colon are among the tumor types that have been associated with the highest relative risk for VTE [21].

Cancer patients undergoing surgery have a two- to fivefold increased risk for postoperative VTE, as compared with non-cancer patients undergoing the same procedures [23]. Regarding perioperative thromboprophylaxis, data show that LMWH have the same efficacy as UFH in oncological surgery. In a large meta-analysis of available randomized trials comparing LMWH, UFH, and placebo or no treatment, LMWH appeared to be as safe and effective as UFH in reducing VTE, in both the general population and a large subgroup of patients with cancer [24, 25]. In addition, the safety, assessed as the rate of bleeding complications, was similar between the two types of heparins. For this and for their other several advantages (i.e., the once-daily administration, the favorable pharmacological profile, and the lower association with heparin-induced thrombocytopenia), LMWH are increasingly used in this area. The standard duration of thromboprophylaxis is about a week after surgery or, in general, until discharge.

Several studies, however, have shown the efficacy of extended prophylaxis to 3–4 weeks after hospital discharge. The prolonged prophylaxis not only reduces the risk of thrombosis during the period of administration of heparin, but the benefits persist beyond 3 months following surgery. In the ENOXACAN II study, patients undergoing surgery for abdominal malignancy received 1 week of LMWH prophylaxis and were then randomized to LMWH or placebo for another 21 days [26]. Bilateral venography performed at the end of treatment period showed a statistically significant reduction in DVT from 12% with placebo to 4.8% with extended prophylaxis. Another study (FAME study) evaluated the efficacy and safety of thromboprophylaxis with LMWH, administered for 28 days after major abdominal surgery compared to a 7-day treatment [27]. The cumulative incidence of VTE was reduced from 16.3% with short-term thromboprophylaxis to 7.3% after prolonged thromboprophylaxis. A third study to test the efficacy and safety of thromboprophylaxis in patients admitted for abdominal or pelvic surgery for cancer is the CANBESURE study. Patients received LMWH once daily for 8 days and were then randomized to receive either LMWH or placebo for 20 additional days [28]. At the end of the double-blind period, VTE occurred in 0.8 and 4.6% patients in the two groups, respectively. The bleeding risk was not increased by extended LMWH prophylaxis.

The American Society of Clinical Oncology (ASCO) guidelines recommend the use of prophylactic anticoagulation in surgical patients. In particular, patients undergoing laparotomy, laparoscopy, or thoracotomy lasting more than 30 min should receive pharmacologic thromboprophylaxis with either low-dose UFH or LMWH unless contraindicated because of ongoing active bleeding or a high risk for it [29]. Since these patients remain at elevated risk for VTE for an extended period of time after hospital discharge, the ASCO panel recommends that prolonged prophylaxis for up to 4 weeks be considered in patients undergoing major abdominal or pelvic cancer surgery with high-risk features, such as residual malignant disease post-resection, obesity, or previous history of VTE [29]. The National Comprehensive Cancer Network (NCCN) guidelines also recommend that all cancer patients with high risk (age $\geq$ 60 years, advanced cancer, operative times more than 2 h, previous VTE, and >3 days of bed rest) undergoing major surgery should be considered for extended VTE prophylaxis [30]. The same recommendations are made by the Italian Society of Medical Oncology (AIOM) (www.aiom.it) and the Italian Society for the Study of Hemostasis and Thrombosis (SISET) [31].

5.5.3 Orthopedic Surgery

Major orthopedic surgery, including total hip replacement (THR), total knee replacement (TKR), and hip fracture surgery (HFS), is associated with a very high risk of VTE. Symptomatic DVT events occur after hospital discharge, and the risk of VTE in this setting remains high for at least 2 months after surgery, in particular after THR [32]. The risk of VTE attributable to the surgical procedure per se is so high that no further risk stratification based on individual risk factors is warranted to decide the optimal thromboprophylaxis.

LMWH and low-dose UFH have been widely investigated in patients undergoing major orthopedic surgery, and their efficacy is well documented, especially following THR and TKR. The ACCP guidelines recommend the routine use of either LMWH, fondaparinux, new anticoagulants (apixaban, dabigatran, rivaroxaban), low-dose UFH, low-dose warfarin, or aspirin for patients undergoing THR, TKR, or HFS (Grade 1B) [33]. LMWH is to be given either preoperatively, that is, started 12 h before surgery according to the European standard of practice, or postoperatively, that is, started 12–24 h after surgery according to the North American standard. Finally, after orthopedic surgery, it is recommended to administer thromboprophylaxis for a minimum of 10 days in all patients and to extend thromboprophylaxis in the outpatient period for up to 35 days. A meta-analysis of six randomized, double-blind trials comparing extended, out-of-hospital thromboprophylaxis with LMWH versus placebo demonstrated that extended out-of-hospital thromboprophylaxis reduces the risk of symptomatic VTE by 64% [34].

Both UFH and LMWH need subcutaneous administration, which is not always convenient for post-discharge use. Conventional anticoagulant therapy with coumarins has some limitations due to short-term adjustment and frequent INR monitoring.

The development of new oral anticoagulant agents, i.e., the direct thrombin inhibitor, dabigatran, and the selective FXa inhibitors, rivaroxaban and apixaban, are approved in many countries for VTE prevention in patients undergoing hip or knee arthroplasty. Thanks to their pharmacodynamic and pharmacokinetic profile, DOAC can be a viable alternative to other anticoagulants: they can be administered at fixed doses, have few interactions with food and other drugs, and do not require monitoring [35].

Large randomized controlled trials have evaluated the efficacy and safety of DOAC for the prevention of VTE. Each of these trials used the same primary outcome measure, a composite of symptomatic or asymptomatic DVT diagnosed by venography, nonfatal PE events, and all-cause mortality. Dabigatran was investigated for prevention of VTE in four Phase III trials, two after THR (RE-NOVATE and RE-NOVATE II) and two after TKR (RE-MODEL and RE-MOBILIZE) [36–39]. RE-MODEL, RE-NOVATE, and RE-NOVATE II have demonstrated non-inferiority versus LMWH for the primary outcome, while RE-MOBILIZE did not demonstrate non-inferiority, although both treatments were similar for the secondary composite outcome. A meta-analysis of the data from these four trials confirmed these findings, showing that dabigatran versus LMWH had a similar efficacy in preventing total VTE and all-cause mortality as well as a similar risk of major bleeding or clinically relevant bleeding [40].

Rivaroxaban was also investigated in four large Phase III trials, two after THR (RECORD 1 and RECORD 2) and two after TKR (RECORD 3 and RECORD 4) [41–44]. All four trials demonstrated the same efficacy of rivaroxaban compared to LMWH for the primary outcome of total VTE and all-cause mortality. There were no significant differences in the rates of major bleeding between the two treatments. A meta-analysis of data from these four trials confirmed these findings [40].

Apixaban was investigated in three large Phase III trials for prevention of VTE after TKR (ADVANCE-1 and ADVANCE-2) and THR (ADVANCE-3) [45–47]. In ADVANCE-1 despite similar efficacy, apixaban did not meet the prespecified, non-inferiority goal because the event rates in the control group were much lower than expected. Major bleeding rates were marginally lower with apixaban (0.7 vs. 1.4% with enoxaparin). In ADVANCE-2 and ADVANCE-3, the same apixaban regimen was as effective as LMWH in reducing total VTE plus all-cause mortality with a similar risk of major bleeding. A meta-analysis of the data from these three trials confirmed these findings with a trend toward a lower risk of major bleeding and a significantly lower risk of clinically relevant bleeding [40].

As dabigatran, rivaroxaban, and apixaban are all partly cleared by renal elimination, their use needs to be carefully considered in patients with renal impairment, which is rather frequent in elderly patients. European guidelines recommend that apixaban and rivaroxaban should not be used in patients with CrCl <15 mL/min, while no dose adjustment is necessary in patients treated with rivaroxaban or apixaban who have mild (CrCl 50–80 mL/min) or moderate renal impairment (CrCl 30–49 mL/min).

The guidelines note the limitations of DOAC, including the possibility of increased bleeding, which may occur with all anticoagulants, but was clearly shown for rivaroxaban, and the lack of long-term safety data with all medications: dabigatran, rivaroxaban, and apixaban.

Conclusions

Many conventional risk factors for VTE established in the young and middle-aged population increase the risk of thrombosis in the elderly. Major surgery, especially oncological or orthopedic, significantly affects that risk. Furthermore, the older the patients undergoing surgery, the more likely that comorbidity exists at the time of intervention; consequently, the risk of VTE increases. Effective VTE prophylaxis for surgical elderly patients at significant risk of thrombosis reduces the burden of VTE and improves outcomes. The current development of VTE stratification models, using the increasing knowledge of the clinical and surgical risk factors of thrombosis, is important for identifying high-risk patients, who can most benefit from thromboprophylaxis, thus reducing VTE-associated morbidity and mortality.

References

1. Heit JA. Venous thromboembolism: disease burden, outcomes and risk factors. J Thromb Haemost. 2005;3(8):1611–7.
2. Goldhaber SZ, Visani L, De Rosa M. Acute pulmonary embolism: clinical outcomes in the international cooperative pulmonary embolism registry (ICOPER). Lancet. 1999;353(9162):1386–9.

3. Janata K, Holzer M, Domanovits H, Mullner M, Bankier A, Kurtaran A, et al. Mortality of patients with pulmonary embolism. Wien Klin Wochenschr. 2002;114(17–18):766–72.
4. Heit JA, Mohr DN, Silverstein MD, Petterson TM, O'Fallon WM, Melton LJ 3rd. Predictors of recurrence after deep vein thrombosis and pulmonary embolism: a population-based cohort study. Arch Intern Med. 2000;160(6):761–8.
5. Baglin T, Luddington R, Brown K, Baglin C. Incidence of recurrent venous thromboembolism in relation to clinical and thrombophilic risk factors: prospective cohort study. Lancet. 2003;362(9383):523–6.
6. Anderson FA Jr, Wheeler HB, Goldberg RJ, Hosmer DW, Patwardhan NA, Jovanovic B, et al. A population-based perspective of the hospital incidence and case-fatality rates of deep vein thrombosis and pulmonary embolism. The Worcester DVT study. Arch Intern Med. 1991;151(5):933–8.
7. Geerts WH, Pineo GF, Heit JA, Bergqvist D, Lassen MR, Colwell CW, et al. Prevention of venous thromboembolism: the seventh ACCP conference on antithrombotic and thrombolytic therapy. Chest. 2004;126(3 Suppl):338S–400S.
8. Falanga A, Russo L. Epidemiology, risk and outcomes of venous thromboembolism in cancer. Hamostaseologie. 2012;32(2):115–25.
9. Silverstein MD, Heit JA, Mohr DN, Petterson TM, O'Fallon WM, Melton LJ 3rd. Trends in the incidence of deep vein thrombosis and pulmonary embolism: a 25-year population-based study. Arch Intern Med. 1998;158(6):585–93.
10. Engbers MJ, van Hylckama VA, Rosendaal FR. Venous thrombosis in the elderly: incidence, risk factors and risk groups. J Thromb Haemost. 2010;8(10):2105–12.
11. Johnson SA, Eleazer GP, Rondina MT. Pathogenesis, diagnosis, and treatment of venous thromboembolism in older adults. J Am Geriatr Soc. 2016;64(9):1869–78.
12. Larsson L, Grimby G, Karlsson J. Muscle strength and speed of movement in relation to age and muscle morphology. J Appl Physiol Respir Environ Exerc Physiol. 1979;46(3):451–6.
13. Gensini GF, Rostagno C, Caciolli S. Treatment options for acute venous thromboembolism in the older patient. Geriatrics. 1998;53(1):34–6. 9–40, 6–7
14. White RH, Gettner S, Newman JM, Trauner KB, Romano PS. Predictors of rehospitalization for symptomatic venous thromboembolism after total hip arthroplasty. N Engl J Med. 2000;343(24):1758–64.
15. Bozzato S, Galli L, Ageno W. Thromboprophylaxis in surgical and medical patients. Semin Respir Crit Care Med. 2012;33(2):163–75.
16. White RH, Zhou H, Romano PS. Incidence of symptomatic venous thromboembolism after different elective or urgent surgical procedures. Thromb Haemost. 2003;90(3):446–55.
17. Caprini JA. Thrombosis risk assessment as a guide to quality patient care. Dis Mon. 2005;51(2–3):70–8.
18. Treasure T, Hill J. NICE guidance on reducing the risk of venous thromboembolism in patients admitted to hospital. J R Soc Med. 2010;103(6):210–2.
19. Gould MK, Garcia DA, Wren SM, Karanicolas PJ, Arcelus JI, Heit JA, et al. Prevention of VTE in nonorthopedic surgical patients: antithrombotic therapy and prevention of thrombosis, 9th ed: American College of Chest Physicians Evidence-Based Clinical Practice Guidelines. Chest. 2012;141(2 Suppl):e227S–77S.
20. Falanga A, Russo L, Milesi V. The coagulopathy of cancer. Curr Opin Hematol. 2014;21(5):423–9.
21. Thodiyil PA, Kakkar AK. Variation in relative risk of venous thromboembolism in different cancers. Thromb Haemost. 2002;87(6):1076–7.
22. Sorensen HT, Mellemkjaer L, Olsen JH, Baron JA. Prognosis of cancers associated with venous thromboembolism. N Engl J Med. 2000;343(25):1846–50.
23. Rickles FR, Levine MN. Epidemiology of thrombosis in cancer. Acta Haematol. 2001;106(1–2):6–12.
24. Mismetti P, Laporte S, Darmon JY, Buchmuller A, Decousus H. Meta-analysis of low molecular weight heparin in the prevention of venous thromboembolism in general surgery. Br J Surg. 2001;88(7):913–30.

25. Kakkar AK, Haas S, Wolf H, Encke A. Evaluation of perioperative fatal pulmonary embolism and death in cancer surgical patients: the MC-4 cancer substudy. Thromb Haemost. 2005;94(4):867–71.
26. Bergqvist D, Agnelli G, Cohen AT, Eldor A, Nilsson PE, Le Moigne-Amrani A, et al. Duration of prophylaxis against venous thromboembolism with enoxaparin after surgery for cancer. N Engl J Med. 2002;346(13):975–80.
27. Rasmussen MS, Jorgensen LN, Wille-Jorgensen P, Nielsen JD, Horn A, Mohn AC, et al. Prolonged prophylaxis with dalteparin to prevent late thromboembolic complications in patients undergoing major abdominal surgery: a multicenter randomized open-label study. J Thromb Haemost. 2006;4(11):2384–90.
28. Kakkar VV, Balibrea JL, Martinez-Gonzalez J, Prandoni P, Group CS. Extended prophylaxis with bemiparin for the prevention of venous thromboembolism after abdominal or pelvic surgery for cancer: the CANBESURE randomized study. J Thromb Haemost. 2010;8(6):1223–9.
29. Lyman GH, Khorana AA, Kuderer NM, Lee AY, Arcelus JI, Balaban EP, et al. Venous thromboembolism prophylaxis and treatment in patients with cancer: American Society of Clinical Oncology clinical practice guideline update. J Clin Oncol Off J Am Soc Clin Oncol. 2013;31(17):2189–204.
30. Farge D, Debourdeau P, Beckers M, Baglin C, Bauersachs RM, Brenner B, et al. International clinical practice guidelines for the treatment and prophylaxis of venous thromboembolism in patients with cancer. J Thromb Haemost. 2013;11(1):56–70.
31. Siragusa S, Armani U, Carpenedo M, Falanga A, Fulfaro F, Imberti D, et al. Prevention of venous thromboembolism in patients with cancer: guidelines of the Italian Society for Haemostasis and Thrombosis (SISET) (1). Thromb Res. 2012;129(5):e171–6.
32. Kearon C. Natural history of venous thromboembolism. Circulation. 2003;107(23 Suppl 1):I22–30.
33. Falck-Ytter Y, Francis CW, Johanson NA, Curley C, Dahl OE, Schulman S, et al. Prevention of VTE in orthopedic surgery patients: antithrombotic therapy and prevention of thrombosis, 9th ed: American College of Chest Physicians Evidence-Based Clinical Practice Guidelines. Chest. 2012;141(2 Suppl):e278S–325S.
34. Hull RD, Pineo GF, Stein PD, Mah AF, MacIsaac SM, Dahl OE, et al. Extended out-of-hospital low-molecular-weight heparin prophylaxis against deep venous thrombosis in patients after elective hip arthroplasty: a systematic review. Ann Intern Med. 2001;135(10):858–69.
35. Pengo V, Crippa L, Falanga A, Finazzi G, Marongiu F, Palareti G, et al. Questions and answers on the use of dabigatran and perspectives on the use of other new oral anticoagulants in patients with atrial fibrillation. A consensus document of the Italian Federation of Thrombosis Centers (FCSA). Thromb Haemost. 2011;106(5):868–76.
36. Eriksson BI, Dahl OE, Rosencher N, Kurth AA, van Dijk CN, Frostick SP, et al. Dabigatran etexilate versus enoxaparin for prevention of venous thromboembolism after total hip replacement: a randomised, double-blind, non-inferiority trial. Lancet. 2007;370(9591):949–56.
37. Eriksson BI, Dahl OE, Huo MH, Kurth AA, Hantel S, Hermansson K, et al. Oral dabigatran versus enoxaparin for thromboprophylaxis after primary total hip arthroplasty (RE-NOVATE II*). A randomised, double-blind, non-inferiority trial. Thromb Haemost. 2011;105(4):721–9.
38. Eriksson BI, Dahl OE, Rosencher N, Kurth AA, van Dijk CN, Frostick SP, et al. Oral dabigatran etexilate vs. subcutaneous enoxaparin for the prevention of venous thromboembolism after total knee replacement: the RE-MODEL randomized trial. J Thromb Haemost. 2007;5(11):2178–85.
39. Committee R-MW, Ginsberg JS, Davidson BL, Comp PC, Francis CW, Friedman RJ, et al. Oral thrombin inhibitor dabigatran etexilate vs north American enoxaparin regimen for prevention of venous thromboembolism after knee arthroplasty surgery. J Arthroplast. 2009;24(1):1–9.
40. Eriksson BI, Quinlan DJ, Eikelboom JW. Novel oral factor Xa and thrombin inhibitors in the management of thromboembolism. Annu Rev Med. 2011;62:41–57.
41. Eriksson BI, Borris LC, Friedman RJ, Haas S, Huisman MV, Kakkar AK, et al. Rivaroxaban versus enoxaparin for thromboprophylaxis after hip arthroplasty. N Engl J Med. 2008;358(26):2765–75.

42. Kakkar AK, Brenner B, Dahl OE, Eriksson BI, Mouret P, Muntz J, et al. Extended duration rivaroxaban versus short-term enoxaparin for the prevention of venous thromboembolism after total hip arthroplasty: a double-blind, randomised controlled trial. Lancet. 2008;372(9632):31–9.
43. Lassen MR, Ageno W, Borris LC, Lieberman JR, Rosencher N, Bandel TJ, et al. Rivaroxaban versus enoxaparin for thromboprophylaxis after total knee arthroplasty. N Engl J Med. 2008;358(26):2776–86.
44. Turpie AG, Lassen MR, Davidson BL, Bauer KA, Gent M, Kwong LM, et al. Rivaroxaban versus enoxaparin for thromboprophylaxis after total knee arthroplasty (RECORD4): a randomised trial. Lancet. 2009;373(9676):1673–80.
45. Lassen MR, Raskob GE, Gallus A, Pineo G, Chen D, Portman RJ. Apixaban or enoxaparin for thromboprophylaxis after knee replacement. N Engl J Med. 2009;361(6):594–604.
46. Lassen MR, Raskob GE, Gallus A, Pineo G, Chen D, Hornick P, et al. Apixaban versus enoxaparin for thromboprophylaxis after knee replacement (ADVANCE-2): a randomised double-blind trial. Lancet. 2010;375(9717):807–15.
47. Lassen MR, Gallus A, Raskob GE, Pineo G, Chen D, Ramirez LM, et al. Apixaban versus enoxaparin for thromboprophylaxis after hip replacement. N Engl J Med. 2010;363(26):2487–98.

Part II

Endocrine Surgery

Thyroid and Parathyroid Diseases in Elderly Patients

6

Silvestro Canonico, Massimo De Falco,
and Giuseppe Santangelo

6.1 Thyroid Diseases

The thyroid undergoes a physiological cellular senescence, involving a progressive weight and volume loss, together with an increase of fibrous components, reduction in follicle size and amount, decrease of colloid production and increase of infiltrating lymphocytes [1–3].

Functional changes occur simultaneously, consisting of increased TSH serum levels and a reduction of T3 and Ft3 circulating levels, likewise increased rT3 levels, which is a metabolically inactive hormone. FT4 and T4 levels are set to be unchanged. Peripheral organs decrease their susceptibility to thyroid hormones, combined with an increasing rate of antithyroid antibodies.

The significance of thyroid hormonal changes in the geriatric population is not perfectly clear yet. It was suggested that they may be a protection mechanism against the physiological catabolism of aging. According to this hypothesis higher TSH levels may be related to a longer lifespan. In conclusion, it is difficult to unequivocally understand laboratory findings of the thyroid function in elderly subjects [1–3].

The clinical suspicion of thyroid disease in geriatric patients is not different from that of younger people. Primary hyperthyroidism consists of an increase of FT3 and FT4 serum levels combined with TSH reduction. On the other hand, primary hypothyroidism consists of a reduction of FT3 and FT4 levels combined with an increased TSH serum concentration [4]. The difficulty in interpreting the results analytically arises from subclinical thyroid dysfunctions in the aim of finding appropriate therapeutic management.

S. Canonico (✉) • M. De Falco • G. Santangelo
Department of Medical, Surgical, Neurological, Metabolic and Geriatric Sciences, University of Campania Region "Luigi Vanvitelli", 81100 Caserta, Italy
e-mail: silvestro.canonico@unicampania.it; massimo.defalco@unicampania.it; giuseppesantangelo@email.it

A. Crucitti (ed.), *Surgical Management of Elderly Patients*,
https://doi.org/10.1007/978-3-319-60861-7_6

Geriatric people are characterized by an increasing rate of patients with high antithyroid antibodies and subclinical hypothyroidism. Subclinical hypothyroidism itself has advantages to the aging human body as the reduction of catabolism. Clinical studies also show that there is no link with the decaying of brain cortical functions: thus, if no symptoms are reported and in cases of moderate subclinical hypothyroidism, no pharmacological treatment would be recommended.

Subclinical hyperthyroidism is classified into two degrees. The first degree is recognized when TSH levels are persistently ranging from 0.1 to 0.39 mIU/L and is related to an increased incidence of atrial fibrillation. In the second degree, TSH levels are always less than 0.1 mIU/L with an increased rate of mortality related to coronary artery disease, increased incidence of atrial fibrillation, heart failure, and fractures [5–9]. So, a first grade of subclinical hyperthyroidism is related to an increased incidence of atrial fibrillation, therefore, subclinical hyperthyroidism in geriatric patients must be treated with antithyroid drugs, or with ^{131}I radio metabolic therapy [5].

6.2 Goiter

The term goiter refers to an abnormal and irreversible enlargement of the thyroid gland. Once diagnosed, goiter reveals its benign nature and can be classified into multinodular (Fig. 6.1) or nodular and toxic or non-toxic goiter. The genesis of a goiter has its roots in genetic, environmental, food and drug factors all combining with each other. Whether in endemic or non-endemic goiter areas the prevalence of a goiter is higher in the geriatric population than in the younger population. Mostly in Western countries, this can be related to several conditions, such as recurrences in patients who had previously undergone partial thyroidectomy, or increased use of instrumental investigations due to other geriatric diseases. A continuous enlarging goiter may become symptomatic over time, and in these cases diagnosis is required.

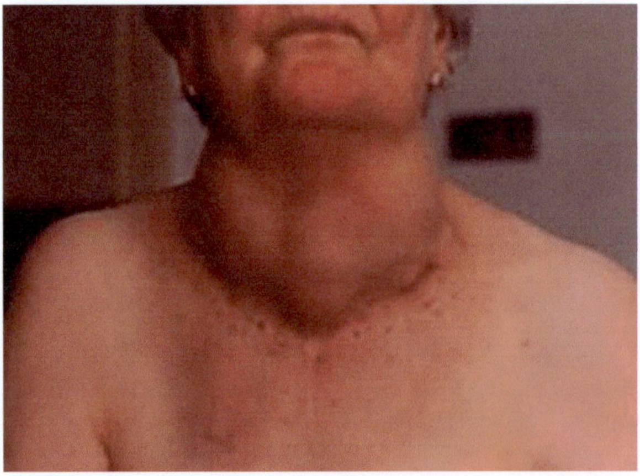

Fig. 6.1 Multinodular goiter in over-65 aged woman

6.2.1 Non-Toxic Goiters

A goiter can be defined as non-toxic when thyroid functional levels range from normal to partly decreased: the second condition may be the consequence of a concurrent autoimmune thyroiditis. Goiter size is likely to be larger in geriatric patients than in young people. A more frequent mediastinal widening also affects older patients [1, 3, 10–12]. Both phenomena are due to the continuous enlargement of the goiter over time.

If a hypothyroidism is recognized, symptoms can be characterized by body-weight gain, asthenia and fatigue, hypersomnia, cold intolerance, myxedema, constipation, skin and appendages disorders, psychiatric depression, altered consciousness or impaired concentration ability, and heart failure. Geriatric patients often report less symptoms than the younger patients with fatigue and asthenia occurring more frequently in the former. Comorbidities as well as the few symptoms related to goiter may be interpreted as expression of non-thyroid primary diseases, delaying the diagnosis of hypothyroidism and resulting in a higher risk of heart failure, atherosclerosis, and insurgent coma. On the other hand, in cases of regular functions, symptoms may only be mechanical, such as dyspnea, dysphagia, and rarely dysphonia [1, 10–12].

Most patients suffering with a goiter, even if affected by an extended goiter, are reported as asymptomatic or fairly paucisymptomatic. This is probably related to a physiological adaptation of the neck tissues to a slow and progressive enlargement of the thyroid gland over time. In fact, many asymptomatic patients suffering from tracheal deviation or compression, due to mediastinal widening, report a subjective feeling of breathing improvement after being treated with total thyroidectomy.

The physiological reduction of sensitivity and possible coexisting respiratory diseases can make it difficult to interpret the real severity of goiter-related symptoms in geriatric patients. Dysphagia, mainly occurring when the left back lobe of the thyroid enlarges, is directly related to the compression of cervical esophagus, but sometimes this diagnosis is difficult in elderly patients. Indeed, a cricopharyngeal dysphagia, linked to a neuromuscular incoordination of the mechanical swallowing process, is not unusual in older patients because it can be generally interpreted as a paraphysiological age-related deficiency, if no other potentially linked neurological, muscular, or vascular pathologies are diagnosed.

Dysphonia has more frequently to be interpreted as a neoplastic infiltration of one of the inferior laryngeal nerves rather than its extrinsic compression. However, in geriatric patients a clinical diagnosis of dysphonia must take into account either a possible primary or secondary larynx disease, or because of a reduced aging-related vocal ability, in absence of other specific diseases.

To assess the thyroid function, the dosage of TSH, FT3, and FT4 is necessary together with the measurement of Ab-hTg and Ab-TPO with the aim of diagnosing a possible concurrent autoimmune chronic thyroiditis [3].

Instrumental diagnosis consists firstly of an US-scan that evaluates the glandular size, the number, location, and features of possible lumps, the evidence of tracheal dislocation, a potential mediastinal widening and the lymphatic state. A chest and thorax CT scan is required in cases of substernal widening. The diagnostic is to be completed by performing a needle biopsy, in cases of solid lumps with suspicious characteristics.

6.2.2 Toxic Goiters

The definition of toxic goiter refers to a pathological condition of thyroid enlargement associated with overproduction of thyroid hormones. According to the presence of lumps in the area of parenchyma, goiters can be classified into diffuse toxic goiters or toxic nodular goiters (uninodular or multinodular) [10–13]. In both geriatric and in young patients, diffuse toxic goiter is also known as Graves Flajani Basedow disease and as a consequence of its genesis, it is autoimmune. In fact, some people are genetically predisposed with anti-TSH receptor auto-antibodies which can bind to their target, the thyroid, and have a stimulatory activity resulting in miming thyrotropin action. There are sub-populations of auto-antibodies which show some differences both in binding affinity and in intrinsic activity, and they are predisposed to differ over time. This explains why the disease can present an erratic intensity over time, both increasing and decreasing. In diffuse toxic goiters, there is a parenchymal compactness, due to an extreme colloidal reduction. The thyroid is more vascularized with lymphocytic infiltration. Toxic nodular goiters can be either uninodular or multinodular. A uninodular thyroid toxic nodule, also called Plummer's disease, typically consists of a single increasing toxic nodule, that produces thyroid hormones, autonomously functioning from the hypothalamic pituitary axis. Such autonomous hyperactivity is conferred to the solitary nodule by a somatic mutation activating the TSH receptor in single cells. The pathogenic mechanism is identical in multinodular toxic goiters. The only difference is the somatic mutation, occurring in one or even more pre-existing nodules, which turns them "autonomous."

Toxic goiter, mainly multinodular, is generally more frequent in elderly patients than in young individuals: the nodular mutation to "autonomously functioning" is more likely to happen in old nodules, that is to say in elderly people. Such a phenomenon is far more frequent in endemic iodine deficiency areas.

Symptomatology of toxic goiters is always functional, but at times can also be mechanical. The most common symptoms are tachycardia, palpitation, weight loss, heat intolerance, tachypnea, tremor, diarrhea, and nervousness; widespread itching, and less frequently urticaria and fever. Patients suffering from Graves-Flajani-Basedow disease can also have ophthalmopathy, acropachia, and pretibial myxedema.

While hyperthyroidism in young patients generally manifests with numerous symptoms, even if variable in their intensity, in geriatric patients only one or two symptoms can be detected. Tachycardia, weight loss, and tachypnea are among the most commonly reported symptoms in the elderly. Furthermore, apathy rather than nervousness appears in about 35% of geriatric patients suffering from hyperthyroidism. The clinical picture, already subtle in itself, should then be interpreted in the light of potential existing co-morbidities and drug treatments, which can make the diagnosis of hyperthyroidism difficult or delayed [1–5, 10, 11]. If present, mechanic symptoms are related to the goiter size and depend on the individual patient's degree of susceptibility: compressive dyspnea, dysphagia, and rarely dysphonia.

The laboratory diagnosis consists of a reduced or annulled TSH dosage with a high FT3 and FT4 dosage. It is important to consider that a condition of low or annulled levels of THS, occurring with high FT3 and T3 levels and normal FT4 levels—also known as T3 toxicosis—is more likely to occur in geriatric patients than in young patients. It is appropriate to add the anti-receptors TSH antibody dosage to the normal one. The former is specifically employed to diagnose Graves-Flajani-Basedow disease, both in its diffuse and nodular versions.

US scan represents the first instrumental exam. It allows assessment of the gland size, potential traces of lumps with their characteristics, the degree of parenchyma and lumps vascularization, and the trachea condition. If a mediastinal extrication is taking place, a chest and thorax CT scan is recommended to complete the second level diagnosis, allowing an optimal evaluation of the goiter's mediastinal portion.

A radiolabel ^{99m}Tc scan enables evaluation of whether the hypercaptation involves all the parenchymal gland or just a portion of one or more lumps. A needle biopsy is required in cases of suspicious scanned lumps. Indeed, it has been proven that 2–6% of patients diagnosed with papillary thyroid carcinomas were also carriers of the TSH receptors mutation. This demonstrates that papillary carcinomas can also manifest as autonomous lumps.

6.2.3 Treatment

Surgical treatment is recommended in cases of mechanical symptoms, tracheal dislocation and mediastinal extrication. The risk related to surgery is as high in geriatric patients as in young patients [10–13]. However, there are some specific age-related complications, in the presence of more enlarged goiter, mediastinal widening, glands hyperactivity, relapse, and thyroiditis. Even when dealing with geriatric patients, a surgical treatment of the multinodular goiter is considered best practice, unless general or local conditions make surgery-related risks higher than the expected benefit.

Surgical options to treat multinodular goiter, in the case of bilateral pathology, are a total or subtotal thyroidectomy. On the other hand, a thyroid lobectomy may be performed in cases of monolateral pathology. The option of a subtotal thyroidectomy prevails when relapse risk is lower because of a reduced lifespan. Such surgical procedure does not entail the risk of a bilateral recurrent paralysis and drastically reduces the risk of iatrogenic hypoparathyroidism [10–13]. When threatening conditions evidently contraindicate a surgical treatment, either totally or partially, the optional alternative treatment is almost always an alcohol injection. Cystic nodules accountable for the mechanic symptomatology or tracheal dislocation can be treated with such procedure. Solid nodules can be reduced by thermoablation, radiofrequency, high-intensity focused ultrasound and microwave [14–17].

Regarding toxic goiters, the primary therapeutic objective is to obtain euthyroidism by the administration of antithyroid drugs, notably methimazole. Obtaining a normal thyroid function is the precondition even in carrying out surgery. In case of contraindications to surgery and if mechanic symptomatology remains, although a normal thyroid functionality is achieved, an ^{131}I radiometabolic therapy would be appropriate. This enables the resolution of the hyperthyroidism state and the reduction of lump volume. Nonetheless, the same options that are considered as appropriate to treat non-toxic goiters can be employed [10–17].

6.3 Malignant Tumors

The cancers that can be generated from the follicular thyroid epithelium are papillary and follicular cancers, presenting some differences, and the anaplastic thyroid cancer. Other forms (lymphomas, miscellaneous tumors, metastatic tumors, non-classified tumors) are rare. Parafollicular cells can instead give rise to medullary cancer. From an etiopathogenetic standpoint, familial predisposition and prior exposure to ionizing radiation of the cervical-mediastinal region are recognized as risk factors. The incidence of malignant thyroid cancers is currently ranging from 5 to 7 cases out of 100.000 people a year, with an F/M ratio corresponding to 3.5/1. According to several contributions, the rate is indeed much higher in the elderly than in young people, the rate being reported as progressively increasing with aging [18, 19]. This is explained by the fact that each isotype has more frequent aggressive variants in elderly people. Anaplastic cancer and its various forms are almost always found in geriatric people, as far as differentiated forms are concerned (papillar and the follicular cancer) these are both characterized by more frequent histologic aggressive variants.

Nearly 80% of malignant thyroid cancers are papillar cancers which constitute the most frequent isotype in all ages, including geriatric people, who have an increase of the most aggressive biological variants (oxyphilic, tall, sclerosing, columnar and insular cells) [20]. The genotype of papillar cancer consists of a great frequency of $BRAF^{V600E}$ somatic mutation and RET/PTC gene rearrangements (notably in patients highly exposed to ionizing radiation). Both older age and $BRAF^{V600E}$ mutation, if detected, combine with a more aggressive biological behavior. Papillar cancer is likely to metastasize via the lymphatic system. Such a process is more frequent in geriatric patients and in children under 14 years together with a possible diffusion to the neck lymph node stations [19]. However, only in geriatric patients does such an element negatively affect the prognosis. Bone and lungs hematogenous metastases are much rarer.

Follicular cancer represents 10% of malignant thyroid cancers, occurs in iodine deficiency areas, and is more likely to metastasize via hematogen, mainly affecting lungs and bones. Slightly differentiated cancer and anaplastic cancer are higher in iodine deficiency areas and they represent near 1% of malignant thyroid cancers, both often being the development of differentiated papillar and follicular untreated forms.

From the genetic viewpoint, a p53 tumor-suppressor gene mutation, which seems to be the determining mutation in the rising of anaplastic cancers, can be added to the common mutations in papillar and follicular forms. Anaplastic cancer has a fast-growing rate, with an early extracapsular extension and the infiltration in all the neck tissues. Its features make it virtually impossible to treat with surgery both radically or even partially. In addition, it is a fast metastasizing cancer either via the lymphatic or hematogenous systems, with neck lymph node metastases, neoplastic venous blood clots, lung and bone lesions. The prognosis is always poor. Exitus is commonly due to obstructive respiratory failure [18–20].

Medullary cancer is a malignant neuroendocrine tumor originating from parafollicular or C cells and represents 5–6% of malignant thyroid cancers. It may be sporadic (in 75% of cases) and familial (25% of cases). Medullary familial cancers together with MEN2A and MEN2B syndromes represent the familial forms but they occur above all in the young and juvenile [18].

On the contrary, medullary cancer is almost always sporadic in geriatric patients and is mostly related to a RET gene somatic mutation. This kind of cancer frequently metastasize through the lymph system all the neck lymph nodes, but also to lungs, liver, and bones through the venous system [18–20].

The cancer biology is documented as more aggressive and the prognosis is much worse in geriatric patients than in young patients. Under 45 years of age and female subjects are historically recognized as positive prognostic factors for thyroid carcinoma. The prognosis gradually gets worse for 45-year-old people thereafter: cancer-specific mortality increases with age regardless of the frequency of anaplastic carcinoma and the scarcely differentiated type. Regarding each isotype, primary tumor size, extracapsular thyroid extension, mortality, disease relapses, and lymph metastases become much higher in geriatric patients in a statistically significant way.

6.3.1 Symptomatology

Thyroid carcinoma is not always symptomatic and it can be accidentally diagnosed when other analyses are being carried out for other purposes. When symptomatic, the carcinoma reveals itself with a swelling in the iodine neck area that can be of higher consistency and hypomobile compared with superficial layers, if infiltrated. In case of lymph node metastases, superficial swallowing combines with lymph node swallowings located in the laterocervical region or in the central compartment. A lymph metastasis may sometimes occur as the first sign of the cancer (precessive metastases). The widening of thyroid swallowing may entail the onset of dysphonic and dysphagic symptomatology compression. Dysphonia can occur if one of the laryngeal nerves is infiltrated. The symptomatology of the anaplastic carcinoma is, on the other hand, very characteristic: an iodine swelling, often increased is present; that swelling may rise extremely quickly in a few days or weeks. The infiltration of the subcutaneous plane makes the cutaneous look translucent with a typical more or less intense livedo. Jugular veins may feel turgid because of extrinsic compression, infiltration or intrasegmental neoplastic clots. Lymph node metastatic swallowing is often associated. The mass is extended, hard, and fixed in comparison with the neighboring organs which are rapidly infiltrated. Dysphagia is frequent while dyspnea is, for the most part, steady and both are linked to the obstructive effect. The rapid infiltration of low laryngeal nerves determines dysphonia and reduction of glottis space with consequent tirage and cornage symptoms.

6.3.2 Diagnosis

The pre-operative laboratory diagnosis can be useful in medullary carcinoma: calcitonin levels are frequently high and have diagnostic susceptibility with specificity significantly increasing as the serum calcitonin levels rise. If the increase in calcitonin levels is modest and not nullifying (notably in cases of an existing therapy with proton pump inhibitors), a pentagastrin-stimulating test may be helpful. Calcitoninemia also represents a great diagnostic element during the follow-up phase. The thyroglobulin dosage administrated during a pre-operative phase is not diagnostic in well-differentiated cancers, but it still remains helpful to assess the post-operative delay on the basis of a possible ^{131}I -based ablation therapy and in light of the follow-up. Anaplastic carcinoma may combine with a CEA elevation, while on the other hand thyroglobulin levels lose their usefulness, even during the follow-up, because, in this case it is about neoplastic undifferentiated cells not able to reproduce any more. US scan is the first level instrumental analysis that consists of evaluating the thyroid nodules and lymphoid state. Suspicious nodular features are hypo echogenicity, feathered edges, presence of micro calcifications, and intranodular vascularity.

The US scan is strongly recommended to carry out an ultrasound-guided thyroid needle biopsy that enables making the diagnosis on the six diagnostical Bethesda classes basis.

In case of suspected medullary carcinoma, the immunocytochemistry calcitonin levels detection-based reveals nullifying. A lymph node needle biopsy is appropriate if a local-regional lymphadenopathy is suspected. If the lymphoid metastasis is cystic, a thyroglobulin dosage on the aspirated liquid may prove diagnostic. Along the preoperative staging, a neck and thorax CT with and without contrast is a second level analysis.

The presence of pulmonary or bone nodules suspected as being relapsed cell thyroid cancer may be further investigated through a ^{99m}Tc o ^{123}I scintigraphic imaging: the possible radiopharmaceutical uptake from some nodules resolves the source. Running a neck MRI, an OctreoScan whole-body scintigraphy, and sometimes a PET-CT may be helpful during the medullary carcinoma staging. A video laryngoscopy enables diagnosis of a vocal cord paralysis if the inferior laryngeal nerve was affected by neoplastic infiltration. Such examination is always appropriate even if dysphonia is not occurring because even during an existing vocal cord paralysis, a vocal compensation will establish, thus allowing good vocal qualities.

6.3.3 Therapy

Both papillar and follicular carcinomas should be treated with total thyroidectomy and therapeutic lymphadenectomy, thus removing all the lymph nodes macroscopically involved. Furthermore, since thyroid malignant neoplasms prove much more aggressive in geriatric patients, a prophylactic lymphadenectomy of the central compartment should be appropriated too [18, 19]. This treatment has no controversies in high-risk forms. According to the stage of papillar carcinoma, three grades of risk are classified: very low, low, and high. An ^{131}I ablation therapy is certainly the appropriate treatment in high-risk patients but it is also recommended in low risk patients. In both cases the L-thyroxin suppression therapy is recommended [18–23].

According to recent guidelines, very low risk papillary neoplasms should be treated only with a lobeistmectomy when no evidence of contralateral pathology is detected despite the chance of the disease being bilateral. Cases involving recidivism should be dealt with surgically and with ^{131}I therapy. In cases, non-susceptible to surgical treatment forms ^{131}I therapy represents the only therapeutic option available when dealing with BRAF negative forms. On the other hand, in BRAF positive forms an adjuvant tyrosine kinase inhibitors drug therapy (Sorafenib, Dabrafenib) can also be employed [18–22].

In cases of follicular carcinoma if a lobeistmectomy was carried out in presence of a single lump there is currently no indication to total thyroidectomy in the presence of a single neoplasia, with positive histotype, smaller than 1 cm in diameter and without wide extracapsular extension. Totalization and adjuvant ^{131}I therapy is recommended when dealing with other forms.

Surgical treatment of medullary carcinoma is mostly sporadic in elderly people; it should be treated with total thyroidectomy, prophylactic lymphadenectomy of the central compartment and therapeutical monolateral or bilateral cervical lymphadenectomy.

Anaplastic carcinoma's surgery rarely has a radical aim mostly because it represents a utopia if the disease is not at an early stage. Surgical treatment only aims for a debulking procedure just to preserve the respiratory and digestive tracts from infiltration. However, the invasion of respiratory tracts and the consequent obstructive respiratory failure are not always prevented after tracheotomy. Chemo and adjuvant radiation current protocols show little progress, with a very low increase in median survivals. The current availability of tracheal and esophageal implants can help to lessen the need for tracheotomy and despite its high cost it enhances substantially the remaining quality of life in patients [21, 22].

6.4 Parathyroid Diseases

Parathyroid glands control the amount of calcium in the blood and within the bones and they can vary in number and position. In most individuals, there are typically four parathyroid glands but they can range from 1 to 12. Regarding their position, superior parathyroid glands are in most cases positioned behind the superior pole of the thyroid gland at the cricothyroidal cartilage junction. On the other side are the inferior parathyroid glands which are positioned at the inferior poles of the thyroid gland near the capsule between the inferior thyroid artery branches. Both superior and inferior parathyroid glands can migrate from their original position. In this case, some disorders in number and position may develop: parathyroid tissue may locate in each point of the neck and mediastinum. The superior parathyroid glands migrate a shorter distance than the inferior glands, which results in a relatively more constant location in the neck [24].

The parathyroid pathologies of surgical interest are those causing hyperparathyroidism conditions as well as carcinoma.

6.5 Hyperparathyroidism

Hyperparathyroidism occurs when there is an excess parathyroid hormone production, which results in an elevated urinary calcium serum level, a reduction in phosphorus and an increasing osteoclast activity. The different forms of hyperparathyroidism are classified: primary, secondary, and tertiary [25–27].

Primary hyperparathyroidism is more frequently due (85% of cases) to a single parathyroid adenoma, even in geriatric patients. Less frequently (15%) it is due to a parathyroid hyperplasia or rarely (0.5%) to parathyroid carcinoma. It has a prevalence of about 0.8% and it may occur predominantly in women aged from 60 to 70. However, it may occur earlier in familial endocrine syndromes and in MEN1 and MEN2A.

Secondary hyperparathyroidism is due to a thyroid hyperplasia, as a consequence of ionized calcium serum deficiency, and is predominantly due to a long-term chronic renal failure, that is more likely to affect elderly people. Tertiary hyperparathyroidism occurs as recurrence after removing the cause of the secondary form, for example after renal transplant. Typically, this is due to an adenoma resulting from a secondary hyperplasia.

6.5.1 Symptomatology

Hyperparathyroidism symptomatology varies according to the length of the disease and the magnitude of hypercalcemia. In 40–50% of cases, notably in secondary hyperparathyroidism with renal failure, the diagnosis is made at a presymptomatic stage for the laboratory detection of the disease.

Nephrourolithiasis in primary hyperparathyroidism causes a symptomatology characterized by urinary tract stones with recurrent colics which are the most predominant symptoms even in geriatric patients; hypercalcemia also entails a myasthenic symptomatology of varying intensity; mood alteration can develop depression and emotional liability. Creativity and attention span are also drastically reduced.

Constipation is one of the gastrointestinal symptoms. Peptic ulcers and dysmetabolic pancreatitis can be potential complications. The altered turn-over of bone mineral metabolism also causes osteoathralgia and severe osteoporosis notably in old women, which results in a higher risk of pathological fractures.

The classical frame of fibrocystic osteitis is more difficult to depict thanks to a better timeliness for the diagnosis than in the past. Geriatric patients suffering from primary hyperparathyroidism are likely to have similar symptoms regardless of the specific pathology, which results in a complex set of symptoms.

A peculiar frame of symptoms is represented by the proteotoxic crisis, occurring in 7–12% of parathyroid carcinoma patients. In this case calcium levels are generally higher than 16 mg/ld, causing severe heart arrhythmias and alteration of consciousness or even coma.

Beyond the possible classical symptoms in secondary hyperparathyroidism, symptomatology is generally mainly represented by osteoathralgia and widespread itching: these symptoms are due to the drastic reduction of calcium salts in soft tissues which causes a histamine release from mast cells. There may be a deposition of calcium salts in noble parenchyma, in parietal and vascular space, perivascular space resulting even in skin or organ necrosis (calciphylaxis).

6.5.2 Diagnosis

Clinical suspicion is confirmed by laboratory analysis. A PTHi increase is detected in each form of hyperparathyroidism. In primary and tertiary hyperparathyroidism cases of hyperparathormonemia combine with hypercalcemia and hypophosphatemia. On the other hand, in secondary hyperparathyroidism calcium levels may experience just a slight increase or even be normal, with phosphorus and PTHi significantly increased. In secondary cases with a chronic renal failure basis, creatinine and alkaline phosphatase are also increased, notably in case of bone involvement.

From an instrumental standpoint, a neck scan enables to detect pathologic parathyroidism, which appears as hypoechogenic, in extracapsular thyroid space, paraesophageal or paracarotid. A ^{99m}Tc and Sestamibi subtraction scintigraphy for parathyroid imaging enables to detect the parathyroid or pathological parathyroid position even when positioned at a mediastinal level. An X-ray test typically depicts the subperiosteal bone reabsorption of the cranial shrine, at a metacarpophalangeal, metacarpal, and metatarsal level. Such a test may also help to detect soft-tissue calcifications if present.

In case of suspicious instrumental images a needle biopsy should be an appropriate further exam. As reported by different authors, this exam helps to analyze the parathyroid nature of the swallowing but its employment remains controversial for two main reasons. The first reason is due to the possibility of the disease to an extracapsular spread, which may cause persistence or post-surgical relapses. The second reason is due to the possible morphologic alterations the exam may have over the gland, thus resulting in a consequently problematic histologic diagnosis.

6.5.3 Therapy

A surgical treatment is the gold standard and currently surgical indications regard patients suffering from symptomatic and asymptomatic hyperparathyroidism. In primary hyperparathyroidism with adenoma a removal of the single adenoma gland or multiple glands, in rare cases of multiple adenomas and in hyperplasia cases a subtotal parathyroidectomy is carried out.

The surgery is generally performed by a cervicotomy, with mini-cervicotomy or by MIVAP technique. If cervicotomy is performed, the surgery should use a gamma probe which facilitates the detection of the hyperfunctioning parathyroid tissue. An intraoperative rapid dosage of PTH is always recommended, because serum level reduction indicates that pathological tissue has now been removed [25–28].

In secondary hyperparathyroidism, the appropriate surgery is a subtotal parathyroidectomy, or a total parathyroidectomy with a subcutaneous or muscular replanting of the parathyroid tissue at a volar forearm level [29–32].

In tertiary hyperparathyroidism, instead, one or more glands are to be removed depending on how many of them were affected by the autonomous evolution. Medical treatment is administrated in cases of parathyrotoxic crisis and should entail hydration of the patient together with a loop diuretics and calcitonin administration [31, 33].

6.6 Parathyroid Carcinoma

Parathyroid carcinoma represents around 1% of hyperparathyroidism and it is a rare form of cancer, representing 0.005% of all malignant cancers. This form of cancer will be sporadic or originate during genetic syndromes (MEN 1 and MEN2A; isolated familial _FIHP hyperparathyroidism; "jaw tumor"— HPTJT hyperparathyroidism). Due to this aspect, no certain determinant mutations were detected, even though a significant number of HRPT2 and p53 mutation cases are involved together with an increased number of copies of the CCND1 gene [34–37].

Symptoms manifest in around 90% of parathyroid carcinomas, while 3–7% of the tumors are not functioning. In these tumors, the symptoms only deal with the detection of a palpable mass with possible compression and or infiltration signs, or local-regional lymphadenopathy metastases (in around 15–30% of cases). Distant lung, hepatic or skeletal metastases are detectable in around one third of the patients.

In functioning tumors, a possible palpable mass adds to a typical hyperparathyroidism symptomatology with urinary stones, myasthenia, psychiatric depression, epigastralgy, osteoarthralgy. In around 7–12% of cases it also manifests a parathyrotoxic crisis which occurs when calcium levels are higher than 16 mg/dL causing severe cardiac arrhythmia, altered consciousness or even coma. No clinical, biochemical, or imaging parameters can help to distinguish a parathyroid pathology from being malignant or benign during a pre-operative stage [36, 38, 39].

The only criteria raising suspicions are: (a) a fast-rising clinical picture and the fast worsening symptomatology; (b) calcium levels higher than 14 mg/dL which are in around 65–75% of cases related to carcinoma; (c) PTHi levels ten times higher than normal (81% predictive value); (d) metastatic outgrowth detected by instrumental exams (US, CT, MRI, scintigraphy, PET).

A needle biopsy procedure only helps to confirm the relapsing nature while it is contraindicated during an early diagnosis, because cytological data are insufficient to distinguish a benign lesion from a malignant lesion. Furthermore, needle biopsy also entails the risk of the mass lesion which would result in a neoplastic dissemination along the exam [40].

As a result, only a histopathological Shantz and Castleman-guided examination gives certainty: trabecular pattern; mitotic figures, tick and fibrous band, capsular and blood vessel invasion. In some cases, an immunohistochemical completion evaluating PTH, GATA3, TTF-1, PAX8, and thyroglobulin may also be helpful.

The therapy consists of an accurate and total surgical removal of the mass related to the peritumoral tissue involved, preserving the capsule integrity, with a lymphadenectomy of the central and/or ipsilateral laterocervical compartment, if a lymph node involvement is reported.

The use of an intraoperative gamma probe technique and the rapid intraoperative PTHi dosage, all together enable documenting of all the excision and therefore, both represent necessary complements. Should the suspicions remain, at an intraoperative stage, an ipsilateral hemithyroidectomy should be carried out, even if the thyroid lobe was not obviously infiltrated, thus preventing a second exploration of the neck which would in turn give rise to a high risk of complications [39].

Relapses in parathyroid carcinoma occur in around 49–60% of cases, normally from 2 to 5 years after the first surgery. Relapsing risk is higher in patients presenting with lymphoid metastases during the diagnosis. Even at the same stage of the disease, geriatric patients undergo a lower relative risk when compared with younger individuals: relapses are predominantly local or regional, while distant metastases would affect lungs, liver, and bones [41–44].

Surgical treatment represents the first therapeutical step to be taken, even in relapsing cases. There are no current multi-center studies documenting the usefulness of adjuvant radiotherapy and chemotherapy to decrease relapses and to improve survival.

References

1. Papaleontiou M, Haymart MR. Approach to and treatment of thyroid disorders in the elderly. Med Clin North Am. 2012;96:297–310.
2. Tabatabaie V, Surks MI. The aging thyroid. Curr Opin Endocrinol Diabetes Obes. 2013;20:455–9.
3. Weissel M. Disturbances of thyroid function in the elderly. Wien Klin Wochenschr. 2006;118:16–20.
4. Ceresini G, Marina M. Approach to geriatric patients with subclinical thyroid disorders. Endocrine. 2014;47:7–8.
5. Biondi B, Bartalena L, Cooper DS, Hegedüs L, Laurberg P, Kahaly GJ. The 2015 European thyroid association guidelines on diagnosis and treatment of endogenous subclinical hyperthyroidism. Eur Thyroid J. 2015;4:149–63.

6. Cappola AR, Fried LP, Arnold AM, et al. Thyroid status, cardiovascular risk, and mortality in older adults. JAMA. 2006;295:1033–41.
7. Ceresini G, Ceda GP, Lauretani F, et al. Thyroid status and 6-year mortality in elderly people living in a mildly iodine-deficient area: the aging in the chianti area study. J Am Geriatr Soc. 2013;61:868–74.
8. Sahin SB, Ayaz T, Sumer F, et al. Bone mineral density in geriatric patients with toxic nodular goiter. Aging Clin Exp Res. 2015;27:221–6.
9. Viniol A, Hickstein L, Walker J, et al. Influence of thyroid hormone therapy on the fracture rate—a claims data cohort study. Bone. 2016;86:86–90.
10. Ríos A, Rodríguez JM, Galindo PJ, et al. Surgical treatment for multinodular goitres in geriatric patients. Langenbeck's Arch Surg. 2005;390:236–42.
11. Passler C, Avanessian R, Kaczirek K, et al. Thyroid surgery in the geriatric patient. Arch Surg. 2002;137:1243–8.
12. Seybt MW, Khichi S, Terris DJ. Geriatric thyroidectomy: safety of thyroid surgery in an aging population. Arch Otolaryngol Head Neck Surg. 2009;135:1041–4.
13. Sullivan MC, Roman SA, Sosa JA. Clinical and economic outcomes of thyroid surgery in elderly patients: a systematic review. J Thyroid Res. 2012;2012:615846.
14. Reddy A, Chand G, Mayilvaganan S. Effectiveness and mechanism of preoperative lugol solution for reducing thyroid blood flow in patients with euthyroid graves' disease. World J Surg. 2017;41:333.
15. Kohlhase KD, Korkusuz Y, Gröner D, et al. Bipolar radiofrequency ablation of benign thyroid nodules using a multiple overlapping shot technique in a 3-month follow-up. Int J Hyperth. 2016;32:511–6.
16. Korkusuz Y, Mader OM, Kromen W, et al. Cooled microwave ablation of thyroid nodules: initial experience. Eur J Radiol. 2016;85:2127–32.
17. Korkusuz H, Fehre N, Sennert M, et al. Volume reduction of benign thyroid nodules 3 months after a single treatment with high-intensity focused ultrasound (HIFU). J Ther Ultrasound. 2015;4:3–4.
18. Kitahara CM, McCullough ML, Franceschi S, et al. Anthropometric factors and thyroid cancer risk by histological subtype: pooled analysis of 22 prospective studies. Thyroid. 2016;26:306–18.
19. Santangelo G, Del Giudice S, Gallucci F, et al. Cancer of the thyroid gland in geriatric age: a single center retrospective study with a 10-year post-operative follow-up. Int J Surg. 2014;12(Suppl 2):S103–7.
20. Dellal FD, Özdemir D, Tam AA, et al. Clinicopathological features of thyroid cancer in the elderly compared to younger counterparts: single-center experience. J Endocrinol Investig. 2016;40(5):471–9.
21. Rao SN, Zafereo M, Dadu R, et al. Patterns of treatment failure in anaplastic thyroid carcinoma. Thyroid. 2017;27(5):672–81. https://doi.org/10.1089/thy.2016.0395.
22. Wendler J, Kroiss M, Gast K, et al. Clinical presentation, treatment and outcome of anaplastic thyroid carcinoma: results of a multicenter study in Germany. Eur J Endocrinol. 2016;175:521–9.
23. Moon JH, Ahn S, Seo J, et al. The effect of long-term thyroid-stimulating hormone suppressive therapy on the cognitive function of elderly patients with differentiated thyroid carcinoma. J Clin Endocrinol Metab. 2014;99:3782–9.
24. Lapps D, Noussios G, Anagnostis P, et al. Location, number and morphology of parathyroid glands: results from a large anatomical series. Anta Sci Int. 2012;87:160–4.
25. Bobang ID, McHenry CR. Is intraoperative parathyroid hormone monitoring necessary for primary hyperparathyroidism with concordant preoperative imaging? Am J Surg. 2016;213(3):484–8. https://doi.org/10.1016/j.amjsurg.2016.11.035.
26. Pitt SC, Panneerselvan R, Chen H, Sippel RS. Secondary and tertiary hyperparathyroidism: the utility of ioPTH monitoring. World J Surg. 2010;34:1343–9.
27. Trinh G, Noureldine SI, Russell JO, et al. Characterizing the operative findings and utility of intraoperative parathyroid hormone (IOPTH) monitoring in patients with normal baseline

IOPTH and normohormonal primary hyperparathyroidism. Surgery. 2017;161:78–86. https://doi.org/10.1016/j.surg.2016.10.001.
28. Jacobs L, Samson MM, Verhaar HJ, et al. Therapeutic challenges in elderly patients with symptomatic hypercalcaemia caused by primary hyperparathyroidism. Neth J Med. 2012;70:35–8.
29. Wong B, Wang X. Treatment of nonagenarians with primary hyperparathyroidism. J Am Geriatr Soc. 2016;64:e112–3.
30. Hendrickson CD, Castro Pereira DJ, Comi RJ. Renal impairment as a surgical indication in primary hyperparathyroidism: do the data support this recommendation? J Clin Endocrinol Metab. 2014;99:2646–50.
31. Wilhelm SM, Wang TS, Ruan DT, et al. The American association of endocrine surgeons guidelines for definitive management of primary hyperparathyroidism. JAMA Surg. 2016;151:959–68.
32. Loncar G, Bozic B, Cvetinovic N, et al. Secondary hyperparathyroidism prevalence and prognostic role in elderly males with heart failure. J Endocrinol Investig. 2016;40(3):297–304.
33. Bollerslev J, Rosen T, Mollerup CL, et al. Effect of surgery on cardiovascular risk factors in mild primary hyperparathyroidism. J Clin Endocrinol Metab. 2009;94:2255–61.
34. Shanttz A, Castleman B. Parathyroid carcinoma: a study of 70 cases. Cancer. 1973;31:600–5.
35. Kumari N, Chaudhary N, Pradhan R, et al. Role of histological criteria and immunohistochemical markers in predicting risk of malignancy in parathyroid neoplasms. Endocr Pathol. 2016;27:87–96.
36. Sharretts JM, Simonds WF. Clinical and molecular genetics of parathyroid neoplasms. Best Pract Res Clin Endocrinol Metab. 2010;24:491–502.
37. Zhao L, Sun LH, Liu DM, et al. Copy number variation in CCND1 gene is implicated in the pathogenesis of sporadic parathyroid carcinoma. World J Surg. 2014;38:1730–7.
38. Busaidy NL, Jimenez C, Habra MA, et al. Parathyroid carcinoma: a 22-year experience. Head Neck. 2004;26:716–26.
39. Harari A, Waring A, Fernandez-Ranvier G, et al. Parathyroid carcinoma: a 43-year outcome and survival analysis. J Clin Endocrinol Metab. 2011;96:3679–86.
40. Norman J, Politz D, Browarsky I. Diagnostic aspiration of parathyroid adenomas causes severe fibrosis complicating surgery and final histologic diagnosis. Thyroid. 2007;17:1251–5.
41. Silverberg SJ, Rubin MR, Faiman C, et al. Cinacalcet hydrochloride reduces the serum calcium concentration in inoperable parathyroid carcinoma. J Clin Endocrinol Metab. 2007;92:3803–8.
42. Calandra DB, Chejfec G, Foy BK, Lawrence AM, Paloyan E. Parathyroid carcinoma: biochemical and pathologic response to DTIC. Surgery. 1984;96:1132–7.
43. Munson ND, Foote RL, Northcutt RC, et al. Parathyroid carcinoma: is there a role for adjuvant radiation therapy? Cancer. 2003;98:2378–84.
44. Talat N, Schulte KM. Clinical presentation, staging and long-term evolution of parathyroid cancer. Ann Surg Oncol. 2010;17:2156–74.

7 Breast Cancer Management in the Older Woman

Marsilio Francucci, Roberto Cirocchi,
and Marina Vinciguerra

> "Comfort me in times of trouble, grant me the serenity to accept the inevitable and lengthen the brevity of my time. Show me that the good of life is not in its duration, but in the use made of it. It is possible, or rather usual, for a man who has lived long to have lived too little"
>
> (Seneca)

7.1 Introduction

In the past, breast cancer in older women has been the subject of scarce attention, despite its high incidence. In effect, 49% of all breast cancers have been reported in women over 65 years of age. Evidence-based management recommendations are limited; in fact, only 9% of elderly patients have been enrolled for randomized clinical trials (RCTs). The absence of high-quality clinical trials regarding geriatric breast surgery has made it difficult to standardize therapeutic strategies [1].

In the late 1980s, the development of geriatric surgery and oncology has significantly increased the interest in cancer treatment for elderly women, in particular, thanks to Ludovico Balducci, Umberto Veronesi, as well as the Italian Society of Geriatric Surgery. In 1993 in Perugia, the international conference "Breast Cancer in Older Women: An Agenda for the 1990s" was organized, which was officially diffused by Rosmary Yancik in *Cancer* journal [2]. Successively, prospective clinical studies focusing on the breast-conserving surgery (BCS) and a lower extension of axillary dissection were designed for the treatment of elderly patients [3, 4].

In 2006, the highly important role of prevention in geriatric patients was recognized at the National Consensus Conference of the Italian Group for Breast Cancer

M. Francucci (✉) • M. Vinciguerra
General Surgery and Day Surgery Unit, Hospital of Terni, Terni, Italy
e-mail: francuccim@aospterni.it

R. Cirocchi
General Surgical and Surgical Oncology Unit, University of Perugia, Perugia, Italy

A. Crucitti (ed.), *Surgical Management of Elderly Patients*,
https://doi.org/10.1007/978-3-319-60861-7_7

Screening (GISMa). The consensus statement was that breast cancer prevention programs for women of over 70 years should be extended [5]. Subsequently, in 2007 the International Society of Geriatric Oncology (SIOG) created a task force with the aim of developing multidisciplinary guidelines for the treatment of breast cancer in elderly women. More recently in 2012, these recommendations were updated by SIOG in association with the European Society of Breast Cancer Specialists (EUSOMA) [1]. In their statements, the SIOG and EUSOMA task force reiterate that elderly patients rarely undergo standardized therapies and have a higher rate of treatment interruption [1].

At the same time, the Italian Association of Medical Oncology (AIOM) added a chapter dealing with the specific treatment of breast cancer in older women, as part of their national clinical practice guidelines for oncology [6].

7.2 Epidemiology

In Italy, breast cancer is the most frequent cancer in women (29% of all cases) [6]: 41% in the age group 0–49 years, 35% in the age group 50–69 years, and 21% in cases of women over 70 years of age [7–9]. In the USA, over 40% of women of 65+ years of age develop breast cancers; in 20% of them, diagnosis is made in women of 75+ years of age [7]. Aging is one of the main risk factors for breast cancer: patients of up to 49 years of age show an incidence rate of 2.4% in the diagnosis of new breast cancer, while those of over 70 years of age show a higher incidence trend of 4.7% [6]. Age is not an independent risk factor for the development of new breast cancer but is a result of the increased period of exposure to carcinogenic factors. As a result of the progressive increase in life expectancy, in the years to come, there will be a consequent significant increase in breast cancer rates in women >80 years of age.

In Italy in 2014, 16% of deaths caused by breast cancer were reported in women 70+ years of age [7]. Breast cancer is also the leading cause of death in women of all age groups: 29% of deaths by cancer before age 50, 21% between 50 and 69 years, and 16% after 70 years [10]. The SEER (Surveillance, Epidemiology, and End Results) study showed that in these women, mortality is not only related to cancer but also related to general comorbidities. In women of over 70 years of age, the deaths were not related to malignancy. In effect 80% of deaths occurred in patients without lymph node involvement (N) conversely and 60% in women with lymph node involvement (N+) [11].

7.3 Biological and Histological Characteristics

Breast cancer in the elderly woman has a prognostic profile more favorable than that of the younger woman; in fact, with aging the risk of local recurrence after surgery decreases [12]. In geriatric patients, the anatomical and pathological features of breast cancer are not significantly different from those of other age groups.

Unfortunately, invasive ductal carcinoma prevails, even if there is a greater frequency in some better prognosis histology. In effect, papillary carcinoma and mucinous carcinoma have a higher incidence after 75 years of age (4–6%) compared to women of childbearing age (1%) [13]. Neoplasms diagnosed in old age are associated with more favorable biological factors as well as a reduced aggressiveness. These characteristics are represented by lower aneuploidy [14] as well as lower expression of HER-2 (20.8%), Ki67 (33.7%), p53 (39.2%), EGF receptors (19.8%) and a greater expression of estrogen receptors (70.5%) and progesterone (56.7%) [15, 16].

In elderly women, breast cancer presents a greater degree of differentiation and a lower cell proliferation index: characteristics, which condition a slower neoplastic doubling time and a reduced tendency to develop both loco-regional recurrence and systemic metastasis [14]. These features seem to be at odds with the higher incidence rates of advanced cancer diagnosed in the elderly. Because of this, there is an erroneous oncologist opinion that these "more aggressive" tumors are associated with a poor prognosis [17]. Conversely, locally advanced tumors are often due to multiple factors including the failure to extend mammography screening to the over 70, along with a generally delayed diagnosis. This high risk of missed or delayed diagnosis is due to the reduced inclination of older women to undergo a breast assessment, even in the presence of clinical signs and symptoms. Another element is the disparity of access to the health-care system (the absence of family stimulus and poor compliance, scarce economic resources, travel difficulties, as well as availability of somebody to accompany them).

7.4 Role of Mammographic Screening

Mammography screening, performed in the age group between 49 and 69 years, has dramatically reduced mortality due to breast cancer [18]; based on this data, the possibility of extending mammographic screening up to 74 years has been suggested [19]. The role of mammographic screening in determining mortality reduction has been clearly shown in women of over 70+ years old who have a life expectancy greater than 10 years and who have a good performance status [14, 20, 21]. Moreover, mammography in geriatric-aged patients presents a sensitivity and specificity similar or greater than in younger patients; consequently, there is a greater predictive value and lower cost for each breast cancer diagnosed in these elderly women.

In 2006, the Italian Group for Breast Cancer Screening (GISMa) organized a national consensus conference on this topic. They recommended the extension of mammographic screening up to 74 years of age, where local health-care resources permit. This screening prolongation is only appropriate for women who had responded to previous screening steps and had a good life expectancy.

As regards the first point, the cost-effective analysis showed that the prolongation of screenings up to 79 years of age would require between $ 8000 and 27,000, considerably lower than the resources necessary ($ 24,000–65,000) for prolongation to

Table 7.1 Life expectancy/age

	Percentage				
Age	10°	25°	50°	75°	90°
50	20.5	21.5	36.5	415	45.5
60	16.5	17.5	26.5	31.5	35.5
65	12.5	12.5	21.5	26.5	30.5
70	9.5	11.5	17.5	22.5	26.5
75	3.5	8.5	12.5	17.5	21.5

40–49 age group [22]. For these reasons, the age limit for mammographic screening has been prolonged to 75 years of age in many European countries and the USA [21]. Although the prolongation of the age range for screening has some critical aspects, with the increase of age, there is a progressively reduced adhesion to screening programs, and the expected benefits of such prevention programs manifest themselves after 6–8 years of their launch (Table 7.1) [23]. Based on this evidence, some Italian regions have prolonged mammographic screening up to 74 years of age:

- The Region of Emilia-Romagna, in January 2010, prolonged screening to women between 45 and 74 years of age.
- The Region of Umbria, in April 2013, prolonged the screening program up to 74 years.
- The Region of Tuscany, in September 2016, prolonged the screening program to women aged 70–74 years, who had participated in one of the two previous calls before the age of 70.
- The Region of Basilicata, in December 2016, prolonged mammography screening to all women from 45 to 74 years old.
- The Region of Lazio offered the opportunity of free mammogram for women between 70 and 74 years, during the "Pink October" festival.
- The ASL of Milan offered the screening program to women aged 50–74 years who are resident in the territory of the ASL Milan.

In cases where age prolongation for mammography screening is not possible, GISMa recommended facilitating access to spontaneous screening or providing specific diagnosis/treatment planning. Here, the family physician, who is familiar with the general health of his/her patients, plays a fundamental role: regulating access to spontaneous screening, implementing clinical breast evaluation during follow-up control, as well as instructing regular self-inspection [19].

7.5 Organizational Models

The EUSOMA recommended targeting women with breast cancer in specialist breast centers (Breast Units). Here, in the light of the heterogeneity of breast cancer, a specific and effective therapy guaranteeing a higher percentage of survival and a better quality of life to every woman is available [24]. In the Breast Unit, all decisions arrived from collaboration between various medical specialists and strictly upon evidence-based medicine (EBM). The patient's point of view plays a critical role here; it is essential for a successful treatment, as well as occupying a critical role in the management of treatment. It has been shown that, in the elderly patient, an accurate information and an active participation in the diagnostic and therapeutic process allow for an increased success and an improved quality of life [12]. Moreover, the Breast Unit plays an important role in facilitating specific diagnosis/treatment planning, as well as reducing surgery waiting time.

In old age, the increased risk of postoperative complications, as well as frequent functional and cognitive decline, requires a greater level of attention in the perioperative period. This higher level of clinical attention can only be guaranteed in geriatric surgical centers. Here surgeons, anesthetists, and nurses will be aware of the specificities and the management of the complexities of aging. This mix of Breast Units and geriatric surgery centers together carries out outpatient diagnosis, admission to hospital, preparation for surgery, and perioperative care, as well as early rehabilitation and follow-up. To this end, the Italian Society of Geriatric Surgery together with the Italian Chapter of the American College of Surgeons (ACS) has contextualized the guidelines of the ACS and AGS (Geriatric Healthcare Professionals) to the Italian health system [25].

Multidisciplinary geriatric assessment, already started in the outpatient phase, serves to clarify the course of treatment, the risks associated with surgery, and the acquisition of consent to treatment by the patient and her family entourage, especially important in women with reduced decision-making capacities. Frequent home polypharmacotherapy represents a critical point typical of old age, due to potential interactions with anesthetic drugs. For this reason, recognition and reconciliation of drug therapy are essential, as recommended by health-care organizations.

In the elderly, the most serious postoperative complication is delirium, caused by prolonged hospital stay. It is responsible for functional decline, higher rate of institutionalization in residential age care centers, as well as higher mortality rates. The delirium rate is reduced by short postoperative hospital stay in designated facilities of day/week surgery, as well as postoperative setup monitoring in order to ensure optimal and early treatment of delirium.

7.6 Role of Preoperative Evaluation

In geriatric patients, it is crucial to undertake a global assessment of health status, through a multidimensional approach aimed at identifying their comorbidities and functional status, cognitive, psychological, and nutritional, to choose the best treatment strategy. The main comorbidities responsible for reduced survival rates are as follows: diabetes, kidney and/or liver failure, stroke, previous diagnosis of cancer, and cigarette smoking. It has been shown that in the age group between 65 and 74 years, there are on average three comorbidities, but in the age group between 75 and 84 years, there are on average four comorbidities, and in ≥85 years there are five comorbidities [26].

Table 7.2 Categories of aging

Patients	Characteristics
Fit	Absence of functional dependence
	No significant comorbidities
Vulnerable	Presence of one or more aspects on the IADL scale
	Stable comorbidities (e.g., stable angina, chronic renal insufficiency, etc.)
Frail	Presence of one or more of the following aspects
	Dependence on one or more of the ADL aspects
	Three or more comorbidities or one uncompensated comorbidity
	One or more geriatric syndromes (depression, dementia, delirium[a], falls[b], poor personal care, inability to put on weight[c], urinary and/or fecal incontinence[d], osteoporosis[e])

IADL instrumental activity of daily living; *ADL* activity of daily living
[a]Severe episodes, possibly evidenced by neurologist or psychiatrist
[b]At least three times a month, particularly in well-known environments, such as the home
[c]Body mass index minor or equal to 20
[d]Irreversible and nonassociated to cancer or radiotherapy/surgical treatment
[e]Disabilities associated with pathological fractures

Geriatric assessment is especially important in frail patients, for whom it is necessary to implement measures aimed at maintaining functional status. In addition to identifying any comorbidities present, multidimensional geriatric evaluation allows us to highlight any psychophysical limitations, the presence or absence of social support, as well allowing for the stabilization of risk factors, thus improving compliance, tolerability to treatment, and quality of life [1, 27]. Global evaluation, using validated scales, allows for the creation of a socio-targeted health intervention plan for each individual patient.

The most frequently used tool for the evaluation of geriatric patient as global assessment is the Comprehensive Geriatric Assessment (CGA), which has a systematic approach aimed at evaluation of multiple aspects: autonomy level, presence or absence of comorbidities, nutritional status, pharmacotherapy, cognitive function, and emotional state [28]. The use of the CGA allows for the categorization of elderly patients into three profiles: fit, vulnerable, and frail (Table 7.2) [29]. In common clinical practice, this assessment is not yet included as a routine test since in the literature concerned there is still no sufficient evidence to consider CGA as a mandatory practice in the management of older women with breast cancer [30]. In geriatric surgical centers involved with the routine use of the CGA, it allows for identification of the most appropriate plan for the specific conditions of individual elderly patients ("made to measure" surgery) [31].

7.7 Therapeutic Strategy

In the past, breast cancer surgery required a more aggressive approach (mastectomy sec. Halsted) to obtain a maximum loco-regional disease control (Fig. 7.1). On the other hand, in the 1980s, Fisher suggested that breast cancer is a systemic disease, requiring less extensive surgery than that associated with improved systemic control by means of chemoradiotherapy [32].

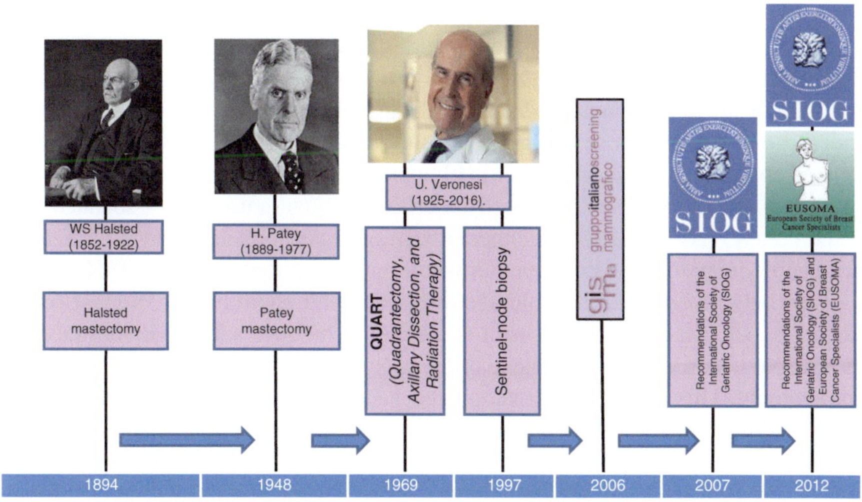

Fig. 7.1 Surgical history of treatment of breast cancer in older women

Over the years, the management of breast cancer in older women used to be very heterogeneous: ranging from radical mastectomy to hormone therapy alone. During this period, various surgical techniques have been proposed: ranging from mastectomy with axillary dissection to simple mastectomy or wide lumpectomy. These changes of treatment options were supported by an alleged minor surgical risk than radical mastectomy, even if the failure to perform a complete axillary lymphadenectomy did not allow an adequate nodal oncological staging [33]. Hormone therapy, especially in women with closely related concomitant conditions of reduced life expectation, was proposed as a wise alternative to surgery.

The absence of a standardized procedure was the result of the lack of scientific evidence from clinical studies. Subsequently the execution of well-organized scientific studies has allowed the development of guidelines based on evidence-based medicine. In fact, in 2007 the guidelines produced by the multidisciplinary task force of the SIOG, subsequently updated in 2012 by SIOG and EUSOMA, suggest that women from 70 years onwards with the absence of significant comorbidities should receive the same surgical treatment as offered to younger patients [6]. Currently, the standard of care is represented by BCS followed by radiation therapy (statement by SIOG and EUSOMA 2012). Mastectomy is advised only in the following selected cases: large or multifocal tumors, which cannot be treated by BCS alone, patients who cannot undergo postoperative radiotherapy, as well as for patients who prefer such intervention rather than BCS (statement by SIOG and EUSOMA 2012) [6].

7.7.1 Surgical Management

Even in older women, the recommended surgical choice is BCS. As reported by Umberto Veronesi, surgical senology has progressed "from the maximum tolerable to the minimum effective treatment" [34].

BCS is followed up by radiotherapy on what remains of the breast, in order to reduce the incidence of loco-regional recurrence. This therapeutic approach is recommended in DCIS (ductal carcinoma in situ), except in the presence of absolute contraindications (previous irradiation of the breast region, multifocal DCIS, microcalcifications of suspicious malignancy nature, as well as mastitis carcinomatosa) or related contraindications (difficulty in obtaining good aesthetic results, poor tumor/breast volume ratio, patient refusal to undertake the quadrantectomy associated with radiotherapy) (AIOM 2016 guidelines) [7]. In such cases, mastectomy is carried out with subsequent breast reconstruction wherever this option is possible [35].

Currently, the opinion that old age does not bring about higher surgical risk is shared by all. Thanks to advances in anesthetic techniques with local anesthesia, it is possible to carry out a wide range of breast surgical techniques, including simple mastectomy. This represents an undoubted benefit for women with a high rate of comorbidities. In 2012, Kaur published a retrospective observational study of 1028 patients aged up to 70 years versus 4207 younger patients; the 30 and 90 postoperative day mortalities were similar in the two groups, respectively, 0.2% in the elderly group versus 0 among younger patients and 0.9% in the elderly group versus 0.05% among younger patients [36].

7.7.2 Reconstructive and Oncoplastic Surgery

NICE guidelines highlight the lack of studies in oncoplastic and reconstructive surgery, which reflects an underutilization of these techniques in geriatric patients. In the literature concerned, few studies report the long-term follow-up of breast reconstruction with the use of prosthesis or with autologous techniques [37]. Since the percentage of cases in which breast reconstruction is offered decreases with age, similarly, it reduces the rate of acceptance by the patients [35]. In fact, breast reconstructive surgery performed in the elderly is not burdened by increased mortality. In women aged less than 65 years, Lipa et al. reported a 10-year survival rate of 91% for those who had undergone reconstruction with implants and 88% for those who had undergone the TRAM procedure [38].

These benefits are also reported in the National Health Service (NHS) guidelines. Women who accept reconstruction are generally satisfied with their treatment and affirm an improved quality of life [35]. James, despite the small number of patients enrolled, feels autologous techniques are safer, in spite of an increased invasiveness and a longer operative time [35]. On the other hand, Selber suggests reconstruction with prosthetic implants to shorten operative time, despite the risk of a higher frequency of postoperative complications [39]. It is recommended that autologous reconstruction should be considered an option only in women with an acceptable risk profile.

NICE guidelines reaffirm that, at the time of the strategy proposal, a therapeutic strategy for older women should not be discriminatory on the basis of chronological age alone. Each woman should receive the most appropriate treatment for her medical condition and comorbidities, over and above the preconception that a woman in geriatric age has a different perception of her aging body (Table 7.3).

Table 7.3 Offer of breast reconstruction. Acceptance percentage by patients

Age (years)	Offered reconstruction (%)	Accepted reconstruction (%)
<40	60	43
50	60	35
60	53	20
70	45	8
80	18	2

In this regard, the UK All-Parliamentary Group on Breast Cancer published the recommendations from its inquiry into breast cancer in older woman and recommends nondiscrimination on the basis of age. To ensure greater compliance of the elderly woman to the therapeutic process, it is essential that at the time of diagnosis and during the briefing, the possibility of breast reconstruction should also be proposed. James, according to his experience and a systematic review of the literature, believes that breast plastic remodeling (oncoplastic) could be considered a viable alternative to mastectomy. In geriatric patients, the oncoplastic option is considered to be a safe procedure and does not determine a greater surgical risk. The incidence of postoperative complications, length of hospital stay, and recovery time do not differ between the different age groups.

The oncoplastic procedure also presents several advantages:

- Wider local breast excision, since it allows a greater probability of obtaining margins free of cancer cells, with a consequent reduction in the number of reoperations for loco-regional recurrence
- Better cosmetic results since the breast of older women has an increased proportion of fat tissue [35]

In conclusion, oncoplastic and reconstructive breast surgical techniques are considered safe even for elderly women.

7.7.3 Axillary Lymphadenectomy

In the past, axillary lymphadenectomy, performed with double diagnostic and therapeutic targets, represented the gold standard to obtain a more complete staging and oncological radicality, ensuring an improved prognosis. Subsequent studies showed that this surgical approach was excessive in both younger and older groups. The Fisher study (NSABP B-04), carried out on patients of all ages, without clinical lymph node involvement, did not show statistically significant differences between radical mastectomy versus simple mastectomy with or without radiotherapy [32]. Similar results, in a retrospective study of 671 patients aged ≥70 years with operable breast cancer and clinically negative axillary lymph nodes, were reported by Martelli; he detected no significant differences in mortality during a follow-up of 15 years between the two groups: axillary dissection versus tamoxifen alone [40].

NICE guidelines recommended that patients with invasive breast cancer, without lymph node involvement on ultrasound or negative lymph node biopsy, should undergo axillary sentinel node biopsy, correlated to lower morbidity than the complete axillary dissection as well as avoiding upper arm lymphedema [41]. Thus, the introduction in common clinical practice of sentinel node biopsy has completely revolutionized axillary management.

The SIOG/EUSOMA guidelines recommended axillary dissection alone for elderly patients with clinically positive or highly suspected nodes; in such patients, sentinel node biopsy should avoid an unnecessary axillary dissection [1, 6].

7.7.4 Radiotherapy after Breast-Conserving Surgery

The role of radiotherapy after breast-conserving surgery in elderly patients is highly controversial.

The CALGB 9343 study was conducted on women aged ≥70 years with ER-positive tumors CT1 CN0 (clinical stage I), undergoing BCS and subsequently randomized for treatment with radiotherapy (WBRT) + tamoxifen versus tamoxifen alone. This RCT showed only an 8% reduction in the loco-regional recurrence rate at 10-year follow-up in-group undergoing radiotherapy, without reduction of the risk of distant metastasis and/or cancer-related mortality [42].

These results seem at odds with other studies, which showed better overall survival rates in radiotherapy groups [1]. Also the Veronesi RCT, which compared quadrantectomy alone with quadrantectomy + radiotherapy, shows lower local recurrence rates in over 55-year-old women than in younger patients not undergoing radiation therapy [43]. Furthermore, the *first* 248 study has reported that in elderly patients undergoing hormone therapy after BCS treatment for low-grade tumors and hormone receptor-positive and receptor-negative axillary lymph nodes, there is a low recurrence rate [44].

For these reasons, the omission of postoperative radiotherapy may be considered a viable treatment option in elderly women, undergoing BCS (clinical nodes negative, ER positive), who are receiving adjuvant hormonal therapy. In this regard, the British Association (BASO) suggested that tamoxifen probably has the same effectiveness as radiation therapy in reducing local recurrence among low-risk women undergoing BCS [45].

7.7.5 Hormonotherapy

In the older woman, hormone therapy alone, due to frequent association with more closely related comorbidities, represents a viable alternative to surgery.

The data resulting from the GRETA study [46] and by the study of Gazet [47] have shown that surgery followed by tamoxifen presents a higher disease-free survival (DFS) rate even though it does not change the overall survival rate. A systematic review and meta-analysis (Cochrane review) confirmed that surgical treatment

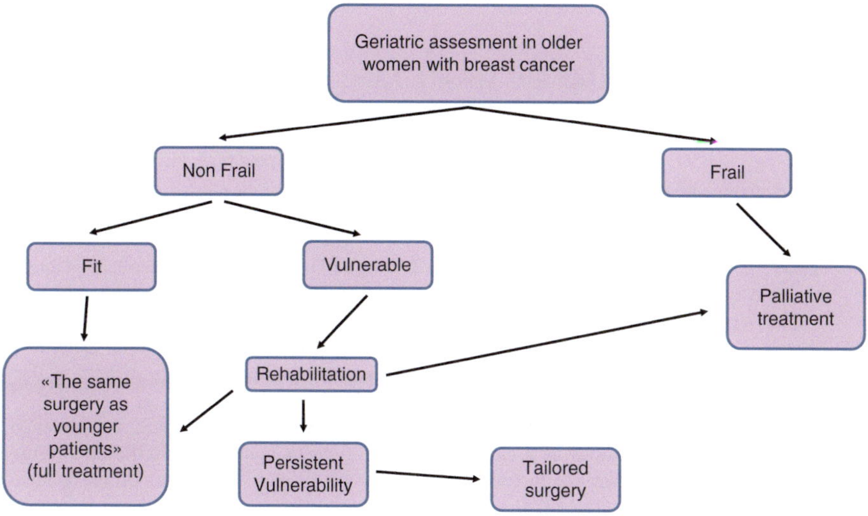

Fig. 7.2 Algorithm of surgical treatment of breast cancer in older women

with or without tamoxifen is superior to tamoxifen alone in terms of overall survival (OS), progression-free survival (PFS), and local recurrence [48].

Since the DFS and the quality of life are the main end points of breast cancer treatment of elderly patients, an endocrine treatment with tamoxifen or aromatase inhibitors can still be considered for older women with ER-positive tumors and poor general condition or those who refuse surgery.

Conclusion

Current opinion shared by the international scientific community (SIOG and EUSOMA) is that the surgical approach to breast cancer in elderly woman should always have the same radical oncological aim, regardless of the chronological age of the patient concerned.

The prevalence of any comorbidities, associated with the aging process, can have a negative impact on major surgical postoperative outcomes, such as 30-day postoperative morbidity and mortality, as well as the length of hospital stay.

For this reason, in order to identify the most appropriate management, an accurate multidimensional evaluation of the health status and life expectancy of the patient is essential from a clinical point of view, in order to avoid undertreatment of breast cancer, which could lead to disease recurrence and death [49].

As a result, treatment should be individualized for each elderly woman in order to perform a "tailored surgery" [31]. BCS is the gold standard of care. Hormone therapy alone should be reserved only for patients with severe comorbidities, the "frail" for surgery, or for those who refuse surgery (Fig. 7.2).

Acknowledgments We thank Nicholas J. Collerton for his collaboration and translation.

References

1. Biganzoli L, Wildiers H, Oakman C, Marotti L, Loibl S, Kunkler I, Reed M, Ciatto S, Voogd AC, Brain E, Cutuli B, Terret C, Gosney M, Aapro M, Audisio R. Management of elderly patients with breast cancer: updated recommendations of the International Society of Geriatric Oncology (SIOG) and European Society of Breast Cancer Specialists (EUSOMA). Lancet Oncol. 2012;13(4):e148–60.
2. Yancik R. Cancer burden in the aged. An epidemiologic and demographic overview. Cancer. 1997;80(7):1273–83.
3. Galante E, Cerrotta A, Martelli G, Del Prato I, Moglia D, Piromalli D. Treatment of breast cancer in elderly women: retrospective analysis of 111 wide lumpectomies performed in a day hospital regimen between 1982 and 1988. Tumori. 1992;78(2):111–4.
4. Martelli G, DePalo G, Rossi N, Coradini D, Boracchi P, Galante E, Vetrella G. Long-term follow-up of elderly patients with operable breast cancer treated with surgery without axillary dissection plus adjuvant tamoxifen. Br J Cancer. 1995;72(5):1251–5.
5. Distante V, Ciatto S, Frigerio A, Naldoni C, Paci E, Ponti A, del Turco MR, Vettorazzi M, Zappa M. Recommendations of a national Italian consensus conference on the opportunity of extending screening service by mammography to 40-49 and 70-74 years of age women. Epidemiol Prev. 2007;31(1):15–22.
6. Wildiers H, Kunkler I, Biganzoli L, et al. Management of breast cancer in elderly individuals: recommendations of the International Society of Geriatric Oncology. Lancet Oncol. 2007;8:1101–15.
7. http://www.aiom.it/C_Common/Download.asp?file=/$Site$/files/doc/LG/2016_LG_AIOM_Mammella.pdf. Accessed 10 Jan 2017.
8. National Cancer Institute (NCI). Surveillance, Epidemiology, and End Results (SEER) program. URL: www.seer.cancer.gov/popdata. Accessed 30 Oct 2014.
9. AIRTUM. I numeri del cancro in Italia 2016. http://www.registri-tumori.it/cms/it/node/4572. Accessed 10 Jan 2017.
10. Shachar SS, Hurria A, Muss HB. Breast cancer in women older than 80 years. J Oncol Pract. 2016;12(2):123–32.
11. Schairer C, Mink PJ, Carroll L, et al. Probabilities of death from breast cancer and other causes among female breast cancer patients. J Natl Cancer Inst. 2004;96:1311–21.
12. Vicini E, Swaminathan V, Audisio RA. Management of breast cancer in elderly patients. Clin Pract. 2014;11(1):59–69.
13. Honma N, Sakamoto G, Akiyama F, Esaki Y, Sawabe M, Arai T, Hosoi T, Harada N, Younes M, Takubo K. Breast carcinoma in women over the age of 85: distinct histological pattern and androgen, oestrogen, and progesterone receptor status. Histopathology. 2003;42(2):120–7.
14. Tesarova P. Specific aspects of breast cancer therapy of elderly women. Biomed Res Int. 2016;2016:1381695.
15. Syed BM, Green AR, Paish EC, Soria D, Garibaldi J, Morgan L, Morgan DA, Ellis IO, Cheung KL. Biology of primary breast cancer in older women treated by surgery: with correlation with long-term clinical outcome and comparison with their younger counterparts. Br J Cancer. 2013;108(5):1042–51.
16. Bergen ES, Tichy C, Berghoff AS, Rudas M, Dubsky P, Bago-Horvath Z, Mader RM, Exner R, Gnant M, Zielinski CC, Steger GG, Preusser M, Bartsch R. Prognostic impact of breast cancer subtypes in elderly patients. Breast Cancer Res Treat. 2016;157(1):91–9.
17. Molino A, Giovannini M, Auriemma A, Fiorio E, Mercanti A, Mandarà M, et al. Pathological, biological and clinical characteristics, and surgical management, of elderly women with breast cancer. Crit Rev Oncol Hematol. 2006;59:226–33.
18. DeSantis C, Siegel R, Bandi P, Jemal A. Breast cancer statistics, 2011. CA Cancer J Clin. 2011;61(6):409–18.
19. Schonberg MA, Li VW, Eliassen AH, Davis RB, LaCroix AZ, McCarthy EP, Rosner BA, Chlebowski RT, Rohan TE, Hankinson SE, Marcantonio ER, Ngo LH. Performance of the

breast cancer risk assessment tool among women age 75 years and older. J Natl Cancer Inst. 2015;108(3):djv348.
20. Cortadellas T, Córdoba O, Gascón A, Haladjian C, Bernabeu A, Alcalde A, Esgueva A, Rodriguez-Revuelto R, Espinosa-Bravo M, Díaz-Botero S, Xercavins J, Rubio IT, Gil-Moreno A. Surgery improves survival in elderly with breast cancer. A study of 465 patients in a single institution. Eur J Surg Oncol. 2015;41(5):635–40.
21. Ecomard LM, Malingret N, Asad-Syed M, Dilhuydy MH, Madranges N, Payet C, Debled M. Breast cancer diagnosis among women aged 75 and over: study on information delivered by organized breast cancer screening agencies to women reaching the limit age. Bull Cancer. 2013;100(7–8):671–6.
22. Barratt AL, Les Irwig M, Glasziou PP, et al. Benefits, harms and costs of screening mammography in women 70 years and over: a systematic review. Med J Aust. 2002;176:266–71.
23. Walter LC, Covinski KE. Cancer screening in elderly patients: a framework for individualized decision-making. JAMA. 2001;285:2750–6.
24. Kesson EM, Allardice GM, George WD, Burns HJG, Morrison DS. Effects of multidisciplinary team working on breast cancer survival: retrospective, comparative, interventional cohort study of 13 722 women. Br Med J. 2012;344:1e9.
25. Crucitti A, Puzziello A, Amato B, editors. American College of Surgeons Gestione Peri-Operatoria Ottimale del Paziente Chirurgico Geriatrico: Rossi Srl; 2016. isbn:978-88-904063-1-7.
26. Rodin MB, Mohile SG. A practical approach to geriatric assessment in oncology. J Clin Oncol. 2007;25:1938–44.
27. Pallis AG, Fortpied C, Wedding U, et al. EORTC elderly task force position paper: approach to the older cancer patient. Eur J Cancer. 2010;46:1502–13.
28. Williamson J, Stokoe IH, Gray S, Fisher M, Smith A, McGhee A, et al. Old people at home. Their unreported needs. Lancet. 1964;1(7343):1117–20.
29. Hamerman D. Toward an understanding of frailty. Ann Intern Med. 1999;130(11):945–50.
30. Parks RM, Lakshmanan R, Winterbottom L, Al Morgan D, Cox K, Cheung KL. Comprehensive geriatric assessment for older women with early breast cancer – a systematic review of literature. World J Surg Oncol. 2012;10:88.
31. Audisio RA. Tailoring surgery to elderly patients with cancer. Br J Surg. 2016;103(2):e10–1.
32. Fisher B, Redmond C, Poisson R, Margolese R, Wolmark N, Wickerham L, Fisher E, Deutsch M, Caplan R, Pilch Y, et al. Eight-year results of a randomized clinical trial comparing total mastectomy and lumpectomy with or without irradiation in the treatment of breast cancer. N Engl J Med. 1989;320(13):822–8.
33. Goldenberg IS, Janus ZL, Bailar JC 3rd, Eisenberg H. Survival patterns of elderly women with breast cancer. Arch Surg. 1969;99(5):649–51.
34. Curigliano G, Cardoso F, Costa A, Galimberti V, Goldhirsch A, Pelicci PG, Veronesi P, Viale G, Orecchia R. From the maximum tolerable to the minimum effective treatment: the Umberto Veronesi's life commitment to breast cancer care. Breast. 2017;31:241–3.
35. James R, McCulley SJ, Macmillan RD. Oncoplastic and reconstructive breast surgery in the elderly. Br J Surg. 2015;102(5):480–8.
36. Kaur P, Santillan AA, McGuire K, Turaga KK, Shamehdi C, Meade T, et al. The surgical treatment of breast cancer in the elderly: a single institution comparative review of 5235 patients with 1028 patients ≥70 years. Breast J. 2012;18(5):428–35.
37. Advanced breast cancer – an integrated view everything NICE as said. https://www.nice.org.uk/guidance/cg80/chapter/1-guidance. Accessed 10 Jan 2017.
38. Lipa JE, Youssef AA, Kuerer HM, Robb GL, Chang DW. Breast reconstruction in older women: advantages of autogenous tissue. Plast Reconstr Surg. 2003;111(3):1110–21.
39. Selber JC, Bergey M, Sonnad SS, Kovach S, Wu L, Serletti JM. Free flap breast reconstruction in advanced age: is it safe? Plast Reconstr Surg. 2009;124(4):1015–22.
40. Martelli G, Miceli R, Daidone MG, et al. Axillary dissection versus no axillary dissection in elderly patients with breast cancer and no palpable axillary nodes: results after 15 years of follow-up. Ann Surg Oncol. 2011;18:125–33.

41. Bromham N, Schmidt-Hansen M, Astin M, Hasler E, Reed MW. Axillary treatment for operable primary breast cancer. Cochrane Database Syst Rev. 2017;1:CD004561. https://doi.org/10.1002/14651858.CD004561.pub3.
42. Hughes KS, Schnaper LA, Bellon JR, et al. Lumpectomy plus tamoxifen with or without irradiation in women age 70 years or older with early breast cancer: long-term follow-up of CALGB 9343. J Clin Oncol. 2013;31:2382–7.
43. Veronesi U, Luini A, del Vecchio M, Greco M, Galimberti V, Merson M, et al. Radiotherapy after breast-preserving surgery in women with localised cancer of the breast. N Engl J Med. 1993;328:1587–91.
44. Kunkler I. Avoiding radiotherapy is an option for some older patients with breast cancer. In: San Antonio Breast Cancer Symposium 2013, San Antonio, 2013.
45. Blamey RW, Bates T, Chetty U, Duffy SW, Ellis IO, George D, et al. Radiotherapy or tamoxifen after conserving surgery for breast cancers of excellent prognosis: British Association of Surgical Oncology (BASO) II trial. Eur J Cancer. 2013;49:2294–302.
46. Mustacchi G, Ceccherini R, Milani S, et al. Tamoxifene alone vs adjuvant tamoxifen for operable breast cancer of the elderly: long-term results of the phase III randomized controlled multicenter GRETA trial. Ann Oncol. 2003;14:414–20.
47. Gazet JC, Ford H, Coombes RC. Prospective randomised trial of tamoxifen versus surgery in elderly patients with breast cancer. Eur J Surg Oncol. 1994;20:207–14.
48. Hind D, Wyld L, Beverley CB, Reed MW. Surgery versus primary endocrine therapy for operable primary breast cancer in elderly women (70 years plus). Cochrane Database Syst Rev. 2006;1:CD004272.
49. Morgan JL, Richards P, Zaman O, Ward S, Collins K, Robinson T, Cheung KL, Audisio RA, Reed MW, Wyld L, Bridging the Age Gap in Breast Cancer Trial Management Team. The decision-making process for senior cancer patients: treatment allocation of older women with operable breast cancer in the UK. Cancer Biol Med. 2015;12(4):308–15.

8 Surgical Approach to Adrenal Diseases in the Elderly

Andrea Valeri, Andrea Polistena, Carlo Bergamini, and Nicola Avenia

8.1 Introduction

Elderly patients can be affected by a wide spectrum of benign and malignant adrenal diseases which can be referred to surgery. They include endocrine disorders which are often the cause of secondary hypertension such as primary aldosteronism (PA) in Conn disease, hypercortisolism in Cushing's syndrome (CS) both sustained by adenomas and hyperplasia, pheochromocytoma (PH), and paragangliomas (PG). Similarly, adrenocortical carcinomas (ACC) and adrenal metastases are usually considered for surgical resection. Adrenal nodules are seen in 9% of the human population, and most of them are incidentally detected during abdominal imaging for other conditions and are defined as incidentalomas. Most of these incidentally detected lesions are benign especially if the patient does not have any endocrine abnormality or malignancy [1].

8.2 Secondary Hypertension

In the United States, one in three adults has hypertension. When no clear etiology has been detected, the hypertension is classified as essential [2]. However, 5–10% of patients present with secondary hypertension, in which an underlying, potentially correctable etiology can be identified. *The prevalence of secondary hypertension*

A. Valeri • C. Bergamini
General, Emergency and Minimally Invasive Surgery Unit, Careggi University Hospital, Florence, Italy
e-mail: valeri@aou-careggi.toscana.it

A. Polistena (✉) • N. Avenia
General and Endocrine Surgery Unit, S. Maria University Hospital, University of Perugia, Terni, Italy
e-mail: andrea.polistena@unipg.it; nicola.avenia@unipg.it

A. Crucitti (ed.), *Surgical Management of Elderly Patients*,
https://doi.org/10.1007/978-3-319-60861-7_8

and the most common etiologies vary by age group [3, 4]. In patients with recent diagnosis of hypertension, specific symptoms (e.g., flushing and sweating observed in PH or tachycardia, cold/heat intolerance, diarrhea in hyperthyroidism), clinical findings (e.g., an abdominal murmur suggestive of renal artery stenosis), or laboratory findings (e.g., hypokalemia suggestive of PA) might require further investigation on the suspicion of a secondary etiology. Secondary hypertension should also be considered in patients with resistant hypertension and early or late onset of hypertension. In young adults, particularly women, renal artery stenosis caused by fibromuscular dysplasia is one of the most common secondary etiologies. In middle-aged adults, PA is the most common secondary cause of hypertension [5]. *However,* in *older adults over 65 years, the most frequent etiologies for secondary hypertension are atherosclerotic renal artery stenosis, renal failure, and thyroid disorders.* Renal artery stenosis should be suspected in patients who develop hypertension after 50 years of age, present with atherosclerotic lesions in other districts and meanwhile present with unexplained renal insufficiency, or have a rapid deterioration in kidney function (i.e., an increase in the serum creatinine level of at least 0.5–1 mg per dL) when started on an angiotensin-converting enzyme inhibitor or angiotensin receptor blocker [6]. Revascularization with surgical or endovascular procedure is not required for all patients since the medical management is as effective as revascularization in high-risk patients [7]. Renal failure and hypertension are closely related since the latter can be a major cause of renal parenchymal damage, *particularly in older adults*, which in turn leads to worsening hypertension. Hypothyroidism can affect mostly the diastolic blood pressure causing an elevation of its value, whereas hyperthyroidism can cause an isolated elevation of systolic blood pressure; there is actually an increased incidence of hypothyroidism with age, peaking in patients over 60 years. Hyperthyroidism is significantly associated with elevated blood pressures in 20–50-year-olds [8, 9].

8.3 Adrenal Secondary Hypertension and Endocrine Adrenal Syndrome in Elderly Patients

Adrenal endocrine disorders usually represent a *cause of secondary hypertension with low frequency in patients over 65 years*, whereas they show a peak of incidence in middle-aged adults (40–64 years of age).

8.3.1 Primary Aldosteronism (PA)

PA, also referred to as hyperaldosteronism, is actually a group of conditions, including aldosterone-producing adenomas and bilateral idiopathic hyperaldosteronism. A severe hypokalemia not related to medication intake should lead to the suspicion of PA, although this abnormality occurs in only 30% of patients. In PA, aldosterone production is inappropriately high, relatively autonomous from the renin-angiotensin system and non-suppressible by sodium loading. This adrenal dysfunction causes cardiovascular damage, suppression of plasma renin, hypertension, sodium retention, and potassium excretion that in the chronic evolution might be associated with significant hypokalemia [10]. PA was once considered to be rare, but with cross-sectional and prospective studies, the incidence among patients with hypertension was found to be approximately 10% [11–14]. PA affects 10–20% of patients with resistant hypertension, making it the most common cause of secondary hypertension in this subgroup [15]. The initial recommended test to detect PA is measurement of the aldosterone/renin ratio (ARR) which is the most sensitive investigation, although approximately 25% of affected patients present normal aldosterone levels [16]. Current indications to investigate PA in patients with hypertension are considered according to the stages defined by the Joint National Commission, specifically stage 2 (>160–179/100–109 mm Hg), stage 3 (>180/110 mm Hg), or drug-resistant hypertension; hypertension and spontaneous or diuretic-induced hypokalemia; hypertension with adrenal incidentaloma; or hypertension and a family history of early-onset hypertension or cerebrovascular accident at a young age (<40 year). All patients with PA should undergo an adrenal computed tomography (CT) scan as the initial study which in the meantime can exclude large masses that may be a suspicion of adrenocortical carcinoma. It is recommend that, when surgical treatment is practicable, the distinction between unilateral and bilateral adrenal disease is obtained by adrenal venous sampling (AVS) [17]. The CT findings on adrenal glands may detect normal-appearing adrenals, unilateral macroadenoma (>1 cm), minimal unilateral adrenal limb thickening, unilateral microadenomas (<1 cm), or bilateral macro- or microadenomas. Adenomas may be visualized as small hypodense nodules (usually <2 cm in diameter) on CT. Aldosterone-producing ACC are usually larger than 4 cm in diameter, but occasionally smaller, and like most ACC present suspicious features on CT [18]. Adrenal CT has several limitations. Unilateral adrenal hyperplasia and microadenomas are more challenging in CT examination which makes it difficult to differentiate unilateral from bilateral forms of PA [17]. For this reason, AVS is essential for a correct diagnosis of localization and therefore for a correct surgical plan in patients with PA candidate to adrenalectomy. The sensitivity and specificity of AVS (95 and 100%, respectively) for detecting unilateral aldosterone excess are superior to that of adrenal CT (78 and 75%, respectively) [19]. In this scenario the use of magnetic resonance imaging (MRI) has no advantage [17]. According to the guidelines of the American Endocrine Society [17], unilateral laparoscopic adrenalectomy must be offered to patients with documented unilateral PA. Therefore, lateralization of PA is of paramount importance to plan the surgical treatment. Surgery following correct localization results in normalization of hypokalemia in all, improvement of hypertension in all, and complete cure in 30–60%. Postoperative plasma aldosterone and renin activity levels are the biochemical markers of response to treatment. In bilateral hyperplasia, unilateral or bilateral adrenalectomy seldom corrects the hypertension and medical therapy is the treatment of choice. Unilateral disease may be treated medically if the patient declines or is at high risk for surgery. If a patient is not suitable or decline to undergo surgery, medical treatment with a mineralocorticoid receptor (MR) antagonist is recommended [17].

8.3.1.1 Adrenal Veins Catheterization

The adrenal veins are catheterized through a percutaneous femoral vein approach, using during the procedure a nonionic contrast medium. AVS is obtained from both adrenal veins and from peripheral veins usually in the cubital fossa and assayed for aldosterone and cortisol concentrations. The venous sample from the left side typically is obtained with the catheter tip at the junction of the inferior phrenic and left adrenal vein. The right adrenal vein may be especially difficult to catheterize because it is short and enters the IVC at an acute angle. The cortisol concentrations from the adrenal veins and peripheral vein are used to confirm successful catheterization. The adrenal/peripheral vein cortisol ratio is typically more than 10:1 with the continuous cosyntropin infusion protocol and more than 3:1 without the use of cosyntropin. With continuous cosyntropin administration, a cutoff of the cortisol-corrected aldosterone ratio from high side to low side of more than 4:1 is used to indicate unilateral aldosterone excess, and a ratio less than 3:1 is suggestive of bilateral disease [19].

8.3.2 Cushing's Syndrome (CS)

Increased production of cortisol by cortical adrenal adenoma represents a rare cause of secondary hypertension. A reliable estimate of the real incidence of CS is limited to two to five cases per 1 million persons per year, but the association of this condition with cardiovascular sequelae is significant since 80% or more of these patients will develop hypertension. The *elderly are rarely affected* [20]. The common causes of CS include cortisol-producing adrenal adenoma and ACTH-secreting pituitary adenoma defined as Cushing's disease (CD) or ectopic ACTH secretion. Thus, differential diagnostic testing and tumor localization studies are fundamental for a successful treatment. In the case of bilateral macronodular adrenal hyperplasia, the disease eventually affects both glands, although it may present initially as an asymmetric unilateral nodule. Bilateral laparoscopic adrenalectomy is generally the surgical treatment of choice, although in older patients some advocate selective removal of the larger adrenal gland. Given the low frequency of Cushing's syndrome, testing should be done only if suggestive clinical features such as buffalo hump, central obesity, moon facies, and striae rubrae are detected at a clinical examination [5]. Options for initial testing include 24-h urinary free cortisol, low-dose dexamethasone suppression, or late-night salivary cortisol tests, although ultimately these patients should be referred to an endocrinologist for a complete evaluation. Unilateral resection is recommended for all cases of benign unilateral disease. Similarly, localizing and resecting ectopic ACTH-secreting tumors with node dissection as appropriate is recommended. As the optimal treatment for CD in pediatric and adult patients, transsphenoidal selective adenomectomy is suggested. In case of bilateral macronodular adrenal hyperplasia, surgical resection of bilateral adrenal disorders and medical therapy to block aberrant hormone receptors are the treatment of choice. For occult or metastatic ectopic ACTH secretion or as a life-preserving emergency treatment in patients with very severe ACTH-dependent disease who cannot be promptly controlled by medical therapy, again bilateral adrenalectomy is the best treatment option. As expected, patients with persistent or recurrent hypercortisolism continue to have higher than expected cardiovascular disease, venous thrombosis, and infections being primary causes of the excess mortality. The treatment of CS and its comorbidities is important therefore to reduce mortality [21].

8.3.3 Pheochromocytoma (PH) and Paragangliomas (PG)

PH is a rare neuroendocrine disorder arising from adrenomedullary chromaffin cells that commonly produce one or more catecholamines, epinephrine, norepinephrine, and dopamine, and which is located in the adrenal gland in 85% of cases, whereas the PG present extra-adrenal location arising from the extra-adrenal chromaffin cells of the sympathetic paravertebral ganglia of thorax, abdomen, and pelvis. Most PHs represent sporadic tumors and about 35% of PHs are of familial origin. Sporadic PHs are usually unicentric and unilateral, while familial PHs are often multicentric and bilateral. PGs also arise from parasympathetic ganglia located along the glossopharyngeal and vagal nerves in the neck and at the base of the skull; these are not catecholamine producing. *This tumor presents a peak of incidence between the third and the sixth decades.* Clinical symptoms and signs characteristic of patients presenting with PH include headache, palpitations, anxiety, nervousness, abdominal/chest pain, nausea, fatigue, dyspnea, dizziness, heat intolerance, visual symptoms, constipation, diarrhea, hypertension (sustained, paroxysmal) and orthostatic hypotension, pallor, flushing, hyperglycemia, vomiting, and convulsion. Attacks of signs and symptoms may occur weekly, several times daily, or as infrequently as once every few months [22]. The main clinical manifestation of PH is arterial hypertension, which is the result of uncontrolled production of catecholamines. PH occurs in about 0.05–0.1% of patients with sustained hypertension. However, this probably accounts for only 50% of persons with PH, when taking into consideration that about half the patients with PH have only paroxysmal hypertension or present normal blood pressure. It must also be considered that the prevalence of sustained hypertension in the adult population of western countries is between 15 and 20%. PH must always be considered because if identified, it can be cured in about 90% cases, whereas if left untreated, the tumor is likely to be fatal due to catecholamine-induced malignant hypertension, heart failure, myocardial infarction, stroke, ventricular arrhythmias, or metastatic disease following malignant transformation [5]. The surgical removal of the tumor, by adrenalectomy, can be challenging because of the hemodynamic instability during the procedure and in the postoperative stages. Development of the anesthesiologic technique and of the medical treatment before surgery significantly improved the outcome of patients operated on for a pheochromocytoma significantly reducing the mortality rate which in recent series decreased to 0 from 2.9% [23]. In the presence of suggestive symptoms, the measurement of metanephrines in a 24-h urine sample or the measurement of plasma-free metanephrines or urinary fractionated metanephrines represents the gold standard of biochemical diagnosis [24]. After initial biochemical testing for diagnosis of PH and PG imaging studies are recommended to locate the tumor. CT rather than MRI is recommended as the first-choice imaging modality because of its excellent spatial resolution for the thorax, abdomen, and pelvis. MRI could be useful in patients with metastatic disease or for detection of skull base and neck paragangliomas, in the presence of an allergy to CT contrast, in childhood, or in pregnant women. The use of ^{123}I-metaiodobenzylguanidine (MIBG) scintigraphy as a functional imaging modality is recommended in patients with metastatic disease detected by other imaging modalities when radiotherapy using ^{131}I-MIBG is planned and occasionally in some patients with an increased risk of metastatic or recurrent disease. ^{123}I-MIBG has better sensitivity than ^{131}I-MIBG for detection of PH and PG, ranging, respectively, between 85 and 88% and between 56 and 75% [25–27]. In metastatic patients the use of 18F-fluorodeoxyglucose (18FFDG) positron emission tomography (PET)/CT scanning is recommended over ^{123}I-MIBG scintigraphy [28]. This criterion is founded on the evidence that PH is either potentially associated with other endocrine diseases in the multiple endocrine neoplasms (MEN) type 2A and MEN type 2B or detected in familial syndromes (von Hippel-Lindau syndrome and neurofibromatosis type 1). In these instances, the tumors are usually diagnosed in young adults. *However, pheochromocytomas also affect children and the elderly, with sporadic cases being more common in older patients particularly those undergoing periodic routine checkup* [29]. *The number of elderly patients who undergo adrenalectomy for pheochromocytoma increased and concerns have arisen regarding the perioperative management of older individuals undergoing this surgery. The elderly are physically more fragile than younger adults, and this evidence implies specific issues in the perioperative management of these patients* [30]. Current medical preparation for surgery includes use of selective alpha-receptor blockers administered preoperatively in all patients. Fluid intake to reverse catecholamine-induced blood volume contraction preoperatively must be also considered in order to prevent severe hypotension after tumor removal [28]. *Some recommendations can be adopted in the management of elderly patients including the use of short-acting selective alpha-blockers, the prevention of hydric and electrolyte disturbances, the containment of the risk of postoperative pulmonary embolism with anticoagulation regimens and earlier postoperative ambulation, and the reduction of postoperative pulmonary complications with intense pulmonary rehabilitation. Elderly patients show a significantly increased likelihood of receiving vasopressors postoperatively, compared to younger patients, and during recovery, older patients had a longer duration of intensive care unit stay and hospitalization with a higher rate of clinical postoperative complications (*60 vs. 18%) *compared to younger individuals* [29]. The incidence of metastatic PH ranges from 3 to 36% or even higher, depending on the genetic background and location of the primary tumor. Location of metastatic lesions appears to affect patient's survival. Short-term survival is usually observed in patients with metastatic lesions in the liver and lungs, whereas better outcome is described for bone metastases. Less than 40% of patients with metastatic PH respond to chemotherapy or ^{131}I-MIBG which is the most effective treatment after surgery. Tumor size reduction ameliorates symptoms, but a survival advantage of debulking surgery has not been established although it is useful for the therapeutic results following radiotherapy or chemotherapy. Generally PGs are sporadic and solitary with almost equal distribution by sex with a maximum frequency in the middle age. Genetic susceptibility occurs in MEN type 2A and 2B syndromes, neurofibromatosis type 1, and von Hippel-Lindau syndrome, and mutations of the succinate dehydrogenase family (SDHB, SDHC, and SDHD) have been associated, with much higher frequency with PH and PG [31]. The surgical treatment includes radical removal associated or not with adrenalectomy, in the case of concomitant adrenal disease or because of proximity, and it includes the open transperitoneal approach which is specifically recommended when the tumor is large, there is suspicion of malignancy, or when multiple sites are evident at preoperative investigation by CT scan and scintigraphy. Wider surgical field, safer control of vascular structures, and easier access to bilateral retroperitoneal tumors are specific advantage of the open approach. Laparoscopic, transperitoneal, anterior, or lateral and retroperitoneoscopic are described and proposed as alternative techniques in center with high volume and specific expertise. Both in open and in minimally invasive surgery, intraoperative ultrasound or gamma probe might be used in the case of difficult localization or multiple lesions [32, 33].

8.4 Adrenocortical Carcinoma (ACC)

ACC is a rare malignant disease presenting an annual incidence between 0.5 and 2 cases per million people with a female-to-male ratio of 1.2–1.5:1. *It typically occurs during middle age, the usual presentation of ACC being in the fifth to sixth decade of life, but onset can also occur in older patients*. The clinical presentation is different depending on the endocrine activity of the tumor, varying from hormonal symptoms to a specific symptoms as abdominal pain and fatigue or to mass or infiltrative effect with poor clinical status in the case of nonfunctioning metastatic carcinoma at the time of presentation with the most common sites of distant metastasis being, in decreasing frequency, the liver, lungs, and bone. In functioning ACC cortisol or its precursor is mostly produced but also elevation of catecholamines and aldosterone with hyperaldosteronism can be observed. Very often ACC is discovered as an adrenal incidentaloma during contrast-enhanced CT being the most sensitive imaging which usually reveals a large, often more than 5 cm, tumor in one of the adrenal glands [34]. A cutoff of 4 cm has a sensitivity of 93% for identifying adrenal carcinoma, and although it is a conservative size cutoff, it should be used due to the aggressive nature of ACC and the importance of early diagnosis. Tumor extension into the vena cava with a tumor thrombus is seen in a proportion of tumors, particularly in right-sided tumors, and is indicative of malignancy [35]. Biopsy of adrenal masses has a low diagnostic accuracy and may promote needle track seeding. Therefore, biopsy in patients scheduled for surgery is not recommended and unnecessarily delays the treatment [36]. Radical surgery which is possible in a few cases is considered the treatment of choice in resectable ACC. In functioning or locally advanced tumor, surgery of primary tumor with debulking purpose is considered as an option to achieve better symptom control even in metastatic patients. Repeated surgery in recurrent tumors is also considered [34]. Mitotane and streptozotocin are the most used drugs for chemotherapy although a combination with etoposide, doxorubicin, and cisplatin on top of mitotane has been proposed as a first-line therapy following the results of a large prospective randomized controlled trial [37]. Radiotherapy is also associated in advanced disease [38]. Adrenalectomy is the only possible cure in ACC, and the overall survival varies significantly according to stage and R1-2 resection at primary surgery. Radical R0 adrenalectomy instead achieves significantly better prognosis with survival of decades after surgery. *As in previous experience, age did not have a great impact on survival and therefore also elderly patients can be cured with radical surgery in non-advanced stages* [34]. Prognosis is usually affected by local recurrence and the more sensitive prognostic factors after repeated surgery were time to first recurrence and radical surgery [39]. Histopathological diagnosis of ACC is based on specific parameters, and among them the classical Weiss score considers the observation of at least three of the nine criteria (grade 3 or 4 nuclear grade with enlarged, oval to lobulated nuclei with coarsely granular to hyperchromatic chromatin and easily discernible, prominent nucleoli; mitotic grade > 5/50 HPFs; atypical mitoses; clear cells comprising 25% or less of the tumor; diffuse architecture greater than one third of the tumor; necrosis; invasion of venous structures; invasion of sinusoidal structures; invasion of the tumor capsule) [40, 41] or in a modified revision only five of them (mitotic grade; percent of clear cells comprising the tumor; abnormal mitoses; necrosis; capsular invasion) [42]. The European Network for the Study of Adrenal Tumors staging system defines stage I, ACC ≤5 cm in the largest diameter and confined to the adrenal gland; stage II, ACC >5 cm without extra-adrenal invasion; stage III, presence of positive lymph nodes, infiltration to the surrounding tissue, or vascular tumor extension; and stage IV, distant metastasis. This staging system was considered prognostically superior to the International Union Against Cancer staging system [43].

8.5 Metastases

The adrenal gland is the fourth most common organ to be involved by metastases after the lung, liver, and bone. Metastases to adrenal glands usually originate from malignancies of the gastrointestinal district, lung, breast, prostate, kidney, liver, and melanoma. Carcinoma is the histological type mostly represented. Isolated metastases to adrenal glands are rare, being adrenal secondarism usually associated with multiple organ metastases. Adrenal metastases appear as soft tissue lesions on CT either replacing the gland or as its diffuse enlargement. Typically adrenal metastases show significant attenuation on unenhanced CT and do not produce signal drop on opposed phase images on MRI. These criteria show a high degree of sensitivity and specificity to permit a diagnostic differentiation from adenomas. Furthermore FDG-PET CT can increase accuracy since usually metastases are hypermetabolic compared to adenomas. Progressive increase in size at short-term follow-up of an indeterminate lesion in a cancer patient is suggestive of metastatic secondarism [44]. The management of adrenal metastases includes surgery, local ablative treatments, radiotherapy, chemotherapy, and palliative treatment. The strategy depends on the different clinical situations, tumor type, stage, synchronous metastases in other organs, and local features of the adrenal secondarism. Surgery presents a specific indication in selected patients with isolated adrenal metastases, and in this setting, a survival benefit after resection has been shown [45]. Laparoscopic adrenalectomy has been shown to improve patients' morbidity and to reduce hospitalization with equivalent oncological outcome compared to the open resection technique for ACC and also for adrenal metastases. It must be considered as the first option approach to adrenal metastases but still has clear contraindications in larger lesions with a 6 cm cutoff [46, 47]. Radiotherapy has been used with palliative intent with good response rates reported and limited toxicity, especially in terms of pain relief. Other therapeutic options include radiofrequency ablation, microwave ablation, and stereotactic body radiation therapy [48].

8.6 Incidentaloma

The current prevalence of unsuspected adrenal masses is approximately 3–4% in abdominal CT scan series. This rate is probably underestimated because adrenal adenomas were found in up to 10% of patients who died without any premortem suspicion of adrenal disease. Incidentaloma is slightly more frequent in women [49, 50]. *While the incidence of incidentalomas increases with age, it can be seen across all age groups with high incidence in fifth and sixth decades* [35]. Although an incidentaloma is nearly always benign with nonfunctioning adenomas being the most common tumors [51], usually malignant adrenal incidentalomas are metastatic in origin [52]. Therefore, accurate diagnosis of malignant adrenocortical tumors, particularly distinguishing ACC from adrenal adenomas, is essential for the management, but correct diagnosis is challenging. Size and heterogeneity remain the most predictive features of malignancy, as more than 4 cm in size and presence of hemorrhage, necrosis, heterogeneous contrast enhancement, and lack of contrast washout favor malignancy. Currently adrenal incidentalomas are considered to be the most common adrenal lesion; increased detection has been attributed to the increased availability of CT and improvements in CT technology enabling detection of even small adrenal lesions. Adrenal incidentalomas are adrenal lesions greater than 1 cm in size detected incidentally on imaging, most commonly CT and occasionally on ultrasound, MRI, or PET-CT. Unenhanced CT is recommended as the initial test with the use of an attenuation value of 10 Hounsfield units to differentiate between adenomas and non-adenomas [51]. Seemingly, nonfunctioning adenomas are usually asymptomatic, but indeed they may present minimal secretory activity which may cause subclinical forms of Cushing's syndrome, catecholamine excess, hyperaldosteronism, or hyperandrogenism. As shown in a large Italian series, often the discovery of an adrenal incidentaloma may lead to the detection of a remarkable number of subclinical hormone-producing tumors and could result in an early cure of clinically silent hypercortisolism, silent catecholamine hypersecretion, and rarely unsuspected hyperaldosteronism. Although patients with Cushing's syndrome have clearly established complications, the morbidity of patients with subclinical disease is less clear, and controversy exists around the risk of progression from subclinical to overt hypercortisolism, but subclinical forms might also be associated with increased risk for hypertension, diabetes, obesity, or osteoporosis. An early diagnosis of pheochromocytoma, by determination of urinary catecholamines in all adrenal masses, is important to avoid future hypertensive complications and an eventual perioperative mortality, which is possible in medically untreated patients with unrecognized pheochromocytoma before surgery. Not all patients with silent hyperaldosteronism had slightly decreased potassium levels, but they might have hypertension and suppressed upright PRA levels [35, 53]. After prevalent nonfunctioning adenomas, other benign masses like cysts, myelolipoma, and hemorrhage also have characteristic imaging features and can be differentiated from the other conditions. However, in a patient with a known underlying malignancy, the probability of incidentaloma being malignant substantially increases, and 50–70% of adrenal masses are likely to be metastases [30, 54].

A *myelolipoma* is an uncommon benign lesion composed of mature fat interspersed with marrow-like hematopoietic tissue. It occurs with a prevalence of 0.08–0.2% and it is usually unilateral and asymptomatic. The size varies from 2 to more than 10 cm, and attenuation depends on the amount of fat with the presence of calcification. On ultrasound myelolipoma is visualized as heterogeneously hyperechoic lesion owing to the presence of variable amounts of fatty and myeloid component. CT remains the diagnostic modality of choice which depicts the presence of fat as low-attenuation areas. The areas of fat are hyperintense on T1- and T2-weighted images on MRI with loss of signal on fat-suppressed sequences. Lipoma and angiomyolipoma are other fat-containing lesions which must be considered for differential diagnosis [55].

Adrenal cysts are incidentally detected lesions and are usually asymptomatic. Ultrasound shows a well-defined lesion with anechoic contents in uncomplicated cysts, and CT demonstrates the exact nature and extent of the lesion. They may appear hyperdense in the case of hemorrhage or infection within and show no enhancement on post contrast scan [56].

Adrenal hemorrhage is usually encountered in patients with blunt abdominal trauma where it affects the right adrenal more than the left. Attenuation on CT depends on the stage of hemorrhage, higher attenuation in the acute stage becoming isodense to hypodense as the clot liquefies and may calcify in the chronic stage [56]. The final diagnosis is most frequently inferred from stability of the adrenal mass over variable periods of observation (at least 6 months). Adrenal incidentaloma is not a uniform disease, and its natural history varies depending on the pathological classification of the adrenal mass. It is obvious that primary malignant adrenal tumors, and pheochromocytomas, can significantly affect patients' health and patients' outcome, and which can be greatly improved by prompt adrenalectomy. Adrenalectomy is usually recommended to all patients with subclinical CS or PH and to all patients without endocrine activity but with mass size >4 cm or a size increasing by >1 cm during the follow-up [53].

8.7 Adrenalectomy in Elderly Patients: Indications and Surgical Technique

In recent years the diagnosis of neoplasms in the elderly has increased because of the rise in life expectancy and the implementation of routine screening exams [30]. Elderly patients are physically fragile due to their attenuated systemic response to surgical stress and the frequent presence of comorbidities. In the elderly the surgery of adrenal glands had been shown to be feasible, but the surgical outcomes may be worse due to the fact that these patients are more prone to postoperative complications and have a slower recovery. It is important to consider that in nonspecialist centers, surgeons may be hesitant to perform surgery in elderly patients because of their higher risk of perioperative complications (due to a reduced breathing capacity, renal function, and resting cardiac output) and death [54, 55] and that this kind of surgery in such fragile patients requires maximum effort, focusing on strict control of comorbidities and complete preoperative care in order to facilitate a quicker surgical recovery with fewer complications.

In the elderly the clinical features of surgical diseases of the adrenal glands do not basically differ from those found in younger patient [56].

The history of adrenal surgery is long-standing. In 1914 the first planned adrenalectomy was performed by Perry Sargent [57]; meanwhile, the first flank approach for pheochromocytoma was performed by Dr. Charles Mayo in 1927. In 1992, instead, Michael Gagner performed the first laparoscopic procedure of the adrenal gland [58] and since then there has been a radical change in the management of adrenal tumors.

With the introduction of laparoscopic adrenalectomy, there was a reduction of the length of hospital stay, healthcare cost, wound complications, and blood loss and an improvement in the patient's outcome [59–61]; in fact, currently the laparoscopic approach is considered the "gold standard" therapy for the majority of adrenal gland tumors.

Different studies [29, 56, 62] have demonstrated the feasibility and the safety of the laparoscopic approach in elderly patients even if this may be associated with postoperative complications or a more frequent open conversion rate [63].

8.8 Indications for Surgery

The indications for adrenalectomy concern the presence of a functional tumor associated with hormone secretion (PA, CS, PH, and PG), the presence of a nonfunctional tumor associated with a suspicion of malignancy or ACC [64], and the presence of adrenal metastases from primary lesions of the lung, kidney, and breast, melanoma, and the gastrointestinal tract and incidentalomas [65].

8.9 Open Adrenalectomy

The open adrenalectomy has been for decades the only surgical approach to adrenal tumors; meanwhile currently it is generally performed in the presence of general contraindications to laparoscopy or in presence of large lesions (>12 cm in diameter) or malignant tumor with an invasion of the adjacent structures. Different accesses are possible in order to perform open adrenalectomy: transperitoneal approach (anterior, median, transverse, subcostal), extrapleural-extraperitoneal approach (lateral, posterior), and transpleural-transdiaphragmatic approach (trans-thoraco-abdominal).

It is important to consider that all approaches that limit the access to the peritoneal cavity decrease the rates of postoperative ileus, while the extraperitoneal approaches are associated with high rates of neuromuscular morbidity such as chronic pain (14%), laxity in flank muscles (30%), and flank numbness (10%) [66].

8.10 Laparoscopic Adrenalectomy

Different laparoscopic approaches have been described, such as the anterior approach (with patient in supine position), the lateral approach (with patient in lateral position), and a retroperitoneoscopic approach (with patient in prone or lateral position) [67–70].

The most widely practiced approach is the lateral transabdominal one because it provides a good exposure of the adrenal gland and surrounding structures and provides the surgeon with the precise anatomic landmark together with a safe control of vascular structures [67, 68].

The anterior transabdominal adrenalectomy is less employed because the conventional abdominal laparoscopic view of the abdomen leads to longer operatory times and greater number of ports used [71, 72].

The retroperitoneoscopic approaches, instead, allow a direct access to the adrenal glands avoiding the peritoneal cavity but have important limitations in tumor size and in longer operating times [73–76].

8.11 Selection of Patients

The "gold standard" treatment for adrenal tumors is laparoscopic adrenalectomy [77], and for this reason, all functional tumors including pheochromocytoma are candidates for a laparoscopic approach in the absence of other contraindications. The open approach is recommended in patients with evidence at preoperative imaging studies of malignancy with local invasion of adjacent structures. Another important parameter is the size of the tumor, but it is not an absolute contraindication to a laparoscopic resection; in actual fact, tumor size greater than 6 cm is not an absolute contraindication to laparoscopy [47, 78].

In the adrenal gland surgery, it is important to consider that a multidisciplinary approach, which comprises surgeons, anesthesiologists, endocrinologists, oncologists, plays an important role in the management of elderly patients and that the success of the procedure is also related to surgeon experience and hospital volume.

Conclusions

Some studies confirmed that laparoscopic adrenalectomy in elderly patients is safe and effective and decreases hospital stays, operative blood loss, and wound complications. Age alone should not be considered a real contraindication to laparoscopic adrenalectomy, while the real contraindications to this technique are represented by large tumors, malignant tumor with an invasion of the adjacent structures, and the general contraindications to laparoscopy, whereas regarding the preoperative care, it is important to adopt several actions in order to facilitate a quicker surgical recovery associated with fewer complications. Usually in the preoperative management of elderly patients, short-acting selective alpha-blockers are preferred in order to avoid prolonged postoperative hypotension [79]. Furthermore, in elderly patients a preoperative bowel preparation is judicious in order to prevent hydric and electrolyte disturbances and to minimize the risks of colonic bacterial translocation [80]. Moreover, it is recommended to introduce an early anticoagulation therapy in order to reduce the risk of postoperative pulmonary embolism and to institute an intense pulmonary rehabilitation in order to reduce the risk of other postoperative pulmonary complications.

In conclusion, a meticulous preparation for surgery is crucial among the elderly patients, and particular attention should be focused on maintaining the balance between the adrenal disease and comorbidities and on the early management of any postoperative complications.

References

1. Taffel M, Haji-Momenian S, Nikolaidis P, Miller FH. Adrenal imaging: a comprehensive review. Radiol Clin N Am. 2012;50:219–43.
2. Fields LE, Burt VL, Cutler JA, Hughes J, Roccella EJ, Sorlie P. The burden of adult hypertension in the United States 1999 to 2000: a rising tide. Hypertension. 2004;44:398–404.
3. Rudnick KV, Sackett DL, Hirst S, Holmes C. Hypertension in a family practice. Can Med Assoc J. 1977;117:492–7.
4. Omura M, Saito J, Yamaguchi K, Kakuta Y, Nishikawa T. Prospective study on the prevalence of secondary hypertension among hypertensive patients visiting a general outpatient clinic in Japan. Hypertens Res. 2004;27:193–202.
5. Viera AJ, Neutze DM. Diagnosis of secondary hypertension: an age-based approach. Am Fam Physician. 2010;82:1471–8.
6. Hirsch AT, Haskal ZJ, Hertzer NR, et al. ACC/AHA 2005 practice guidelines for the management of patients with peripheral arterial disease (lower extremity, renal, mesenteric, and abdominal aortic): a collaborative report from the American Association for Vascular Surgery/Society for Vascular Surgery; Society for Cardiovascular Angiography and Interventions; Society for Vascular Medicine and Biology; Society of Interventional Radiology; ACC/AHA task force on practice guidelines (writing committee to develop guidelines for the management of patients with peripheral arterial disease); endorsed by the American Association of Cardiovascular and Pulmonary Rehabilitation; National Heart, Lung, and Blood Institute;

Society for Vascular Nursing; TransAtlantic inter-society consensus; vascular disease foundation. Circulation. 2006;113:1474–547.

7. Wheatley K, Ives N, Gray R, Kalra PA, Moss JG, Baigent C, Carr S, Chalmers N, Eadington D, Hamilton G, Lipkin G, Nicholson A, Scoble J, ASTRAL Investigators. Revascularization versus medical therapy for renal-artery stenosis. N Engl J Med. 2009;361:1953–62.
8. Klein I, Danzi S. Thyroid disease and the heart. Circulation. 2007;116:1725–35.
9. Prisant LM, Gujral JS, Mulloy AL. Hyperthyroidism: a secondary cause of isolated systolic hypertension. J Clin Hypertens. 2006;8:596–9.
10. Mulatero P, Stowasser M, Loh KC, Fardella CE, Gordon RD, Mosso L, Gomez-Sanchez CE, Veglio F, Young WF Jr. Increased diagnosis of primary aldosteronism, including surgically correctable forms, in centers from five continents. J Clin Endocrinol Metab. 2004;89: 1045–50.
11. Loh KC, Koay ES, Khaw MC, Emmanuel SC, Young WF Jr. Prevalence of primary aldosteronism among Asian hypertensive patients in Singapore. J Clin Endocrinol Metab. 2000;85:2854–9.
12. Mosso L, Carvajal C, Gonzalez A, Barraza A, Avila F, Montero J, Huete A, Gederlini A, Fardella CE. Primary aldosteronism and hypertensive disease. Hypertension. 2003;42:161–5.
13. Rossi GP, Bernini G, Caliumi C, Desideri G, Fabris B, Ferri C, Ganzaroli C, Giacchetti G, Letizia C, Maccario M, Mallamaci F, Mannelli M, Mattarello MJ, Moretti A, Palumbo G, Parenti G, Porteri E, Semplicini A, Rizzoni D, Rossi E, Boscaro M, Pessina AC, Mantero F. A prospective study of the prevalence of primary aldosteronism in 1,125 hypertensive patients. J Am Coll Cardiol. 2006;48:2293–300.
14. Schwartz GL, Turner ST. Screening for primary aldosteronism in essential hypertension: diagnostic accuracy of the ratio of plasma aldosterone concentration to plasma renin activity. Clin Chem. 2005;51:386–94.
15. Eide IK, Torjesen PA, Drolsum A, Babovic A, Lilledahl NP. Low-renin status in therapy-resistant hypertension: a clue to efficient treatment. J Hypertens. 2004;22:2217–26.
16. Myint KS, Watts M, Appleton DS, Lomas DJ, Jamieson N, Taylor KP, Coghill S, Brown MJ. Primary hyperaldosteronism due to adrenal microadenoma: a curable cause of refractory hypertension. J Renin-Angiotensin-Aldosterone Syst. 2008;9:103–6.
17. Funder JW, Carey RM, Fardella C, Gomez-Sanchez CE, Mantero F, Stowasser M, Young WF Jr, Montori VM. Case detection, diagnosis, and treatment of patients with primary aldosteronism: an Endocrine Society clinical practice guideline. J Clin Endocrinol Metab. 2008;93: 3266–81.
18. Young WF Jr. Clinical practice. The incidentally discovered adrenal mass. N Engl J Med. 2007;356:601–10.
19. Daunt N. Adrenal vein sampling: how to make it quick, easy, and successful. Radiographics. 2005;25:S143–58.
20. Magiakou MA, Smyrnaki P, Chrousos GP. Hypertension in Cushing's syndrome. Best Pract Res Clin Endocrinol Metab. 2006;20:467–82.
21. Nieman LK, Biller BM, Findling JW, Murad MH, Newell-Price J, Savage MO, Tabarin A, Endocrine Society. Treatment of Cushing's syndrome: an endocrine society clinical practice guideline. J Clin Endocrinol Metab. 2015;100:2807–31.
22. Lenders JW, Eisenhofer G, Mannelli M, Pacak K. Phaeochromocytoma. Lancet. 2005;366:665–75.
23. Bruynzeel H, Feelders RA, Groenland TH, van den Meiracker AH, van Eijck CH, Lange JF, de Herder WW, Kazemier G. Risk factors for hemodynamic instability during surgery for pheochromocytoma. J Clin Endocrinol Metab. 2010;95:678–85.
24. Lenders JW, Pacak K, Walther MM, Linehan WM, Mannelli M, Friberg P, Keiser HR, Goldstein DS, Eisenhofer G. Biochemical diagnosis of pheochromocytoma: which test is best? Biochemical diagnosis of pheochromocytoma: which test is best? JAMA. 2002;287:1427–34.
25. Furuta N, Kiyota H, Yoshigoe F, Hasegawa N, Ohishi Y. Diagnosis of pheochromocytoma using [123I]-compared with [131I]-metaiodobenzylguanidine scintigraphy. Int J Urol. 1999;6:119–24.

26. Nakatani T, Hayama T, Uchida J, Nakamura K, Takemoto Y, Sugimura K. Diagnostic localization of extra-adrenal pheochromocytoma: comparison of (123)I-MIBG imaging and (131) IMIBG imaging. Oncol Rep. 2002;9:1225–7.
27. Lev I, Kelekar G, Waxman A, Yu R. Clinical use and utility of metaiodobenzylguanidine scintigraphy in pheochromocytoma diagnosis. Endocr Pract. 2010;16:398–407.
28. Lenders JW, Duh QY, Eisenhofer G, Gimenez-Roqueplo AP, Grebe SK, Murad MH, Naruse M, Pacak K, Young WF Jr, Society E. Pheochromocytoma and paraganglioma: an endocrine society clinical practice guideline. J Clin Endocrinol Metab. 2014;99:1915–42.
29. Srougi V, Chambo JL, Tanno FY, Soares IS, Almeida MQ, Pereira MA, Srougi M, Fragoso MC. Presentation and surgery outcomes in elderly with pheochromocytoma: a comparative analysis with young patients. Int Braz J Urol. 2016;42:671–7.
30. Zenilman ME. Surgery in the elderly. Curr Probl Surg. 1998;35:99–179.
31. Novosel A, Heger A, Lohse P, Schmidt H. Multiple pheochromocytomas and paragangliomas in a young patient carrying a SDHD gene mutation. Eur J Pediatr. 2004;163:701–3.
32. Polistena A, Cavallaro G, Cotesta D, Petramala L, Letizia C, Basile U, Filetti S, Cavallaro A, De Toma G. Surgical management of extra-adrenal abdominal paragangliomas report of three cases and review of the literature. Endocrinologist. 2010;20:63–5.
33. Polistena A, D'Angeli L, Cavallaro G, Izzo L, Cotesta D, Petramala L, Letizia C, Cavallaro G, De Toma G. Surgical treatment of extra-adrenal abdominal paragangliomas. Am Surg. 2009;75:1153–5.
34. Calissendorff J, Calissendorff F, Falhammar H. Adrenocortical cancer: mortality, hormone secretion, proliferation and urine steroids - experience from a single centre spanning three decades. BMC Endocr Disord. 2016;16:15.
35. Mantero F, Terzolo M, Arnaldi G, Osella G, Masini AM, Ali A, Giovagnetti M, Opocher G, Angeli A. A survey on adrenal incidentaloma in Italy. J Clin Endocrinol Metab. 2000;85:637–44.
36. Bilimoria KY, Shen WT, Elaraj D, Bentrem DJ, Winchester DJ, Kebebew E, Sturgeon C. Adrenocortical carcinoma in the United States: treatment utilization and prognostic factors. Cancer. 2008;113:3130–6.
37. Fassnacht M, Terzolo M, Allolio B, Baudin E, Haak H, Berruti A, Welin S, Schade-Brittinger C, Lacroix A, Jarzab B. Combination chemotherapy in advanced adrenocortical carcinoma. N Engl J Med. 2012;366:2189–97.
38. Lebastchi AH, Kunstman JW, Carling T. Adrenocortical carcinoma: current therapeutic state-of-the-art. J Oncol. 2012;2012:234726.
39. Erdogan I, Deutschbein T, Jurowich C, Kroiss M, Ronchi C, Quinkler M, Waldmann J, Willenberg HS, Beuschlein F, Fottner C. The role of surgery in the management of recurrent adrenocortical carcinoma. J Clin Endocrinol Metab. 2013;98:181–91.
40. Weiss LM, Medeiros J, Vickery AL. Pathologic features of prognostic significance in adrenocortical carcinoma. Am J Surg Pathol. 1989;13:202–6.
41. Lau SK, Weiss LM. The Weiss system for evaluating adrenocortical neoplasms: 25 years later. Hum Pathol. 2009;40:757–68.
42. Aubert S, Wacrenier A, Leroy X, Devos P, Carnaille B, Proye C, Wemeau JL, Lecomte-Houcke M, Leteurtre E. Weiss system revisited: a clinicopathologic and immunohistochemical study of 49 adrenocortical tumours. Am J Surg Pathol. 2002;26:1612–9.
43. Lughezzani G, Sun M, Perrotte P, Jeldres C, Alasker A, Isbarn H, Budaus L, Shariat SF, Guazzoni G, Montorsi F. The European network for the study of adrenal tumours staging system is prognostically superior to the international union against cancer-staging system: a North American validation. Eur J Cancer. 2010;46:713–9.
44. Dhamija E, Panda A, Das CJ, Gupta AK. Adrenal imaging (part 2): medullary and secondary adrenal lesions. Indian J Endocrinol Metab. 2015;19:16–24.
45. Zheng QY, Zhang GH, Zhang Y, Guo YL. Adrenalectomy may increase survival of patients with adrenal metastases. Oncol Lett. 2012;3:917–20.
46. Strong VE, D'Angelica M, Tang L, Prete F, Gönen M, Coit D, Touijer KA, Fong Y, Brennan MF. Laparoscopic adrenalectomy for isolated adrenal metastasis. Ann Surg Oncol. 2007;14:3392–400.

47. Henry JF, Sebag F, Iacobone M, Mirallie E. Results of laparoscopic adrenalectomy for large and potentially malignant tumours. World J Surg. 2002;26:1043–7.
48. Ippolito E, D'Angelillo RM, Fiore M, Molfese E, Trodella L, Ramella S. SBRT: a viable option for treating adrenal gland metastases. Rep Pract Oncol Radiother. 2015;20:484–90.
49. Glazer HS, Weyman PJ, Sagel SS, Levitt RG, McClennan BL. Nonfunctioning adrenal masses: incidental discovery on computed tomography. Am J Roengtenol. 1982;139:81–5.
50. Kloos RT, Gross MD, Francis IR, Korobkin M, Shapiro B. Incidentally discovered adrenal masses. Endocr Rev. 1995;16:460–84.
51. Boland GW, Blake MA, Hahn PF, Mayo-Smith WW. Incidental adrenal lesions: principles, techniques, and algorithms for imaging characterization. Radiology. 2008;249:756–75.
52. Johnson PT, Horton KM, Fishman EH. Adrenal mass imaging with multidetector CT: pathologic conditions, pearls, and pitfalls. Radiographics. 2009;29:1333–51.
53. Terzolo M, Stigliano A, Chiodini I, Loli P, Furlani L, Arnaldi G, Reimondo G, Pia A, Toscano V, Zini M, Borretta G, Papini E, Garofalo P, Allolio B, Dupas B, Mantero F, Tabarin A, Italian Association of Clinical Endocrinologists. AME position statement on adrenal incidentaloma. Eur J Endocrinol. 2011;164:851–70.
54. Damhuis RA, Meurs CJ, Meijer WS. Postoperative mortality after cancer surgery in octogenarians and nonagenarians: results from a series of 5,390 patients. World J Surg Oncol. 2005;3:71.
55. New classification of physical status. American Society of Anaesthesiologists. Anaesthesiology. 1963;24:111.
56. Chung TL, Van Heerden JA, Grant CS, Soreide JA, Warner MA, Ilstrup DM. Adrenal surgery in the elderly: too risky? World J Surg. 1996;20:368–74.
57. Prager G, Heinz-Peer G, Passler C, Kaczirek K, Schindl M, Scheuba C, et al. Surgical strategy in adrenal masses. Eur J Radiol. 2002;41:70–7.
58. Gagner M, Lacroix A, Prinz RA, Bolte E, Albala D, Potvin C. Early experience with laparoscopic approach for adrenalectomy. Surgery. 1993;114:1120–4.
59. Gagner M, Pomp A, Heniford BT, Pharand D, Lacroix A. Laparoscopic adrenalectomy: lessons learned from 100 consecutive procedures. Ann Surg. 1997;226:238–46.
60. Brunt LM, Moley JF, Doherty GM, Lairmore TC, DeBenedetti MK, Quasebarth MA. Outcomes analysis in patients undergoing laparoscopic adrenalectomy for hormonally active adrenal tumors. Surgery. 2001;130:625–9.
61. Heslin MJ, Winzeler AH, Weingarten JO, Diethelm AG, Urist MM, Bland KI. Laparoscopic adrenalectomy and splenectomy are safe and reduce hospital stay and charges. Am Surg. 2003;69:377–81.
62. Kuriansky J, Sáenz A, Astudillo E, Ardid J, Cardona V, Fernández-Cruz L. Laparoscopic adrenalectomy in the elderly. J Laparoendosc Adv Surg Tech. 1999;9:317–20.
63. Fried GM, Cías D, Meakins JL. Minimally invasive surgery in the elderly patient. Surg Clin North Am. 1994;74:375–86.
64. Zeiger MA, Thompson GB, Duh QY, Hamrahian AH, Angelos P, Elaraj D, et al. The American Association of Clinical Endocrinologists and American Association of endocrine surgeons medical guidelines for the management of adrenal incidentalomas. Endocr Pract. 2009;15:1–20.
65. Abrams HL, Spiro R, Goldstein N. Metastases in carcinoma analysis of 1000 autopsied cases. Cancer. 1950;3:74–85.
66. Thompson GB, Grant CS, van Heerden JA, Schlinkert RT, Young WF Jr, Farley DR, Ilstrup DM. Laparoscopic versus open posterior adrenalectomy: a case-control study of 100 patients. Surgery. 1997;122:1132–6.
67. Henry JF. Minimally invasive adrenal surgery. Best Pract Res Clin Endocrinol Metab. 2001;15:149–60.
68. Gumbs AA, Gagner M. Laparoscopic adrenalectomy. Best Pract Res Clin Endocrinol Metab. 2006;20:483–99.
69. Mercan S, Seven R, Ozarmagan S, et al. Endoscopic retroperitoneal adrenalectomy. Surgery. 1995;118:1071–6.

70. Walz MK, Alesina PF, Wenger FA, et al. Posterior retroperitoneoscopic adrenalectomy results of 560 procedures in 520 patients. Surgery. 2006;140:943–50.
71. Perretta S, Campagnacci R, Guerrieri M, Paganini AM, De Sanctis A, Sarnari J, Rimini M, Lezoche E. Sub-mesocolic access in laparoscopic left adrenalectomy. Surg Endosc. 2005;19:977–80.
72. Lezoche E, Guerrieri M, Crosta F, Lezoche G, Baldarelli M, Campagnacci R. Flank approach versus anterior sub-mesocolic access in left laparoscopic adrenalectomy: a prospective randomized study. Surg Endosc. 2008;22:2373–8.
73. Lin Y, Li L, Zhu J, Qiang W, Makiyama K, Kubota Y. Experience of retroperitoneoscopic adrenalectomy in 195 patients with primary aldosteronism. Int J Urol. 2007;14:910–3.
74. Suzuki K, Kageyama S, Hirano Y, Ushiyama T, Rajamahanty S, Fujita K. Comparison of 3 surgical approaches to laparoscopic adrenalectomy: a nonrandomized, background matched analysis. J Urol. 2001;166:437–43.
75. Terachi T, Yoshida O, Matsuda T, Orikasa S, Chiba Y, Takahashi K, Takeda M, Higashihara E, Murai M, Baba S, Fujita K, Suzuki K, Ohshima S, Ono Y, Kumazawa J, Naito S. Complications of laparoscopic and retroperitoneoscopic adrenalectomies in 370 cases in Japan: a multi-institutional study. Biomed Pharmacother. 2000;54:211s–4s.
76. Gagner M, Lacroix A, Bolte E, Pomp A. Laparoscopic adrenalectomy: the importance of a flank approach in the lateral decubitus position. Surg Endosc. 1994;8:135–8.
77. Smith CD, Weber CJ, Amerson JR. Laparoscopic adrenalectomy: new gold standard. World J Surg. 1999;23:389–96.
78. Parnaby CN, Chong PS, Chisholm L, et al. The role of laparoscopic adrenalectomy for adrenal tumours of 6 cm or greater. Surg Endosc. 2008;22:617–21.
79. Weismann D, Fassnacht M, Weinberger F, Hamelmann W, Diehl S, Lorenz K, et al. Intraoperative haemodynamic stability in patients with phaeochromocytoma—minimally invasive vs conventional open surgery. Clin Endocrinol. 2006;65:352–8.
80. Compagna R, Aprea G, De Rosa D, Gentile M, Cestaro G, Vigliotti G, et al. Fast track for elderly patients: is it feasible for colorectal surgery? Int J Surg. 2014;12:S20–2.

Pancreatic Neuroendocrine Tumors (pNETs)

9

Alessandro Sanguinetti, Andrea Polistena,
Louis Banka Johnson, and Nicola Avenia

9.1 Epidemiology

Originally called islet cell tumors, pNETs were redesignated by the World Health Organization (WHO) in 2010. These tumors are rare, with an incidence of 0.43 per 100,000 according to the National Cancer Institute's Surveillance, Epidemiology, and End Results (SEER) registry; however, this rate has more than doubled in the last 20–30 years [1, 2]. This increase is due, at least in part, to increased physician awareness, improvements in diagnostic imaging, and the overall increased use of CT scans. However, autopsy studies have found the prevalence of pNETs ranges from 0.8 to 10% [3–5], suggesting that the vast majority of them are clinically silent. There is a slight male predominance (55% male vs. 45% female). Most patients present in their 50s, although patients with functional tumors present earlier than patients with nonfunctional tumors (mean age of presentation 55 vs. 59 years) [6]. The vast majority of these patients are Caucasian (84 vs. 16%) [3]. Overall, pNETs comprise 1–2% of all pancreatic tumors and 7% of NETs in general, second only to gastrointestinal carcinoid [2, 7–9]. The majority of pNETs arise sporadically, but approximately 10% are associated with an underlying genetic syndrome such as multiple endocrine neoplasia type I (MEN1) and type IV (MEN4), von Hippel-Lindau disease (VHL), neurofibromatosis type I (NF1), or tuberous sclerosis complex (TSC) [10]. pNETs are most prevalent in MEN1 with nearly all individuals having multiple nonfunctional adenomas on autopsy, predominantly microadenomas (<5 mm in diameter) [10, 11]. The prevalence of clinically significant pNETs increases with age with roughly 50% of patients being diagnosed by age 50 and most having multiple pNETs [11–14]. The

A. Sanguinetti (✉) • A. Polistena • N. Avenia
Unit of Endocrine Surgery, Department of Surgical Sciences, School of Medicine University of Perugia, Azienda Ospedaliera "S. Maria, Via Tristano di Joannuccio 1, 05100 Terni, Italy

L.B. Johnson
Department of Colorectal Surgery, University Hospital of Malmoe-Lund, SUS, Lund, Sweden

A. Crucitti (ed.), *Surgical Management of Elderly Patients*,
https://doi.org/10.1007/978-3-319-60861-7_9

most common type of pNET in MEN1 is a nonfunctional tumor; however, the majority of MEN1 patients will develop symptomatic lesions, with around 50% developing Zollinger-Ellison (ZE) syndrome from an underlying gastrinoma, roughly 20% developing symptoms of an insulinoma, and 3–5% developing VIPomas or glucagonomas [8, 10–16]. Overall, the result is that 25% of all gastrinomas and 4% of all insulinomas are linked to MEN1 [8]. Patients with MEN1 will also develop NETs in other organs; however, development of a pNET is a poor prognostic factor. pNETs are the most common underlying cause of MEN1-associated mortality, and these patients have a reduced life expectancy of 69 years compared to 77 years for MEN1 patients without a pNET [10, 14, 17]. Recently, MEN4, which is caused by a mutation in CDKN1B which codes for p27, was discovered in a subset of patients with MEN1-like syndromes without identifiable MEN1 mutations. These patients are prone to MEN1-associated tumors in addition to adrenal, renal, gonadal, and thyroid tumors. Given its recent discovery, the prevalence and natural history of pNETs in this genetic syndrome are unclear [18, 19]. Pancreatic neoplasms in general are common in VHL with 35–77% of patients developing lesions. The majority of these are benign, with serous cystadenomas being the most common. Only 10–17% of patients with VHL will develop a true pNET, almost always nonfunctional [8, 10]. The incidence of pNET in NF1 is 0–10%, comprised of almost exclusively somatostatinomas. pNETs are also rare in TSC, with an incidence of <1%, usually associated with TSC type I [8, 10].

9.2 Pathogenesis

The endocrine function of the pancreas is carried out by pockets of cells designated as the islets of Langerhans. These cells secrete many key hormones, including insulin, glucagon, somatostatin, vasoactive intestinal peptide (VIP), and others. These are hormones commonly produced by functional pNETs. Originally, it was thought that pNETs arose from the islets of Langerhans, but more recent investigation has suggested they arise from pluripotent stem cells in the pancreatic ductal/acinar system [20]. However, pNETs demonstrate important genetic differences from pancreatic adenocarcinomas. Recent pNET exome sequencing demonstrated that gene mutations typical for adenocarcinoma, such as KRAS, are absent in pNETs. Furthermore, pNETs appear to commonly involve distinct mutations from adenocarcinoma, particularly MEN1 in 44% of tumors, DAXX in 25% of tumors, ATRX in 18% of tumors, and mTOR pathway genes in 16% of tumors [21]. MEN1 codes for menin, which has an essential function in chromatin remodeling regulation, and its role in NET development have long been known due to its involvement in the MEN1 syndrome. The serine-threonine kinase mTOR is at the center of an oncogenic pathway involved in cell growth and proliferation [21]. Interestingly DAXX and ATRX mutations have not been previously associated with cancer. DAXX and ATRX participate in chromatin remodeling at telomeres and other genomic sites and appear to be associated with pNETs through development of a telomerase-independent telomere maintenance process termed alternative lengthening of telomeres (ALT) [22–25]. The ALT phenotype is found in immortalized cell lines and has been implicated in some human cancers. In one series, 61% of pNETs had abnormal telomeres consistent with ALT, and there was a perfect correlation between these tumors and DAXX/ATRX mutations or loss of nuclear expression of these genes [22]. Loss of DAXX/ATRX and development of ALT appear to occur late in pNET development, being found in larger tumors (>2–3 cm) and metastatic lymph nodes [23]. DAXX/ATRX mutations are also a poor prognostic sign and are associated with earlier recurrence and decreased disease-specific survival [24]. Furthermore, the DAXX/ATRX pathway appears to be unique to pNETs among other gastrointestinal NETs. In one series of gastrointestinal carcinoid tumors, only 4% demonstrated the ALT phenotype, and the presence of ALT has been proposed as a method to predict the site of origin of NET liver metastases with unknown primary [25]. These recent discoveries, particularly the mutations in the mTOR pathway genes, suggest exciting possibilities for targeted molecular therapy.

9.3 Pathology/Staging

The history of classification and staging of pNETs is complex and has undergone a great number of changes in the last 10–15 years. Currently, the WHO, European Neuroendocrine Tumor Society (ENETS), and American Joint Committee on Cancer (AJCC) have each proposed a formal staging system for pNETs [25–27]. The 2010 WHO classification system is based on the proliferative activity of the tumor as measured by mitotic count and the expression of nuclear antigen Ki-67, a marker for cellular proliferation. Grade 1 tumors have fewer than 2 mitoses per 10 high power fields and less than or equal to 3% Ki-67 staining. Grade 2 tumors have 2–10 mitoses per 10 high power fields or 3–20% Ki-67 staining. Grade 3 tumors have greater than 20 mitoses per 10 high power fields or greater than 20% Ki-67 staining. Grade 1 and 2 lesions are well differentiated and classified as NETs (90% of tumors), while Grade 3 lesions are poorly differentiated and classified as neuroendocrine carcinomas (10% of tumors). The WHO classification system is summarized in Table 9.1 [26]. The ENETS staging system is based on TNM classification (Table 9.2), while the AJCC staging system is taken from the TNM staging system developed for pancreatic adenocarcinoma (Table 9.3) [26, 27]. Most head-to-head comparisons of the ENETS and the AJCC staging systems have shown no statistical difference in their ability to predict survival [28, 29]; however, one cohort study did find a slight advantage favoring the ENETS system [30]. In the face of three

Table 9.1 2010 WHO grading system for pNETs

	Grade 1 (G1)	Grade 2 (G2)	Grade 3 (G3)
Ki-67 index	<3%	3–20%	>20%
Mitotic count	<2/10 HPF	2–20/10 HPF	>20/10 HPF
Differentiation	Well differentiated	Well differentiated	Poorly differentiated
Five-year survival rate	85%	78%	9%

Survival data from Ellison TA et al. [28]. *WHO*, World Health Organization; *HPF*, high power field; *pNETs*, pancreatic neuroendocrine tumors

Table 9.2 2006 ENETS staging system for pNETs

Stage	Tumor	Node	Metastasis	Stage specific	Five-year survival
I	T1	N0	M0	Stage I	97%
IIA	T2	N0	M0	Stage II	87%
IIB	T3	N0	M0	Stage III	73%
IIIA	T4	N0	M0	Stage IV	56%
IIIB	Any T	N1	M0		
IV	Any T	Any N	M1		

Survival data from Ellison TA et al. [28]. *ENETS*, European Neuroendocrine Tumor Society; *pNETs*, pancreatic neuroendocrine tumors. *T1*, <2 cm but limited to the pancreas; *T2*, 2–4 cm but limited to the pancreas; *T3*, >4 cm but limited to the pancreas or invading the duodenum or common bile duct; *T4*, tumor invading adjacent structures or large vessels; *N0*, no regional lymph node metastases; *N1*, regional lymph node metastases; *M0*, no distant metastases; *M1*, distant metastases

Table 9.3 2010 AJCC staging system for pNETs

Stage	Tumor	Node	Metastasis	Stage specific	Five-year survival
I	T1	N0	M0	Stage IA	96%
IIA	T2	N0	M0	Stage IB	92%
IIB	T3	N0	M0	Stage IIA	76%
IIIA	T4	N0	M0	Stage IIB	73%
IIIB	Any T	N1	M0	Stage III	–
IV	Any T	Any N	M1	Stage IV	56%

Survival data from Ellison TA et al. [28]. *SMA*, superior mesenteric artery; *AJCC*, American Joint Committee on Cancer; *pNETs*, pancreatic neuroendocrine tumors. *T1*, <2 cm but limited to the pancreas; *T2*, >2 cm but limited to the pancreas; *T3*, tumor extends beyond the pancreas but not involving the celiac axis or SMA; *T4*, tumor involves celiac axis or SMA; *N0*, no regional lymph node metastases; *N1*, regional lymph node metastases; *M0*, no distant metastases; *M1*, distant metastases

different staging systems, work toward a single, comprehensive, accurately predictive model continues. Recently, one retrospective analysis suggested that combining the WHO grading system using Ki-67 expression rates with the lesser known Hochwald grading system, which divides tumors into two stages based on tumor necrosis and mitotic rates, is more predictive of survival than any of the current staging systems [28]. Similarly, another series out of Johns Hopkins found that Ki-67 expression rates have a linear relationship with mortality, calling into question the validity of breaking Ki-67 rates into categories as the WHO system does. They proposed a nomogram based on age, gender, and Ki-67 labeling as a continuous variable that appears to be both simpler and more prognostic than either the ENETS or AJCC systems [29]. The staging of pNETs will continue to evolve in the coming years as our understanding increases.

9.4 Presentation

pNETs are divided into functional versus nonfunctional tumors with about 90% being classified as nonfunctional. Commonly, tumors are defined as nonfunctional if the patient does not suffer from symptoms due to hormone hypersecretion, even if hormone levels are elevated on laboratory evaluation. Most nonfunctional pNETs present with symptoms due to mass effect, such as jaundice, weight loss, abdominal pain, palpable mass, nausea/emesis, pancreatitis, or back pain, and mimic the presentation of pancreatic adenocarcinoma.

9.4.1 Natural History

Most PNETs are indolent but have malignant potential. The true natural history of PNETs has not been studied systemically. PNETs in MEN1 grow slowly and remain stable for years, at least when they are small [31, 32]. Whether the natural history of PNETs in MEN1 is representative of that of sporadic, PNETs is unknown. If untreated, most PNETs grow and eventually metastasize to the liver; extensive liver metastasis is the most common cause of death for patients with PNETs [33, 34]. The biological behavior of an individual PNET is unpredictable; a higher tumor grade, lymph node, and liver metastasis and a larger primary tumor generally portend a less favorable prognosis [35, 36]. Molecular markers that predict PNET behavior are necessary to improve clinical decision-making. Most patients survive many years after diagnosis. PNETs are classified as functioning or nonfunctioning depending on whether they cause hormonal hypersecretion syndrome.

Functioning PNETs result in hormonal hypersecretion syndromes, as elaborated below (Table 9.4).

Nonfunctioning PNETs cause nonspecific symptoms, such as vague abdominal pain, and can be an incidental finding.

The distinction between functioning and nonfunctioning PNETs is based on clinical presentation, and there is no absolute difference in hormone expression between functioning and nonfunctioning PNETs. For example, the tumor cells in a small PNET may express glucagon, resulting in a borderline elevation of glucagon levels; clinically, however, this PNET is classified as nonfunctioning because the slight elevation of glucagon is not sufficient to cause glucagonoma syndrome. Through immunochemical examination, most PNETs express numerous hormones. Some hormones are expressed in normal islets (e.g., insulin, glucagon, somatostatin, and pancreatic polypeptide), and others (e.g., gastrin, vasoactive intestinal peptide (VIP), serotonin, adrenocorticotropin (ACTH), corticotropin-releasing hormone (CRH), parathyroid hormone-related peptide (PTHrp), parathyroid hormone (PTH), growth hormone-releasing hormone (GHRH), growth hormone (GH), calcitonin,

Table 9.4 Functioning pancreatic neuroendocrine tumor (PNET) syndromes

Tumor	Symptom(s)
Insulinoma	Hypoglycemia
Gastrinoma	Severe peptic ulceration
VIPoma	Watery diarrhea, hypokalemia, achlorhydria (WDHA syndrome)
Glucagonoma	Glucose intolerance, necrolytic migratory erythema, stomatitis/ glossitis, hypoaminoacidemia
Somatostatinoma	Hyperglycemia, cholelithiasis, steatorrhea, achlorhydria

ghrelin, human choriogonadotropin (hCG), and renin) that are not normally expressed in the islets are expressed by PNETs. The expressed hormones may or may not be secreted or biologically active, and the hormone expression profile of each tumor can change over time. It is common that an initially nonfunctioning PNET later triggers hormonal hypersecretion syndrome [37–39].

9.5 Functioning PETs

9.5.1 Insulinomas

Patients with insulinomas present with the symptoms of hyperinsulinemic hypoglycemia, i.e., the Whipple's triad, consisting of mental confusion, weakness, fatigue, and seizures while fasting, blood glucose levels below 50 mg/dL, and immediate relief of symptoms following ingestion of glucose. Most patients have documented weight gain. The serum insulin levels are inappropriately elevated for the prevailing plasma glucose concentration, and there is usually a higher ratio of proinsulin than normally found. Insulinomas may also arise in the pancreas of non-insulin-dependent diabetics and can lead to an improvement in the symptoms [40]. Insulinomas are the most frequent functioning pancreatic endocrine tumors and have been diagnosed over a wide range, but the peak incidence is found between 40 and 60 years [41, 42]. Neonates and infants with persistent hyperinsulinemic hypoglycemia most often suffer from inappropriate insulin secretion caused by inactivation of the potassium ion channels of beta cells of the endocrine pancreas due to various point mutations of the channel proteins. Morphologically, diffuse or focal nesidioblastosis is found [43, 44]. Diffuse nesidioblastosis may also occur, although very rarely, in the adult [45, 46]. Virtually all insulinomas are found in the pancreas. They are distributed almost evenly throughout the pancreas or are attached to it. Reports convincingly demonstrating insulin production and hypoglycemic symptoms in neuroendocrine tumors located outside the pancreas are rare. So far such tumors have been observed in the duodenum [47], ileum [48, 49], lung [50], cervix [51], and ovary [52]. Between 85 and 99% of insulinomas are benign, solitary, and less than 2.5 cm in diameter when detected [53]. Insulinomas that turn out to be malignant usually have a diameter of over 3 cm, and about one-third have metastasized at the time of diagnosis. Multiple insulinomas, occurring synchronously or metachronously, are found in 2–7% of patients and MEN1-associated insulinomas in 6%. Immunocytochemically, insulin- and proinsulin-producing cells can be identified in all insulinomas. Strong positivity for insulin (at the basal pole of the cell) and proinsulin (in the perinuclear region) is usually seen in well-differentiated insulinomas with a trabecular growth pattern [54]. By contrast, insulinomas with a solid pattern may show only a weak reaction and diffuse cytoplasmic distribution of proinsulin and insulin. Insulinomas also commonly express islet amyloid polypeptide (IAPP) [55, 56], and in approximately 5% of these tumors, IAPP may be precipitated as amyloid in the tumor stroma [57]. IAPP is normally released by the pancreatic beta cells together with insulin; it has also been named amylin. Massive secretion of IAPP from a malignant pancreatic tumor has been reported [58]. Insulinomas, irrespective of whether they are benign or malignant, may also express hormones other than insulin. Electron microscopically, well-granulated cells with typical beta granules; cells with atypical, sometimes pleomorphic granules; and scarcely granulated cells have been described. In addition, cells with typical alpha and PP granules may be identified. Based on the different ultrastructural features of neoplastic beta cells, three working classifications of insulinomas have been advanced [59–61], which can, to some degree, be related to the proportion of proinsulin secreted by these insulinomas (e.g., related to varying degrees of conversion of proinsulin to insulin). In the non-tumorous endocrine pancreas of patients with insulinomas, the islet content of immunoreactive insulin may be decreased. This might be due to an adaptive response of the normal beta cells to prolonged hypoglycemia [62].

9.5.2 Gastrinomas

Inappropriate gastrin secretion by gastrinomas causes the Zollinger-Ellison syndrome (ZES). This is characterized by gastric acid hypersecretion, intractable peptic ulceration, and occasionally severe diarrhea [63, 64]. Between 60 and 75% of patients with ZES are found to have the syndrome as an isolated disease (sporadic ZES); in the remaining patients, ZES is part of the MEN1 syndrome [65]. The term pseudo-ZES (also called ZES type 1, as opposed to ZES type 2 caused by a gastrinoma) was coined for a syndrome with symptoms similar to ZES that appears to be caused by antral G-cell hyperfunction and G-cell hyperplasia [66, 67]. The fact that this syndrome has no longer been described in recent years raises questions as to its existence. In rare cases the syndrome of recurrent and intractable peptic ulceration may be found in association with a pancreatic endocrine tumor that does not produce and secrete gastrin [68]. The factor causing peptic ulceration in these patients has yet to be identified [69]. Gastrinomas are second only in incidence to insulinomas and are most often malignant. The peak incidence of gastrinomas lies between 40 and 50 years; children (5–15 years of age) are rarely affected. Approximately 50–70% of the gastrinomas associated with the sporadic form of ZES occur in the pancreas, particularly in its head, while the remainder are mainly found in the duodenum. The predominant location of gastrinomas within the anatomic area comprising the head of the pancreas and the first and second portions of the duodenum has been called the gastrinoma triangle [70]. Unusual sites of gastrinomas are the stomach [71], jejunum [72, 73], biliary tract, liver, and kidney [74]. Ovarian or pancreatic mucinous cystic tumors that contain a sufficient number of active endocrine cells with gastrin production may also cause ZES, but are uncommon [75, 76]. Around 90% of the gastrinomas associated with the MEN1 syndrome reside in the duodenum. These tumors are usually smaller than 1 cm, are multicentric, and arise from gastrin cell precursor lesions [77]. Because of their small size, they are, like sporadic duodenal gastrinomas, difficult to detect. Pancreatic gastrinomas associated with MEN1 are rare [78], although the pancreas of these patients usually contains multiple endocrine tumors. These tumors, however, virtually never produce detectable amounts of gastrin. Sporadic gastrinomas, occurring either in the pancreas or in the duodenum, are apparently solitary tumors. In the pancreas, they usually have a diameter of 2 cm or more, whereas in the duodenum their diameter is most often less than 1 cm [79]. Metastasis to regional lymph nodes is found in approximately 60% of patients with pancreatic gastrinomas [80] and at an even higher percentage in patients with duodenal gastrinomas. Because duodenal gastrinomas can metastasize while still very small, they may give rise to periduodenal lymph node metastases which are larger than the primary. It has therefore been suggested that so-called peripancreatic and periduodenal lymph node gastrinomas may be metastases of duodenal microgastrinomas that were overlooked during surgery, rather than true primary tumors [81, 82]. In contrast to the distribution of lymph node metastases, duodenal gastrinomas, whether sporadic or associated with MEN1, seem to give rise to liver metastases in a smaller percentage of cases than pancreatic gastrinomas. Thus 10-year survival rates have been shown to be higher in patients with duodenal gastrinomas (84%) than in patients with pancreatic gastrinomas (57%) [83]. Histologically, gastrinomas most often show a trabecular or pseudoglandular pattern. Immunocytochemically, gastrin can be demonstrated in almost all tumors. Approximately 50% of gastrinomas are multihormonal and contain PP, glucagons, and/or insulin in addition to gastrin. Islet hyperplasia and nesidioblastosis have repeatedly been described in the non-neoplastic pancreas of patients with gastrinomas, but these findings could not be confirmed by morphometry [84]. Recently, however, morphometrically defined PP-cell hyperplasia has been described in the ventrally derived region of the pancreatic head [85]. So far it has not been definitely established what influence hypergastrinemia may have on these changes. In the gastric mucosa, however, sustained hypergastrinemia induces parietal cell hyperplasia with thickened mucosal folds and gastric acid hypersecretion. In addition, the number of enterochromaffin-like (ECL) cells is increased in the fundic mucosa [86, 87]. ECL cell tumors in the fundus of the stomach, which are a well-known complication in patients suffering from pernicious anemia with chronic type A gastritis, appear to be very uncommon in patients with sporadic ZES. They have, however, been reported in patients with ZES and MEN1. In these instances, they probably represent another neoplastic manifestation of the MEN1 syndrome rather than merely the result of a trophic effect of gastrin [86].

9.5.3 Glucagonomas

This syndrome includes a skin rash known as necrolytic migratory erythema, mild glucose intolerance, normochromic normocytic anemia, weight loss, depression, and a tendency to develop deep vein thrombosis [87]. This symptomatology is thought to reflect the catabolic action of highly elevated glucagon serum concentrations [88]. The syndrome has not been convincingly described in extrapancreatic glucagon-producing tumors. Functionally active glucagonomas are rather large (size range 2–35 cm), commonly occur in the distal portion of the pancreas or attached to the pancreas, and are most often malignant. Tumors containing glucagon-producing cells that are not associated with the glucagonoma syndrome are often benign and are usually found as small neoplasms at autopsy or in a MEN1 pancreas [89, 90]. Immunocytochemically, glucagonomas often stain weakly for glucagon, but also show reactivity for peptides derived from proglucagon (glicentin, glucagon-like peptides 1 and 2) [91]. In addition, numerous PP cells can often be identified. Electron microscopically, readily identifiable A-cell granules may be recognized in functionally silent glucagon-producing tumors, whereas atypical secretory granules predominate in glucagonomas associated with the syndrome.

9.5.4 VIPomas

Inappropriate secretion of vasoactive intestinal polypeptide (VIP) by VIPomas causes the watery diarrhea, hypokalemia, and achlorhydria (WDHA) syndrome, also called Verner-Morrison syndrome [92]. Although VIP is the most likely mediator of the WDHA syndrome, other hormonelike substances such as the peptide histidine methionine may also be involved. In the adult, the vast majority of VIPomas are of pancreatic origin. Exceptions are some rare VIP-producing pheochromocytomas [93, 94] and intestinal endocrine tumors [95]. In children, WDHA syndromes have been reported in association with VIP-secreting ganglioneuromas and ganglioneuroblastomas [96, 97]. The WDHA syndrome has also been attributed to islet hyperplasia [98, 99]. These reports are difficult to interpret because, in the normal adult human pancreas, VIP is only present in autonomic nerves but not in islet cells. Pancreatic VIPomas are usually solitary large tumors (mean size 4–5 cm), occur often in the pancreas tail (approximately 50%), and are malignant in at least 80% of cases. Immunocytochemically, VIP can be visualized in well-preserved tissue routinely fixed with formalin or in freeze-dried and vapor-fixed specimens. Tissue with suboptimal fixation may lose its VIP reactivity. It is sometimes advantageous to look for mRNA by using in situ hybridization. VIP-producing tumor cells have also been shown to express PHM-27, a protein sharing with VIP a common big precursor peptide (prepro-VIP/PHM-27). In addition, they commonly express PP74 and, less commonly, calcitonin and neurotensin [100].

9.5.5 Somatostatinomas

Patients with a pancreatic somatostatinoma may have a syndrome thought to be attributable to the widespread inhibitory effects of somatostatin. It consists of diabetes mellitus, cholelithiasis, steatorrhea, indigestion, hypochlorhydria, and, occasionally, anemia [101]. Pancreatic somatostatinomas are very rare. They are virtually always malignant, and occasionally they may contain psammomatous calcifications [102]. Extrapancreatic somatostatinomas occur most often in the second portion of the duodenum, often at the site of the papilla of Vater or in close proximity to it, and are sometimes associated with NF1 (von Recklinghausen's disease) and pheochromocytomas.

9.6 Functioning Tumors Producing Ectopic Hormones or Multiple Hormones

Among the syndromes infrequently observed with pancreatic endocrine tumors and caused by ectopic hormones are those due to the production of ACTH (Cushing's syndrome) [103, 104], serotonin (carcinoid syndrome) [105], growth hormone-releasing factor (acromegaly) [106, 107], paraneoplastic hypercalcemia (PTH)-related protein (PTHrP) mimicking the action of PTH [108, 109], and calcitonin (diarrhea in 50% of cases). Most of the neoplasms associated with syndromes caused by ectopic hormones are malignant and of large size. Their microscopic patterns are usually the same as in other pancreatic endocrine tumors. Exceptions are some neoplasms producing growth hormone-releasing factor and causing acromegaly, which may show a distinct paraganglioma-like microlobular pattern [110] and spindle-shaped cells. Combinations of various hormonal syndromes or transitions from one syndrome to another have been described. They appear to be uncommon. The known associations are ZES and hypercalcemia [111], ZES and Cushing's syndrome [112, 113], hypoglycemia and Cushing's syndrome [114], and hypoglycemia with ZES [115], or carcinoid syndrome [116, 117]. In some rare cases, the glucagonoma syndrome followed a hypoglycemic syndrome after cytostatic therapy [118]. It should be emphasized that a number of patients with combined clinical syndromes, in particular ZES and Cushing's syndrome, have been shown to suffer from MEN1.

9.7 Nonfunctioning Tumors

Nonfunctioning neoplasms become clinically apparent (abdominal pain, jaundice, weight loss) due either to their large size, to invasion of adjacent organs, or to the occurrence of metastases. Infrequently they may present as pancreatitis [119] or in association with hematologic changes such as pancytopenia [120] or eosinophilic infiltration of the skin [121]. There are various explanations for the lack of hormonally induced syndromes, even in the presence of immunocytochemically detectable hormones: (1) the amount of hormone (s) produced and released may be too low to cause symptoms; (2) the principal hormone synthesized and secreted by the tumor does not induce any specific clinical signs although it is released in excess, as is the case with PPomas and neurotensinomas [122]; (3) the tumor secretes a precursor hormone or a hormonelike substance that is functionally inert; or (4) the hormonal product of the tumor has not yet been identified. The majority of surgically removed nonfunctioning tumors are >5 cm in diameter and show malignant behavior [123]. Their symptoms are related either to the appearance of metastases or to their size and site. Immunocytochemically, about 10% of the tumors are virtually agranular, with only sparse hormone-positive cells. The agranularity of these tumors is reflected by very weak or absent chromogranin staining, while synaptophysin positivity is preserved. In chromogranin A-reactive positive nonfunctioning tumors, PP is frequently found. Because PP is sometimes the predominant hormone, these neoplasms have been called PPomas, although they do not represent a clinical entity. Among the extrapancreatic tumors rich in PP cells are the majority of gangliocytic paragangliomas of the duodenum [124] and some rectal neuroendocrine tumors [125]. A few nonfunctioning malignant tumors have been shown immunocytochemically to produce serotonin [126, 127]. Tumors described as neurotensinomas and calcitoninomas or those producing bombesin [127] are either hormonally silent or are associated with syndromes that are difficult to relate to the effects of these hormones.

9.8 Pancreatic Endocrine Tumors in MEN1

Pancreatic tumors are part of a tumor spectrum that involves the parathyroid glands (80–98% of patients), the anterior pituitary (9–40%), and the duodenum (40–85%) [128, 129], but occasionally also the stomach, ileum, lung, or thymus [130, 131]. The outstanding feature of the pancreatic lesions in MEN1 is diffuse microdenomatosis in association with one or several macrotumors (>0.5 cm in diameter) [132]. Histologically, most of the small tumors display a distinct trabecular pattern and may show a connective tissue capsule. Multihormonality is a consistent finding in these tumors, with one hormone usually prevailing. Most frequent are glucagonomas and PPomas, followed by insulinomas. Serum PP has therefore been recommended as a screening hormone in MEN1 patients [133], although subsequent data suggested a wider distribution of hormone type [134]. In MEN1 patients with hypoglycemia, it was noted that, despite the presence of multiple tumors, usually only one of the macrotumors produced insulin. Removal of this tumor relieved the patients' hypoglycemic syndrome. In MEN1 patients with ZES, which occurs in approximately 60% of MEN1 patients, pancreatic gastrinomas are surprisingly uncommon, although the pancreas of these patients may be studded with tumors of varying sizes producing other hormones. The gastrinomas in these patients reside predominantly in the proximal part of the duodenum, are usually <1 cm in diameter, and show multicentricity (see section on gastrinomas, above). The occurrence of WDHA syndrome, glucagonoma syndrome, [132, 133] or acromegaly due to a tumor-secreting growth hormone-releasing factor is very rare in the setting of MEN1.

9.9 Mixed Endocrine-Exocrine Tumors

True mixed endocrine-exocrine tumors (i.e., ductal endocrine or acinar-endocrine tumors) of the pancreas, in which both components are clearly demonstrated, are exceedingly rare [134]. Arguments supporting the endocrine-exocrine nature of tumors are the presence of both elements in both the primary tumor and its metastases and the ultrastructural identification of cells containing both hormone granules and zymogen or mucin granules. The inclusion of normal ducts within endocrine tumors (so-called ductulo-insular tumors) or the occurrence of endocrine cells attached to the neoplastic glands of ductal adenocarcinomas of the pancreas cannot be regarded as evidence that a tumor is truly endocrine-exocrine in nature.

9.10 Diagnosis/Staging

9.10.1 History and Physical

A detailed history and physical is essential in these patients. The history should focus on signs of mass effect or metastasis, evaluate for symptoms of an endocrine syndrome, and screen for family history suggestive of genetic syndromes associated with pNETs. Physical exam should look for jaundice and abdominal masses.

9.10.2 Laboratory Evaluation

If a functional tumor is suspected, workup should include biochemical assessment for the appropriate syndrome. Seventy two-hour fast is the gold standard for diagnosis of an insulinoma, with measurement of glucose and insulin levels at the time of symptoms. It is also important to measure C-peptide to rule out surreptitious insulin use [135]. With gastrinoma, an elevated fasting serum gastrin level is usually the first test, and a level greater than ten times the limits of normal is virtually diagnostic of this disease. Proton pump inhibitors elevate serum gastrin levels, and it is important to draw labs after holding these drugs for 1 week due to their long-acting nature. ZE syndrome is usually confirmed with a secretin stimulation test, but gastric acid secretion studies are sometimes required [136, 137]. Migratory necrotizing dermatitis, while highly suggestive of a glucagonoma, can also occur in celiac disease, cirrhosis, or pancreatitis, and the diagnosis must be confirmed by elevated glucagon levels [138–140]. VIPoma and somatostatinoma are confirmed by elevated levels of VIP and somatostatin, respectively [141, 142]. A variety of tumor markers have been proposed for functional and nonfunctional pNETs. The most common of these is chromogranin A (CgA), an acid-soluble protein that is found in secretory granules of neuroendocrine cells, although others, such as neuron-specific enolase (NSE), pancreatic polypeptide, pancreastatin, and human chorionic gonadotropin, have been proposed. CgA is the most sensitive of these, with elevated levels present in 72–100% of patients. However, CgA levels are highly variable, limiting specificity to 50–80% [55, 56]. Furthermore, proton pump inhibitor use, impaired renal function, liver disease, and inflammatory bowel disease can all cause an increase in CgA leading to false-positive results. Higher CgA levels correlate with increased tumor burden and metastatic disease and may be most useful in assessing response to therapy [55, 56]. The sensitivity of NSE as a tumor marker is low at 30–40%, but its specificity is almost 100% [57]. Using a combination of CgA and NSE levels improves the sensitivity of using either alone [58].

9.10.3 Imaging

Localization and staging of the tumor are essential to appropriate therapy for pNET. A variety of imaging modalities exist to assist the clinician, including computed tomography (CT), magnetic resonance imaging (MRI), somatostatin receptor scintigraphy (SRS), positron-emission tomography (PET), and endoscopic ultrasonography (EUS). In the rare case that the tumor cannot be located with these modalities, angiography with selective arterial stimulation and venous sampling may be employed. If the tumor cannot be located prior to surgery, bimanual palpation with intraoperative ultrasound often discovers the lesion as a last resort. This is a situation seen most often with small insulinomas that are only a few millimeters in size.

9.11 CT

CT is the most common initial imaging study in the evaluation of patients with pNETs. Triple-phase contrast CT is the optimal study as pNETs are typically best visualized during the arterial phase. They usually appear as spherical, hyper-dense, and hyper-vascular mass that rarely obstruct the pancreatic duct. The reported sensitivity of CT ranges from 62 to 83% with a specificity of 83–100%, although it varies with the size of the lesion [59, 60]. Although most pNETs are solid lesions, about 10% will present as cystic lesions with smooth margins and peripheral enhancement on both arterial and portal phases. Overall, it is difficult to differentiate cystic pNETs from other cystic pancreatic lesions on cross-sectional imaging with a misdiagnosis rate of 43% in a recent series [61].

9.12 MR

pNETs are usually well visualized on MR. The MR signal is typically low in T1-weighted sequences and high in T2-weighted sequences. Again, pNETs are best visualized during the arterial contrast phase. The sensitivity of MR ranges from 85 to 100% with a specificity of 75–100% [59, 62]. In one recent series of 55 patients, the sensitivity of MR was 95%, rivaling that of EUS [63]. Not as commonly used as CT, MR is most often ordered when lesions are too small to be visualized on CT. In detecting and following liver metastases, MR has been suggested to be superior to CT [62, 64, 65].

9.13 SRS

SRS (somatostatin receptor scintigraphy) uses radiolabeled somatostatin analogs and relies on somatostatin receptors expressed by pNETs. This leads to an important caveat that insulinomas, in which somatostatin receptors are present only at low levels or absent entirely, are not well visualized with this technique. However, for other functional pNETs and nonfunctional pNETs, the ability of SRS to localize the tumor is good, with sensitivities ranging from 75 to 100% [62, 66]. SRS is often used when a functional pNET is suspected and conventional cross-sectional imaging fails to localize the tumor. It can be particularly helpful with glucagonoma as this have a greater propensity to present outside of the pancreas than other functional NETs [59]. SRS has an advantage over other imaging modalities in evaluating patients for sufficient uptake for targeted radiation therapy using radiolabeled somatostatin analogs. SRS is also typically useful in evaluating the burden of metastatic disease.

9.14 PET

Standard PET imaging with 18F-fluorodeoxyglucose (FDG) does not visualize pNETs well, given that most pNETs are well differentiated with a low metabolic rate. However, it can detect poorly differentiated pNETs and FDG avidity correlates with early tumor progression and increased mortality [67, 68]. Alternatively, PET imaging has increasingly utilized 68Ga-labeled somatostatin analogs with excellent results. PET imaging with this utilization has been shown to be superior to both SRS and conventional cross-sectional imaging [69, 70]. The results from fusion of PET with CT images are better than either modality individually with sensitivities of 94–100% [71]. In one series, use of fused PET/CT images changed treatment decisions in 59.6% of patients compared to CT or MRI alone.

9.15 EUS

EUS (endoscopic ultrasound) has become an invaluable tool in the evaluation of pancreatic lesions. In addition to radiologic examination of the pancreas, EUS offers the additional benefit of obtaining biopsies for diagnosis. EUS has an 82% sensitivity and a 92% specificity in identifying pNETs, although EUS is more sensitive in the head of the pancreas than the tail and results are operator dependent [72, 73]. EUS is most useful in identifying small insulinomas, as these lesions infrequently express somatostatin receptors and are not well visualized on SRS or PET. EUS has the added benefit of being able to tattoo smaller lesions for easier intraoperative identification, facilitating laparoscopic resection [73].

9.16 Surgical Management

9.16.1 General Principles for Surgical Management of pNETs

Pancreatic NETs should ideally be managed in a multidisciplinary setting. In choosing the appropriate therapy, physicians should adopt an individualized, patient-focused medical management strategy at centers with an interest in the disease, expertise in treating it, and a multidisciplinary approach to patient care. Surgery with curative intent should be considered in all cases if clinically appropriate and technically feasible. Enucleation for small (B2 cm) G1 pNETs is an acceptable approach. Larger G1 and G2 pNETs and NECs require the same oncologic principles as those applied to pancreatic adenocarcinomas.

9.17 Surgical Approaches

9.17.1 Functioning Disease

Functioning PNETs primarily include insulinomas and gastrinomas, with an incidence of 70–80% and 20–25% of all PNETs and an incidence of malignancy of <10% and 50–60%, respectively [9]. Insulinomas are generally solitary, benign, and curable with surgery [74–76]. Recurrence after resection occurs in about 3% [77, 78]. The procedures of choice are enucleation for small and isolated insulinomas and partial pancreatectomy for large and potentially malignant insulinomas [143, 144]. Besides enucleation, middle pancreatectomy is an alternative parenchyma-sparing technique for this tumor entity [79]. Also, laparoscopic management of insulinoma in the body and tail of the pancreas, with distal pancreatectomy or enucleation, is feasible and safe [80]. In the case of occult insulinoma, blind distal pancreatectomy should be avoided [81]. However, explorative surgery with intraoperative ultrasound may be indicated in cases where preoperative diagnostics could not reveal any pancreatic lesions, as this is an excellent method for identifying occult insulinoma [82]. Gastrinoma is associated with gastric ulcerations due to overproduction of gastrin [145]. The clinical presentation of gastrinoma is referred to as Zollinger-Ellison syndrome. With the introduction of proton pump inhibitors, which prevent ulcer formation, surgery changed from being symptomatic to curative treatment in patients with Zollinger-Ellison syndrome. All patients with Zollinger-Ellison syndrome without multiple neuroendocrine neoplasia type 1 or metastatic disease should be offered surgical exploration for a possible cure [146]. Routine use of duodenotomy in cases of pancreatic gastrinoma increases short- and long-term cure rates due to a higher detection rate of duodenal gastrinomas, as multiple gastrinomas are relatively common [147]. The incidences of other functioning PNETs, such as vasoactive intestinal peptide-producing tumors (VIPoma), glucagonoma, and somatostatinoma, are very low. These patients should undergo tumor resection to correct the severe hormonally caused metabolic derangements.

9.17.2 Neuroendocrine Carcinoma

Neuroendocrine carcinomas (NECs) are defined as neuroendocrine tumors with a Ki-67 index above 20%, according to the WHO 2010 classification. Such tumors are highly malignant and typically invade adjacent structures or metastasize before the diagnosis is made [148]. NECs of the pancreas are very rare and account for only about 2–3% of all PNETs [149, 150]. The outcome is generally poor and most patients die within 5 years after diagnosis [151]. However, curative resections have been reported in single cases [149]. Therefore, radical surgery should be attempted in localized disease [152, 153], while surgery in metastatic disease is not recommended.

9.17.3 Locally Advanced Disease

Locally advanced disease extends beyond the limits of the pancreas directly into surrounding organs or tissue, involves regional lymph nodes, or fulfills both of these criteria. As many PNETs are nonfunctioning and slow-growing, a large proportion of these present with locally advanced disease. Resection for locally advanced PNETs is in general technically feasible and can result in favorable disease-free and overall survival in selected patients [154]. However, most patients will develop recurrence [155]. When not operated, patients with locally advanced PNETs may suffer from complications related to local mass effect and infiltrative growth, including gastrointestinal bleeding, vascular/intestinal/biliary obstruction, and occlusion of the superior mesenteric (SMV) or portal vein (PV) [156]. Hill et al. found that resection of the primary tumor in patients with PNETs is associated with improved survival across all stages of disease [157]. Based on this, surgery of locally advanced PNET without metastasis should be attempted. Interestingly, R1 resections of PNET are not associated with a worse overall survival compared to R0 resections [158].

9.17.4 Metastatic Disease

PNETs commonly metastasize to the liver. This is especially true for nonfunctioning tumors as these are generally diagnosed at a late stage. In selected patients, resection of the primary PNET in the setting of unresectable but limited hepatic metastases may be indicated [159, 160] as this may prolong survival [161, 162]. As mentioned earlier, it has been shown that resection of the primary tumor in patients with PNETs is associated with improved survival across all stages of disease. However, there is currently no clear answer to when and whether resection of the primary tumor should be performed in metastatic disease [163]. Surgical resection with curative intent or palliative debulking of more than 90% of liver metastases from nonfunctioning PNETs provides favorable oncologic outcomes, despite a high recurrence rate [164, 165]. Patients with metastatic disease in the liver may profit from liver resection with long-term palliation and possibly cure in one-third of the patients [166]. Number, size, and localization of tumor sites seem less important than performing a complete resection of metastatic tissue from PNETs [167]. Patients with hormonally active liver metastases without prior extrahepatic or synchronous disease have the greatest survival benefit from surgery. Two-stage procedures for synchronous bilobar liver metastases from NET, including portal vein embolization, enable complete resection and good long-term outcome in selected patients [168]. Debulking extends survival although recurrence is expected [169, 170]. Surgical treatment of metastatic PNET should be performed in specialized centers and managed with a multidisciplinary approach [171].

9.18 Technical Remarks

9.18.1 Resection Versus Enucleation

Standard surgical approaches to PNETs include pancreaticoduodenectomy and distal or subtotal pancreatectomy. Middle segment pancreatectomy is an alternative in the management of PNETs located in the neck or body of the pancreas [172]. A general risk of major pancreatic resections is functional impairment of the organ due to loss of parenchyma, resulting in exocrine and/or endocrine insufficiency. Thus, parenchyma-sparing surgical techniques should be attempted when possible. Enucleation is a feasible procedure for the radical treatment of benign and borderline pancreatic neoplasms [173] and is associated with long-term survival, despite a relatively high risk of pancreatic fistula formation [174, 175]. Before enucleating a PNET, it is important to consider where the tumor is located in relation to the main pancreatic duct, as enucleations of tumors located very close to this may result in damage to the pancreatic duct and subsequent pancreatic leakage. Decisions regarding enucleations are highly individual compared to standard resections, underlining the importance of treatment in experienced high-volume institutions. Tumor enucleation is associated with shorter operative time, less intraoperative blood loss, and shorter hospital stay compared to pancreaticoduodenectomy and distal pancreatectomy [173].

9.18.2 Open Versus Laparoscopic Surgery

Over the last decade, there has been a trend toward more parenchyma-sparing and minimally invasive techniques in the management of PNETs. This shift has not increased morbidity or compromised survival [176]. Laparoscopic surgery for small and solitary PNETs is feasible and safe [177, 178]. Advantages of the minimally invasive approach are less intraoperative bleeding [179], faster postoperative recovery [180], shorter hospital stay [181, 182], and improved cosmesis, compared to the open approach. Laparoscopic distal pancreatectomy (LDP) is today an established procedure at several institutions worldwide [183]. The procedure provides similar short- and long-term oncologic outcomes as open distal pancreatectomy and a selective use of it also seems to be a cost-efficient alternative to open distal pancreatectomy. LDP with preservation of the spleen is feasible with a moderate risk of postoperative splenic infarction [184]. However, the significance of spleen preservation on oncologic outcome in patients with PNET remains unclear. Besides LDP of PNET in the pancreatic body and tail, laparoscopic enucleation of nonfunctioning PNETs in the pancreatic head [185] and laparoscopic pylorus-preserving pancreatoduodenectomy are feasible procedures that can be considered in selected cases [186]. When performing laparoscopic pancreatic surgery for PNET, intraoperative laparoscopic ultrasound should always be applied, as this allows safe tumor dissection and excision. If the tumor cannot be identified precisely by laparoscopic ultrasound, conversion to open surgery should be considered [187]. Laparoscopic pancreatic surgery demands a high level of surgical skills in minimally invasive surgery and should be performed in specialized centers [188].

9.18.3 Lymph Node Sampling

From studies performed on pancreatic ductal adenocarcinoma, it is known that lymph node status is an important prognostic factor in resectable disease [189, 190]. This has also been demonstrated in studies on PNET, where lymph node ratio is a significant predictor of recurrence after curative resection for malignant PNETs [191], and lymph node metastases in PNETs are related to better survival [192]. In many surgical specimens of PNETs, lymph nodes are not evaluated by the pathologist [125]. This may result in understaging of patients with potentially inadequate resection. It is of great importance to know to what extent parenchyma-sparing and minimally invasive pancreatic surgery can provide sufficient lymph node sampling for optimal oncologic outcome. When compared to open surgery, there are studies concluding with a clear limitation of LDP as well as studies concluding with a comparable lymph node sampling after LDP. Enucleations are associated with a low lymph node sampling rate compared with standard resections. Lymph node sampling should be performed routinely when performing parenchyma-preserving or minimally invasive removal for small PNETs, to avoid understaging. Moreover, frozen section examination should be performed, and when malignancy is confirmed, oncologically appropriate lymph node dissection is recommended.

9.18.4 Vascular Reconstruction

Surgery for locally advanced PNETs with vascular involvement is controversial. Vascular reconstruction has already been established in the treatment of locally advanced pancreatic adenocarcinoma [193]. Several case reports [194, 195] suggest that a similar approach is feasible and beneficial in selected patients with PNETs. In most cases, even if the radiological evaluation suggests vascular involvement and at surgery the PNET is found to partially encase or involve the vessel, the tumor can be removed with careful dissection without requiring vascular reconstruction. Conventional contraindications to surgical resection of pancreatic malignancy, such as superior mesenteric vein invasion, should be reconsidered in patients with locally advanced PNETs [196].

9.19 Medical Management

In addition to surgery, diverse types of medical treatment are used in the management course for patients with pancreatic NETs as well as gastrointestinal NETs. The main aim of the treatment should be clearly defined before choosing treatment; there are two main aims of treatment: to ameliorate hormonal symptoms and to improve the survival. Observation without any agents might be the best management for patients with stable disease for a long time or the elderly patients.

9.19.1 Medical Treatment of Functioning Pancreatic NETs

In patients with functioning NETs, medical management can often provide release symptoms by inhibition of the secretion of bioactive agents. Administration of diazoxide [197, 198] or long-acting somatostatin analogs (octreotide, lanreotide) [199, 200] can control hypoglycemic symptoms in about 50% of patients with insulinoma. Histamine H2-receptor antagonists and proton pump inhibitors can control the acid hypersecretion in most patients with ZES [201]. For patients with other functioning pancreatic NETs, long-acting somatostatin analogs are generally successful in the initial management [202, 203].

9.19.2 Medical Treatment with Molecular-Targeted Therapy

Tumor grading is paramount for selecting patients who should receive chemotherapy, and platinum-based chemotherapy is recommended in patients with NEC G3 [204]. In some patients with NET G1/G2, molecular-targeted treatment or chemotherapy may provide a benefit. The European Society for Medical Oncology (ESMO) 2012 guidelines recommended use of molecular-targeted agents in advanced pancreatic NETs G1/G2 [205]. According to the North American Neuroendocrine Tumor Society (NANETS) guidelines, the level of recommendation is listed as "consider" to use of everolimus in metastatic functioning NETs because there has been no sufficient evidence to recommend routine use of it [206]. Everolimus, an oral inhibitor of mammalian target of rapamycin (mTOR) [207], and sunitinib, an inhibitor of VEGF and platelet-derived growth factor receptors [208], are now registered worldwide for the treatment of pancreatic NETs. These two agents have similar tumor-stabilizing effects in pancreatic NETs. Since there has been no trial that compared the two agents directly, choice of the agent in each case could be suggested in perspective of side effects. For example, in patients with poorly controlled hormonal symptoms, congestive heart failure, poorly controlled hypertension, high risk of gastrointestinal bleed, or a history of myocardial infarction or stroke, everolimus is thought to be the preferred agent of choice. In patients with poorly controlled diabetes mellitus, pulmonary disease, or high risk of infection, sunitinib would be a more appropriate choice [209]. To evaluate the response of these agents, several biomarkers have been investigated. It has been suggested that chromogranin A and neuron-specific enolase are useful as prognostic markers in patients with advanced pNET treated with everolimus [210]. Soluble vascular endothelial growth factor receptor 2 and 3, interleukin-8, and stromal cell-derived factor 1-alpha have been reported to have a potential as biomarkers associated with response to sunitinib.

References

1. Fraenkel M, Kim MK, Faggiano A, et al. Epidemiology of gastroenteropancreatic neuroendocrine tumours. Best Pract Res Clin Gastroenterol. 2012;26:691–703.
2. Lawrence B, Gustafsson BI, Chan A, et al. The epidemiology of gastroenteropancreatic neuroendocrine tumors. Endocrinol Metab Clin N Am. 2011;40:1–18.
3. Halfdanarson TR, Rubin J, Farnell MB, et al. Pancreatic endocrine neoplasms: epidemiology and prognosis of pancreatic endocrine tumors. Endocr Relat Cancer. 2008;15:409–27.
4. Yao JC, Hassan M, Phan A, et al. One hundred years after "carcinoid": epidemiology of and prognostic factors for neuroendocrine tumors in 35,825 cases in the United States. J Clin Oncol. 2008;26:3063–72.
5. Kimura W, Kuroda A, Morioka Y. Clinical pathology of endocrine tumors of the pancreas: analysis of autopsy cases. Dig Dis Sci. 1991;36:933–42.
6. Halfdanarson TR, Rabe KG, Rubin J, et al. Pancreatic neuroendocrine tumors (PNETs): incidence, prognosis and recent trend toward improved survival. Ann Oncol. 2008;19:1727–33.
7. Yao JC, Eisner MP, Leary C, et al. Population-based study of islet cell carcinoma. Ann Surg Oncol. 2007;14:3492–500.
8. Metz DC, Jensen RT. Gastrointestinal neuroendocrine tumors: pancreatic endocrine tumors. Gastroenterology. 2008;135:1469–92.
9. Rindi G, Bordi C. Highlights of the biology of endocrine tumours of the gut and pancreas. Endocr Relat Cancer. 2003;10:427–36.
10. de Wilde RF, Edil BH, Hruban RH, et al. Well differentiated pancreatic neuroendocrine tumors: from genetics to therapy. Nat Rev Gastroenterol Hepatol. 2012;9:199–208.
11. Perren A, Anlauf M, Henopp T, et al. Multiple endocrine neoplasia type 1 (MEN1): loss of one MEN1 allele in tumors and monohormonal endocrine cell clusters but not in islet hyperplasia of the pancreas. J Clin Endocrinol Metab. 2007;92:1118–28.
12. Massironi S, Sciola V, Peracchi M, et al. Neuroendocrine tumors of the gastro-entero-pancreatic system. World J Gastroenterol. 2008;14:5377–84.
13. Ehehalt F, Saeger HD, Schmidt CM, et al. Neuroendocrine tumors of the pancreas. Oncologist. 2009;14:456–67.
14. Triponez F, Dosseh D, Goudet P, et al. Epidemiology data on 108 MEN 1 patients from the GTE with isolated nonfunctioning tumors of the pancreas. Ann Surg. 2006;243:265–72.
15. Oberg K. Genetics and molecular pathology of neuroendocrine gastrointestinal and pancreatic tumors (gastroenteropancreatic neuroendocrine tumors). Curr Opin Endocrinol Diabetes Obes. 2009;16:72–8.
16. Alexakis N, Connor S, Ghaneh P, et al. Hereditary pancreatic endocrine tumours. Pancreatology. 2004;4:417–33. discussion 434-5.
17. Dean PG, van Heerden JA, Farley DR, et al. Are patients with multiple endocrine neoplasia type I prone to premature death? World J Surg. 2000;24:1437–41.
18. Pellegata NS. MENX and MEN4. Clinics (Sao Paulo). 2012;67(Suppl 1):13–8.
19. Thakker RV. Multiple endocrine neoplasia type 1 (MEN1) and type 4 (MEN4). Mol Cell Endocrinol. 2014;386:2–15.
20. Vortmeyer AO, Huang S, Lubensky I, et al. Nonislet origin of pancreatic islet cell tumors. J Clin Endocrinol Metab. 2004;89:1934–8.
21. Jiao Y, Shi C, Edil BH, et al. DAXX/ATRX, MEN1, and mTOR pathway genes are frequently altered in pancreatic neuroendocrine tumors. Science. 2011;331:1199–203.

22. Heaphy CM, de Wilde RF, Jiao Y, et al. Altered telomeres in tumors with ATRX and DAXX mutations. Science. 2011;333:425.
23. Singh R, Basturk O, Klimstra DS, et al. Lipid-rich variant of pancreatic endocrine neoplasms. Am J Surg Pathol. 2006;30:194–200.
24. Marinoni I, Kurrer AS, Vassella E, et al. Loss of DAXX and ATRX are associated with chromosome instability and reduced survival of patients with pancreatic neuroendocrine tumors. Gastroenterology. 2014;146:453–60.
25. Klimsta DS, Armold R, Capella C, et al. Neuroendocrine neoplasms of the pancreas. In: Bosman F, Carneiro F, Hruban RH, et al., editors. WHO classification of tumours of the digestive system. Lyon: IARC Press; 2010. p. 322–6.
26. Rindi G, Kloppel G, Alhman H, et al. TNM staging of foregut (neuro)endocrine tumors: a consensus proposal including a grading system. Virchows Arch. 2006;449:395–401.
27. Exocrine and endocrine pancreas. AJCC cancer staging manual. New York, NY: Springer; 2010. p. 241–9.
28. Ellison TA, Wolfgang CL, Shi C, et al. A single institution's 26-year experience with nonfunctional pancreatic neuroendocrine tumors: a validation of current staging systems and a new prognostic nomogram. Ann Surg. 2014;259:204–12.
29. Liu TC, Hamilton N, Hawkins W, et al. Comparison of WHO classifications (2004, 2010), the Hochwald grading system, and AJCC and ENETS staging systems in predicting prognosis in locoregional well-differentiated pancreatic neuroendocrine tumors. Am J Surg Pathol. 2013;37:853–9.
30. Rindi G, Falconi M, Klersy C, et al. TNM staging of neoplasms of the endocrine pancreas: results from a large international cohort study. J Natl Cancer Inst. 2012;104:764–77.
31. Sakurai A, Katai M, Yamashita K, et al. Long term follow-up of patients with multiple endocrine neoplasia type 1. Endocr J. 2007;54:295–302.
32. Davì MV, Boninsegna L, Dalle Carbonare L, et al. Presentation and outcome of pancreaticoduodenal endocrine tumors in multiple endocrine neoplasia type 1 syndrome. Neuroendocrinology. 2011;94:58–65.
33. Broder LE, Carter SK. Pancreatic islet cell carcinoma. I. Clinical features of 52 patients. Ann Intern Med. 1973;79:101–7.
34. Cubilla AL, Hajdu SI. Islet cell carcinoma of the pancreas. Arch Pathol. 1975;99:204–7.
35. La Rosa S, Klersy C, Uccella S, et al. Improved histologic and clinicopathologic criteria for prognostic evaluation of pancreatic endocrine tumors. Hum Pathol. 2009;40:30–40.
36. Schmitt AM, Anlauf M, Rousson V, WHO, et al. Criteria and CK19 are reliable prognostic markers in pancreatic endocrine tumors. Am J Surg Pathol. 2004;2007(31):1677–82.
37. Zhu L, Domenico DR, Howard JM. Metastatic pancreatic neuroendocrine carcinoma causing Cushing's syndrome. ACTH secretion by metastases 3 years after resection of nonfunctioning primary cancer. Int J Pancreatol. 1996;19:205–8.
38. Milanesi A, Yu R, Geller SA, et al. Concurrent primary hyperparathyroidism and humoral hypercalcemia of malignancy in a patient with multiple endocrine neoplasia type 1. Pancreas. 2011;40:634–7.
39. Miehle K, Tannapfel A, Lamesch P, et al. Pancreatic neuroendocrine tumor with ectopic adrenocorticotropin production upon second recurrence. J Clin Endocrinol Metab. 2004;89:3731–6.
40. Heik SCW, Klöppel G, Krone W, et al. Hypoglykämie durch Insulinom bei Diabetes mellitus. Dtsch Med Wochenschr. 1988;113:1714–7.
41. Mann JR, Rayner PH, Gourevitch A. Insulinoma in childhood. Arch Dis Child. 1969;44:435–42.
42. Lo CY, Lam KY, Kung AW, et al. Pancreatic insulinomas. A 15-year experience. Arch Surg. 1997;132:926–30.
43. Sempoux C, Guiot Y, Dahan K, et al. The focal form of persistent hyperinsulinemic hypoglycemia of infancy: morphological and molecular studies show structural and functional differences with insulinoma. Diabetes. 2003;52:784–94.
44. Reinecke-Lüthge A, Koschoreck F, Klöppel G. The molecular basis of persistent hyperinsulinemic hypoglycemia of infancy and its pathologic substrates. Virchows Arch. 2000;436:1–5.
45. Keller A, Stone AM, Valderrama E, et al. Pancreatic nesidioblastosis in adults. Report of a patient with hyperinsulinemic hypoglycemia. Am J Surg. 1983;145:412–6.

46. Anlauf M, Wieben D, Perren A, et al. Persistent hyperinsulinemic hypoglycemia in 15 adults with diffuse nesidioblastosis: diagnostic criteria, incidence and characterization of β-cell changes. Am J Surg Pathol. 2005;29:524–33.
47. Miyazaki K, Funakoshi A, Nishihara S, et al. Aberrant insulinoma in the duodenum. Gastroenterology. 1986;90:1280–5.
48. Adamson AR, Grahame-Smith DG, Bogomoletz V, et al. Malignant argentaffinoma with carcinoid syndrome and hypoglycaemia. Br Med J. 1971;3:93–4.
49. Pelletier G, Cortot A, Launay JM, et al. Serotonin-secreting and insulin-secreting ileal carcinoid tumor and the use of in vitro culture of tumoral cells. Cancer. 1984;54:319–22.
50. Shames JM, Dhurandhar NR, Blackard WG. Insulin-secreting bronchial carcinoid tumor with widespread metastases. Am J Med. 1968;44:632–7.
51. Kiang DT, Bauer GE, Kennedy BJ. Immunoassayable insulin in carcinoma of the cervix associated with hypoglycemia. Cancer. 1973;31:801–5.
52. Ashton MA. Strumal carcinoid of the ovary associated with hyperinsulinaemic hypoglycaemia and cutaneous melanosis. Histopathology. 1995;27:463–7.
53. Liu TH, Tseng HC, Zhu Y, et al. Insulinoma. An immunohistochemical and morphologic analysis of 95 cases. Cancer. 1985;56:1420–9.
54. Roth J, Klöppel G, Madsen OD, et al. Distribution patterns of proinsulin and insulin in human insulinomas: an immunohistochemical analysis in 76 tumors. Virchows Arch B Cell Pathol. 1992;63:51–61.
55. Paik WH, Ryu JK, Song BJ, et al. Clinical usefulness of plasma chromogranin a in pancreatic neuroendocrine neoplasm. J Korean Med Sci. 2013;28:750–4.
56. Vinik AI, Silva MP, Woltering EA, et al. Biochemical testing for neuroendocrine tumors. Pancreas. 2009;38:876–89.
57. Bajetta E, Ferrari L, Martinetti A, et al. Chromogranin A, neuron specific enolase, carcinoembryonic antigen, and hydroxyindole acetic acid evaluation in patients with neuroendocrine tumors. Cancer. 1999;86:858–65.
58. Oberg K. Circulating biomarkers in gastroenteropancreatic neuroendocrine tumours. Endocr Relat Cancer. 2011;18(Suppl 1):S17–25.
59. Anders S. Radiological and nuclear medicine imaging of gastroenteropancreatic neuroendocrine tumors. Best Pract Res Clin Gastroenterol. 2012;26:803–18.
60. Herwick S, Miller FH, Keppke AL. MRI of islet cell tumors of the pancreas. AJR Am J Roentgenol. 2006;187:W472–80.
61. Singhi AD, Chu LC, Tatsas AD, et al. Cystic pancreatic neuroendocrine tumors: a clinicopathologic study. Am J Surg Pathol. 2012;36:1666–73.
62. Sundin A, Vullierme MP, Kaltsas G, et al. ENETS consensus guidelines for the standards of care in neuroendocrine tumors: radiological examinations. Neuroendocrinology. 2009;90:167–83.
63. Caramella C, Dromain C, De Baere T, et al. Endocrine pancreatic tumors: which are the most useful MRI sequences? Eur Radiol. 2010;20:2618–27.
64. Oberg K. Diagnostic work-up of gastroenteropancreatic neuroendocrine tumors. Clinics (Sao Paulo). 2012;67:109–12.
65. Joseph S, Wang YZ, Boudreaux JP, et al. Neuroendocrine tumors: current recommendations for diagnosis and surgical management. Endocrinol Metab Clin N Am. 2011;40:205–31.
66. de Herder WW, Kwekkeboom DJ, Valkema R, et al. Neuroendocrine tumors and somatostatin: imaging techniques. J Endocrinol Investig. 2005;28:132–6.
67. Garin E, Le Jeune F, Devillers A, et al. Predictive value of 18F-FDG PET and somatostatin receptor scintigraphy in patients with metastatic endocrine tumors. J Nucl Med. 2009;50:858–64.
68. Binderup T, Knigge U, Loft A, et al. 18F-fluorodeoxyglucose positron emission tomography predicts survival of patients with neuroendocrine tumors. Clin Cancer Res. 2010;16: 978–85.
69. Gabriel M, Decristoforo C, Kendler D, et al. 68 Ga- DOTA-Tyr3-octreotide PET in neuroendocrine tumors: comparison with somatostatin receptor scintigraphy and CT. J Nucl Med. 2007;48:508–18.

70. Naswa N, Sharma P, Kumar A, et al. Gallium-68-DOTANOC PET/CT of patients with gastroenteropancreatic neuroendocrine tumors: a prospective single-center study. AJR Am J Roentgenol. 2011;197:1221–8.
71. Frilling A, Sotiropoulos GC, Li J, et al. Multimodal management of neuroendocrine liver metastases. HPB (Oxford) 2010;12:361-79. 69. Kim MK. Endoscopic ultrasound in gastroenteropancreatic neuroendocrine tumors. Gut Liver. 2012;6:405 10.
72. Atiq M, Bhutani MS, Bektas M, et al. EUS-FNA for pancreatic neuroendocrine tumors: a tertiary cancer center experience. Dig Dis Sci. 2012;57:791–800.
73. Lennon AM, Newman N, Makary MA, et al. EUS-guided tattooing before laparoscopic distal pancreatic resection (with video). Gastrointest Endosc. 2010;72:1089–94.
74. Fendrich V, Waldmann J, Bartsch DK, Langer P. Surgical management of pancreatic endocrine tumors. Nat Rev Clin Oncol. 2009;6(7):419–28.
75. Grant CS. Surgical management of malignant islet cell tumors. World J Surg. 1993;17(4):498–503.
76. Grama D, Eriksson B, Martensson H, et al. Clinical characteristics, treatment and survival in patients with pancreatic tumors causing hormonal syndromes. World J Surg. 1992;16(4):632–9.
77. Crippa S, Zerbi A, Boninsegna L, et al. Surgical management of insulinomas: short- and long-term outcomes after enucleations and pancreatic resections. Arch Surg. 2012;147(3):261–6.
78. Rothmund M, Angelini L, Brunt LM, et al. Surgery for benign insulinoma: an international review. World J Surg. 1990;14(3):393–9.
79. Falconi M, Zerbi A, Crippa S, et al. Parenchyma-preserving resections for small nonfunctioning pancreatic endocrine tumors. Ann Surg Oncol. 2010;17(6):1621–7.
80. Zhao YP, Zhan HX, Zhang TP, et al. Surgical management of patients with insulinomas: result of 292 cases in a single institution. J Surg Oncol. 2011;103(2):169–74.
81. Hirshberg B, Libutti SK, Alexander HR, et al. Blind distal pancreatectomy for occult insulinoma, an inadvisable procedure. J Am Coll Surg. 2002;194(6):761–4.
82. Norton JA, Shawker TH, Doppman JL, et al. Localization and surgical treatment of occult insulinomas. Ann Surg. 1990;212(5):615–20.
83. Wolfe MM, Alexander RW, McGuigan JE. Extrapancreatic, extraintestinal gastrinoma: effective treatment by surgery. N Engl J Med. 1982;306:1533–6.
84. Thompson JC, Lewis BG, Wiener I, et al. The role of surgery in the Zollinger–Ellison syndrome. Ann Surg. 1983;197:594–607.
85. Schwarting H, Osse G, Sippel M, et al. Morphometry of the pancreatic islets in patients with insulinomas and gastrinomas. In: Mutt V, Uvnäs-Moberg K, editors. Regulatory peptides. Abstracts of the 4th international symposium on gastrointestinal hormones. Amsterdam: Elsevier; 1983. p. 129.
86. Martella EM, Ferraro G, Azzoni C, et al. Pancreatic-polypeptide cell hyperplasia associated with pancreatic or duodenal gastrinomas. Hum Pathol. 1997;28:149–53.
87. Mallinson CN, Bloom SR, Warin AP, et al. A glucagonoma syndrome. Lancet. 1974;304:1–5.
88. Fujita J, Seino Y, Ishida H, et al. A functional study of a case of glucagonoma exhibiting typical glucagonoma syndrome. Cancer. 1986;57:860–5.
89. Ruttman E, Klöppel G, Bommer G, et al. Pancreatic glucagonoma with and without syndrome. Immunocytochemical study of 5 tumour cases and review of the literature. Virchows Arch A Pathol Anat. 1980;388:51–67.
90. Bordi C, Ravazzola M, Baetens D, et al. A study of glucagonomas by light and electron microscopy and immunofluorescence. Diabetes. 1979;28:925–36.
91. Hamid QA, Bishop AE, Sikri KL, et al. Immunocytochemical characterization of 10 pancreatic tumours, associated with the glucagonoma syndrome, using antibodies to separate regions of the pro-glucagon molecule and other neuroendocrine markers. Histopathology. 1986;10:119–33.
92. Trump DL, Livingston JN, Baylin SB. Watery diarrhea syndrome in an adult with ganglioneuroma-pheochromocytoma: identification of vasoactive intestinal peptide, calcitonin, and catecholamines and assessment of their biologic activity. Cancer. 1977;40:1526–32.
93. Mendelsohn G, Eggleston JC, Olson JL, et al. Vasoactive intestinal peptide and its relationship to ganglion cell differentiation in neuroblastic tumors. Lab Investig. 1979;41:144–9.

94. Capella C, Polak JM, Buffa R, et al. Morphologic patterns and diagnostic criteria of VIP-producing endocrine tumors. A histologic, histochemical, ultrastructural and biochemical study of 32 cases. Cancer. 1983;52:1860–74.
95. Udall JN Jr. Diarrhea due to hormone-secreting tumours. In: Lebenthal E, editor. Textbook of gastroenterology and nutrition in infancy. 2nd ed. New York: Raven; 1989. p. 1193–205.
96. Long RG, Bryant MG, Mitchell SJ, et al. Clinicopathological study of pancreatic and ganglioneuroblastoma tumours secreting vasoactive intestinal polypeptide (vipomas). Br Med J (Clin Res Ed). 1981;282:1767–71.
97. Verner JV, Morrison AB. Endocrine pancreatic islet disease with diarrhea. Report of a case due to diffuse hyperplasia of nonbeta islet tissue with a review of 54 additional cases. Arch Intern Med. 1974;133:492–9.
98. Tomita T, Kimmel JR, Friesen SR, et al. Pancreatic polypeptide cell hyperplasia with and without watery diarrhea syndrome. J Surg Oncol. 1980;14:11–20.
99. Ooi A, Kameya T, Tsumuraya M, et al. Pancreatic endocrine tumours associated with WDHA syndrome. An immunohistochemical and electron microscopic study. Virchows Arch A Pathol Anat. 1985;405:311–23.
100. Krejs GJ, Orci L, Conlon JM, et al. Somatostatinoma syndrome. Biochemical, morphologic and clinical features. N Engl J Med. 1979;301:285–92.
101. Vinik AI, Gonzales MR. New and emerging syndromes due to neuroendocrine tumors. Endocrinol Metab Clin North Am. 2011;40:19–63, vii.
102. Sessa F, Arcidiaco M, Valenti L, et al. Metastatic psammomatous somatostatinoma of the pancreas causing severe ketoacedotic diabetes cured by surgery. Endocr Pathol. 1997;8:327–33.
103. Heitz PU, Klöppel G, Polak JM, et al. Ectopic hormone production by endocrine tumors: localization of hormones at the cellular level by immunocytochemistry. Cancer. 1981;48:2029–37.
104. Melmed S, Yamashita S, Kovacs K, et al. Cushing's syndrome due to ectopic proopiomelanocortin gene expression by islet cell carcinoma of the pancreas. Cancer. 1987;59:772–8.
105. Wilander E, El-Salhy M, Willén T, et al. Immunocytochemistry and electron microscopy of an argentaffin endocrine tumor of the pancreas. Virchows Arch A Pathol Anat. 1981;392:263–9.
106. Sano T, Asa SL, Kovacs K. Growth hormone-releasing hormoneproducing tumors: clinical, biochemical, and morphological manifestations. Endocr Rev. 1988;9:357–73.
107. Bostwick DG, Quan R, Hoffman AR, et al. Growth-hormonereleasing factor immunoreactivity in human endocrine tumors. Am J Pathol. 1984;117:167–70.
108. Rasbach DA, Hammond JM. Pancreatic islet cell carcinoma with hypercalcemia. Primary hyperparathyroidism or humoral hypercalcemia of malignancy. Am J Med. 1985;78:337–42.
109. Broadus AE, Mangin M, Ikeda K, et al. Humoral hypercalcemia of cancer. Identification of a novel parathyroid hormone-like peptide. N Engl J Med. 1988;319:556–63.
110. Saeger W, Schulte HM, Klöppel G. Morphology of a GHRH producing pancreatic islet cell tumor causing acromegaly. Virchows Arch A Pathol Anat. 1986;409:547–54.
111. Cryer PE, Hill GJ. Pancreatic islet cell carcinoma with hypercalcemia and hypergastrinemia: response to streptozotocin. Cancer. 1976;38:2217–21.
112. Hammar S, Sale G. Multiple hormone producing islet cell carcinomas of the pancreas. A morphological and biochemical investigation. Hum Pathol. 1975;6:349–62.
113. Maton PN, Gardner JD, Jensen RT. Cushing's syndrome in patients with the Zollinger–Ellison syndrome. N Engl J Med. 1986;315:1–5.
114. Sadoff L, Gordon J, Goldman S. Amelioration of hypoglycemia in a patient with malignant insulinoma during the development of the ectopic ACTH syndrome. Diabetes. 1975;24:600–3.
115. Wynick D, Williams SJ, Bloom SR. Symptomatic secondary hormone syndromes in patients with established malignant pancreatic endocrine tumors. N Engl J Med. 1988;319:605–7.
116. Gloor F, Pletscher A, Hardmeier T. Metastasierendes Inselzelladenom des Pankreas mit 5-Hydroxytryptamin- und Insulin-Produktion. Schweiz Med Wochenschr. 1964;94:1476–80.
117. Appleyard TN, Losowsky MS. A pancreatic tumor with carcinoid syndrome and hypoglycemia. Postgrad Med J. 1970;46:159–71.
118. Ohneda A, Otsuki M, Fujiya H, et al. A malignant insulinoma transformed into a glucagonoma syndrome. Diabetes. 1979;28:962–9.

119. Simpson WF, Adams DB, Metcalf JS, et al. Nonfunctioning pancreatic neuroendocrine tumors presenting as pancreatitis: report of four cases. Pancreas. 1988;3:223–31.
120. Aabo K, Romond E, Dimitrov NV, et al. Pancreatic islet cell carcinoma associated with multiple hormone secretion and pancytopenia. Evidence of a serum factor suppressing hematopoiesis. Cancer. 1983;51:1691–6.
121. Kniffin WD Jr, Spencer SK, Memoli VA, et al. Metastatic islet cell amphicrine carcinoma of the pancreas. Association with an eosinophilic infiltration of the skin. Cancer. 1988;62:1999–204.
122. Feurle GE, Helmstaedter V, Tischbirek K, et al. A multihormonal tumor of the pancreas producing neurotensin. Dig Dis Sci. 1981;26:1125–33.
123. Eckhauser FE, Cheung PS, Vinik AI, et al. Nonfunctioning malignant neuroendocrine tumors of the pancreas. Surgery. 1986;100:978–88.
124. Perrone T, Sibley RK, Rosai J. Duodenal gangliocytic paraganglioma. An immunohistochemical and ultrastructural study and a hypothesis concerning its origin. Am J Surg Pathol. 1985;9:31–41.
125. Parekh JR, Wang SC, Bergsland EK, et al. Lymph node sampling rates and predictors of nodal metastasis in pancreatic neuroendocrine tumor resections: the ucsf experience with 149 patients. Pancreas. 2012;41(6):840–4.
126. Alumets J, Alm P, Falkmer S, et al. Immunohistochemical evidence of peptide hormones in endocrine tumors of the rectum. Cancer. 1981;48:2409–15.
127. Kanavaros P, Hoang C, Le Bodic MF, et al. Serotonin-producing pancreatic endocrine tumour. Histological, ultrastructural and immunohistochemical study of a case. Histol Histopathol. 1990;5:325–8.
128. Padberg B, Schröder S, Capella C, et al. Multiple endocrine neoplasia type 1 (MEN 1) revisited. Virchows Arch. 1995;426:541–8.
129. Samaan NA, Ouais S, Ordóñez NG, et al. Multiple endocrine syndrome type I. Clinical, laboratory findings, and management in five families. Cancer. 1989;64:741–52.
130. Duh QY, Hybarger CP, Geist R, et al. Carcinoids associated with multiple endocrine neoplasia syndromes. Am J Surg. 1987;154:142–8.
131. Anlauf M, Schlenger R, Perren A, et al. Microadenomatosis of the endocrine pancreas in patients with and without the multiple endocrine neoplasia type 1 syndrome. Am J Surg Pathol. 2006;30:560–74.
132. Friesen SR. Tumors of the endocrine pancreas. N Engl J Med. 1982;306:580–90.
133. Le Bodic MF, Heymann MF, Lecomte M, et al. Immunohistochemical study of 100 pancreatic tumors in 28 patients with multiple endocrine neoplasia, type I. Am J Surg Pathol. 1996;20:1378–84.
134. Warner TF, Block M, Hafez GR, et al. Glucagonomas. Ultrastructure and immunohistochemistry. Cancer. 1983;51:1091–6.
135. Grant CS. Insulinoma. Best Pract Res Clin Gastroenterol. 2005;19:783–98.
136. Berna MJ, Hoffmann KM, Serrano J, et al. Serum gastrin in Zollinger-Ellison syndrome: I. Prospective study of fasting serum gastrin in 309 patients from the National Institutes of Health and comparison with 2229 cases from the literature. Medicine (Baltimore). 2006;85:295–330.
137. Milan SA, Yeo CJ. Neuroendocrine tumors of the pancreas. Curr Opin Oncol. 2012;24:46–55.
138. van Beek AP, de Haas ER, van Vloten WA, et al. The glucagonoma syndrome and necrolytic migratory erythema: a clinical review. Eur J Endocrinol. 2004;151:531–7.
139. Mullans EA, Cohen PR. Iatrogenic necrolytic migratory erythema: a case report and review of nonglucagonomaassociated necrolytic migratory erythema. J Am Acad Dermatol. 1998;38:866–73.
140. Appetecchia M, Ferretti E, Carducci M, et al. Malignant glucagonoma. New options of treatment. J Exp Clin Cancer Res. 2006;25:135–9.
141. Nikou GC, Toubanakis C, Nikolaou P, et al. VIPomas: an update in diagnosis and management in a series of 11 patients. Hepato-Gastroenterology. 2005;52:1259–65.

142. Ghaferi AA, Chojnacki KA, Long WD, et al. Pancreatic VIPomas: subject review and one institutional experience. J Gastrointest Surg. 2008;12:382–93.
143. Vaidakis D, Karoubalis J, Pappa T, Piaditis G, Zografos GN. Pancreatic insulinoma: current issues and trends. Hepatobiliary Pancreat Dis Int. 2010;9(3):234–41.
144. Sa Cunha A, Rault A, Beau C, Collet D, Masson B. Laparoscopic central pancreatectomy: single institution experience of 6 patients. Surgery. 2007;142(3):405–9.
145. Ellison EC, Sparks J, Verducci JS, et al. 50-year appraisal of gastrinoma: recommendations for staging and treatment. J Am Coll Surg. 2006;202(6):897–905.
146. Norton JA, Fraker DL, Alexander HR, et al. Surgery to cure the Zollinger-Ellison syndrome. N Engl J Med. 1999;341(9):635–44.
147. Norton JA, Alexander HR, Fraker DL, et al. Does the use of routine duodenotomy (DUODX) affect rate of cure, development of liver metastases, or survival in patients with Zollinger-Ellison syndrome? Ann Surg. 2004;239(5):617–26.
148. Panzuto F, Boninsegna L, Fazio N, et al. Metastatic and locally advanced pancreatic endocrine carcinomas: analysis of factors associated with disease progression. J Clin Oncol. 2011;29(17):2372–7.
149. Kinoshita K, Minami T, Ohmori Y, Kanayama S, Yoshikawa K, Tsujimura T. Curative resection of a small cell carcinoma of the pancreas: report of a case of long survival without chemotherapy. J Gastroenterol Hepatol. 2004;19(9):1087–91.
150. Reyes CV, Wang T. Undifferentiated small cell carcinoma of the pancreas: a report of five cases. Cancer. 1981;47(10):2500–2.
151. Nilsson O, Van Cutsem E, Delle Fave G, et al. Poorly differentiated carcinomas of the foregut (gastric, duodenal and pancreatic). Neuroendocrinology. 2007;84(3):212–5.
152. Kolby L, Nilsson O, Ahlman H. Gastroduodenal endocrine tumours. Scand J Surg. 2004;93(4):317–23.
153. Akerstrom G. Management of carcinoid tumors of the stomach, duodenum, and pancreas. World J Surg. 1996;20(2):173–82.
154. Abu Hilal M, McPhail MJW, Zeidan BA, Jones CE, Johnson CD, Pearce NW. Aggressive multi-visceral pancreatic resections for locally advanced neuroendocrine tumours. Is it worth it? J Pancreas. 2009;10(3):276–9.
155. Norton JA, Kivlen M, Li M, et al. Morbidity and mortality of aggressive resection in patients with advanced neuroendocrine tumors. Arch Surg. 2003;138(8):859–66.
156. Hellman P, Andersson M, Rastad J, et al. Surgical strategy for large or malignant endocrine pancreatic tumors. World J Surg. 2000;24(11):1353–60.
157. Hill JS, McPhee JT, McDade TP, et al. Pancreatic neuroendocrine tumors. Cancer. 2009;115(4):741–51.
158. Glazer ES, Tseng JF, Al-Refaie W, et al. Long-term survival after surgical management of neuroendocrine hepatic metastases. HPB. 2010;12(6):427–33.
159. Bruzoni M, Parikh P, Celis R, et al. Management of the primary tumor in patients with metastatic pancreatic neuroendocrine tumor: a contemporary single-institution review. Am J Surg. 2009;197(3):376–81.
160. Cho CS, Labow DM, Tang L, et al. Histologic grade is correlated with outcome after resection of hepatic neuroendocrine neoplasms. Cancer. 2008;113(1):126–34.
161. Chen H, Hardacre JM, Uzar A, Cameron JL, Choti MA. Isolated liver metastases from neuroendocrine tumors: does resection prolong survival? J Am Coll Surg. 1998;187(1):88–92.
162. Que FG, Nagorney DM, Batts KP, Linz LJ, Kvols LK. Hepatic resection for metastatic neuroendocrine carcinomas. Am J Surg. 1995;169(1):36–43.
163. Capurso G, Bettini R, Rinzivillo M, Boninsegna L, Fave GD, Falconi M. Role of resection of the primary pancreatic neuroendocrine tumour only in patients with unresectable metastatic liver disease: a systematic review. Neuroendocrinology. 2011;93(4):223–9.
164. Mayo SC, De Jong MC, Pulitano C, et al. Surgical management of hepatic neuroendocrine tumor metastasis: results from an international multi-institutional analysis. Ann Surg Oncol. 2010;17(12):3129–36.

165. Cusati D, Zhang L, Harmsen WS, et al. Metastatic nonfunctioning pancreatic neuroendocrine carcinoma to liver: surgical treatment and outcomes. J Am Coll Surg. 2012;215(1):117–24.
166. Dousset B, Saint-Marc O, Pitre J, Soubrane O, Houssin D, Chapuis Y. Metastatic endocrine tumors: medical treatment, surgical resection, or liver transplantation. World J Surg. 1996;20(7):908–15.
167. Elias D, Lasser P, Ducreux M, et al. Liver resection (and associated extrahepatic resections) for metastatic welldifferentiated endocrine tumors: a 15-year single center prospective study. Surgery. 2003;133(4):375–82.
168. Kianmanesh R, Sauvanet A, Hentic O, et al. Two-step surgery for synchronous bilobar liver metastases from digestive endocrine tumors: a safe approach for radical resection. Ann Surg. 2008;247(4):659–65.
169. Sarmiento JM, Heywood G, Rubin J, Ilstrup DM, Nagorney DM, Que FG. Surgical treatment of neuroendocrine metastases to the liver: a plea for resection to increase survival. J Am Coll Surg. 2003;197(1):29–37.
170. Thompson GB, Van Heerden JA, Grant CS, Carney JA, Ilstrup DM. Islet cell carcinomas of the pancreas: a twenty-year experience. Surgery. 1988;104(6):1011–7.
171. Grazi GL, Cescon M, Pierangeli F, et al. Highly aggressive policy of hepatic resections for neuroendocrine liver metastases. Hepato-Gastroenterology. 2000;47(32):481–6.
172. Bassi C. Middle segment pancreatectomy: a useful tool in the management of pancreatic neoplasms. J Gastrointest Surg. 2007;11(4):421–4.
173. Hackert T, Hinz U, Fritz S, et al. Enucleation in pancreatic surgery: indications, technique, and outcome compared to standard pancreatic resections. Langenbeck's Arch Surg. 2011;396:1197–203.
174. Crippa S, Bassi C, Salvia R, Falconi M, Butturini G, Pederzoli P. Enucleation of pancreatic neoplasms. Br J Surg. 2007;94(10):1254–9.
175. Dedieu A, Rault A, Collet D, Masson B, Sa Cunha A. Laparoscopic enucleation of pancreatic neoplasm. Surg Endosc Other Intervent Tech. 2011;25(2):575–6.
176. DiNorcia J, Lee MK, Reavey PL, et al. One hundred thirty resections for pancreatic neuroendocrine tumor: evaluating the impact of minimally invasive and parenchyma-sparing techniques. J Gastrointest Surg. 2010;14(10):1536–46.
177. Assalia A, Gagner M. Laparoscopic pancreatic surgery for islet cell tumors of the pancreas. World J Surg. 2004;28(12):1239–47.
178. Gagner M, Pomp A, Herrera MF, et al. Early experience with laparoscopic resections of islet cell tumors. Surgery. 1996;120(6):1051–4.
179. Limongelli P, Belli A, Russo G, et al. Laparoscopic and open surgical treatment of left-sided pancreatic lesions: clinical outcomes and cost-effectiveness analysis. Surg Endosc Other Intervent Tech. 2012;26(7):1830–6.
180. Kim SC, Park KT, Hwang JW, et al. Comparative analysis of clinical outcomes for laparoscopic distal pancreatic resection and open distal pancreatic resection at a single institution. Surg Endosc Other Intervent Tech. 2008;22(10):2261–8.
181. Baker MS, Bentrem DJ, Ujiki MB, Stocker S, Talamonti MS. A prospective single institution comparison of peri-operative outcomes for laparoscopic and open distal pancreatectomy. Surgery. 2009;146(4):635–45.
182. Kooby DA, Hawkins WG, Schmidt CM, et al. Curative laparoscopic resection for pancreatic neoplasms: a critical analysis from a single institution. J Am Coll Surg. 2010;210(5):779–85.
183. Fernández-Cruz L, Cosa R, Blanco L, Levi S, Lopez-Boado MA, Navarro S. Curative laparoscopic resection for pancreatic neoplasms: a critical analysis from a single institution. J Gastrointest Surg. 2007;11(12):1607–22.
184. Butturini G, Inama M, Malleo G, et al. Perioperative and long-term results of laparoscopic spleen-preserving distal pancreatectomy with or without splenic vessels conservation: a retrospective analysis. J Surg Oncol. 2012;105(4):387–92.
185. Singh N, Lo CY, Chan WF. Laparoscopic enucleation of a nonfunctioning neuroendocrine tumor at the head of the pancreas. JSLS. 2006;10(2):259–62.

186. Kim SC, Song KB, Jung YS, et al. Short-term clinical outcomes for 100 consecutive cases of laparoscopic pylorus-preserving pancreatoduodenectomy: improvement with surgical experience. Surg Endosc. 2012;27(1):95–103.
187. Fernandez-Cruz L, Cesar-Borges G. Laparoscopic strategies for resection of insulinomas. J Gastrointest Surg. 2006;10(5):752–60.
188. Toniato A, Meduri F, Foletto M, Avogaro A, Pelizzo M. Laparoscopic treatment of benign insulinomas localized in the body and tail of the pancreas: a single-center experience. World J Surg. 2006;30(10):1916–9.
189. Murakami Y, Uemura K, Sudo T, et al. Number of metastatic lymph nodes, but not lymph node ratio, is an independent prognostic factor after resection of pancreatic carcinoma. J Am Coll Surg. 2010;211(2):196–204.
190. Pomianowska E, Westgaard A, Mathisen O, et al. Prognostic relevance of number and ratio of metastatic lymph nodes in resected pancreatic, ampullary, and distal bile duct carcinomas. Ann Surg Oncol. 2012;20(1):233–41.
191. Boninsegna L, Panzuto F, Partelli S, et al. Malignant pancreatic neuroendocrine tumour: lymph node ratio and Ki67 are predictors of recurrence after curative resections. Eur J Cancer. 2012;48(11):1608–15.
192. Tomassetti P, Campana D, Piscitelli L, et al. Endocrine pancreatic tumors: factors correlated with survival. Ann Oncol. 2005;16(11):1806–10.
193. Ouaissi M, Hubert C, Verhelst R, et al. Vascular reconstruction during pancreatoduodenectomy for ductal adenocarcinoma of the pancreas improves resectability but does not achieve cure. World J Surg. 2010;34(11):2648–61.
194. Akatsu T, Aiura K, Shimazu M, et al. Successful pancreatectomy with En-bloc resection of the celiac artery and portal vein for pancreatic endocrine carcinoma. Hepato-Gastroenterology. 2007;54(76):1269–71.
195. Sakamoto E, Hasegawa H, Ogiso S, et al. Curative resection for a pancreatic endocrine carcinoma involving the portal vein. Hepato-Gastroenterology. 2004;51(60):1849–51.
196. Norton JA, Harris EJ, Chen Y, et al. Pancreatic endocrine tumors with major vascular abutment, involvement, or encasement and indication for resection. Arch Surg. 2011;146(6):724–32.
197. Gill GV, Rauf O, MacFarlane IA. Diazoxide treatment for insulinoma: a national UK survey. Postgrad Med J. 1997;73:640–1.
198. Goode PN, Farndon JR, Anderson J, et al. Diazoxide in the management of patients with insulinoma. World J Surg. 1986;10:586–92.
199. Vezzosi D, Bennet A, Rochaix P, et al. Octreotide in insulinoma patients: efficacy on hypoglycemia, relationships with Octreoscan scintigraphy and immunostaining with anti-sst2A and anti-sst5 antibodies. Eur J Endocrinol. 2005;152:757–67.
200. Jensen RT. Peptide therapy. Recent advances in the use of somatostatin and other peptide receptor agonists and antagonists. In: Lewis JH, Dubois A, editors. Current clinical topics in gastrointestinal pharmacology. Malden: Blackwell Science, Inc.; 1997. p. 144–223.
201. Lew EA, Pisegna JR, Starr JA, et al. Intravenous pantoprazole rapidly controls gastric acid hypersecretion in patients with Zollinger-Ellison syndrome. Gastroenterology. 2000;118:696–704.
202. Plöckinger U, Wiedenmann B. Neuroendocrine tumors. Biotherapy. Best Pract Res Clin Endocrinol Metab. 2007;21:145–62.
203. Oberg K, Kvols L, Caplin M, et al. Consensus report on the use of somatostatin analogs for the management of neuroendocrine tumors of the gastroenteropancreatic system. Ann Oncol. 2004;15:966–73.
204. Costa FP, Gumz B, Pasche B. Selecting patients for cytotoxic therapies in gastroenteropancreatic neuroendocrine tumours. Best Pract Res Clin Gastroenterol. 2012;26:843–54.
205. Öberg K, Knigge U, Kwekkeboom D, et al. Neuroendocrine gastro-entero-pancreatic tumors: ESMO clinical practice guidelines for diagnosis, treatment and follow-up. Ann Oncol. 2012;23(Suppl 7):vii124–30.
206. Kunz PL, Reidy-Lagunes D, Anthony LB, et al. Consensus guidelines for the management and treatment of neuroendocrine tumors. Pancreas. 2013;42:557–77.

207. Yao JC, Shah MH, Ito T, et al. Everolimus for advanced pancreatic neuroendocrine tumors. N Engl J Med. 2011;364:514–23.
208. Raymond E, Dahan L, Raoul JL, et al. Sunitinib malate for the treatment of pancreatic neuroendocrine tumors. N Engl J Med. 2011;364:501–13.
209. Yao J, Phan AT. Optimising therapeutic options for patients with advanced pancreatic neuroendocrine tumours. Eur Oncol Haematol. 2012;8:217–23.
210. Yao JC, Pavel M, Phan AT, et al. Chromogranin a and neuron-specific enolase as prognostic markers in patients with advanced pNET treated with everolimus. J Clin Endocrinol Metab. 2011;96:3741–9.
211. Carstens PH, Cressman FK Jr. Malignant oncocytic carcinoid of the pancreas. Ultrastruct Pathol. 1989;13:69–75.

Part III

Gastrointestinal System

Esophageal Cancer

10

Di Martino Natale and Monaco Luigi

10.1 Introduction

Over recent decades, the percentage of elderly people in the world's population has progressively increased, and while representing percentages in the order of 5% in countries with high population growth, such as Brazil and China, it reaches percentages of approximately 20% in countries such as Germany, Japan, and Italy as well.

For many patients, in particular for esophageal cancer, surgery is still the main treatment. Esophagectomy is the major surgical procedure although burdened by a high incidence of morbidity and mortality.

However, the effect of age on the outcome of these patients is still controversial. In the early 1990s, Fentiman (1990) published an interesting review in the Lancet analyzing the treatment of older oncological patients showing that these patients received treatments, both medical and surgical, that were considered suboptimal. That observation, according to the author, was secondary to the fact that these patients presented a reduced long-term survival and that the procedures to which they were subjected had a high postoperative mortality and morbidity [1, 2].

Over the last decades, however, this trend has been significantly reversed, and at the root of these changes, there is evidence that not all elderly patients have the same surgical risk. The wider clinical heterogeneity of over 65-year-old subjects, in fact, even with an equal chronological age, requires that eligibility for a particular type of antineoplastic treatment should not rely solely on the registry data.

D.M. Natale (✉)
Division of General and Gastroenterologic surgery, University of Campania "Luigi Vanvitelli", Naples, Italy
e-mail: natale.dimartino@unina2.it

M. Luigi
General and Laparoscopic Surgery, Nursing Home Villa Esther Avellino, Avellino, Italy

A. Crucitti (ed.), *Surgical Management of Elderly Patients*,
https://doi.org/10.1007/978-3-319-60861-7_10

These considerations have allowed recruitment of a greater number of fit for surgery older patients demonstrating, in recent years, a morbidity and postoperative mortality comparable to those of young patients [3–5].

10.2 Epidemiology and Risk Factor

Over the last decades, esophageal tumors have shown a significant increase in incidence around the world, and the demographical increase in elderly patients, also in relation to higher life expectancies, has led to an increase of over 65-year-old patients coming to the observation suffering with cancer.

In the 1960s the incidence of esophageal adenocarcinoma (EAC) began to increase, and in the 1990s esophageal cancer was predominant in the USA, but, worldwide, the squamous cell carcinoma (SCC) is still predominant [5, 6]. These differences in incidence are to be related to different ethnic groups, different geographical areas, genetic factors, and lifestyles that all seem to play a fundamental role in the development of the EAC or SCC [7–9].

In particular, SCC is predominant in East Asia, Eastern and Southern Africa, and Southern Europe.

Tobacco is the major cause of SCC, and the risk of SCC is higher in current smokers and those who smoked >30 packs/year [10].

Other important risk factors are alcohol consumption, and it has been observed that more than 170 g of alcohol intake per week increases the risk of SCC [11].

Gastroesophageal reflux disease (GERD) is not clearly associated with SCC nor body mass index (BMI), but BMI is associated with high blood pressure, and this correlates to an increased risk of SCC [12].

EAC is predominant in Northwestern Europe and North America and shows a high incidence in the UK, France, Ireland, and the Netherlands [13].

Several risk factors participate in the development of EAC but first of all GERD. Symptoms of GERD that occur weekly increase the risk of EAC by approximately fivefold. GERD is associated to EAC through a cascade of events that lead from erosive esophagitis to Barrett's esophagus [14, 15], but not all the cohort of Barrett patients develop EAC probably because this evolution occurred in predisposed subjects [16, 17].

BMI is associated with an increased risk of EAC, and the risk increases proportionally to BMI probably because obesity increases hiatal hernia, GERD, and the incidence of Barrett's esophagus [18].

Smoking is a risk factor for the development of both Barrett's esophagus and EAC, and continuing to smoke increases the risk of EAC by about twofold [19].

All correlations between risk factors and esophageal cancer are summarized in Table 10.1.

Table 10.1 Risk factor related to squammous cell carcinoma (SCC) and adenocarcinoma of the esophagus

	SCC	ADC
Tobacco	+++	++
Alcohol	+++	---
Barrett's esophagus	---	++++
Weekly reflux	---	+++
Obesity	---	++
Achalasia	+++	---
Caustic lesions	++++	---
Plummer-vinson syndrom	++++	---
Head and neck cancer	++++	---
RT For breast cancer	+++	+++
Hot drink	+	---
Poor life condition	++	---

10.3 Symptoms

In the early stage, unfortunately esophageal cancer is poorly symptomatic, and when symptoms occur, the cancer is in an advanced stage. In any case, the typical symptom of esophageal cancer is dysphagia, and initially it is experienced when ingesting solid food but eventually progresses to include liquids. This symptom is typically localized in the neck only when the cancer is cephalic, but when the cancer occurs in the distal esophagus, the patient is not usually able to localize the site describing difficulty in a point as far cephalic as the sternal notch.

Besides dysphagia, esophageal cancer may present unexpected weight loss which represents the second most common symptom and occurs in more than 50% of patients.

Bleeding, epigastric or retrosternal pain, hoarseness caused by invasion of the laryngeal nerve, and a persistent cough represent other symptoms of esophageal cancer, and they are correlated with advanced disease. In fact, less than 25% of patients with esophageal cancer have localized disease at the time of presentation [20].

10.4 Preoperative Assessment

The management of esophageal cancer is mainly based on exhaustive preoperative assessment, and in particular in elderly patients, the accuracy of diagnosis and staging is as important as the evaluation of the performance status of the patients.

In fact, there were no significant differences in tumor location and size, histological type, and differentiation between the elderly and younger patients [21], but the differences in postoperative morbidity and mortality were related to the performance status of patients and the presence of many comorbidities [22].

The procedure for identification of elderly people at higher risk is not yet standardized. The impairment of the muscular and nervous systems resulting in impaired motor function of the lower limbs appears to be a determining factor. The events triggering disability can be varied and include a reduction in lean body mass, poor nutrition, cognitive impairment, lack of social support, immobilization, acute diseases, and aggressive treatments [4].

In geriatric oncology there is an operational definition of *frailty* given by Balducci that can be obtained when one or more of the following parameters are present: the presence of at least one geriatric syndrome and/or dependence in at least one ADL and/or >3 comorbidities and/or age > 85 years.

The evaluation of the performance status of the elderly patient (*Karnofsky score, ECOG score, EHO score, Lansky score*) must also be associated to a series of parameters such as cognition, emotional condition, geriatric syndromes, nutrition, the use of drugs, socioeconomic conditions, and finally, but no less important, the evaluation of lung, kidney, and heart function and the presence of any additional comorbidities. Still today, though, conventionally and widely used in the literature, the elderly are defined as patients over the age of 70 years, and yet there are few trials that evaluate the elderly not in relation to the anagraphical age but to the biological age that helps to classify these patients as *fragile* and *non-fragile*, the latter with a significantly higher life expectancy than those classified as *fragile* [23].

Both in elderly and younger patients, a proper diagnosis and staging is mandatory for the planning of the most suitable therapeutic strategy, and it appears to be the main key to decreased morbidity and improved long-term survival.

The endoscopy with biopsy is the gold standard for diagnosis. In particular, it is able to show localized tumors and to detect the tumor's location and the proximal and distal extents of the mass and their relationship to the cardias. In fact, according to the Siewert classification, type 1 and 2 tumors are treated as esophageal tumors and type 3 as gastric tumors.

EUS is more accurate than cross-sectional imaging techniques (CT or PET) to assess the depth of invasion (T status), but for superficial cancer (T1a or T1b), EUS can over-stage the lesion, and for T1b tumors, where endoscopic treatment should be indicated, the endoscopic mucosal resection (EMR) should be included in the staging [24]. EUS associated to fine needle biopsy is the best modality for assessing involvement of loco-regional lymph nodes [25]. EUS shows limits in the assessment of tumors with strictures that prevent passage and in the posttreatment (CRT) assessment due to fibrosis.

In the assessment of esophageal tumors, there are numerous imaging techniques, and their role is to study and to stage distant metastasis. In particular, CT scan is used to study thoracic and abdominal metastasis and associated to positron emission tomography (PET) can detect more accurately the distant metastasis, but this technique shows less sensitivity to study low-depth invasion (T1a or T1b) compared to EUS [26]. PET is also used to evaluate posttreatment reassessment and to appraise the response to neoadjuvant therapy [27].

To detect brain metastasis, MRI should be considered because PET/CT is not effective for studying tissue with high glucose uptake.

In the study of patients with esophageal cancer, diagnostic laparoscopy has a role in directing patients with subcarinal tumors to chemotherapy [28], particularly those with liver subcapsular metastases and/or peritoneal carcinomatosis [29].

For retrocarenal neoplasms, the tracheobronchoscopy allows patients to be excluded from surgery in which radical resection (R0) would be scarcely attainable and admits a significant number of patients to be directed to neoadjuvant therapy [30].

10.5 Staging

Staging is an essential prerequisite for the long-term success of the therapy and in particular of surgical therapy, and proper staging is intended to exclude patients with metastatic disease from surgery and identify subgroups for adjuvant or neoadjuvant therapy, ensuring comparability of case studies and quality controls for clinical trials.

Proper staging is the most important factor in improving long-term survival in patients with esophageal cancer because the treatment options are mainly driven by the stage of the disease. In fact, if intramucosal tumors (T1a) have a small percentage of or no lymph node invasion, this percentage increases significantly for tumors that invade the deeper layers (T1b).

From the anatomical, topographical, and endoscopic point of view, the esophagus is divided into cervical esophagus, thoracic esophagus (upper-middle-lower), and gastroesophageal junction (crossing point between squamous epithelium and glandular epithelium).

The latter, from the anatomical and topographical point of view, according to the classification of Siewert, is divided into three types [31]:

- Type 1: the center of the tumor is located at 1–5 cm above the cardias.
- Type 2: the center of the tumor is located between 1 cm above and 2 cm below the cardias.
- Type 3: the center of the tumor is localized to 2–5 cm below the cardias.

Siewert type 1 and type 2 should be classified and staged as esophageal tumors, and type 3 should be classified and staged as gastric cancers.

The esophageal wall is composed of successive layers, the mucosa, consisting in turn of epithelium, lamina propria, and muscularis mucosae; the submucosa, which is separated from the mucosa by a layer called the basal membrane; the muscularis propria; and, more externally, the adventitia.

The EAC and SCC are staged according to the AJCC (American Joint Committee on Cancer). This staging system, updated in 2010 (seventh edition), for the first time stages esophageal adenocarcinoma and squamous cell carcinoma separately [32] (Table 10.2a, b).

Neoplasms affecting mucosal layers are defined as intramucose and represent the T1a, and those invading the submucosa represent T1b. Invasion reaching the deeper layers is classified into T2 when they invade the muscularis propria and in T3 when

Table 10.2 AJCC classification of squamous cell carcinoma (a) and adenocarcinoma of the esophagus (b) according to 7th edition 2010

(a) Squamous cell carcinoma						(b) Adenocarcinoma				
Stage	T	N	M	Grade	Tumor location	Stage	T	N	M	Grade
0	Tis (HGD)	N0	M0	1	Any	0	Tis (HGD)	N0	M0	1
IA	T1	N0	M0	1	IA	T1	N0	M0	1–2	
IB	T1	N0	M0	2–3	Any	IB	T1	N0	M0	3
	T2-3	N0	M0	1	Lower		T2	N0	M0	1–2
IIA	T2-3	N0	M0	1	Upper, middle	IIA	T2	N0	M0	3
	T2-3	N0	M0	2–3	Lower	IIB	T3	N0	M0	Any
IIB	T2-3	N0	M0	2–3	Upper, middle		T1-2	N1	M0	Any
	T1-2	N1	M0	Any	Any	IIIA	T1-2	N2	M0	Any
IIIA	T1-2	N2	M0	Any	Any		T3	N1	M0	Any
	T3	N1	M0	Any	Any		T4a	N0	M0	Any
	T4a	N0	M0	Any	Any	IIIB	T3	N2	M0	Any
IIIB	T3	N2	M0	Any	Any	IIIC	T4a	N1-2	M0	Any
IIIC	T4a	N1-2	M0	Any	Any		T4b	Any	M0	Any
	T4b	Any	M0	Any	Any		Any	N3	M0	Any
	Any	N3	M0	Any	Any	IV	Any	Any	M1	Any
IV	Any	Any	M1	Any	Any					

they exceed the adventitia. As for the tumors classified as T4, i.e., malignancies that invade organs or periesophageal structures, they should be divided into T4a when they invade structures such as the pleura, pericardium, or diaphragm; despite the invasion of adjacent structures, they can still be regarded as potentially resectable and divided into T4b, i.e., neoplasms that affect structures, such as the aorta, vertebral bodies, or trachea, which therefore are not resectable.

10.6 Treatment Option

Although in the last few decades, there has been an increase in long-term survival for cancer of the esophagus, for patients treated, altogether it still stands at around 20% at 5 years, and, unfortunately, more than 50% of the patients who come to observation present with locally advanced or non-resectable tumors [33]. The aging of the population and a longer life expectancy have led to a significant increase in elderly patients being referred for treatment.

For these reasons the multimodality therapy has become the foundation for treatment of the majority of patients with cancer of the esophagus and cardias. The treatment approach depends on several factors and requires a team of specialists including gastroenterologists, pathologists, radiologists, surgeons, oncologists, radiotherapists, and also nutritionists and support staff. The right treatment strategy, therefore, must be guided by the stage of disease and the patient's condition, and as previously highlighted, the treatment options can range from endoscopic treatment for early-stage cancer, multimodal treatment for locally advanced or metastatic, up to salvage therapies for relapsing tumors or, finally, purely palliative for non-resectable tumors or for patients unfit for surgery or unfit for CT and/or RT.

10.6.1 Chemotherapy and Radiotherapy

Studies of analysis of the results of chemotherapy and radiotherapy in esophageal cancer are often characterized by difficulties in interpretation dependent on heterogeneity of the histological types in the different case studies, such as patient selection, difficulty to attribute the primitiveness (esophageal or gastric) to adenocarcinomas of the junction, different surgical techniques adopted, response criteria, different radiotherapy schedules (doses and fractionation), and different chemotherapy regimens.

Numerous studies, recent guidelines and in particular clinical trials, show that the sole use of chemotherapy or, worse still, radiation therapy alone has little or no success in the treatment of esophageal cancer compared to surgery alone [34, 35].

On the contrary, many reviews on clinical trials published over the last 20 years have shown that unlike the sequential use, the combined use of chemotherapy and radiotherapy before surgical treatment (neoadjuvant trimodality therapy) indicated that this protocol is important to understage disease and optimize surgery [36], and it also leads to the optimization of benefits of each treatment reducing the cancer burden, removing persistent microscopic disease after chemoradiation, and increasing pathologic complete resection rate with negative circumferential margins, and it has an adjuvant effect on micrometastatic disease with pathological complete response (pCR) ranging from 20 up to 40% (Table 10.3); in fact, it is the latter that is the most important prognostic factor. Obtaining a complete pathologic response is,

Table 10.3 Summary of the most important articles comparing CRT and surgery vs surgery alone

						Survival	
Authors	Treatment	Pts (N)	RT (Gy)	R0 rate (%)	pCR (%)	Median (mo)	Overall
Walsh	Cisplatin/5-FU	58	40	NS	25	16	3-Y 32%
	Surgery	55				11	3-Y 6%
Urba	Cisplatin/5-FU/Vnb	50	HFX, 45	45	24	16,9	3-Y 30%
	Surgery	40		45		17,6	3-Y 6%
Bosset	Cisplatin	143	SC, 37		26	18,6	
	Surgery	139				18,6	
Burmeister	Cisplatin/5-FU	128	35	80	16	22,2	NS
	Surgery	128		59		27,3	NS
Lee	Cisplatin/5-FU	51	HFX, 45,6	68	43	28,2	2-Y 49%
	Surgery	50		84		27	2-Y 57%
Tepper	Cisplatin/5-FU	30	50,4	NS	40	54	5-Y 39%
	Surgery	26				21,6	3-Y 16%
van Hagen	Carboplatin/Ptx	175	41,4	92	29	49	3-Y 59%
	Surgery	188		69		24	3-Y 48%

Modified from Orditura et al. [36]
5-FU Fluoruracil, *Vnb* Vinorebine, *Ptx* Paclitaxel, *SC* Short Course, *HFX* Hyperfractionated

in fact, the main goal of neoadjuvant therapy and is the prerequisite for control of the disease over time.

In the study CROSS, published in 2012, which used a scheme with carboplatin and weekly paclitaxel combined with RT 41.4Gy, survival was superior to that with surgery alone. More specifically, in patients with unresectable carcinoma (T2-3N0-1M0) of the esophagus and gastroesophageal junction (75% AC, 23% SCC), the preoperative chemoradiotherapy branch showed statistically significant benefits compared to surgery alone with a survival average (49 vs. 24 months), short- and medium-term survival (47 vs. 34% at 5 years), and surgical radical R0 resection (92 vs. 69%). The complete pathologic response was greater for patients with squamous cell carcinoma compared to that obtained in adenocarcinomas (49 vs 23% $p = 0.008$), but the histological type was not a prognostic factor for survival. Although combined chemoradiotherapy treatment was generally well tolerated (toxicity gr. 3–4 23%), it should be pointed out that the average age of the patients corresponded to 69 years (range 36–79 years), and also not having been conducted a specific sub-analysis by age group, it is therefore complex to generalize the efficacy, results, and tolerability in the elderly population [37].

Patients with good performance status with adenocarcinoma of the esophagus and gastroesophageal junction may be referred to a three-drug chemotherapy treatment, adding epirubicin or a taxane to a brace cisplatin (oxaliplatin) and fluorouracil (oral fluoropyrimidine).

The most used protocols (level of evidence 1 ++) are represented by cisplatin 75–100 mg/m^2, fluorouracil + 750–1000 mg/m^2 continuous infusion × 96 h every 28 days concomitant with radiotherapy 50–50.4 Gy (1.8 Gy/die−2 Gy/day) [36], or carboplatin AUC 2 + paclitaxel 50 mg/m^2 weekly × 5 weeks concomitant with radiotherapy 41.4 Gy (1.8 Gy/day) [37].

Finally, there are many new chemotherapeutic agents that might play a role in the control of micrometastases including paclitaxel, irinotecan, and gemcitabine that are also potent radiation sensitizers.

10.6.2 Target Therapy

At present, new medical treatment modes are being evaluated to improve long-term survival through the use of monoclonal antibodies. In particular, encouraging results have been reported from the use of antibodies to the VEGF ligand, Anti-HER2, and TK1s [38].

10.6.3 Esophagectomy

Surgery is the main option to get local control of the disease, and the esophagectomy represents the best chance for treatment in localized and locally advanced tumors [47] although it appears to be still one of the more difficult operations and still burdened by significant postoperative mortality.

Progress in pre-, intra-, and postoperative managing has significantly improved results in terms of morbidity and mortality. The improvement of anesthetic techniques, adequate preparatory and intraoperative assessment, and better postoperative pain control have certainly increased the number of patients, especially the elderly, eligible for surgical therapy. Though, in relation to younger patients, the number of fit-for-surgery elderly patients is still significantly lower, this is related to the fact that eligibility for esophagectomy must consider several parameters, in particular the presence of comorbidities that are significantly greater in elderly patients.

Although the role of surgery appears to be clear, there is still debate on what is the most appropriate surgical treatment, particularly for elderly patients, and, for esophageal resection, several approaches have been described.

The surgical procedures for esophagectomy are represented by:

- *Transhiatal esophagectomy* which requires abdominal access and a neck incision. The esophagus is mobilized and prepared, abdominally through the esophageal hiatus the medial and lower portion of the esophagus and the upper portion of the neck. An anastomosis is performed in the neck. This procedure has the disadvantage of not allowing a perfect exposition of the medial esophageal cancer and does not guarantee a complete lymph node dissection in the chest.
- *Tri-incisional esophagectomy* provides in addition to the transhiatal esophagectomy a thoracic access to adequately prepare the medial esophagus and a large thoracic lymphadenectomy.
- *Abdominothoracic esophagectomy* (*Ivor-Lewis procedures*) implies an abdominal phase to prepare the esophagus and a left thoracotomy for preparation of the thoracic esophagus to the superior segment where the anastomosis is performed. Thanks to this procedure is possible to have a good mediastinal lymphadenectomy, a good exposure of the tumor, and provides intrathoracic anastomosis. Minimally invasive esophagectomy (MIE) has recently been proposed requiring an Ivor-Lewis procedure to be performed with laparoscopic access for abdominal phase and a thoracoscopic access to the thoracic phase.

Which approach is chosen depends on tumor location and the surgeon's ability to obtain a curative R0 resection and adequate lymphadenectomy. In fact, some authors propose transhiatal esophagectomy as the treatment of choice for older patients because it ensures lower morbidity and better short-term results; others, on the contrary, prefer to extend esophagectomy with a two-field lymphadenectomy in all patients with cancer of the esophagus in order to achieve maximum cancer control and reduce the risk of local recurrence, although there is no level 1 evidence that any of these different approaches increases survival time [39].

Many studies, homogeneous in terms of patients analyzed, showed that the elderly (i.e., patients aged >70 year) have a higher morbidity and mortality than younger patients (Table 10.4) but, adjusted for comorbidities, the outcomes are similar across the group with no significant differences in morbidity and in mortality rate [5].

Another topic that was discussed and is still discussed is how much the lymphadenectomy (i.e., two- and three-field lymphadenectomy) should be extended. The CROSS trial [37] showed that patients treated with surgery alone had a better

Table 10.4 Results of Esophagectomy in the elderly and Young patients: Summary of some of the most important articles

Author	Age (years)	No. of patients	Morbidity (%)	30-day mortality rate (%)	In-hospital mortality rate (%)	Overall survival rate (%)
Ellis	>70	147	37.5	4.5	5.3	24.1
	<70	358	32.3	1.25	2.4	22.4
Alexiou	>70–86	186	34.4	–	6.4	21.2
	<70	337	24.7	–	4.7	25.1
Poon	>70	167	>39.5	7.2	18.0	26.0
	<70	570	>28.1	3.0	14.4	35.0
Joungon	>70	89	24.7	–	7.5	13.3
	<70	451	26.8	–	5.3	20.7
Thomas	>70	56	50.0	8.9	10.7	17.0
	<70	330	57.3	7.9	11.2	18.9
Naunheim	>70	38	68	–	18	13
Fang	>70	79	65.8	3.3	8.9	40.9
	<70	362	61.6	0.3	3.8	48.1
Morita	>80	16	25	0	0	9
	70–79	158	42	8	2	28
	<70	494	32	7	3	39
Moskovitz	>80	31	>32	–	6	16.8 mo
	70–79	207	>22	–	15	29.1 mo
Ruol	>70	165	49.1	1.9	1.9	35.4
	<70	599	48.6	1.9	2.7	33.6
Alibakhshi	>70	165	23.5	3		
	<70	315	22.1	2.8		

Modified from Alibakhshi et al. [57]

long-term survival when a more extensive lymph node dissection was carried out, but as evidenced by Noordmann and Van Lanshot, advantage was annulled in patients treated with neoadjuvant therapy. At present, according to the most recent guidelines, adequate lymph node dissection should include at least 18 negative nodes with a total number of lymph nodes removed >25 [40].

10.7 Treatment Decision

Proper treatment planning for cancer of the esophagus is influenced by numerous factors represented in the first instance by the stage, grading, and location of the tumor and, in the case of elderly patients, the patient's general condition and the presence of comorbidities taking a role of primary importance to the operability of the patient and postoperative outcome.

The most appropriate treatment protocol must first of all take into account the involvement of the wall which appears to be strongly associated with the presence of lymph node involvement and distant metastases in order to plan the most appropriate therapeutic approach which would guarantee the best results in terms of morbidity and survival in relation to the patient's performance status (Figs. 10.1, 10.2, and 10.3).

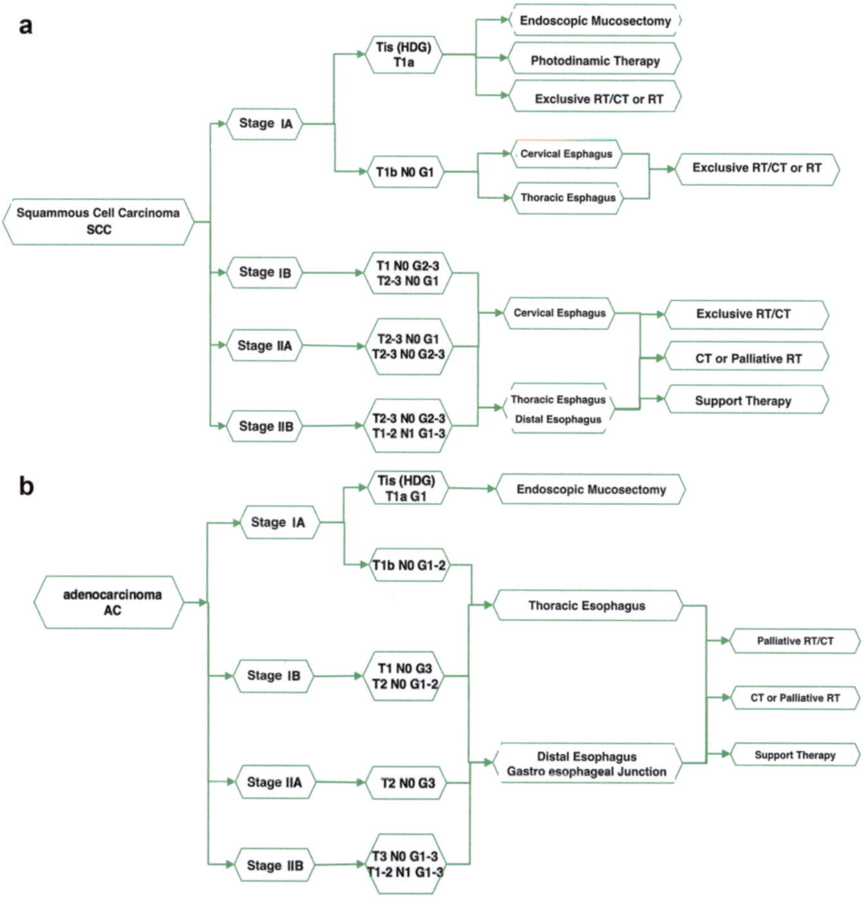

Fig. 10.1 Treatment protocol for stage IA-IIB squamous cell carcinoma (**a**) and Adenocarcinoma (**b**) tumors in Patients in poor clinical condition (ECOG>2) unfit for surgery

10.7.1 Intramucosal Tumor (Tis–T1a)

The intramucosal tumors have an extremely low nodal spread estimated at between 0 and 2%, unlike T1b tumors that can present a nodal involvement at more than 20% [40]. Given the low propensity of lymph node involvement of the intramucosal cancer, endoscopic treatment can find a potentially curative role.

Endoscopic treatment is mainly represented by the endoscopic resection that can be made either by band ligation methods, cap-and-snare methods, or with endoscopic submucosal resection (ESR). Other endoscopic techniques are represented by radiofrequency ablation (RFA), argon plasma coagulation (APC), and photodynamic therapy; nowadays, there are no reliable data on the real advantage of one technique over the other [41].

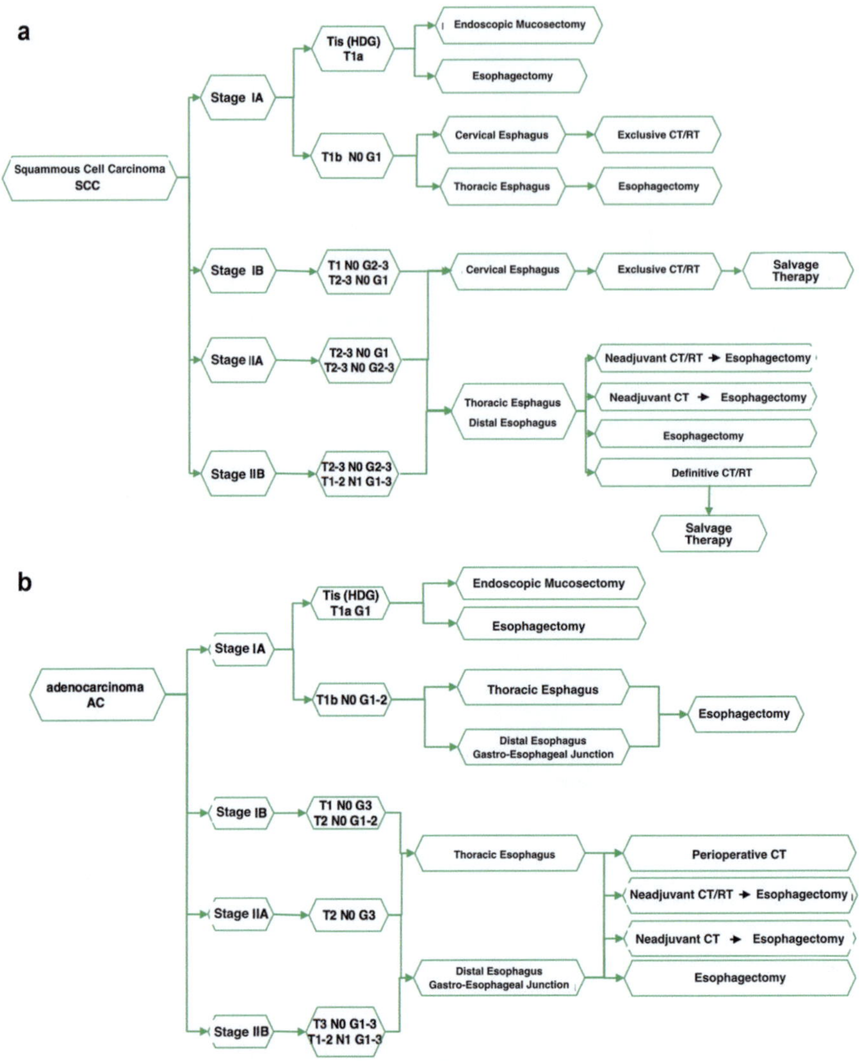

Fig. 10.2 Treatment protocol for stage IA-IIB squammous cell carcinoma (**a**) and Adenocarcinoma (**b**) resectable tumors in Patients in good clinical condition (ECOG<2) fit for surgery

According to the most recent guidelines, in relation to the low sensitivity of EUS to accurately discriminate between lesions T1a and T1b, submucosal endoscopic resection appears to offer the greatest benefits for these tumors, in particular in elderly patients, and, in addition, offers a histological sample useful in accurately assessing the margins of resection and the real depth of invasion of the esophageal wall [42]. In case of high-grade dysplasia (HDG) in Barrett's esophagus, ESD should always be followed by a complete eradication of Barrett because it is shown that patients with Barrett who developed adenocarcinoma, if not eradicated, will develop a relapse in about 30% of cases [43, 44].

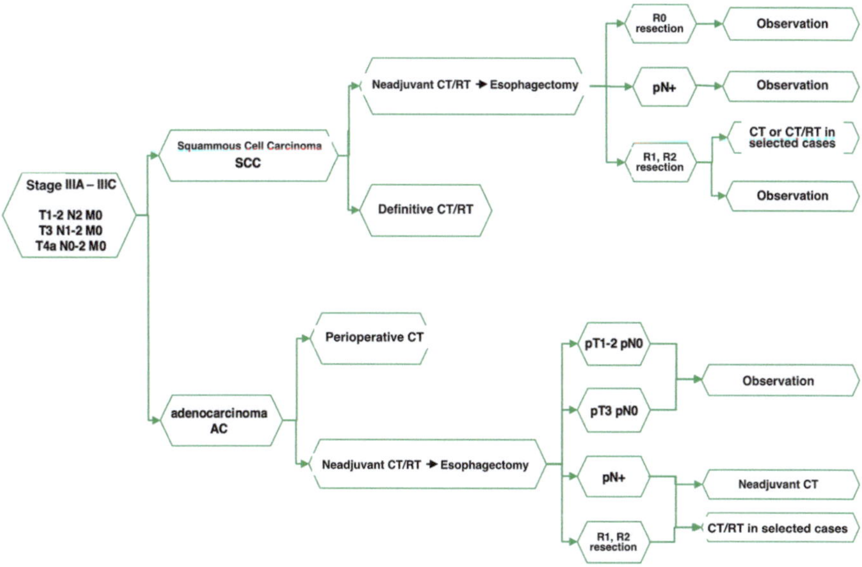

Fig. 10.3 Treatment protocol for locally Advanced disease, partially reswctable (stage IIIA-IIIC) squammous cell carcinoma and Adenocarcinoma in Patients in good clinica condition (ECOG<2) fit for CT/RT and surgery

Furthermore, according to recent guidelines, for patients fit for surgery, in good clinical condition, esophagectomy has an important role in the curative treatment of these malignancies, particularly when associated with motor abnormalities [45, 46].

10.7.2 Invasive Cancer (T1b–T2)

Invasive tumors, meaning those tumors involving the submucosa (sm T1b 1–3) and extending to the muscularis propria without exceeding it (T2) unlike intramucosal lesions, have a significantly higher percentage of lymph node involvement that can vary from 20 to 50% [40–46].

T1b lesions sm1 G1 can find a valid therapeutic option in ESD that can also be applied in combination to adjuvant therapy in fit-for-CRT patients but who are unfit for surgery [47–49]. In lesions sm 2–3, which may present even greater lymph node involvement, the esophagectomy in patients fit for surgery remains indicated [40].

The invasion of the submucosal layer by the tumor is, therefore, to be considered an indication for esophagectomy and should be addressed directly to surgery, even in patients where the EMR was found to be incomplete or not executable. We must also consider that patients with T2 tumors are upstaged in more than 60% of the cases. For these patients and for patients properly staged, surgical therapy may be considered as the definitive treatment, while understaged patients should be directed to an adjuvant therapy [50].

10.7.3 Locally Advanced Tumor (T3–T4)

Locally advanced tumors are considered tumors whose wall invasion is invasion of the adventitia (T3) and up to tumors that exceed the adventitia and are infiltrating the pleura, pericardium, or diaphragm but are still resectable (T4a) or malignancies with involvement of locoregional lymph nodes T1 with a wall involvement in T4a. These malignancies still represent the majority of cancers in patients who seek treatment, especially elderly patients who, very often, do not fall into public screening programs.

These malignancies, either squamous or adenocarcinoma tumors, still present margins for resectability and find the best treatment in esophagectomy with radical lymphadenectomy in order to get local control of the disease. Unfortunately, performed in the first instance, this is still burdened by a poor long-term survival and significant local recurrence. In addition, elderly patients are especially burdened by high perioperative morbidity and mortality [51].

Numerous studies in the literature have evaluated the disease-free survival time and long-term survival, comparing patients treated with surgery alone and patients treated with surgery preceded by neoadjuvant therapy whether CT or RT. Patients undergoing neoadjuvant treatment present a long-term survival and a rate of R0 resections significantly greater than in patients treated with surgery alone. In particular, numerous studies have shown that long-term survival is significantly increased in patients treated with CRT followed by surgery and that the complete pathologic response highlighted in the histological examination was found to be the most important positive prognostic factor [52, 53].

In SCC, in the evidence of a pCR, CRT treatment could be considered as definitive therapy in elderly subjects. As reported in a recent retrospective study conducted in China on patients with esophageal squamous cell carcinoma of age > 70 years undergoing chemoradiotherapy, an average survival of 22.3 months with toxicity gr. 3–4 only in 17% of cases was observed [34].

10.7.4 Metastatic Disease or Unresectable Cancer

In patients that cannot be treated in a curative manner with surgery or cannot undergo surgery, CRT or CT is the definitive therapy. In these patients, it was observed that the combination of chemotherapy and radiotherapy offers, compared to the standard chemotherapy, survival rates of approximately 15% at 5 years [34–54].

Endoscopic treatment in these patients takes on a purely palliative intent and may consist of expansion (with balloon or bougie) to improve dysphagia or, when possible, endoscopic resection which in addition to improving dysphagia can allow the placement of stents [55, 56].

Conclusion

Esophageal cancer is still a leading cause of cancer-related death in the world, and, in recent decades, the increase in life expectancy has led to a significant increase of elderly patients with cancer of the esophagus or cardia being referred for treatment.

Even today, however, most of the patients, especially the elderly, who are first observed, present metastatic or locally advanced malignancies, and this figure has emphasized the need for a multimodal approach to this pathology for a significant improvement of survival, although, at present, it still amounts to approximately 20% at 5 years [33].

For the therapeutic schedule, appropriate timing for the patient and a correct preoperative staging are fundamental to predict long-term survival.

Endoscopic techniques, which represent the gold standard in the diagnosis of esophageal lesions (EGD and EUS), are also useful in pure palliation particularly to improve dysphagia (balloon, bougie, stent). With therapeutic intent, however, endoscopic methods are indicated, represented mainly by endoscopic mucosectomy, in intramucose or in HGD lesions of Barrett with good results in terms of survival and excellent results on quality of life.

Surgery is still the treatment of choice for patients with cancer of the esophagus or esophagogastric junction and, despite being one of the most challenging in cancer surgery, when performed by experienced surgeons and centers with large volumes, with proper indication and in selected patients, offers definite advantages in the local control of the disease and quality of life of patients with an acceptable morbidity and mortality.

In addition, with the improvement of anesthetic techniques and postoperative pain control and, especially, the introduction into clinical practice of assessing the "fragility" of the elderly patient, it has allowed the enlistment, even in aggressive treatment protocols, of a growing number of elderly patients with results in terms of morbidity (especially pulmonary complications) and mortality, similar to those of younger patients [5–57].

In the literature, there is no evidence of benefits in terms of long-term survival of any particular surgical technique compared one with the other, but certainly in the last few years, a minimally invasive approach, in particular, the Ivor-Lewis, can offer advantages in terms of recovery and postoperative morbidity while respecting the fundamental surgical radicality parameter in improving the long-term survival of these patients.

Certainly, an R0 resection and lymphadenectomy with removal of at least 18 negative nodes would seem to offer better survival than in patients with fewer blocks of lymph nodes [58].

Neoadjuvant chemotherapy is the main cornerstone in improving the outcome of patients with SCC and AEC, locally advanced and especially in metastatic cancer or in patients unfit for surgery. In the latter, it is the definitive therapy allowing, in the case of disease recurrence, the possibility to make a salvage esophagectomy however, this is also burdened by a significantly greater morbidity and mortality than elective surgery.

Latest chemoradiotherapeutic protocols represented by the combination of cisplatin or its derivatives in combination with fluorouracil represent the reference regimen for both histologies, squamous and adenocarcinoma. Their use in neoadjuvant treatments has certainly resulted in improved survival rate not only helping to understage disease and optimize surgery but, above all, increasing the rate of complete pathological response that, at present, is the most important prognostic factor in increasing disease-free survival and the overall survival rate [59, 60].

Finally, the study of monoclonal antibodies might allow the planning of a tailored therapy, in patients with genetically mutated receptors, and represent, as it does now for colorectal and lung cancers, the future therapeutic strategy for locally advanced esophageal cancer.

References

1. Fentiman IS, Tirelli U, Monfardini S, Schneider M, Festen J, Cognetti F, Aapro MS. Cancer in the elderly: why so badly treated? Lancet. 1990;335(8696):1020–2.
2. O'Connel JB, Maggard MA, Ko CY. Cancer-direct surgery for localized disease: decreased use in the elderly? Ann Surg Oncol. 2004 Nov;11(11):962–9.
3. Internullo E, Moons J, Nafteux P, Coosemans W, Decker G, De Leyn P, et al. Outcome after esophagectomy for cancer of the esophagus and GEJ in patients aged over 75 years. Eur J Cardiothorac Surg. 2008;33:1096–104.
4. Walter LC, et al. Cancer screening in elderly patients a framework for individualized decision making. JAMA. 2001;285:2750–6.
5. Ruol A, Portale G, Zaninotto G, Cagol M, Cavallin F, Castoro C, et al. Results of esophagectomy for esophageal cancer in elderly patients: age has little influence on outcome and survival. J Thorac Cardiovasc Surg. 2007;133:1186–92.
6. Simard EP, Ward EM, Siegel R, Jemal A. Cancers with increasing incidence trends in the United States: 1999 through 2008. CA Cancer J Clin. 2012;62:118–28.
7. Bosetti C, Levi F, Ferlay J, et al. Trends in oesophageal cancer incidence and mortality in Europe. Int J Cancer. 2008;122:1118–29.
8. Falk GW. Risk factors for esophageal cancer development. Surg Oncol Clin N Am. 2009;18:469–85.
9. Pickens A, Orringer MB. Geographical distribution and racial disparity in esophageal cancer. Ann Thorac Surg. 2003;76:S1367–9.
10. Pandeya N, Olsen CM, Whiteman DC. Sex differences in the proportion of esophageal squamous cell carcinoma cases attributable to tobacco smoking and alcohol consumption. Cancer Epidemiol. 2013;37:579–84.
11. Pandeya N, Williams G, Green AC, Webb PM, Whiteman DC, Australian CS. Alcohol consumption and the risks of adenocarcinoma and squamous cell carcinoma of the esoph- agus. Gastroenterology. 2009;136:1215–24. e1211ee1212
12. Lindkvist B, Johansen D, Stocks T, et al. Metabolic risk factors for esophageal squamous cell carcinoma and adenocarcinoma: a prospective study of 580,000 subjects within the me-can project. BMC Cancer. 2014;14:103.
13. Bosetti C, Levi F, Ferlay J, et al. Trends in oesophageal cancer incidence and mortality in Europe. Int J Cancer. 2008;122:1118–29.
14. Monaco L, Brillantino A, Torelli F, Schettino M, Izzo G, Cosenza A, Di Martino N. Prevalence of bile reflux in gastroesophageal reflux disease patients not responsive to proton pump inhibitors. World J Gastroenterol. 2009;15(3):334–8.
15. Nason KS, Wichienkuer PP, Awais O, et al. Gastro- esophageal reflux disease symptom severity, proton pump inhibitor use, and esophageal carcinogenesis. Arch Surg. 2011;146: 851–8.
16. Corley DA, Kubo A, Zhao W. Abdominal obesity and the risk of esophageal and gastric cardia carcinomas. Cancer Epidemiol Biomark Prev. 2008;17:352–8.
17. Brillantino A, Monaco L, Schettino M, Torelli F, Izzo G, Cosenza A, Marano L, Di Martino N. Prevalence of pathological duodenogastric reflux and the relationship between duodenogastric and duodenogastrooesophageal reflux in chronic gastrooesophageal reflux disease. Eur J Gastroenterol Hepatol. 2008;20(12):1136–43.
18. Hoyo C, Cook MB, Kamangar F, et al. Body mass index in relation to oesophageal and oesophagogastric junction adenocarcinomas: a pooled analysis from the international BEACON consortium. Int J Epidemiol. 2012;41:1706–18.

19. Cook MB, Kamangar F, Whiteman DC, et al. Cigarette smoking and adenocarcinomas of the esophagus and esophagogastric junction: a pooled analysis from the international BEACON consortium. J Natl Cancer Inst. 2010;102:1344–53.
20. Ma J-Y, Wu Z, Wang Y, Zhao Y-F, Liu L-X, Kou Y-L, Zhou Q-H. Clinicopathologic characteristics of esophagectomy for esophageal carcinoma in elderly patients. World J Gastroenterol. 2006;12(8):1296–9.
21. Monson K, et al. Surgery in the aged population. Arch Surg. 2003;138(10):1061–7.
22. Feder G, Cryer C, Donovan S, Carter Y. Guidelines for the prevention of falls in people over 65. The Guidelines' development group. BMJ. 2000;321:1007–11.
23. Robinson TN, et al. Simple frailty score predicts post-operative complications across surgicall specialties. Am J Surg. 2013;206(4):544–50.
24. Young PE, Gentry AB, Acosta RD, et al. Endoscopic ultrasound does not accurately stage early adenocarcinoma or high-grade dysplasia of the esophagus. Clin Gastroenterol Hepatol. 2010;8:1037–41.
25. Smith BR, Chang KJ, Lee JG, et al. Staging accuracy of endoscopic ultrasound based on pathologic analysis after minimally invasive esophagectomy. Am Surg. 2010;76:1228–31.
26. Rebollo Aguirre AC, Ramos-Font C, Villegas Portero R, et al. 18F- fluorodeoxiglucose positron emission tomography for the evaluation of neoadjuvant therapy response in esophageal cancer: systematic review of the literature. Ann Surg. 2009;250:247–54.
27. Sjoquist KM, Burmeister BH, Smithers BM, et al. Survival after neoadjuvant chemotherapy or chemoradiotherapy for resectable oesophageal carcinoma: an updated meta- analysis. Lancet Oncol. 2011;12:681–92.
28. Bonavina L, Bona D, Binyom P, Peracchia A. A laparoscopy-assisted surgical approach to esophageal carcinoma. J Surg Res. 2004;117:52–7.
29. Luketich JD, Meehan M, Nguyen NT, et al. Minimally invasive surgical staging for esophageal cancer. Surg Endosc. 2000;4:700.
30. Baisi A, Bonavina L, Peracchia A. Bronchoscopic staging of squamous cell carcinoma of the upper thoracic esophagus. Arch Surg. 1999;132:140–3.
31. Siewert JR, Stein HJ. Classification of adenocarcinoma of the oesophagogastric junction. Br J Surg. 1998;85:1457–9.
32. Edge SB, American Joint Committee on Cancer, Amer- ican Cancer Society. AJCC cancer staging handbook from the AJCC cancer staging manual. New York: Springer; 2010.
33. Siegel RL, Miller KD, Jemal A. Cancer statistics, 2015. CA Cancer J Clin. 2015;65(1):5–29.
34. Al-Sarraf M, Martz K, Herskovic A, et al. Progress report of combined chemoradiotherapy versus radiotherapy alone in patients with esophageal cancer: an intergroup study. J Clin Oncol. 1997;15:277–2.
35. Philip PA, Ajani JA. Has combined modality therapy improved the outlook in carcinoma of the esophagus? Oncology. 1994;8:37–42.
36. Orditura M, Galizia G, Fabozzi A, Lieto E, Gambardella V, Morgillo F, Del Genio GM, Fei L, Di Martino N, Renda A, Ciardiello F, De Vita F. Preoperative treatment of locally advanced esophageal carcinoma (review). Int J Oncol. 2013;43(6):1745–53.
37. Van Hagen P, Hulshof MC, van Lanschot JJ, et al. Preoperative chemoradiotherapy for esophageal or junctional cancer. N Engl J Med. 2012;366:2074–84.
38. Ajani JA. Current status of new drugs and multidisciplinary approaches in patients with carcinoma of the esophagus. Chest. 1998;113(Suppl):S112–9.
39. Cools-Lartigue J, Spicer J, Ferri LE. Current status of management of malignant disease: current management of esophageal cancer. J Gastrointest Surg. 2015;19:964–72.
40. Leers JM, DeMeester SR, Oezcelik A, et al. The prevalence of lymph node metastases in patients with T1 esophageal adenocarcinoma a retrospective review of esophagectomy specimens. Ann Surg. 2011;253:271–8.
41. Semlitsch T, Jeitler K, Schoe R, et al. A systematic review of the evidence for radiofrequency ablation for Barrett's esophagus. Surg Endosc. 2010;24:2935–43.
42. Chennat J, Waxman I. Endoscopic treatment of Barrett's esophagus: from metaplasia to intramucosal carcinoma. World J Gastroenterol. 2010;16:3780–5.

43. Ell C, May A, Gossner L, et al. Endoscopic mucosal resection of early cancer and high-grade dysplasia in Barrett's esophagus. Gastroenterology. 2000;118:670–7.
44. May A, Gossner L, Pech O, et al. Local endoscopic therapy for intraepithelial high-grade neoplasia and early adenocarcinoma in Barrett's oesophagus: acute-phase and intermediate results of a new treatment approach. Eur J Gastroenterol Hepatol. 2002;14:1085–91.
45. Pech O, Bollschweiler E, Manner H, et al. Comparison between endoscopic and surgical resection of mucosal esophageal adenocarcinoma in Barrett's esophagus at two high-volume centers. Ann Surg. 2011;254:67–72.
46. Sepesi B, Watson TJ, Zhou D, et al. Are endoscopic therapies appropriate for superficial submucosal esophageal adenocarcinoma? An analysis of esophagectomy specimens. J Am Coll Surg. 2010;210:418–27.
47. Manner H, May A, Pech O, et al. Early Barrett's carcinoma with "low-risk" submucosal invasion: long-term results of endoscopic resection with a curative intent. Am J Gastroenterol. 2008;103:2589–97.
48. Peters FP, Brakenhoff KP, Curvers WL, et al. Histologic evaluation of resection specimens obtained at 293 endoscopic resections in Barrett's esophagus. Gastrointest Endosc. 2008;67:604–9.
49. Manner H, Pech O, Heldmann Y, et al. Efficacy, safety, and long-term results of endoscopic treatment for early stage adenocarcinoma of the esophagus with low-risk sm1 invasion. Clin Gastroenterol Hepatol. 2013;11:630–5. quiz e45
50. Rice TW, Mason DP, Murthy SC, et al. T2N0M0 esophageal cancer. J Thorac Cardiovasc Surg. 2007;133:317–24.
51. Ronellenfitsch U, Schwarzbach M, Hofheinz R, et al. Preoperative chemo(radio)therapy versus primary surgery for gastroesophageal adenocarcinoma: systematic review with meta-analysis combining individual patient and aggregate data. Eur J Cancer. 2013;49:3149–58.
52. Markar SR, Karthikesalingam A, Penna M, et al. Assessment of short-term clinical outcomes following salvage esophagectomy for the treatment of esophageal malignancy: systematic review and pooled analysis. Ann Surg Oncol. 2014;21:922–31.
53. Teoh AY, Yan Chiu PW, Wong TC, et al. Functional performance and quality of life in patients with squamous esophageal carcinoma receiving surgery or chemoradiation: results from a randomized trial. Ann Surg. 2011;253:1–5.
54. Herskovic A, Martz K, Al-Sarraf M, et al. Combined chemotherapy and radiotherapy compared with radio- therapy alone in patients with cancer of the esophagus. N Engl J Med. 1992;326:1593–8.
55. Manner H, May A, Rabenstein T, et al. Prospective evaluation of a new high-power argon plasma coagulation system (hp-APC) in therapeutic gastrointestinal endoscopy. Scand J Gastroenterol. 2007;42:397–405.
56. Abdel-Wahab M, Gad-Elhak N, Denewer A, et al. Endoscopic laser treatment of progressive dysphagia in patients with advanced esophageal carcinoma. Hepatogastroenterology. 1998;45:1509–15.
57. Alibakhshi A, Aminian A, Mirsharifi R, Jahangiri Y, Dashti H, Karimian F. The effect of age on the outcome of esophageal cancer surgery. Ann Thorac Med. 2009;4(2):71–4.
58. Greenstein AJ, Litle VR, Swanson SJ, et al. Effect of the number of lymph nodes sampled on postoperative survival of lymph node-negative esophageal cancer. Cancer. 2008;112(6):1239–46.
59. Orditura M, Galizia G, Morgillo F, Martinelli E, Lieto E, Vitiello F, Di Martino N, Pacelli R, Renda A, Ciardiello F, De Vita F. Complete response to preoperative chemoradiation and survival in esophageal cancer: a pooled analysis of three single-institution phase II trials. Dis Esophagus. 2012;25(2):130–6.
60. Orditura M, Galizia G, Di Martino N, Ancona E, Castoro C, Pacelli R, Morgillo F, Rossetti S, Gambardella V, Farella A, Laterza MM, Ruol A, Fabozzi A, Napolitano V, Iovino F, Lieto E, Fei L, Conzo G, Ciardiello F, De Vita F. Effect of preoperative chemoradiotherapy on outcome of patients with locally advanced esophagogastric junction adenocarcinoma-a pilot study. Curr Oncol. 2014;21(3):125–33.

Cancer of the Stomach

11

Roberto Vergari, Vanessa Polenta, and Cristina Marmorale

11.1 Epidemiology

In recent decades, socioeconomic habits and new medical knowledge have improved average life expectancy and quality of life as well. As a direct consequence, the geriatric population is progressively expanding, as is the risk of developing cancer.

Gastric tumour represents the fourth most common malignancy worldwide, after cancers of the lung, breast and colorectum.

The worldwide incidence of gastric neoplasm has declined rapidly over the last few decades [1]. Part of the decline may be due to the recognition of certain risk factors such as *Helicobacter pylori* and other dietary and environmental risks. Refrigerators have improved the storage of food, thereby reducing salt-based preservation of food and preventing bacterial and fungal contamination.

Despite the decrease in the global incidence of this disease, in endemic areas, such as Japan and Latin American countries, gastric cancer is still a major cause of mortality.

According to the Italian Network of Cancer Registries [2], gastric cancer is currently in sixth place in order of incidence among both men and women (4% of all cancers in males and 4% in females), and in 2016 new cases are expected to be nearly 13,000. This distribution is almost entirely attributable to the incidence in older age (over 70 years). Gastric tumour is considered a disease of the old age with a peak of incidence in the seventh decade of life. Although there is not a standard

R. Vergari • V. Polenta
Clinica Chirurgica—Ospedali Riuniti di Ancona, Ancona, Italy

C. Marmorale (✉)
Formazione in Chirurgia Generale—Ospedali Riuniti di Ancona, Ancona, Italy

Direttrice della Scuola di Specialità in Chirurgia Generale—Università Politecnica delle Marche, Ancona, Italy
e-mail: c.marmorale@univpm.it

A. Crucitti (ed.), *Surgical Management of Elderly Patients*,
https://doi.org/10.1007/978-3-319-60861-7_11

definition of "elderly", the most scientific papers fix the age of 70 as the threshold. The average human life expectancy is increasing worldwide and with it also the proportion of elderly people. This is predicted to continue to increase in the coming decades [3]. As a consequence, also the incidence of gastric carcinoma in elderly patients is becoming more frequent. In Italy, the 5 years overall survival is 32.4%, higher than the European average (25.1%). The overall survival in elderly patients is lower than in non-elderly ones: 22.1 versus 41.0% [2].

11.2 Risk Factors

The entire process of gastric carcinogenesis involves several factors, such as, gender, age, diet, tobacco and alcohol consumption, *H. pylori* infections, chronic gastritis, pernicious anaemia, some type of stomach polyps and previous gastric surgery.

Stomach cancer is more common in men than in women, and, as already discussed, there is a sharp increase in people over the age of 70. An increased risk of stomach cancer is seen in people with diets that have large amounts of smoked foods, salted fish and meat and pickled vegetables. Nitrates and nitrites are substances commonly found in cured meats; they can be converted into compounds that have been shown to cause stomach cancer in lab animals. A reduced consumption of fresh fruit and vegetables is another dietary behaviour implicated in gastric carcinogenesis. The rate of stomach cancer is about doubled in smokers and is related to the duration and intensity of smoking. Smoking increases stomach cancer risk, particularly for cancers of the upper portion of the stomach, near the oesophagus [4]. On the other hand, several studies suggest that alcohol consumption increases the risk of cancer in the lower stomach.

It is demonstrated that *H. pylori* infection is frequent in areas of high gastric cancer incidence. Infection with *H. pylori* bacteria seems to be a major cause of stomach cancer, especially cancers located in the distal part of the stomach. On the contrary, this infection seems not to be related with tumours of the gastroesophageal junction. Chronic gastritis associated with pernicious anaemia is related with gastric malignancy. Chronic gastritis is often associated with intestinal metaplasia and mucosal dysplasia which are frequently observed in the mucosa adjacent to gastric cancer. Pernicious anaemia is a disease characterized by fundic mucosal atrophy, loss of parietal and chief cells, hypochlorhydria and hypergastrinemia, and it is present in 3% of people over 60 years. Polyps are growths on the lining of the stomach, and most types, such as hyperplastic polyps or inflammatory polyps, do not seem to increase the risk of gastric cancer. Endoscopic removal is a sufficient treatment; subsequent surveillance is also not necessary. In contrast, adenomatous polyps, also called adenomas, can sometimes develop into cancer; in fact dysplasia and carcinoma in situ develop inside these growths. The carcinogenesis risk has been estimated at 10–20%, and it is higher for polyps of more than 2 cm in diameter.

Gastric cancer is more likely to develop in people who have undergone previous partial gastrectomy, for example, due to a gastric ulcer. This condition is called "remnant gastric cancer". The effective mechanism is unknown, but the potential factors seem to be the decrease of luminal pH, bacterial overgrowth with increased productions of N-nitroso carcinogens and reflux of bile acids into the stomach.

Another known risk factor is obesity, probably because of the high incidence of chronic gastroesophageal reflux disease found in obese subjects.

11.3 Clinicopathological Features

The clinicopathological features of gastric cancer in elderly patients are different from those of non-elderly patients [5].

11.3.1 Gender

Many studies have shown a male predominance in elderly patients with gastric cancer, both in endemic and nonendemic areas [6]. The meaning of this is not clear, but the prolonged exposure of the elderly male population to environmental carcinogens may play a significant role. In young patients, most authors suggest a female predominance, maybe because of the influence that oestrogens have on this pathology [7].

11.3.2 Location

Gastric cancer can develop both in the proximal and the distal regions. These represent two distinct entities from an epidemiological, biological, genetical and clinical point of view. Proximal tumours are more common in younger people and include tumours of the cardia and gastroesophageal junction, which currently represent about 40% of all gastric tumours. Epidemiological and morphological data shows that the majority of adenocarcinomas of the gastroesophageal junction have characteristics more similar to tumours of the oesophagus than those of the stomach. On the other hand, the majority of studies have documented; the predominance of lower or distal third gastric cancer in the elderly has been significantly more frequent than that observed in younger patients [8].

11.3.3 Macroscopic Features

Gastric cancer can be divided into two main entities: early and advanced gastric cancer. Early gastric cancer is defined as a tumour whose growth is confined to the mucosa and the submucosa regardless of the presence or absence of metastatic disease in the perigastric lymph nodes. The presence of lymph node metastasis is closely related to the depth of local invasion. With the submucosal invasion, lymph nodes are involved in 15–20% of cases, whereas when lesions are confined to the mucosa, lymph node involvement is uncommon (≤3%) [9]. A tumour having passed through the submucosa is defined as advanced. Macroscopic appearance, of both early and advanced stages, of gastric cancer seems to be influenced by age. According to the Japanese endoscopic classification of early gastric cancer, the most common macroscopic type in elderly people is the superficial depressed (IIc), followed by type IIa (superficial elevated) and polypoid type (I). Following Borrmann's classification of advanced gastric cancer (type I for polypoid growth, type II for fungating growth, type III for ulcerating growth and type IV for diffusely infiltrating growth which is also referred to as linitis plastica), the most prevalent type in elderly patients is the type III.

Many studies show a significant difference regarding mean tumour size, which tends to be larger in elderly patients than in younger patients [8].

11.3.4 Histological Features

Gastric cancer occurs in two distinct histological subtypes, intestinal and diffuse, as described in Lauren's classification. In the intestinal form, the malignant cells tend to form glands, and it is often associated with chronic atrophic gastritis, intestinal metaplasia and dysplasia. This subtype is more common in populations at high risk, and it occurs with increased frequency in men and older patients. For the other type, the diffuse form, the gland-forming growth is not proven, and it is prevalent in younger patients, in women and in populations with a relatively low incidence of gastric cancer. According to the criteria described by Ming and Esaky, the well-differentiated form of gastric adenocarcinoma is the predominant type in elderly patients. On the other hand, in younger patients the most common pattern is a poorly differentiated tumour. Many studies have suggested in elderly people a progression from a differentiated tumour to an undifferentiated neoplasia, whereas, in younger patients, gastric cancer manifests as an undifferentiated tumour at the initial stage [10].

11.3.5 Clinical Presentation

Symptoms in gastric cancer are unfortunately not specific, and they can usually closely mimic those associated with a number of non-neoplastic gastroduodenal diseases, especially benign gastric ulcer. One of the most common symptoms in the early stage of gastric cancer is epigastric pain, which is present in over 70% of patients and consists of a constant, nonradiating pain which is unrelieved by food ingestion. Symptoms as anorexia, nausea and weight loss are characteristic of the advanced stage. Dysphagia is present in 20% of patients with proximal gastric lesions. Gastrointestinal haemorrhage is present in only 5% and perforation is rare (1%). Cachexia, abdominal mass, hepatomegaly and supraclavicular adenopathy usually indicate metastatic disease. In elderly patients, the onset of symptoms is commonly related to an advanced stage of the disease. A study has shown that gastric cancer incidence in individuals without alarm symptoms is very low [11].

11.3.6 Family History

Familial gastric cancer is generated by a germline mutation of CDH1 gene which encodes the adhesion molecule E-cadherin, inherited by the autosomal dominant mode; it is generally associated to a poorly differentiated, infiltrative and diffuse histotype adenocarcinoma and is more common in younger patients.

11.3.7 Comorbidities

As shown by several studies, elderly patients have significantly more preoperative comorbidities such as cardiovascular disease, including hypertension, atrial fibrillation, ischemic heart disease, heart failure and valvular heart pathology than their younger counterparts [12]. Elderly people are characterized by a loss of renal cortical mass that reflects on a decline of renal function, the homeostatic reserve and electrolyte disorders [13, 14]. Serum creatinine may remain stable masking the underlying progressive loss of renal function. Regarding ageing modifications of pulmonary function, it is demonstrated that forced expiratory volume 1 and vital capacity, blood O_2 level and lung elastic recoil are decreased. Older patients tend to have a poorer preoperative nutritional status shown by low levels of albumin in blood. Preoperative albumin levels have been shown to predict postoperative outcomes [15], and preoperative nutritional support with intravenous hyperalimentation is essential in these patients.

11.3.8 Synchronous Carcinomas

With regard to the incidence of multiple synchronous gastric carcinomas, many studies suggest that they are more prevalent among elderly patients and their incidence increases with advancing age [5]. Endoscopically these tumours are predominantly located in the lower third of the stomach; they are elevated, well-differentiated histological type, and they present the tendency to collide, forming single giant lesions.

11.3.9 Patterns of Metastasis and Staging

Regarding the pattern of metastasis, many studies demonstrate that glandular/well-differentiated/intestinal gastric cancer, which is the predominant histological type in old patients, is usually associated with haematogenous metastasis predominantly involving the liver via the tumour spreading through the portal vein. The peritoneal invasion occurs less frequently. Regarding the incidence of lymph node metastasis, observations are controversial, but it seems to be less frequent in the elderly as compared to younger patients, and this is confirmed by the examination of autopsy cases of fatal gastric cancer.

11.4 Diagnoses

Cancer of the stomach is difficult to diagnose before it has spread. There are no specific symptoms in the early stages, and often in elderly patients they result less clear. If stomach cancer is suspected by symptoms, tests will be needed to confirm the diagnosis. Clinical stage is determined through physical examination, blood chemistry, faecal occult blood test (FOBT), gastroscopy and ultrasonography, biopsy and imaging tests. Gastroscopy is the most definitive diagnostic method when gastric neoplasm is suspected. In the initial stages, gastric cancers can appear polypoid, flat, plaque-like lesions or as shallow ulcers. Generally advanced lesions are typically ulcerated. Although gastroscopy is important to identify a lesion, differentiation of benign from malignant gastric ulcers can only be made definitively by biopsy. When the definitive histologic diagnosis is reached, it is important to evaluate the extent of the disease in order to plan the optimal therapeutic choice of treatment.

The aim of the preoperative staging of gastric cancer is to evaluate the depth of tumour infiltration (T-stage), the extent or number of lymph nodes involved (N-stage) and distant metastasis (M-stage) before surgery. Traditional methods of preoperative staging for gastric cancer are usually imaging diagnostic techniques, such as computed tomography (CT), endoscopic ultrasonography (EUS), positron emission tomography (PET) and laparoscopic exploration.

CT is usually used as a diagnostic method to confirm gastric cancer presence, and it can reliably demonstrate infiltration of the gastric wall by tumour, gastric ulceration and the presence of distal metastasis, more frequently involving the liver. Moreover, this method is less reliable in demonstrating the invasion of adjacent organs or the presence of lymphatic metastasis. EUS is a useful tool of preoperative evaluation for locoregional staging of gastric cancer and to investigate the assessment of gastric wall involvement and the presence of infiltrated paragastric lymph nodes. Moreover, another application of EUS is to delineate subepithelial lesions that may be confused with gastric cancer and to guide biopsy of submucosal tumours within the wall of the stomach [16]. A meta-analysis including 22 studies evaluated the usefulness of EUS in stomach cancer, and it has shown that the sensitivity and specificity by stage were 88.1 and 100% for T1, 82.3 and 95.6% for T2, 89.7 and 94.7% for T3 and 99.2 and 96.7% for T4 staging, respectively [17, 18]. The accuracy of EUS presurgical N-stage evaluation is approximately 65–95% [19]. A study has suggested that in patients with locally advanced gastric cancer, PET scan is the most sensitive noninvasive imaging modality for detecting hepatic metastasis [20] and provides better diagnostic accuracy for detection of distant lymph node metastasis and bone metastasis in patients with untreated advanced gastric cancer [21]. However, especially when tumour deposits are small, the ability of radiologic imaging to detect metastatic disease is limited. The surface of the liver, the omentum and the peritoneal surfaces are common sites for gastric cancer metastasis that are difficult to evaluate preoperatively by imaging. In this case, diagnostic laparoscopy is superior to preoperative CT in detection of peritoneal, hepatic or lymphatic metastasis.

11.5 Treatment

11.5.1 Surgical Treatment

The indications for surgical treatment in elderly patients with stomach cancer have been gradually expanded. This is because the morbidity and mortality rates from postoperative complications have continued to decrease over time as a result of the improvement of anaesthesiologic techniques, intensive care, surgical devices and less invasive surgical procedures, consequently improving short-term outcomes in elderly patients. Surgical resection is the only hope for cure in gastric cancer, even if an advanced stage of disease at the time of diagnosis precludes curative resection for most patients. Radical resection (R0) represents the only treatment modality which offers possible long-term survival [5]. Data in literature regarding elderly patients with gastric cancer seems to be limited and sometimes conflicting for several reasons.

First of all, elderly patients often have age-associated physiologic problems such as decreased organ reserve and concomitant comorbidities: hypertension, diabetes mellitus, ischemic heart disease, cerebrovascular disease and renal, liver and respiratory dysfunction. Several studies have demonstrated that preoperative risk, evaluated by the ASA score (American Society of Anaesthesiologists), is significantly higher in elderly gastric cancer patients than younger patients, mainly because of the higher rate of concomitant diseases [22].

Secondly, older patients often suffer from different grades of malnutrition, reflected by a low albumin level in blood. A recent Japanese study has shown that preoperative hypoalbuminemia is an independent risk factor of postoperative morbidity and mortality. Furthermore, the important thing to note is that initial hypoalbuminemia can affect early surgical outcomes irrespective of the replacement of albumin [23]. Another study suggests that less invasive surgery should be indicated for patients with serum albumin levels below the 2.9 g/dL cutoff [14]. This serum albumin test could be a reasonably simple and cost-effective method for identifying at-risk patients.

Moreover, gastric cancer in the elderly is often diagnosed at an advanced stage; this may be attributed to the lack of symptoms in the elderly population and to the absence of a mass screening programme for this tumour.

For all these reasons, it is sometimes difficult to treat elderly patients with gastric cancer according to the guidelines [24].

With regard to early gastric cancer, endoscopic resection is performed in selected cases, when there is no evidence of lymph node metastasis. The indication criteria are mucosal cancer of any size without ulceration, mucosal cancer with ulcerations sized less or equal to 30 mm or submucosal cancer less than 30 mm and confined to the upper 0.5 mm of the submucosa without lymph-vascular invasion [25]. In endoscopic resection, the typical sequential procedure included marking, mucosal incision and submucosal dissection with simultaneous haemostasis. With this approach, postoperative bleeding or perforation has been reported in 5%, and in 17%, histological examination revealed submucosal invasion that required further operative treatment [26].

For advanced cancer, the surgical procedure in the elderly must be decided carefully by assessing the patient's tolerance of surgical stress because, as already shown, elderly patients have declining organ capacity and the quality of life may suffer postoperatively [27].

Although guidelines indicate that gastrectomy associated with D2 lymph node dissection is the gold standard radical treatment for resectable advanced gastric cancer without any exception regarding age or comorbidities, the dominant trend among surgeons is to perform limited surgery such as subtotal gastrectomy [5, 22] in older patients.

The choice of a surgical procedure must guarantee both the control of the disease and a good result in terms of postoperative mortality and survival as well as quality of life, mainly in an aged population with a shorter life expectancy. In fact, total gastrectomy and D2 resection in this age group have been associated with higher rates of postoperative morbidity and mortality as compared to subtotal gastrectomy and D1 resection [28]. Performing a subtotal gastrectomy in the elderly, when technically feasible, is certainly related to a lower mortality and to a 5-year survival rate at least as good as after total gastrectomy, offering a better quality of life.

The suitability of subtotal gastrectomy for elderly patients is also related to the significantly shorter postoperative hospital stay for patients submitted to subtotal gastrectomy than total gastrectomy. Total gastrectomy frequently leads to considerable changes in dietary intake and absorption, which have a decisive influence on the postoperative nutrition status.

Takeshita et al. have shown that R0 resection with at least limited lymph node dissection should be considered as the treatment of first choice for elderly patients with gastric cancer, especially those between the ages of 80 and 84 years [29]. Similarly, splenectomy or combined resections of adjacent organs are less frequently performed in this group.

According to several studies about the extension of lymph node resection, D1 resection is more frequently performed than D2 resection, especially in patients with comorbidities, while D3 or greater is never performed. Surgical resection accompanied by dissection of a minimum of 14 and optimal 25 lymph nodes is the only modality that is potentially curative [5].

Egushi et al. reported that extended lymphadenectomy in elderly patients did not positively influence the 5-year survival, while it resulted in higher mortality (10 vs 1%) and morbidity rate (57 vs 27%) as compared to limited lymphadenectomy [30]. Another study confirms that after extended nodal dissection, the overall survival in highly comorbid elderly patients, even with nodal involvement, does not show clear benefits owing to the high risk of perioperative complications [31].

11.5.2 Postoperative Complications

Intraabdominal abscesses and pancreatic fistulae have been reported as major complications after total gastrectomy. They are thought to be associated with lymph node dissection around the pancreas that is why surgeons usually avoid lymph node dissection around the pancreas, particularly among the oldest patients.

Other possible postoperative complications include anastomotic leakage, wound infection, postoperative bleeding that required surgical or endoscopic treatment, anastomotic stenosis, ileus and respiratory and cardiac complications. These could prolong medical hospitalization, increasing costs and wasteful uses of human resources.

In elderly patients, it is not infrequent to see the onset of a postoperative delirium which can cause unexpected medical accidents, such as dementia, that prolong hospital stays and which may be associated with an unfavourable prognosis. It has been reported that 10–50% of elderly patients who undergo surgical treatment develop delirium postoperatively [32]. Although the mechanisms of delirium remain unclear, multiple factors are known to be involved; for example, systemic stress and inflammatory response may play important roles in the development of this condition [33]. Therefore, it is important to reduce perioperative stress to minimize the occurrence of delirium in elderly patients.

Although several reports have indicated that the incidence of postoperative complications increases in elderly patients, the applicability of these results to older patients with gastric cancer is arguably limited.

In fact, according to other research, no significant differences in complications, morbidity and hospital stay duration after surgery were found between patients younger and those older than 80 years [6, 34, 35]. This could be explained by a less invasive surgical procedure performed on these patients.

In order to prevent postoperative complications in the elderly, it is important to evaluate the overall preoperative status and to apply postoperative care depending on the type of surgery tailored to the patient's condition. Besides surgical complications, it is important to prevent geriatric clinical complications, first and foremost, and pulmonary infections, and nowadays respiratory rehabilitation programmes are emphasized.

A linear relationship is reported between postoperative complications and the number of preoperative abnormal parameters.

11.5.3 Long-Term Outcomes

Many studies have specifically compared the long-term outcome of gastric cancer in elderly patients with that in younger or middle-aged patients. Some found no significant difference in survival between them [22]. However, most studies confirmed that the prognosis of elderly patients was poorer than that of younger and middle-aged patients [36, 37]. According to a Chinese study, patients aged ≥70 years had a significantly lower 5-year overall survival rate than younger and middle-aged patients [8]. In general, the poor prognosis of elderly patients can be attributed to the delay in diagnosis, advanced tumour stage and also the preoperative condition of the patients.

11.5.4 Multimodality Treatment for Elderly Gastric Cancer

The use of neoadjuvant chemotherapy may have several potential benefits including the early eradication of micro metastasis and downstaging the disease with the possibility of a curative resection. A recent meta-analysis about neoadjuvant chemotherapy in elderly patients has shown a slightly improved survival rate with no significant increase in operative complications or perioperative mortality [38]. According to ESMO Guidelines working group, adjuvant chemotherapy and radiotherapy are recommended for elderly patients with high risk gastric cancer in an attempt to reduce local or distant recurrence and to improve survival after curative resection [24]. In the past, the majority of oncologists were hesitant to prescribe adjuvant chemotherapy to elderly patients because of the high risk of complications and for the toxicity of drugs due to changes in pharmacodynamic features in these patients. However, it has been demonstrated that there are no significant differences in terms of overall survival and pharmacological toxicity between younger and older patients without any severe comorbidity. Although the addition of adjuvant chemotherapy after curative gastrectomy for gastric cancer in general shows potential survival benefit, the need for such treatment in elderly patients should be determined by considering the conditions of individual patients and their life expectancies. However, patients should be strongly involved in decision making in undergoing or in discontinuing adjuvant chemotherapy: they may be more interested in quality than duration of life. For patients who cannot undergo surgical treatment because of relapsed or metastatic gastric cancer, palliative chemotherapy can provide palliation of symptoms, improving the quality of life. In conclusion, data clearly shows that age alone is not sufficient to estimate the general performance status of an elderly patient and their eligibility for curative or palliative treatment.

References

1. Zhu A, Sonnenberg A. Is gastric cancer again rising? J Clin Gastroenterol. 2012;46(9):804–6.
2. [Internet]. Available from: http://www.registri-tumori.it/PDF/AIOM2016/I_numeri_del_cancro_2016.pdf.
3. Nashimoto A, Akazawa K, Isobe Y, Miyashiro I, Katai H, Kodera Y, et al. Gastric cancer treated in 2002 in Japan: 2009 annual report of the JGCA nationwide registry. Gastric Cancer. 2012;16(1):1–27.
4. Moy K, Fan Y, Wang R, Gao Y, Yu M, Yuan J. Alcohol and tobacco use in relation to gastric cancer: a prospective study of men in shanghai, China. Cancer Epidemiol Biomark Prev. 2010;19(9):2287–97.
5. Saif M, Makrilia N, Zalonis A, Merikas M, Syrigos K. Gastric cancer in the elderly: an overview. Eur J Surg Oncol. 2010;36(8):709–17.
6. Kunisaki C, Akiyama H, Nomura M, Matsuda G, Otsuka Y, Ono H, et al. Comparison of surgical outcomes of gastric cancer in elderly and middle-aged patients. Am J Surg. 2006;191(2):216–24.
7. Kim H, Kim J, Lim B, Kim H, Kim H, Park J, et al. Sex disparity in gastric cancer: female sex is a poor prognostic factor for advanced gastric cancer. Ann Surg Oncol. 2016;23(13):4344–51.
8. Liang Y, Liang Y, Deng J, Guo H, Ding X, Wang X, Wang B, Zhang L, Liang H. Characteristics and prognosis of gastric cancer in patients aged ≥ 70 years. World J Gastroenterol. 2013;19(39):6568.
9. Uedo N, Takeuchi Y, Ishihara R. Endoscopic management of early gastric cancer: endoscopic mucosal resection or endoscopic submucosal dissection: data from a Japanese high-volume center and literature review. Ann Gastroenterol. 2012;25(4):281–90.

10. Arai T, Esaki Y, Inoshita N, Sawabe M, Kasahara I, Kuroiwa K, et al. Pathologic characteristics of gastric cancer in the elderly: a retrospective study of 994 surgical patients. Gastric Cancer. 2004;7(3):154–9.
11. Fransen G, Janssen M, Muris J, Laheij R, Jansen J. Meta-analysis: the diagnostic value of alarm symptoms for upper gastrointestinal malignancy. Aliment Pharmacol Ther. 2004;20(10):1045–52.
12. Pisanu A, Montisci A, Piu S, Uccheddu A. Curative surgery for gastric cancer in the elderly: treatment decisions, surgical morbidity, mortality, prognosis and quality of life. Tumori. 2007;93(5):478–84.
13. Phoon R. Chronic kidney disease in the elderly - assessment and management. Aust Fam Physician. 2012;41(12):940–4.
14. Takama T, Okano K, Kondo A, Akamoto S, Fujiwara M, Usuki H, et al. Predictors of post-operative complications in elderly and oldest old patients with gastric cancer. Gastric Cancer. 2014;18(3):653–61.
15. Kim S, Brooks A, Groban L. Preoperative assessment of the older surgical patient: honing in on geriatric syndromes. Clin Interv Aging. 2015;10:13–27.
16. Papanikolaou IS, Triantafyllou M, Triantafyllou K, Rösch T. EUS in the management of gastric cancer. Ann Gastroenterol Q Publ Hellenic Soc Gastroenterol. 2015;24(1):9–15.
17. Cho J. The role of Endosonography in the staging of gastrointestinal cancers. Clin Endosc. 2015;48(4):297.
18. Puli S. How good is endoscopic ultrasound for TNM staging of gastric cancers? A meta-analysis and systematic review. World J Gastroenterol. 2008;14(25):4011.
19. Holt B, Rösch T, Peter S. EUS in the evaluation of gastric tumors. In: Hawes RH, Fockens P, Varadarajulu S, editors. Endosonography. Philadelphia: Saunders; 2015. p. 129–50.
20. Kinkel K, Lu Y, Both M, Warren R, Thoeni R. Detection of hepatic metastasis from cancers of the gastrointestinal tract by using noninvasive imaging methods (US, CT, MR imaging, PET): a meta-analysis. Radiology. 2002;224(3):748–56.
21. Kawanaka Y, Kitajima K, Fukushima K, Mouri M, Doi H, Oshima T, et al. Added value of pre-treatment 18F-FDG PET/CT for staging of advanced gastric cancer: comparison with contrast-enhanced MDCT. Eur J Radiol. 2016;85(5):989–95.
22. Orsenigo E, Tomajer V, Palo S, Carlucci M, Vignali A, Tamburini A, et al. Impact of age on postoperative outcomes in 1118 gastric cancer patients undergoing surgical treatment. Gastric Cancer. 2007;10(1):39–44.
23. Kang S, Kim H, Kim M. Low serum albumin level, male sex, and Total Gastrectomy are risk factors of severe postoperative complications in elderly gastric cancer patients. J Gastric Cancer. 2016;16(1):43.
24. De Manzoni G, Roviello F, Siquini W. Surgery in the multimodal management of gastric cancer. 1st ed. Milan: Springer; 2012.
25. Park H, Ahn J, Jung H, Lee J, Jung K, Kim D, et al. Clinical characteristics and outcomes of gastric cancer patients aged over 80 years: a retrospective case-control study. PLoS One. 2016;11(12):e0167615.
26. Ono H, Kondo H, Gotoda T, Shirao K, Yamaguchi H, Saito D, Hosokawa K, Shimoda T, Yoshida S. Endoscopic mucosal resection for treatment of early gastric cancer. Gut. 2001;48(2):225–9.
27. Sakurai K, Muguruma K, Nagahara H, Kimura K, Toyokawa T, Amano R, et al. The outcome of surgical treatment for elderly patients with gastric carcinoma. J Surg Oncol. 2015;111(7):848–54.
28. Wu C, Lo S, Shen K, Hsieh M, Lui W, P'eng F. Surgical mortality, survival, and quality of life after resection for gastric cancer in the elderly. World J Surg. 2000;24(4):465–72.
29. Takeshita H, Ichikawa D, Komatsu S, Kubota T, Okamoto K, Shiozaki A, et al. Surgical outcomes of Gastrectomy for elderly patients with gastric cancer. World J Surg. 2013;37(12):2891–8.
30. Eguchi YT, Masahito IT. Is extended lymph node dissection necessary for gastric cancer in elderly patients? Eur J Surg. 2000;166(12):949–53.
31. Rausei S, Ruspi L, Rosa F, Morgagni P, Marrelli D, Cossu A, et al. Extended lymphadenectomy in elderly and/or highly co-morbid gastric cancer patients: a retrospective multicenter study. Eur J Surg Oncol. 2016;42(12):1881–9.

32. Deiner SJ. Postoperative delirium and cognitive dysfunction. Br J Anaesth. 2009;103(Supplement 1):i41–6.
33. Field RR, Wall MH. Delirium: past, present, and future. Semin Cardiothorac Vasc Anesth. 2013 Sep;17(3):170–9.
34. Yamada H, Kojima K, Inokuchi M, Kawano T, Sugihara K. Laparoscopy-assisted gastrectomy in patients older than 80. J Surg Res. 2010;161(2):259–63.
35. Mikami K, Hirano K, Futami K, Maekawa T. Department of surgery, Fukuoka University Chikushi Hospital 1-1-1 Zokumyoin, Chikushino City, Fukuoka: Japan; p. 818–8502.
36. Saito H, Osaki T, Murakami D, Sakamoto T, Kanaji S, Tatebe S, Tsujitani S, Ikeguchi M. Effect of age on prognosis in patients with gastric cancer. ANZ J Surg. 2006;76:458–61.
37. Sasada S, Ikeda Y, Saitsu H, Saku M. Characteristics of gastric cancer in patients over 80-years-old. Hepato-Gastroenterology. 2008;55(86–87):1931–4.
38. Liu K, Wan J, Yu G, Bei Y, Chen X, Lu M. The recommended treatment strategy for locally advanced gastric cancer in elderly patients aged 75 years and older: a surveillance, epidemiology, and end results database analysis. J Cancer Res Clin Oncol. 2016;143(2):313–20.

Surgical Treatment of Inflammatory Bowel Diseases in the Elderly

12

Francesco Colombo, Gianluca Pellino, Gianluca Sampietro, Francesco Selvaggi, Silvestro Canonico, and Diego Foschi

12.1 Introduction

Ulcerative colitis (UC) and regional ileitis were first described by Hale-White and Crohn, respectively, mainly in patients under 60 years of age [1]. Regional ileitis was subsequently defined as Crohn's disease (CD). For a long time, UC and CD—which are the two main inflammatory bowel diseases (IBD)—have been considered conditions typical of young people, but in the last 30 years, an increasing number of patients have been diagnosed with IBD after 60 years of age. Although there is no general agreement about the threshold of age for defining the "elderly" IBD patient, currently about 10–15% of the patients affected by UC and CD are over 65 years. This change in the epidemiology of IBD has several implications in the clinical course and evolution of UC and CD. The main differences between young and elderly patients are being related to the drugs used for medical therapy and the indications to surgery. Elderly patients have clinical characteristics, related to their profile of frailty that may affect medical and surgical treatment. Therefore, the surgical management of elderly patients with IBD needs to be carefully considered and must rely on adequate knowledge.

F. Colombo • G. Sampietro • D. Foschi (✉)
General Surgery, Department of Medical Sciences L. Sacco, University of Milan, Milan, Italy
e-mail: diego.foschi@unimi.it

G. Pellino • F. Selvaggi • S. Canonico
Unit of General and Geriatric Surgery, I Policlinico, Università degli Studi della Campania "Luigi Vanvitelli", Naples, Italy

A. Crucitti (ed.), *Surgical Management of Elderly Patients*,
https://doi.org/10.1007/978-3-319-60861-7_12

12.2 Epidemiology

The incidence and prevalence of IBD in the last 30 years show a worldwide increase with a west-east and north-south gradient. The incidence of UC in Europe is 24.3/100,000 person-year and 19.2 in North America, whereas the incidence of CD is higher in North America than in Europe: 20.2 versus 12.7/100,000 person-year. The highest reporte prevalence for both UC and CD is observed in Europe [2]. In Italy, the incidence of IBD is lower than in North Europe and USA, with higher values for UC than CD [3]. Although different thresholds of age have been proposed to consider patients with IBD as "elderly" (60 vs 65 years) [4, 5], about 15% of the patients receive diagnosis of IBD after 65 years of age [6]. Time-related trends demonstrate that both population ageing and late-onset of IBD contribute to the increased prevalence [7]. Loftus et al. [8] analysed the epidemiology of IBD in the Olmsted County, Minnesota, from 1940 to 2000. Over the last 20 years, UC incidence decreased (−7%) and CD increased (+31%), mainly in patients over 60 years. In the Netherlands [7], late onset (>60 years) of IBD had more than doubled from 1991 to 2011, increasing from 11.71 to 23.66/100,000 person-year. In the USA [9] patients older than 65 years accounted for 25% of IBD-related hospitalizations. A multicentre retrospective study from Italy [10] found that late-onset UC accounts for about 25% of cases.

Several factors caused these epidemiological changes. Either late-onset IBD could be a distinct entity, with a better and long-lasting course, or the increase of life expectancy and the improvement of medical and surgical treatment could have resulted in a decrease of the complication/death rate, allowing more IBD patients to live beyond 65 years of age.

12.3 Disease Presentation and Evolution

The spectrum of symptoms at presentation is the same in young and elderly patients with IBD, but the diagnosis in the latter population is more difficult due to the potential coexistence of other bowel-related conditions (e.g. infectious colitis, ischemic colitis, segmental colitis associated to diverticular disease and nonsteroidal anti-inflammatory drug-associated colitis) [11, 12]. A careful clinical evaluation and endoscopy with biopsies are very important tools to obtain diagnosis and to classify the lesions and disease activity.

Family history and genetic alterations occur less frequently in the elderly than in young patients [13, 14]. Gender distribution varies in the different populations, but female prevalence is typical of CD, and male prevalence is typical of UC [7, 15, 16]. Elderly patients with IBD have intestinal bleeding, anaemia and malnutrition more frequently than young patients [9]. Furthermore, they have higher Charlson's index and more comorbidities [17], including diabetes, chronic pulmonary diseases and cardiac and cerebrovascular disease.

Elderly patients with CD are more likely to have colonic disease [18]. Non-stricturing, non-penetrating patterns are more frequent when the small bowel is involved. Contradictory results have been reported concerning the rate of perianal CD involvement in the elderly [4, 12, 16, 19, 20].

UC late-onset patients are more frequently male, complaining of paradoxical constipation and rectal bleeding [18]. They are more likely to have left-sided colitis than proctitis or extensive colitis. However, in elderly patients with a previous diagnosis of UC, the distribution of the lesions is the same as in young patients, with higher incidence of pancolitis (45.9%) than left-sided colitis (14.3%). Extraintestinal manifestations are less common [4, 10, 13, 16, 21].

Progression of both UC and CD in elderly patients seems to be slower than in young patients [4, 13], and the behaviour of CD remains stable with time. Lesions tend to extend only in a few patients. In the AGED-study [10], the most frequent pattern was late disease onset and subsequent mild or no activity. However, the risk of infections and related complications is higher in elderly IBD patients [22, 23], but the time to develop dysplasia and rectal cancer is shorter. Close follow-up and surveillance of the patients are warranted [24, 25]. Mortality is higher in elderly CD than in UC, higher risk being associated with fistulising or active stricturing disease [9, 17]. Surgery is a protective factor reducing the risk for mortality, but surgical operations are less frequently performed than in young patients, probably because comorbidities and complications contraindicate them [9].

12.4 Medical Treatment

The main goals of the medical therapy of IBD are the same in young and elderly patients, including (1) induction and maintenance of remission, (2) prevention of IBD-related complications and (3) safety of treatment with improvement in the quality of life [12, 26]. Although drug efficacy trials in elderly patients are lacking [27], indirect evidence suggests that there is no difference in the response rate to the pharmacological treatment among the elderly and young patients with IBD [28, 29], without any change in the prescription strategy [12]. 5-Aminosalicylate (ASA)-class drugs are used for the treatment of mild-to-moderate activity IBD patients, corticosteroids for acute flare and severe cases, cyclosporine for rescue therapy of severe UC, immune-modifying agents for maintenance therapy and anti-TNF agents for severe UC, in steroid dependent/resistant patients [12].

ASA-class drugs are prescribed in about 50–80% of elderly patients affected by UC and CD [13, 30]. Corticosteroids are used in about 30% and immunomodulators in 10–20% of cases [12]. Biologics are used in 1% of UC and 9% of CD elderly patients [13], although the efficacy of anti-TNF agents is the same as in young patients [10, 31]. Age-related frailty, comorbidities, geriatric conditions (e.g. cognitive impairment and cardiovascular diseases), the low compliance of the patients to polypharmacy, possible drug interactions and the increased risk of infectious complications are the main factors explaining the current treatment approach in elderly patients with IBD.

12.5 Indications to Surgery

Indications to surgery for IBD mainly include unresponsiveness to treatment, complications and cancer. The operation rates in late-onset IBD at 1 and 10 years after diagnosis are 18% and 32%, respectively, in CD and 4 and 8% in UC [13]. Nguyen et al. suggested that elderly-onset UC patients were more likely to undergo surgery than young patients [17]. Early colectomy (within 90 days from the diagnosis) is more frequent in elderly patients with UC at their first presentation [32]. The risk of surgery is the same in elderly and young patients affected by CD [33], but long-standing CD with inflammation and strictures, which could underlie constipation in elderly IBD patients, harbours cancer in 3.5% of the cases [34] and is a further indication to surgery. Therefore, we think that careful attention should be paid in the preoperative workup and assessment of these patients to choose the correct approach.

Perioperative optimization is crucial in the elderly. Concomitant diseases should be controlled when possible, and patients may benefit from perioperative nutritional treatment [35]. In elderly patients presenting with stricturing CD, strictureplasties should be discouraged or carefully considered, especially in long-standing disease and in patients who do not fulfil the criteria for postoperative short bowel syndrome [36, 37]. When feasible, laparoscopy is a good alternative in CD of the elderly, especially in patients requiring primary surgery for remitting-relapsing disease involving the large bowel or localized to the terminal ileum. Minimally invasive surgery in patients with previous midline laparotomy or with extensive small bowel involvement should be selectively advocated, because the recovery advantages may not be maintained when compared with open surgery [38]. Moreover, laparoscopy requires longer operative times, which should be considered in the case of multiple comorbidities. A survey of Italian colorectal surgeons promoted by the Italian Society of Colorectal Surgery (SICCR) showed moderate agreement when considering laparoscopy in other-than-localized CD [39].

In elderly patients with UC, the decision between a colectomy with end ileostomy and a restorative proctocolectomy should be made after considering several variables. It has been suggested that elderly patients without significant comorbidities, who are able to mobilize independently and are self-sufficient, can be considered candidates to restorative proctocolectomy with ileal pouch and pouch anal anastomosis (IPAA). Concerning functional results, patients without clinical impairments of sphincter function may not require routine instrumental testing of the sphincter complex. However, patients should be able to understand the impact and extent of the procedure. IPAA involves either two-stage surgery ((1) proctocolectomy with ileal pouch and loop ileostomy, (2) ileostomy reversal) in elective treatment or three-stage approach ((1) subtotal colectomy with long rectal stump secured to the abdominal wall with terminal ileostomy, (2) completion proctectomy with ileal pouch and loop ileostomy, (3) ileostomy reversal) in emergency settings or in patients with prolonged exposure to biologic drugs [40]. One-stage surgery in elderly patients should never be considered [41, 42]. Routine pre-reversal pouchogram to assess the anastomosis is a safe option in elderly patients. Laparoscopic subtotal colectomy should be encouraged in emergency settings in patients who can tolerate the procedure.

Elderly patients show similar responses to rescue therapy [10], suggesting that this should be attempted. However, the threshold for surgery should be lower in the elderly, because postoperative complications (i.e. toxic megacolon, intra-abdominal septic complications and mortality) are more common when surgery is delayed. Prompt surgery achieves a dramatic reduction in mortality in elderly patients [43]. When patients received biologics, it is safer to defer pouch formation to a later stage irrespective of disease activity at surgery, in order to reduce the risks of postoperative pelvic sepsis [40]. The rectal stump should be either secured to the abdominal wall or used to create a fistula in frail patients [44]. This measure avoids pelvic collections in the event of rectal stump suture leak and eases subsequent surgery. Importantly, patients must accept undergoing scheduled follow-ups and adhere to the surveillance pathway including endoscopy. The risk of pouch-related adenocarcinoma is lower than colorectal cancer risk in the general population [45]. Endoscopic follow-up is not recommended after IPAA in patients without high-risk features for cancer according to the Guidelines of the European Crohn's and Colitis Organisation (ECCO) [46]. Long-standing disease and cancer/dysplasia on the specimen increases the risk of pouch-related cancer by eight times irrespective of mucosectomy [45, 47]. In addition, some patients may be diagnosed with CD later in life or develop other-than-adenocarcinoma pouch cancers without systemic symptoms [48, 49], suggesting that scheduled follow-up with flexible pouchoscopy is a safe choice in elderly patients.

12.6 Surgery in UC

Elderly patients with UC tend to have a less severe disease and more commonly require surgery for premalignancy complications (dysplasia/DALM). Rarely, do they present with an acute setting (haemorrhage, toxic megacolon or perforation) requiring urgent surgery.

Theoretically, three different surgical options are available in elderly patients, similarly to young patients, including (1) proctocolectomy with definitive terminal ileostomy, (2) colectomy with ileorectal anastomosis (IRA) in the presence of spared rectum and (3) IPAA (Fig. 12.1).

IRA is very rarely considered for elderly patients because of poor functional results and disease recurrence, hence reducing the actual alternatives to proctocolectomy with ileostomy and IPAA.

In the past, the complexity of the surgical procedure and the high complication rate, combined with the risk of poor functional outcome, have induced surgeons to perform pouch surgery very rarely in the older population. The low frequency of IPAA in elderly patients has probably been more influenced by prudence than by proven evidence, based on the assumption that they have higher comorbidities and worse sphincter function. A growing body of evidence shows that age itself may not

Treatment	PRO	CAVEAT	CONTRA
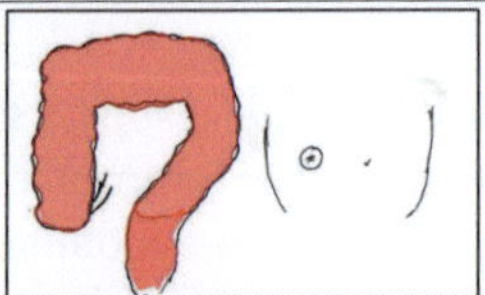 PROCTOCOLECTOMY WITH END ILEOSTOMY	- Removal of entire disease - No endoscopy at follow-up - Often one-stage procedure	- Stoma management (devices/siting) - Stoma-related disorders (electrolyte imbalance/ rare hernia-prolapse-retraction)	- No restoration of bowel continuity - Body image
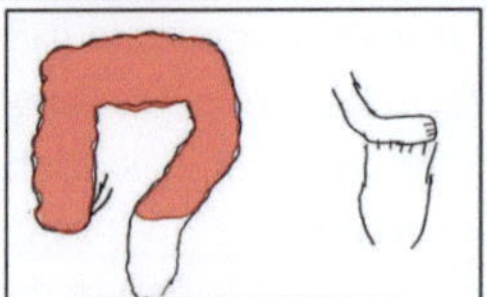 ILEORECTAL ANASTOMOSIS (IRA)	- No pelvic surgery - No sphincter manipulation - Removal of diseased bowel - Transanal defecation preserved - One-stage procedure	- "False" rectal sparing (topical agents may mask proctitis) - Risk of cancer on the residual rectum - Risk of repeated surgery - Flares can jeopardise function	- Need for scheduled follow-up with endoscopy - Need for further medical treatment for recurrent proctitis - Persistence of some extra-intestinal manifestations
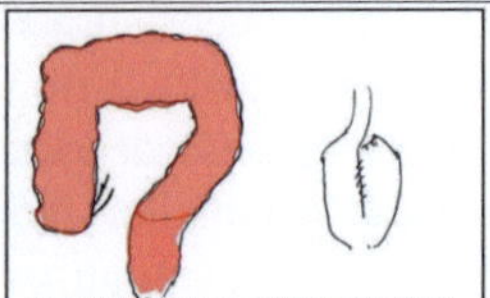 ILEAL POUCH ANAL ANASTOMOSIS (IPAA)	- Removal of entire disease - Transanal defecation preserved	- Complex procedure - Septic complications may impair function and require further complex surgery - Close monitoring for potential complications of diversion ileostomy during maturation - Cuffitis/Pouchitis	- At least two-stage surgery - Longer operative time/anaesthesia - Need to adapt to changed bowel anatomy and function - Follow-up with endoscopy

Fig. 12.1 Advantages and disadvantages of surgical approaches for Ulcerative Colitis in the Elderly

be an accurate predictor of surgical risk in UC because disease severity is a more important contributor to perioperative morbidity and mortality [46].

Frailty is an emerging alternative to age for estimating surgical risk. It describes a state of reduced physiological reserve assessing cognition, function, nutrition and comorbidities. There is no current consensus on the appropriate measure of frailty in elderly IBD patients and which characteristics should be considered when evaluating patient suitability for IPAA [26].

The ideal candidate should be independent, with normal anal sphincter function, and should be able to understand risks and problems associated with IPAA. Elderly patients with UC need to take several medications and may experience complications from drug interactions (e.g. increased risk of leucopoenia and anaemia when azathioprine is combined with ACE inhibitors) or prolonged drug intake (e.g. increased risk of cancer with immunomodulators). Proctocolectomy offers a protective effect on these potential complications and allows for the elimination of the use of drugs for UC-related symptoms.

The physiological reduction of perceived thirst represents another typical problem of elderly patients. Elderly carriers of an ileostomy, especially in case of diversion ileostomy, are at increased risk of dehydration and electrolyte imbalance due to the loss of high quantity of fluids from the stoma or inadequate fluid intake. Therefore, it is highly important to follow up patients after IPAA during the interval between IPAA construction and loop ileostomy reversal (Fig. 12.1). Patients may need a scheduled blood test in outpatient settings and should be promptly readmitted for rehydration and correction of electrolyte or renal function derangements. In staged IPAA, stoma reversal should be performed as soon possible in the elderly, based on a balance between IPAA "maturation" and clinical status.

There are insufficient data that compare treatment safety and efficacy in young and elderly patients, and the total number of patients over 65 treated with IPAA is very small.

Short-term results after IPAA in elderly patients show that perceived quality of life is good enough to overcome some hesitancy in performing IPAA in patients older than 60–65 years [50]. Results in patients aged over 70 are not inferior to those of younger counterparts, provided that patients are carefully selected and strictly followed up [50–52]. The principles of surgical therapy in elderly patients do not differ widely from those of younger patients who need pouch surgery, but some aspects need to be considered.

As expected and previously reported, elderly patients present with a higher incidence of comorbidities. Some authors suggested that comorbidities justify an increased incidence of postoperative complications and longer hospital stay and operating time, but more recent reports showed no increase in surgical morbidity and mortality after IPAA [26].

The incidence of anastomotic leaks, pouch-related complications and pouch failure rates did not differ between young and elderly patients undergoing surgery for UC at the Cleveland Clinic, a high-volume pouch centre [53, 54]. In our experience, elderly patients may need admission to the intensive care unit more frequently than young patients, suggesting that complications may manifest showing a more serious picture, despite similar overall complication rates between the two groups [51, 52, 55]. Notwithstanding, midterm functional results are comparable to that of younger patients, even if a higher proportion of elderly patients tend to take antidiarrheal medications [51, 52, 55].

A physiological decrease of anal sphincter function is expected in elderly patients, and this condition can impair faecal continence [43, 56]. Clinical sphincter disorders justify a total proctocolectomy with permanent ileostomy with significantly better outcomes and quality of life compared with an IPAA which would be fated to fail due to an unbearably poor function.

Stryker et al. suggested that elderly patients are more likely to have difficulty with the daily management of their stoma, although their overall quality of life is equal to or superior to that of younger patients with terminal ileostomy [57].

It is crucial to assess accurately the sphincter function without overestimating incontinence. Elderly patients who need surgery in acute settings or with severe pancolitis tend to present with several fresh-blood evacuations and frequent soiling. Adequate treatment usually removes these symptoms. Therefore, it is important to discriminate between soiling/perianal irritation due to disease activity and an actual deterioration of the continence. Surgeons with expertise in IBD can usually assess the patients adequately with preoperative digital examination.

Indeed, the double-stapled technique and recent advances in technological instrumentation lead to a much better functional outcome compared to hand-sewn anastomosis also in patients over 50–55 years [58, 59].

Furthermore, little is known about the impact of laparoscopy in this patient population, but the mini-invasive approach during IPAA may provide significant benefits and should be offered as first-line treatment [55, 60, 61].

Concluding, the choice of surgical procedure for UC in elderly patients requires a careful evaluation of the “pro” and “contra” of each approach (Fig. 12.1). In elderly patients with preserved sphincter function, IPAA should be the preferred choice. In selected, motivated elderly patients, IPAA surgery has significant benefits with a high rate quality of life and functional outcomes comparable with younger patients. A careful selection and counselling of the patients are mandatory to avoid postoperative complications with detrimental quality of life. It is important to consider that a well-functioning ileostomy is preferable to a malfunctioning IPAA.

12.7 Surgery in CD

As the cumulative lifetime risk of mortality related to IBD seems to be negligible, we are facing two different types of elderly patients with CD, those patients with a diagnosis at a young age and having aged with CD and those developing it in the old age [12]. These two different clinical characteristics are not marginal, since the disease location, behaviour and the need for surgery seem to be different between the two groups. The need for surgery should be lower in elderly onset, with less common recurrence rate but shorter time to recurrence. Older patients have less frequently penetrating CD but are less likely to be operated on with laparoscopy; they have more systemic and local complications (including anastomotic leakage) and longer hospital stay [12, 26, 62].

When surgery is necessary for CD complications, peri- and intraoperative strategies are no different for younger patients. Laparoscopy is the preferred surgical approach whenever technically possible. However, both in CD and UC, many elderly patients have already received abdominal surgery, related or not to IBD, making laparoscopy extremely difficult if not contraindicated [38, 63–72].

Accurate staging of all disease locations is mandatory when planning abdominal surgery for complicated CD, including ileocolonoscopy and cross-sectional imaging. However, intraoperative identification and characterization of all disease locations are essential to tailor a “per-segment” approach, on the basis of the features of every single intestinal diseased segment [73–80].

The need for surgical treatment of upper gastrointestinal involvement is very limited. Gastro-oesophageal and duodenal locations of CD can be approached with Roux-en-Y bypass or strictureplasties, but in elderly patients, it is essential to exclude the presence of neoplasia. Vagotomy is generally contraindicated in CD patients [81–89].

Surgery should be considered as the first option in patients with localised CD of the small or the large intestine with obstructive symptoms. Furthermore, in patients with fistulizing disease, early surgery should be favoured over anti-TNF therapy. Abdominal abscesses should be drained percutaneously and resection be delayed. Strictureplasties are a safe and appealing alternative to resection, but many authors prefer resection for patients with late onset of the disease and at a low risk of developing short bowel syndrome. On the contrary, strictureplasties should be indicated for those patients with a diagnosis in childhood and repeated intestinal resections in their clinical history. Among the vast repertoire of strictureplasties, the two main techniques that general surgeons need to know consist of Heineke-Mikulicz strictureplasty, for stenotic segments up to 6–8 cm, and ileoileal, isoperistaltic, side-to-side strictureplasty (also known as the "Michelassi strictureplasty"), for long stenotic segments or multiple and close strictures [90–99].

When intestinal resection is necessary, a minimal bowel resection is indicated, with no need of microscopically disease-free margins and extended mesentery dissection [100]. Strong evidence shows that stapled, wide-lumen, functional end-to-end anastomosis is the best technique for reconstruction [101, 102].

In colonic CD, conservative surgery is contraindicated. Selected cases of balloon dilatation have been reported, but malignancy must be categorically excluded. A maximum of two segmental colonic resections can be considered in case one or two separate segments of the colon are involved; otherwise a subtotal colectomy with IRA is advised. In very selected and motivated elderly CD patients with isolated colonic location, IPAA has been successfully attempted, but in case of failure, redo pouch is contraindicated [73, 103–110].

Small bowel adenocarcinoma is a rare condition that affects CD patients, with 33-fold higher risk than in the general population but with minimal differences in incidence over decades. Unfortunately, preoperative diagnosis is extremely difficult, and intraoperative findings are suggestive only in half of the cases. The treatment of choice is a wide ileal resection with adequate removal of the mesentery [47, 111–114].

In case of colorectal cancer (CRC), it is essential to address some important aspects. Does the patient have a history of active pancolitis? Arc there any proximal small bowel CD locations? Is CRC associated with segmental colonic CD, or is it a sporadic CRC in a patient without colonic involvement?

In the case of pancolitis (whether it is active or not at the time of operation), a total colectomy or proctocolectomy, with oncologic principles in all colonic segments, is strongly suggested. The possibility of performing IPAA depends on the sphincter conditions and the absence of small bowel disease. The presence of active CD proximal to the colon should be considered for synchronous resection at the moment of surgery for the CRC, since future adjuvant therapy is likely to be compromised by active CD. Sporadic CRC in CD should be treated as in the general population, but the presence of active CD must be excluded, and reactivation during adjuvant therapy is accurately monitored [47, 115–119].

Age has a clear impact on surgical presentation and postoperative course in elderly patients. The overall complication rate is similar to that of young patients but is more serious and more frequently requires admission to intensive care units with a longer hospital stay. Specific complications related to anastomosis and deep venous thrombosis are more frequent in the elderly. As reported in the section dealing with UC, how to measure the frailty of elderly patients with IBD remains an unanswered question. In fact, all the various scales of frailty are not able to discriminate between problems related to ageing and those related to a chronic intestinal condition such as IBD [62, 120, 121].

References

1. Hawkins C. Historical review. In: Allan RN, Keighley MRB, Alexander-Williams J, Hawkins C, editors. Inflammatory bowel diseases. Edinburgh: Churchill Livingstone Pub; 1983. p. 1–7.
2. Molodecky NA, Soon IS, Rabi DM, et al. Increasing incidence and prevalence of inflammatory bowel diseases with time, based on systematic review. Gastroenterology. 2012;142:46–54.
3. Tragnone A, Corrao G, Miglio F, et al. Incidence of inflammatory bowel disease in Italy: a nation-wide population-based study. Gruppo italiano per lo studio del colon e del retto (GISC). Int J Epidemiol. 1996;25:1044–52.
4. Lakatos P, David G, Pandur T. IBD in the elderly population: results from a population based study in western Hungary. 1997–2008. J Crohns Colitis. 2011;5:5–13.
5. Shivananda S, Lennard Jones J, Logan R, et al. Incidence of inflammatory bowel disease across Europe: is there a difference between north and south? Results of the European collaborative study on inflammatory bowel disease (EC-IBD). Gut. 1996;39:690–7.
6. Stepaniuk P, Bernstein CN, Targownik LE, Singh H. Characterization of inflammatory bowel disease in elderly patients: a review of epidemiology, current practices and outcomes of current management strategies. Can J Gastroenterol Hepatol. 2015;29:327–33.
7. Jeuring SFG, Van den Henvel TRA, Zeegers MP. Epidemiology and long-term outcome of inflammatory bowel disease diagnosed at elderly age- an increasing distinct entity. Inflamm Bowel Dis. 2016;22:1425–34.
8. Loftus CG, Loftus EV, Scott Harmsen W, et al. Update on the incidence and prevalence of Crohn's disease and ulcerative colitis in Holmsted County. Minnesota 1940–2000. Infl Bowel Dis. 2007;13:254–61.
9. Ananthakrishnan AN, McGinley EL, Binion DG. Inflammatory bowel disease in the elderly is associated with worse outcomes: a national study of hospitalizations. Inflammm Bowel Dis. 2009;15:182–9.
10. Fries W, Viola A, Manetti N, et al. Disease patterns in late-onset ulcerative colitis: results from the IG-IBD "AGED study". Dig Liver Dis. 2017;49:17–23.
11. Del Val JH. Old age inflammatory bowel disease onset: a different problem? World J Gastroenterol. 2011;17:2734–9.
12. Taleban S, Colombel JF, Mohler MJ, Fain MJ. Inflammatory bowel disease and the elderly: a review. J Crohns Colitis. 2015;9:507–15.
13. Charpentier C, Salleron J, Savoye G, et al. Natural history of elderly-onset inflammatory bowel disease: a population-based cohort study. Gut. 2014;63:423–32.
14. DeRidder L, Weersma RK, Dijkstra G, et al. Genetic susceptibility has a more important role in pediatric-onset Crohn's disease than in adult-onset Crohn's disease. Inflamm Bowel Dis. 2007;13:1083–92.
15. Bitton A, Vutcovici M, Paternande V, et al. Epidemiology of inflammatory bowel disease in Quebec: recent trends. Inflamm Bowel Dis. 2014;20:1770–6.
16. Gower-Rousseau C, Vasseur F, et al. Epidemiology of inflammatory bowel diseases: new insights from a French population-based registry (EPIMAD). Dig Liver Dis. 2013;45:89–94.
17. Nguyen GC, Bernstein C, Benchimol EI. Risk of surgery and mortality in elderly-onset inflammatory bowel disease: a population-based cohort study. Inflamm Bowel Dis. 2017;23:218–23.
18. Katz S, Pardi DS. Inflammatory bowel disease of the elderly: frequently asked questions (FAQs). Am J Gastroenterol. 2011;106:1889–97.
19. Freeman HJ. Age-dependent phenotypic clinical expression of Crohn's disease. J Clin Gastroenterol. 2005;39:774–7.
20. Quezada SM, Steinberger EK. Association of age at diagnosis and Crohn's disease phenotype. Age Ageing. 2013;42:102–6.

21. Juneja M, Baidoo L, Schwartz MB, et al. Geriatric inflammatory bowel disease: phenotipic presentation, treatment patterns, nutritional status, outcomes and comorbidity. Dig Dis Sci. 2012;57:1408–15.
22. Brassard P, Bittou A, Suisse A, et al. Oral corticosteroids and the risk of serious infections in patients with elderly-onset inflammatory bowel disease. Am J Gastroenterol. 2014;109:1795–802.
23. Gisbert JP, Chaparro M. Systematic review with metanalysis: inflammatory bowel disease in the elderly. Alim Pharmacol Ther. 2014;39:459–77.
24. Baars JE, Kuipers EJ, van Haastent M, et al. Age at diagnosis of inflammatory bowel disease influences early development of colorectal cancer in inflammatory bowel disease. A nationwide, long-term survey. J Gastroenterol. 2012;47:1308–22.
25. Brackmann S, Andersen SN, Aamodt G, et al. Relationship between clinical parameters and the colitis-colorectal cancer interval in a cohort of patients with colorectal cancer in inflammatory bowel disease. Scand J Gastroenterol. 2009;44:46–55.
26. Sturm A, Maaser C, Mendall M, et al. European Crohn's and colitis organisation topical review on IBD in the elderly. J Crohns Colitis. 2016;11(3):263–73.
27. Travis S. Is IBD different in the elderly? Inflamm Bowel Dis. 2008;14:S12–3.
28. Chaparro M, Ordas I, Cabre E, et al. Safety of thiopurine therapy in inflammatory bowel disease: long-term follow-up study of 3931 patients. Inflamm Bowel Dis. 2013;19:1404–10.
29. Gisbert JP, Marin AC, Chaparro M. Systematic review: factors associated with relapse of inflammatory bowel disease after discontinuation of anti-TNF therapy. Alim Pharmacol Ther. 2015;42:391–405.
30. Lichtenstein GR, Feagan BG, Cohen RD, et al. Drug therapies and the risk of malignancies: results from the TREAT registry. Am J Gastroenterol. 2010;105:501–23.
31. Cottone M, Kohn A, Deperno M, et al. Advance age is an independent risk factor for severe infections and mortality in patients given anti-tumor necrosis factor therapy for inflammatory bowel disease. Clin Gastroenterol Hepatol. 2011;9:30–5.
32. Targownik LE, Singh H, Nugent Z, et al. The epidemiology of colectomy in ulcerative colitis: results from a population-based cohort. Am J Gastroenterol. 2012;107:1228–35.
33. Ananthakrishnan AN, Shi HY, Tang W, et al. Systematic review and meta-analysis: phenotype and clinical outcomes of older onset inflammatory bowel disease. J Crohns Colitis. 2016;10:1224–36.
34. Fumery M, de Chambrun GP, Stefanescu C, et al. Detection of dysplasia or cancer in 3.5% of patients with inflammatory bowel disease and colonic strictures. Clin Gastroenterol Hepatol. 2015;13:1770–5.
35. Ikeuchi H, Yamamura T, Nakano H, Kosaka T, Shimoyama T, Fukuda Y. Efficacy of nutritional therapy for perforating and non-perforating Crohn's disease. Hepato-Gastroenterology. 2004;51:1050–2.
36. Rieder F, Latella G, Magro F, Yuksel ES, Higgins PD, Di Sabatino A, de Bruyn JR, Rimola J, Brito J, Bettenworth D, van Assche G, Bemelman W, d'Hoore A, Pellino G, Dignass AU. European Crohn's and colitis organisation topical review on prediction, diagnosis and Management of Fibrostenosing Crohn's disease. J Crohns Colitis. 2016;10:873–85.
37. Uchino M, Ikeuchi H, Bando T, Matsuoka H, Takahashi Y, Takesue Y, Matsumoto T, Tomita N. Risk factors for short bowel syndrome in patients with Crohn's disease. Surg Today. 2012;42:447–52.
38. Aytac E, Stocchi L, Remzi FH, Kiran RP. Is laparoscopic surgery for recurrent Crohn's disease beneficial in patients with previous primary resection through midline laparotomy? A case-matched study. Surg Endosc. 2012;26:3552–6.
39. Pellino G, Selvaggi F, Ghezzi G, Corona D, Riegler G, Delaini GG. A think tank of the Italian society of colorectal surgery (SICCR) on the surgical treatment of inflammatory bowel disease using the Delphi method: Crohn's disease. Tech Coloproctol. 2015;19:639–51.

40. Selvaggi F, Pellino G, Canonico S, Sciaudone G. Effect of preoperative biologic drugs on complications and function after restorative proctocolectomy with primary ileal pouch formation: systematic review and meta-analysis. Inflamm Bowel Dis. 2015;21(1):79–92.
41. Lovegrove RE, Tilney HS, Remzi FH, Nicholls RJ, Fazio VW, Tekkis PP. To divert or not to divert: a retrospective analysis of variables that influence ileostomy omission in ileal pouch surgery. Arch Surg. 2011;146:82–8.
42. Pellino G, Sciaudone G, Canonico S, Selvaggi F. Role of ileostomy in restorative proctocolectomy. World J Gastroenterol. 2012;18:1703–7.
43. Vavricka SR, Rogler G. Treatment of severe ulcerative colitis: differences in elderly patients? Dig Dis. 2009;27:315–21.
44. Selvaggi F, Pellino G, Ghezzi G, Corona D, Riegler G, Delaini GG. A think tank of the Italian Society of Colorectal Surgery (SICCR) on the surgical treatment of inflammatory bowel disease using the Delphi method: ulcerative colitis. Tech Coloproctol. 2015;19(10):627–38. https://doi.org/10.1007/s10151-015-1367-5.
45. Selvaggi F, Pellino G, Canonico S, Sciaudone G. Systematic review of cuff and pouch cancer in patients with ileal pelvic pouch for ulcerative colitis. Inflamm Bowel Dis. 2014;20(7):1296–308.
46. Øresland T, Bemelman WA, Sampietro GM, Spinelli A, Windsor A, Ferrante M, Marteau P, Zmora O, Kotze PG, Espin-Basany E, Tiret E, Sica G, Panis Y, Faerden AE, Biancone L, Angriman I, Serclova Z, de Buck van Overstraeten A, Gionchetti P, Stassen L, Warusavitarne J, Adamina M, Dignass A, Eliakim R, Magro F, D'Hoore A, European Crohn's and Colitis Organisation (ECCO). European evidence based consensus on surgery for ulcerative colitis. J Crohns Colitis. 2015;9:4–25.
47. Annese V, Beaugerie L, Egan L, Biancone L, Bolling C, Brandts C, et al. European evidence-based consensus: inflammatory bowel disease and malignancies. J Crohns Colitis. 2015;9(11):945–65.
48. Derikx LA, Nissen LH, Oldenburg B, Hoentjen F. Controversies in pouch surveillance for patients with inflammatory bowel disease. J Crohns Colitis. 2016;10:747–51.
49. Pellino G, Kontovounisios C, Tait D, Nicholls J, Tekkis PP. Squamous cell carcinoma of the anal transitional zone after Ileal pouch surgery for ulcerative colitis: systematic review and treatment perspectives. Case Rep Oncol. 2017;10:112–22.
50. Cohen JL, Strong SA, Hyman NH, et al. Standards practice task force American Society of Colon and Rectal Surgeons. Practice parameters for the surgical treatment of ulcerative colitis. Dis Colon Rectum. 2005;48:1997–2009.
51. Pellino G, Sciaudone G, Candilio G, Camerlingo A, Marcellinaro R, Rocco F, De Fatico S, Canonico S, Selvaggi F. Complications and functional outcomes of restorative proctocolectomy for ulcerative colitis in the elderly. BMC Surg. 2013;13(Suppl 2):S9.
52. Pellino G, Sciaudone G, Candilio G, De Fatico GS, Landino I, Canonico S, Selvaggi F. Restorative proctocolectomy with ileal pouch-anal anastomosis is safe and effective in selected very elderly patients suffering from ulcerative colitis. Int J Surg. 2014;12(Suppl 2):S56–9.
53. Delaney CP, Fazio VW, Remzi FH, et al. Prospective, age-related analysis of surgical results, functional outcome, and quality of life after ileal-pouch-anal anastomosis. Ann Surg. 2003;238:221–8.
54. Fazio VW, Tekkis PP, Remzi F, et al. Quantification of risk for pouch failure after ileal pouch anala anastomosis surgery. Ann Surg. 2003;238:605–14.
55. Colombo F, Sahami S, de Buck Van Overstraeten A, et al. Restorative proctocolectomy in elderly IBD patients: a multicentre comparative study on safety and efficacy. J Crohns Colitis. 2016;11(6):671–9.
56. Holubar SD, Privitera A, Cima RR, et al. Minimally invasive total proctocolectomy with Brooke ileostomy for ulcerative colitis. Inflamm Bowel Dis. 2009;15:1337–42.
57. Stryker SJ, Pemebrton JH, Zinsmeister AR. Long-term results of ileostomy in older patients. Dis Colon Rectum. 1985;28:844–6.

58. Bauer JJ, Gorfine SR, Gelernt IM, et al. Restorative proctocolectomy in patients older than fifty years. Dis Colon Rectum. 1997;40:562–5.
59. Lewis WG, Sagar PM, Holdsworth PJ, et al. Restorative proctocolectomy with end to end pouch-anal anastomosis in patients over the age of fifty. Gut. 1993;34:948–52.
60. Ahmed Ali U, Keus F, Heikens JT, et al. Open vs laparoscopic (assisted) ileo-pouch-anal anastomosis for ulcerative colitis and familial adenomatous polyposis. Cochrane Database Syst Rev. 2009;1:CD006267.
61. Buskens CJ, Sahami S, Tanis PJ, Bemelman WA. The potential benefits and disadvantages of laparoscopic surgery for ulcerative colitis: a review of current evidence. Best Pract Res Clin Gastroenterol. 2014;28:19–27.
62. Argeny S, Stift A, Mittlbock M, et al. Advanced age impacts surgical characteristics and postoperative course in patients with Crohn's disease. Int J Surg. 2016;33:182–6.
63. Bemelman WA, Allez M. The surgical intervention: earlier or never? Best Prac Res Clin Gastroenterol. 2014;28(3):497–503.
64. Eshuis EJ, Polle SW, Slors JF, Hommes DW, Sprangers MA, Gouma DJ, et al. Long-term surgical recurrence, morbidity, quality of life, and body image of laparoscopic-assisted vs. open ileocolic resection for Crohn's disease: a comparative study. Dis Colon Rectum. 2008;51(6):858–67.
65. Eshuis EJ, Slors JF, Stokkers PC, Sprangers MA, Ubbink DT, Cuesta MA, et al. Long-term outcomes following laparoscopically assisted versus open ileocolic resection for Crohn's disease. Br J Surg. 2010;97(4):563–8.
66. Lesperance K, Martin MJ, Lehmann R, Brounts L, Steele SR. National trends and outcomes for the surgical therapy of ileocolonic Crohn's disease: a population-based analysis of laparoscopic vs. open approaches. J Gastrointest Surg. 2009;13(7):1251–9.
67. Maartense S, Dunker MS, Slors JF, Cuesta MA, Pierik EG, Gouma DJ, et al. Laparoscopic-assisted versus open ileocolic resection for Crohn's disease: a randomized trial. Ann Surg. 2006;243(2):143–9. discussion 50-3
68. Milsom JW, Hammerhofer KA, Bohm B, Marcello P, Elson P, Fazio VW. Prospective, randomized trial comparing laparoscopic vs. conventional surgery for refractory ileocolic Crohn's disease. Dis Colon Rectum. 2001;44(1):1–8. discussion -9
69. Polle SW, Wind J, Ubbink DT, Hommes DW, Gouma DJ, Bemelman WA. Short-term outcomes after laparoscopic ileocolic resection for Crohn's disease. A systematic review. Dig Surg. 2006;23(5–6):346–57.
70. Schmidt CM, Talamini MA, Kaufman HS, Lilliemoe KD, Learn P, Bayless T. Laparoscopic surgery for Crohn's disease: reasons for conversion. [erratum appears in Ann Surg 2001 Aug; 234(2):following table of contents]. Ann Surg. 2001;233(6):733–9.
71. Stocchi L, Milsom JW, Fazio VW. Long-term outcomes of laparoscopic versus open ileocolic resection for Crohn's disease: follow-up of a prospective randomized trial. Surgery. 2008;144(4):622–7. discussion 7-8
72. Tilney HS, Constantinides VA, Heriot AG, Nicolaou M, Athanasiou T, Ziprin P, et al. Comparison of laparoscopic and open ileocecal resection for Crohn's disease: a metaanalysis. Surg Endosc. 2006;20(7):1036–44.
73. Gionchetti P, Dignass A, Danese S, On behalf of ECCO, et al. 3rd European. 3rd European evidence-based consensus on the diagnosis and Management of Crohn's disease 2016: part 2: surgical management and special situations. J Crohns Colitis. 2016;11(2):1–16. https://doi.org/10.1093/ecco-jcc/jjw169.
74. Maconi G, Carsana L, Fociani P, Sampietro GM, Ardizzone S, Cristaldi M, et al. Small bowel stenosis in Crohn's disease: clinical, biochemical and ultrasonographic evaluation of histological features. Aliment Pharmacol Ther. 2003;18(7):749–56.
75. Maconi G, Sampietro GM, Parente F, Pompili G, Russo A, Cristaldi M, et al. Contrast radiology, computed tomography and ultrasonography in detecting internal fistulas and intra-abdominal abscesses in Crohn's disease: a prospective comparative study. Am J Gastroenterol. 2003;98(7):1545–55.

76. Maconi G, Sampietro GM, Sartani A, Bianchi Porro G. Bowel ultrasound in Crohn's disease: surgical perspective. Int J Color Dis. 2008;23(4):339–47.
77. Parente F, Greco S, Molteni M, Anderloni A, Sampietro GM, Danelli PG, et al. Oral contrast enhanced bowel ultrasonography in the assessment of small intestine Crohn's disease. A prospective comparison with conventional ultrasound, x ray studies, and ileocolonoscopy. Gut. 2004;53(11):1652–7.
78. Parente F, Greco S, Molteni M, Cucino C, Maconi G, Sampietro GM, et al. Role of early ultrasound in detecting inflammatory intestinal disorders and identifying their anatomical location within the bowel. Aliment Pharmacol Ther. 2003;18(10):1009–16.
79. Parente F, Maconi G, Bollani S, Anderloni A, Sampietro G, Cristaldi M, et al. Bowel ultrasound in assessment of Crohn's disease and detection of related small bowel strictures: a prospective comparative study versus x ray and intraoperative findings. Gut. 2002;50(4):490–5.
80. Rimola J, Rodriguez S, Cabanas ML, Ayuso C, Panes J, Cuatrecasas M. MRI of Crohn's disease: from imaging to pathology. Abdom Imaging. 2012;37(3):387–96.
81. Clarke BW, Cassara JE, Morgan DR. Crohn's disease of the esophagus with esophagobronchial fistula formation: a case report and review of the literature. Gastrointest Endosc. 2010;71(1):207–9.
82. De Felice KM, Katzka DA, Raffals LE. Crohn's disease of the Esophagus: clinical features and treatment outcomes in the biologic era. Inflamm Bowel Dis. 2015;21(9):2106–13.
83. Decker GA, Loftus EV Jr, Pasha TM, Tremaine WJ, Sandborn WJ. Crohn's disease of the esophagus: clinical features and outcomes. Inflamm Bowel Dis. 2001;7(2):113–9.
84. Fichera A, Michelassi F. Surgical treatment of Crohn's disease. J Gastrointest Surg. 2007;11(6):791–803.
85. Poggioli G, Stocchi L, Laureti S, Selleri S, Marra C, Salone MC, et al. Duodenal involvement of Crohn's disease: three different clinicopathologic patterns. Dis Colon Rectum. 1997;40(2):179–83.
86. Remes-Troche JM, Martinez-Benitez B, Valdovinos-Diaz MA. Crohn's disease of the esophagus. Gastroenterology. 2006;130(4):1029. 376
87. Rieder F, Hamer O, Gelbmann C, Scholmerich J, Gross V, Feuerbach S, et al. Crohn's disease of the esophagus: treatment of an esophagobronchial fistula with the novel liquid embolic polymer "onyx". Zeitschrift fur Gastroenterologie. 2006;44(7):599–602.
88. Shapiro M, Greenstein AJ, Byrn J, Corona J, Greenstein AJ, Salky B, et al. Surgical management and outcomes of patients with duodenal Crohn's disease. J Am Coll Surg. 2008;207(1):36–42.
89. van Hogezand RA, Witte AM, Veenendaal RA, Wagtmans MJ, Lamers CB. Proximal Crohn's disease: review of the clinicopathologic features and therapy. Inflamm Bowel Dis. 2001;7(4):328–37.
90. Alexander-Williams J. The technique of intestinal strictureplasty. Int J Color Dis. 1986;1(1):54–7.
91. Cristaldi M, Sampietro GM, Danelli PG, Bollani S, Bianchi Porro G, Taschieri AM. Long-term results and multivariate analysis of prognostic factors in 138 consecutive patients operated on for Crohn's disease using "bowel-sparing" techniques. Am J Surg. 2000;179(4):266–70.
92. Di Abriola GF, De Angelis P, Dall'oglio L, Di Lorenzo M. Strictureplasty: an alternative approach in long segment bowel stenosis Crohn's disease. J Pediatr Surg. 2003;38(5):814–8.
93. Fazio VW, Galandiuk S. Strictureplasty in diffuse Crohn's jejunoileitis. Dis Colon Rectum. 1985;28(7):512–8.
94. Hotokezaka M, Ikeda T, Uchiyama S, Hayakawa S, Tsuchiya K, Chijiiwa K. Side-to-side-to-end strictureplasty for Crohn's disease. Dis Colon Rectum. 2009;52(11):1882–6.
95. Lee EC, Papaioannou N. Minimal surgery for chronic obstruction in patients with extensive or universal Crohn's disease. Ann R Coll Surg Engl. 1982;64(4):229–33.
96. Michelassi F, Taschieri A, Tonelli F, Sasaki I, Poggioli G, Fazio V, et al. An international, multicenter, prospective, observational study of the side-to-side isoperistaltic strictureplasty in Crohn's disease. Dis Colon Rectum. 2007;50(3):277–84.

97. Sampietro GM, Cristaldi M, Maconi G, Parente F, Sartani A, Ardizzone S, et al. A prospective, longitudinal study of nonconventional strictureplasty in Crohn's disease. J Am Coll Surg. 2004;199(1):8–20. discussion -2
98. Sampietro GM, Cristaldi M, Porretta T, Montecamozzo G, Danelli P, Taschieri AM. Early perioperative results and surgical recurrence after strictureplasty and miniresection for complicated Crohn's disease. Dig Surg. 2000;17(3):261–7.
99. Tonelli F, Fazi M, Di Martino C. Ileocecal strictureplasty for Crohn's disease: long-term results and comparison with ileocecal resection. World J Surg. 2010;34(12):2860–6.
100. Fazio VW, Marchetti F, Church M, Goldblum JR, Lavery C, Hull TL, et al. Effect of resection margins on the recurrence of Crohn's disease in the small bowel. A randomized controlled trial. Ann Surg. 1996;224(4):563–71. discussion 71-3
101. Choy PY, Bissett IP, Docherty JG, Parry BR, Merrie A, Fitzgerald A. Stapled versus handsewn methods for ileocolic anastomoses. Cochrane Database Syst Rev. 2011;9:CD004320.
102. Simillis C, Jacovides M, Reese GE, Yamamoto T, Tekkis PP. Meta-analysis of the role of granulomas in the recurrence of Crohn disease. Dis Colon Rectum. 2010;53(2):177–85.
103. Andersson P, Olaison G, Hallbook O, Sjodahl R. Segmental resection or subtotal colectomy in Crohn's colitis? Dis Colon Rectum. 2002;45(1):47–53.
104. de Oca J, Sanchez-Santos R, Rague JM, Biondo S, Pares D, Osorio A, et al. Long-term results of ileal pouch-anal anastomosis in Crohn's disease. Inflamm Bowel Dis. 2003;9(3):171–5.
105. Kiran RP, Nisar PJ, Church JM, Fazio VW. The role of primary surgical procedure in maintaining intestinal continuity for patients with Crohn's colitis. Ann Surg. 2011;253(6):1130–5.
106. Martel P, Betton PO, Gallot D, Malafosse M. Crohn's colitis: experience with segmental resections; results in a series of 84 patients. J Am Coll Surg. 2002;194(4):448–53.
107. Panis Y, Poupard B, Nemeth J, Lavergne A, Hautefeuille P, Valleur P. Ileal pouch/anal anastomosis for Crohn's disease. Lancet. 1996;347(9005):854–7.
108. Polle SW, Slors JF, Weverling GJ, Gouma DJ, Hommes DW, Bemelman WA. Recurrence after segmental resection for colonic Crohn's disease. Br J Surg. 2005;92(9):1143–9.
109. Prudhomme M, Dehni N, Dozois RR, Tiret E, Parc R. Causes and outcomes of pouch excision after restorative proctocolectomy. Br J Surg. 2006;93(1):82–6.
110. Tekkis PP, Purkayastha S, Lanitis S, Athanasiou T, Heriot AG, Orchard TR, et al. A comparison of segmental vs subtotal/total colectomy for colonic Crohn's disease: a meta-analysis. Color Dis. 2006;8(2):82–90.
111. Cahill C, Gordon PH, Petrucci A, Boutros M. Small bowel adenocarcinoma and Crohn's disease: any further ahead than 50 years ago? World J Gastroenterol. 2014;20(33):11486–95.
112. Canavan C, Abrams KR, Mayberry J. Meta-analysis: colorectal and small bowel cancer risk in patients with Crohn's disease. Aliment Pharmacol Ther. 2006;23(8):1097–104.
113. Dossett LA, White LM, Welch DC, Herline AJ, Muldoon RL, Schwartz DA, et al. Small bowel adenocarcinoma complicating Crohn's disease: case series and review of the literature. Am Surg. 2007;73(11):1181–7.
114. Widmar M, Greenstein AJ, Sachar DB, Harpaz N, Bauer JJ, Greenstein AJ. Small bowel adenocarcinoma in Crohn's disease. J Gastrointest Surg. 2011;15(5):797–802.
115. Connelly TM, Koltun WA. The surgical treatment of inflammatory bowel disease-associated dysplasia. Expert Rev Gastroenterol Hepatol. 2013;7(4):307–21. quiz 22
116. Kavanagh DO, Carter MC, Keegan D, Doherty G, Smith MJ, Hyland JM, et al. Management of colorectal cancer in patients with inflammatory bowel disease. Tech Coloproctol. 2014;18(1):23–8.
117. Kiran RP, Nisar PJ, Goldblum JR, Fazio VW, Remzi FH, Shen B, et al. Dysplasia associated with Crohn's colitis: segmental colectomy or more extended resection? Ann Surg. 2012;256(2):221–6.
118. Maser EA, Sachar DB, Kruse D, Harpaz N, Ullman T, Bauer JJ. High rates of metachronous colon cancer or dysplasia after segmental resection or subtotal colectomy in Crohn's colitis. Inflamm Bowel Dis. 2013;19(9):1827–32.

119. Van Cutsem E, Nordlinger B, Cervantes A, Group EGW. Advanced colorectal cancer: ESMO clinical practice guidelines for treatment. Ann Oncol. 2010;21(Suppl 5):v93–7.
120. Stallmach A, Hagen S, Gharbi A, et al. Medical and surgical therapy of inflammatory bowel disease in the elderly – prospects and complications. J Crohns Colitis. 2011;5:177–88.
121. Rieder F, Latella G, Magro F, Yuksel ES, Higgins PD, Di Sabatino A, et al. European Crohn's and Colitis Organisation topical review on prediction, diagnosis and management of fibrostenosing Crohn's disease. J Crohns Colitis. 2016;10:873–5.

Diverticulosis and Diverticulitis 13

Binda Gian Andrea, Cassini Diletta, Gianandrea Baldazzi,
and Nascimbeni Riccardo

13.1 Definitions

According to the currently accepted definition, "diverticulosis" is merely the presence of colonic diverticula; "diverticular disease (DD)" is defined as clinically significant and symptomatic diverticulosis. Diverticular disease may be subclassified into symptomatic uncomplicated diverticular disease (SUDD) and symptomatic complicated diverticular disease (perforation, fistula, obstruction, bleeding) [1]. Diagnosis and treatment of colonic diverticulitis in older patients may be more difficult than in young patients because of more frequent comorbidities. Precise diagnosis and accurate treatment of colonic diverticular disease are important topics in geriatric clinical practice [2].

13.2 Epidemiology

Diverticulosis of the colon is one of the most common diseases of the digestive tract, and its frequency increases with age. The prevalence of diverticulosis and diverticular disease is increasing in Western countries in parallel with increased

B.G. Andrea (✉)
Department of Surgery, Galliera Hospital, Genoa, Italy
e-mail: gian.andrea.binda@galliera.it

C. Diletta • G. Baldazzi
Department of General Minimally-invasive and Robotic Surgery, Policlinic of Abano Terme, Padua, Italy

N. Riccardo
Department of Molecular & Translational Medicine, University of Brescia, Brescia, Italy

A. Crucitti (ed.), *Surgical Management of Elderly Patients*,
https://doi.org/10.1007/978-3-319-60861-7_13

life expectancy; several studies confirmed these data. This is particularly true in industrialized Western countries where the incidence of diverticular disease increases with age; the disease is uncommon in those under the age of 40, the prevalence of which is estimated at approximately 5%; this increases to 65% in those over 65 years of age [3]. A recent, large study on 1091 patients who underwent CT colonography for various reasons has demonstrated a steady increase of the disease prevalence parallel with ageing and, moreover, has found that age was the strongest predictor of diverticula. The diverticula incidence appears to be higher than expected without significant differences according to gender. As regards anatomic distribution, in the Western population, right colon diverticula do not appear to be an uncommon finding, with their prevalence again increasing with patient age. In asymptomatic patients, the highest prevalence of severe diverticulosis was found in the left-sided colon in the sixth and seventh decades. In particular, prevalence was 17.5–20.8% in the sigmoid colon, 15.7–16.2% in the descending colon, 9.7–8.7% in the transverse colon, 6.7–9.8% in the ascending colon and 6.7–7.5% in the caecum [4].

An epidemiological study in the USA has shown that frequency of diverticulitis and diverticular bleeding increases with age [5]. According to another study, age was associated with an increased risk of local and systemic complications [6].

13.2.1 Hospitalization

Diverticular disease and its complications are a relevant cause of hospitalization and not without mortality, particularly in elderly patients [7]. An epidemiological study in the USA has shown that diverticular disease imposes an impressive clinical burden. According to the data from the 2004 National Hospital Discharge Survey, it is responsible for 312,000 admissions and 1.5 million days of inpatient care per year [1]. The annual cost of treatment within the USA is estimated at over 2.6 billion dollars per year [2]. Nowadays whereas the overall number of hospitalizations is declining, the hospitalizations due to diverticular disease and diverticulitis are rising, especially in younger patients [8, 9]. Etzioni et al. reported a 26% increase in admissions coded as acute diverticulitis from 1998 to 2005 (120,500–151,000 admissions). The greatest increase in admissions was in the age ranges of 15–44 and 45–64 years [8]. A further study of NIS data from 1998 to 2005 reported an overall age-adjusted increase in hospital admissions from 61.8 per 100,000 to 75.5 per 100,000 hospitalizations, with equal gender and age distribution [9].

On the other hand, the temporal trends of prevalence of hospitalization for diverticulitis and its complications among elderly patients have been stable during the last decade, except those for bleeding which is becoming more frequent especially among octogenarians [5].

13.3 Pathogenesis

13.3.1 Diverticulosis and Diverticular Disease

As regards pathogenesis, it is well known that diverticula develop at well-defined points of weakness, which correspond to where the vasa recta enter the circular muscle layer of the colon. Change in the extracellular matrix and altered collagen structure with age partly explains this pattern. In addition, emerging evidence suggests that vascular smooth muscle cell behaviour is modified by age. Abnormal colonic motility is another important predisposing factor in the development of diverticula. On this basis, several authors speculate that ageing could be a prominent risk factor for both cardiovascular disease and diverticulosis [10].

Higher prevalence of diverticulosis in older subjects is consistent with several observations. Changes in traditional lifestyle and diet of Western populations probably play some role, of course under the influence of genetic factors [7], but to date, the inherent genetic risk remains unknown [11].

Another risk factor called into play is the Western toilet, described as an unnatural method of defecation [12]. Moreover, current studies have demonstrated a strong association between smoking and symptomatic diverticular disease. In his Swedish cohort study on 4209 individuals with a diagnosis of symptomatic diverticular disease, Humes [13] demonstrated that smoking is associated with symptomatic diverticular disease with an increased risk of developing complicated diverticular disease. In fact, heavy smokers (≥15 cigarettes a day) had a 1.6-fold increased risk of developing symptomatic diverticular disease compared with nonsmokers.

About cardiovascular disease as a risk factor, several studies have provided evidence suggesting a link between diverticular disease and cardiovascular disease. The pathogeneses of diverticular disease and cardiovascular disease are multifactorial and complex. Chronic inflammation contributes to both diseases, particularly in the elderly. As regards physiologic changes, Aldoori et al. [14] found that overall physical inactivity was associated with the risk of diverticular disease, while Williams et al. [15] demonstrated that vigorous physical activity was inversely associated with the risk of incident diverticular disease among older men and women. Obesity is also a significant risk factor for diverticulitis and diverticular bleeding. The Health Care Professionals Follow-Up Study demonstrated after an 18-year follow-up that subjects with a BMI >30 kg/m^2 had a significantly increased risk of developing diverticulitis or diverticular bleeding compared with those with a BMI of <21 kg/m^2 [16]. Moreover, a Swedish study confirmed that a BMI > 30 kg/m^2 increased the risk of being hospitalized with symptomatic diverticular disease over a 28-year follow-up [17].

As regards comorbidity, atherosclerosis is considered the main cause of diverticular bleeding, but also cerebrovascular disease and hyperuricemia are significant predictors of diverticular bleeding [18].

A recent meta-analysis has demonstrated that various medications of common use, especially in aged persons, are implicated in complications of diverticular disease, with pooled data showing significantly increased odds of perforation and abscess formation with steroids (OR: 9.08), opioids (OR: 2.52) and NSAIDs (OR: 2.49). Increased odds of diverticular bleeding from NSAIDs (OR = 2.69), aspirin (OR = 3.24) and calcium-channel blockers (OR = 2.50) were also demonstrated [19].

All factors associated with the development of diverticulitis and complications should be explored in subjects presenting with symptoms of diverticulitis, as they may facilitate diagnosis and suggest possible evolution of disease. Intuitively in aged persons, these roles harbour an enhanced meaning and should be carefully weighed together with outcome predictors.

13.3.2 Complicated Diverticular Disease

In general, of patients with diverticula, 80–85% remain asymptomatic, while, for unknown reasons, only three-fourths of the remaining 15–20% of patients develop symptomatic diverticular disease comparatively. It is estimated that 10–30% of patients with diverticulosis will suffer from complications such as diverticulitis and gastrointestinal bleeding, and the associated mortality is estimated at 23,600 deaths per year in Europe [20].

Elderly patients are traditionally thought to be most commonly affected not only by diverticulosis but also by diverticular disease and its complications. The increased risk of diverticulitis, of its septic complications and bleeding in the elderly has been associated with several factors inherent to physiologic changes, comorbidities and chronic medical treatments typical of advanced age.

Moreover, older patients with diverticulitis and complications are at a higher risk of poor outcome [6]. Even if in several studies the impact of age may have been confounded by comorbidity, a large population study, based on the English “Hospital Episode Statistics” database between 1996 and 2006, has demonstrated that age per se is an important predictor of mortality, extended length of stay and early readmission [21]. More specifically, the authors showed that the largest number of admissions was in the 70–79 age group, but the worst outcomes were in the oldest over 80 patients. Further independent predictors of poor outcomes were comorbidity, as measured by the Charlson Index, emergency admission and emergency surgery. The authors concluded that these factors should be identified, allowing management modification to optimize outcomes. Another population study in Olmsted County, Minnesota, found that among people with diverticulitis, the risk of death was greater in older people (HR per decade 2.12; 95% CI, 2.00–2.25, $p < 0.001$) [6].

In accordance with the overall risk of mortality of older patients with diverticulitis, emergent colorectal surgery in the elderly is associated with significant morbidity and mortality [22]. In octogenarians, up to sixfold higher mortality rate has been reported after emergency colorectal surgery [23]. According to these studies, identification of high-risk individuals, aggressive resuscitation and prompt treatment may help in optimizing the outcome of elderly patients undergoing emergency colorectal surgery.

13.4 Elective Surgery

13.4.1 Indications

The indications for elective colectomy following diverticulitis are debated. Guidelines drawn up in the 1990s recommended performing an elective sigmoid resection after two episodes of acute diverticulitis, after a single episode in young patients or in case of chronic complications, such as stenosis or fistulas. These guidelines were based on the following wrong assumptions:

1. Recurrence rate after every episode is at least 33%;
2. Every recurrence means a higher risk of perforation and other acute complications.
3. Complicated diverticulitis is associated with high morbidity and mortality [24]. Therefore, an elective sigmoid resection could prevent mortality and permanent colostomy.

More recently, these recommendations have been challenged because a new data on the natural history of diverticulitis have shown that most severe complications, such as free perforation, do not occur after recurrences but at the first attack of acute diverticulitis. In fact, the rate of diverticulitis recurrence after resection (5–11%) is similar to the rate of recurrent hospitalized events (4–13%) for those who did not have elective resection [25]. Modelled analyses have shown that elective colectomy has little value as a prophylactic measure since its rising rate does not correlate with decreases in emergency hospitalization and colectomy [8, 26]. Recent studies have confirmed that the risk of emergency colectomy is greatest at the initial episode of diverticulitis, with 80–90% of emergency procedures being performed in patients without prior hospitalization [27]. Furthermore, conservative management of recurrent nonperforated diverticulitis is associated with low rates of morbidity and mortality [28] advocating a more individualised and conservative approach [29].

Currently it seems clear that those patients treated conservatively for acute diverticulitis but still complaining of symptoms that are well correlated to colonic stenosis or fistulas to hollow organs are good candidates for elective surgery. An elective sigmoid resection should be performed also in patients with recurrent diverticular bleeding.

When surgery is contemplated, the number of attacks of acute diverticulitis seems less important than the severity of the complaints and patient-related risk factors.

Despite these recommendations leading to increasing support for nonoperative management of uncomplicated diverticulitis, early elective surgery still appears to be a common practice. In a recent retrospective cohort of hospitalized diverticulitis, Simianu [30, 31] and coworkers found that 56.3% of elective resections for diverticulitis occurred in patients with fewer than three episodes, confirming that the incidence of elective colectomy has more than doubled [8], despite suggestions from actual guidelines [29, 32–34].

As regards patient-related factors, age and certain comorbid conditions may be associated with a more hazardous course of diverticular disease. Patients older than 70 years have higher mortality rates, although this does not seem to be an independent factor [35].

Moreover, the presence of other comorbidities, such as chronic renal failure, diabetes, collagen-vascular diseases or use of steroids and NSAIDs (nonsteroidal anti-inflammatory drugs), has been associated with an increased risk of perforation and mortality in diverticular disease [27].

Several authors postulated that the threshold to recommend and undergo surgical resection for diverticulitis might be lowered by the availability of laparoscopy. This hypothesis originated from evidence that in the USA and in other countries, the widespread practice of laparoscopic resection has been associated with higher rates of elective surgery for diverticulitis [36, 37]. A recent large cohort suggests that the number of previous episodes should not drive the decision whether or not to approach resection for diverticulitis laparoscopically [38].

Given the substantial discrepancies in how episodes are counted, a better approach to determining the actual clinical burden of diverticulitis on patients may be evaluation of the healthy time between episodes. A normal interval between episodes has not yet been described. Similarly, a time-based interval definition of smouldering diverticulitis has not been proposed. Rather, this recognised entity is defined by rebound symptoms when the treatment is withdrawn or a more rapid recurrence of diverticulitis occurs in typical patients. This debate is particularly relevant because most elderly patients with newly diagnosed diverticulitis do not have recurrences and do not undergo operations for their disease.

Lidor et al. [39] followed 16,048 individuals after an episode of diverticulitis for an average of 19.2 months; their mean age was 77.8 years, 14.0% of them underwent surgery, and 82.5% had no further recurrences. Of patients initially managed nonoperatively, 97% did not have surgery. Individuals treated as outpatients upon first presentation and patients ≥80 were significantly less likely to have recurrent episodes and were less likely to require an operation. Authors concluded that the majority of elderly patients newly diagnosed with diverticulitis did not require surgery nor experience recurrent episodes. The apparent benign course of this disease in this population suggests that a conservative approach to the management may be appropriate. Accordingly, a recent consensus in Italy concludes that there is no role for prophylactic interval colectomy after one or more episodes of acute diverticulitis, and the decision to perform elective resection after one or more episodes of AD should be undertaken on a "case-by-case" basis statement (EL 2b—RG B) [7, 34].

On the other hand, the Sigma trial and previous studies have demonstrated very low mortality rates after elective resection for diverticular disease even in such high-risk patients, who should be thus considered good candidates for an elective sigmoid resection when responding to individualized criteria mentioned above [40]. Patient's quality of life and anxiety about future episodes may also be considered as important factors in decision making related to early, elective surgery.

13.4.2 Principles of Surgical Technique

As far as timing is concerned, in order to minimize the risk of intraoperative complications, caused by oedema, acute inflammation, adhesions causing difficulty in identifying the right planes and ureter and any resulting perioperative complications (fistula, leakage, haematoma or abscess), it is important to choose the optimal time for elective surgery. A prospective comparison of early and late laparoscopic resection showed a significantly higher rate of anastomotic leak, abdominal abscess, hospital stay and conversion rate during early elective surgery [41]. Similar results have been reported by Zingg et al. [42].

Surgical technique does not differ greatly from the standard open approach to the minimally invasive approach. As this is for a benign disease, the dissection should be close to the colonic wall, to avoid ureteric injury. Consideration should be given to preoperative (or intraoperative) ureteric stenting if a diverticular phlegmon or colo-vesical fistula is suspected. In order to avoid recurrence, resection should be extended to the upper rectum [43]. Sacrifice of the inferior mesenteric artery or superior rectal artery has not been shown to affect rates of anastomotic leak [44, 45]; however, patients may have a better functional outcome if the vessels are preserved [46, 47]. Mobilisation of the splenic flexure may be required to allow for a tension-free anastomosis [48].

A left colic resection for diverticular disease must provide for the resection of all the sigmoid tract, a resection that can be extended proximally if it involves inflammation of the descending colon. The simple presence of diverticula is not an indication for a more proximal extension of the resection.

The vascular time may foresee the conservation of the left colic artery or even the whole mesenteric and rectal arteries with bindings exclusively of sigmoid arteries. The ligation of the inferior mesenteric artery is not mandatory in elective sigmoidectomy for diverticulitis but can facilitate identification of the ureter in complex diverticulitis: however, its preservation may improve the blood supply of the anastomosis and avoid damage to the pre-aortic nerves. In a recent meta-analysis [45], the leak rate was 7.3% in the patients with preservation of the inferior mesenteric artery versus 11.3% in the ligation group, a difference which was not statistically significant. For this reason, there is limited evidence that there may be a benefit in preserving the inferior mesenteric artery.

A colorectal anastomosis is then performed using a circular stapler of adequate size (at least 2.8 cm) introduced to the transanal way after having positioned the anvil of the stapler in the descending colon prior to packaging a colonic suture.

At the end of the procedure, a pneumatic test can be performed, by introducing air through the anus, having first filled the pelvic cavity with water: if bubbles appear, a simple suture of the hole, if clearly visible, or a protective ostomy can be performed. The intervention concludes with the positioning of drainage in the pelvic cavity and the closure to anatomical layers of the abdominal wall.

Laparoscopic access for elective colon resection could be recommended for uncomplicated diverticulitis, but it has to be performed by well-trained surgeons. Laparoscopy has short-term advantages over open surgery in terms of blood loss, post-operative ileus, morbidity, hospital stay and overall costs (1B) [34]. Two randomised controlled trials [49, 50] demonstrated less blood loss, less pain (fewer analgesic requirements), shorter hospital stay and improved quality of life. Conversion rates are in the order of approximately 9% but may be much lower in expert hands. The results of the Sigma trial [40] suggested a 15.4% reduction in major complications and a 27% reduction in major morbidity with no difference in late outcomes at 6-month follow-up.

A recent meta-analysis comprising 19 studies (2383 patients) comparing open and laparoscopic sigmoid colectomy demonstrates that laparoscopic sigmoid resection is safe and has fewer post- operative surgical complications in terms of wound infection, post-operative ileus, transfusion requirements and incisional hernia (3%) [51, 52]. A systematic review of case-control studies [53] reports the findings of the above RCTs with lower overall morbidity and fewer minor complications in the laparoscopic group. A retrospective review of ACS-NSQIP data demonstrates a lower risk of complications (major wound, respiratory, cardiovascular and sepsis) in patients undergoing laparoscopic resection with primary anastomosis [54].

Hand-assisted laparoscopic surgery maintains the advantages of laparoscopy in complicated disease while avoiding conversion to open surgery in very inflamed and laparoscopically challenging operative fields. A systematic review of hand-assisted laparoscopic surgery in colonic surgery [55] suggests it may be useful especially in complicated diverticular disease [56, 57]. Compared to open surgery, hand-assisted laparoscopic surgery colectomy is associated with shorter hospital stay, smaller incision lengths, faster recovery of gastrointestinal function, less analgesic requirements, less blood loss and lower post-operative pain scores [58].

Single-incision laparoscopic surgery for diverticular disease has been performed although the evidence is limited to small case series demonstrating feasibility and safety of the technique [59, 60].

Actually, there is little experience and few papers about the use of the robotic approach in diverticulitis, but there are some reasons to use that approach: to simplify a challenging situation, lower conversion rate, simplify pelvic stitch (fistula), avoid ureter injury (0.3–1.5%) and improve sexual and urinary outcomes [61]. The conversion rate is 6% in laparoscopic approach versus 2% with robotic technique, considering that the degree of inflammation and BMI [62] are the most important risk factors. In surgery for fistula as well, conversion rate is higher in laparoscopic (14–61%) versus robotic (0–4%) procedures [63]. Robotic colorectal surgery in diverticulitis is a safe and feasible option, but longer operation time and high costs are the main actual limitations to employing it.

13.5 Treatment of Diverticulitis, Diverticular Bleeding and Septic Complications in Elderly Patients

13.5.1 Outpatient Treatment of Acute Uncomplicated Diverticulitis

Between 1998 and 2005 in the USA, there have been 323,097 hospital admissions for diverticulitis, and more than 50% of them were in elderly patients [64].

While outpatient treatment of patients with uncomplicated acute diverticulitis appears to be safe in younger patients [65], in elderly ones it is still a matter of debate. The following parameters should be considered in making this decision: patient's presentation, ability to tolerate oral intake, comorbidity and adequate outpatient support. Based on these criteria, elderly patients have a high probability of needing hospital admission for adequate treatment. Hence, hospitalization for uncomplicated diverticulitis is recommended if the patient is over 75 years of age, especially if she/he has comorbidity [66]. According to several other authors, however, treatment of elderly patients with uncomplicated diverticulitis at home may be safe and effective even in the presence of associated but stabilized comorbidity (cardiopathy, diabetes, renal failure, etc.) [67]. This may be facilitated by the presence of Hospital at Home or other outpatient support services.

In patients with uncomplicated diverticulitis who are clinically stable and able to tolerate fluids, outpatient treatment is based on broad-spectrum antibiotics covering anaerobes and gram-negative rods for 7–10 days and a clear liquid diet. Patients should improve within 48–72 h, at which time solid foods may be cautiously introduced. Close follow-up is considered crucial: patients experiencing increasing pain, fever or inability to tolerate oral fluids should be promptly hospitalized [66].

13.5.2 In-Hospital Treatment of Acute Uncomplicated Diverticulitis

Hospitalization is recommended if patients show signs of significant inflammation, are unable to take oral fluid, are over 75 years of age or have significant comorbidity (diabetes, chronic renal failure, malignant haematological diseases, HIV infection, chemotherapy, steroid therapy, transplant). Treatment options are triaged according to severity of clinical and radiologic findings.

Contrast-enhanced computer tomography with multi-detector technology is the first-line colonic examination [7] and offers a comprehensive evaluation of uncomplicated and complicated forms [68]. The severity of diverticulitis on CT scan is also statistically predictive of the risk of medical treatment failure during the acute phase and of the chances of bad secondary outcome after a successful medical treatment of the first episode [69].

In case of acute uncomplicated diverticulitis, as in patients with acute complicated diverticulitis who do require emergency surgery, bowel rest, intravenous antibiotics and intravenous fluid support are mandatory. Improvement of symptoms should be expected within 2–4 days, at which point a solid diet can be progressively reintroduced. If improvement continues, patients may be discharged to complete a 7–10-day oral antibiotics course. Those not responding within 2–4 days require surgical consultation.

13.5.3 Management of Septic Complications

Septic complications of diverticulitis include abscess and free perforation with peritonitis. They are among the most frequent causes of severe abdominal sepsis in elderly patients, which accounts for a mortality rate ranging from 54 to over 90%. Recently, Ukkonen and coworkers have shown that hospital and 1-year mortality rates of patients with abdominal sepsis increased with age, being over 90% in subjects aged 80 years or more. The mortality was higher in patients with comorbidities including cardiac, chronic pulmonary and chronic renal diseases and in those on cancer chemotherapy [70].

Moreover, it is estimated that 22–28% of patients with diverticular disease [25], presenting with septic complications, will require an urgent operation. These complications are associated not only with increased mortality and need for surgery but also with prolonged hospital stays, increased intensive care requirements and increased costs.

Even if specific outcome data and evidence-based indications in the elderly are scarce, it is widely recognised that rapid diagnosis, proper treatment with both antibiotics and supportive therapy and source control are crucial. In the elderly, however, physiological aspects and poor cooperation may interfere with the diagnostic and therapeutic process.

When there is a suspicion of intra-abdominal sepsis, an urgent CT study reduces diagnostic delay and guides the appropriate measures in order to rapidly control the source of infection.

13.5.4 Treatment of Diverticular Abscesses

Diverticular abscesses are associated with an acute mortality of 5–10% [71] but are also associated with a high risk of recurrences and further disease complications [72]. Patients with a CT diagnosis of diverticular abscess have three treatment options: (a) diverticular abscesses with a diameter of 3–4 cm or less should be medically treated with broad-spectrum antibiotics, (b) diverticular abscesses with a diameter of 4 cm or larger should undergo percutaneous-guided drainage (PGD) and (c) diverticular abscesses not amenable of or not responding to nonoperative treatment (including PGD) should undergo surgery with bowel resection.

In 2014, a systematic review showed that percutaneous drainage was successful in 49% of patients (diameter > 3 cm) and antibiotic therapy in 14% of patients. An urgent surgery during the index hospitalization was performed in 30% of patients, elective resection in 36% and no surgery in 35%. Recurrence rates were as high as 39% in patients awaiting elective resection and 18% in the non-surgery group, with an overall recurrence rate of 28%. Of the whole cohort, only 28% had no surgery and no recurrence during follow-up [71]. A recent series confirmed that recurrences after medical treatment are frequent and may be more severe than the index presentation [72]. On the other hand, previous retrospective studies have shown that percutaneous CT-guided (or US-guided) drainage of diverticular abscesses is safe and effective in treating acute intra-abdominal sepsis, bridging patients to elective single-stage resection [73–76].

The size of the abscesses is an important determinant of success of treatment: those of 4 cm or more in diameter are less likely to be associated with successful antibiotic treatment alone and more likely to be amenable to percutaneous-guided drainage [73–75]. Besides the size of abscess, other factors may influence the risk of nonoperative treatment failure, but the evidence is mostly based on small retrospective series. Factors associated with PGD failure have been ASA 4 (OR: 11.6) [77], pelvic location of abscess [76], systemic features of inflammation [75], immunosuppression and chronic kidney disease [78]. Age per se has not been associated to PGD failure.

Once it is evident that percutaneous drainage has failed, there are two options: positioning a new drain or proceeding to surgery. Both have drawbacks that must be carefully considered, especially in elderly persons. First, the number of drainage attempts is directly correlated to the risk of urgent Hartmann' resection [79]. Second, drainage failure and older age are associated with increased post-operative morbidity [77]. An elderly patient presenting with a diverticular abscess should be treated according to the criteria applied in younger subjects, and age should not dissuade surgeons from urgent action when indicated.

A controversial issue, with substantial meaning in the aged frail person, is the need of subsequent elective colectomy after a first episode of diverticular abscess, successfully treated medically or with PGD. The high risk of recurrence and further disease complications after successful nonoperative treatment advocates for an interval elective colectomy [77], whereas an expectant management is supported particularly in patients with comorbidities and a high risk for mortality [80].

Case-by-case decision making is mandatory, balancing on one side, the risk of recurrence based on the above-mentioned factors, including comorbidities and polypharmacy, and on the other side the risk of elective surgery in the aged person.

13.5.5 Treatment of Diffuse Peritonitis

Diverticular perforation and diffuse peritonitis are life-threatening conditions with a mortality rate of up to 13% for purulent contamination and 43% for fecal contamination [28, 81–85]. It requires emergency surgery, independently of patient's age. The choice of procedure to perform is based primarily on severity of peritonitis, which is most commonly graded according to Hinchey classification. Further factors that should influence the decision-making process are age, comorbidities, steroid or immunosuppressant treatments.

Resection and primary anastomosis with or without proximal fecal diversion and non-restorative sigmoid resection, namely, Hartmann's procedure, peritoneal laparoscopic lavage and less invasive stepwise strategies including damage control surgery constitute the main available armamentarium. At present time, the Hartmann's procedure remains the surgical gold standard for many surgeons as it provides removal of septic source with relative ease and safety [86, 87].

However, as far as *purulent peritonitis* is concerned, two recent, prematurely interrupted RCTs [88, 89], along with data from previous studies with weaker design [90–99], plus systematic reviews [100–102], have indicated that resection and primary anastomosis with or without proximal fecal diversion are not inferior to Hartmann's procedure, in terms of surgical efficacy and safety.

Moreover, reversal of colostomy after Hartmann's procedure adds a challenging operation, associated with relevant morbidity and mortality; as such it will never be performed in a wide proportion of patients leaving them with a permanent stoma [85, 88]. Even if ageing exerts a significant influence on physical health-related quality of life independently of single-staged or staged resection for complicated diverticulitis [100], age and comorbidities are determinants of non-reversal of Hartmann's procedure [95]. Accordingly, generally speaking resection with primary anastomosis is considered a preferable approach in most patients with purulent peritonitis, reserving the Hartmann's procedure to cases at increased risk of anastomotic leakage [103, 104]. A propensity score analysis has indicated that factors influencing the choice between Hartmann's and primary anastomosis are body mass index >30 kg/m^2, Mannheim peritonitis index >10, operative urgency and Hinchey stage >II [105]. A subsequent decision-analysis suggests that central to the operative strategy decision is an accurate calculation of the risk of complications using validated prediction models, as well as determination of patient attitudes towards complications and reversal operations [38]. Furthermore, surgical specialization remains a potent predictor of operation performed in the setting of severe acute diverticulitis [106].

Recently *laparoscopic peritoneal lavage (LPL)* with drainage and antibiotics has been introduced into the surgical practice for purulent peritonitis from diverticular colonic perforation, with the aim to decrease the rate of HP [107, 108]. In 2009, Toorenvliet's systematic review identified 231 patients with acute diverticulitis who underwent LPL, drainage and antibiotics therapy [109]. In 95.7% of patients this minimally invasive procedure permitted adequate control of the abdominal and systemic sepsis, with low rates of mortality (1.7%), morbidity (10.4%) and stoma (1.7%). Most patients subsequently had a delayed elective laparoscopic PRA. Patients who did not undergo subsequent resection had a long recurrence-free period. The authors concluded that LPL was an effective and safe treatment of peritonitis secondary to perforated diverticulitis [109]. However, the use of peritoneal lavage without primary resection in generalised peritonitis originating from perforated diverticulitis remains controversial. Recently three RCT (DILALA-trial, Scandiv-trial, LADIES trial) including a total of 343 participants (178 in the lavage group versus 175 in the resection group) have been published on this topic [110–112].

Five meta-analyses of these RCT trials have been published [113–117] that failed to demonstrate significant benefits. Overall, the quality of evidence was low due to serious concern regarding the risk of bias and imprecisions. A significantly increased rate of intra-abdominal abscess formation (RR = 2.54, 95% CI 1.34–4.83) (moderate quality of evidence) was seen with this approach. However, LPL does not appear inferior to traditional surgical resection and may achieve reasonable outcomes (lower rate of post-operative wound infections, R = 0.10, 95% CI 0.02–0.51) and less hospital resources (shorter duration of post-operative hospital stay during index admission, WMD = −2.03, 95% CI − 2.59−−1.47).

Fecal peritonitis is usually a polymicrobial infection with a high bacterial load due to the high density of Bacteroides spp., Enterobacteriaceae, and enterococci. As such, it is frequently a cause of sepsis and is associated with high mortality rates. A recent study [118] on a large cohort of patients with fecal peritonitis admitted to the European ICUs found a 6-month mortality of 31.6%. As reported in previous series of patients with abdominal sepsis [119, 120], the most significant prognostic factor in this study was increased age. In the elderly undergoing gastrointestinal surgery with severe sepsis, Ukkonen et al. reported an in-hospital mortality of 47.9% and a 1-year mortality of 64.4%, including 31.6% of the discharged patients [70].

Limited data are available to sustain a specific surgical strategy in diffuse fecal peritonitis.

In most retrospective series, the Hartmann's procedure is the first choice in patients with diverticular perforation and fecal peritonitis [100–102]. In fact, even if resection with primary anastomosis has shown similar results in terms of efficacy, when considering feculent peritonitis, the number of accrued patients is still inadequate to challenge the established use of non-restorative surgery [88, 89].

Diverticular perforation with diffuse peritonitis and severe sepsis is an extreme often-fatal infectious event, especially in an elderly subject. Patients have poor pre- and intraoperative conditions (septic shock and organ failure) and are haemodynamically unstable with a significant need for catecholamines. The ICU scoring systems (APACHE, SAPS and SOFA) and elevated lactate levels predict increased mortality, and a rapid control of source of infection is mandatory. In the past, patients deemed at high risk for the Hartmann's procedure underwent a three-stage procedure with colostomy as first stage.

A recent alternative for these "extreme" cases has been introduced as *damage control surgery* [121]. It is based on a fast procedure with peritoneal lavage, limited resection of the perforated segment with blind ending of bowel stumps or closure of the perforation site by suture, limited intestinal mobilisation and abdominal closure by vacuum-assisted systems. The decision to restore continuity or create a colostomy is postponed to an elective second-look laparotomy 24–48 h afterwards, following resuscitation at the intensive care unit. Accordingly, the decision-making process takes place in a haemodynamically stable patient with the possibility to consider the clinical course (deterioration or improvement), the comorbidities and other risk factors and to re-evaluate the local peritoneal and colonic conditions. This strategy offers the advantages of a rapid source control and a "delayed" reconstruction of bowel continuity with reduction of ostomy rate. Data are still scarce, and no specific evidence in elderly patients has been published so far, but Kafka-Ritsch have reported their 5-year experience in 2012 [122]. They showed an in-hospital mortality rate of 9.8% which compares favourably with general and peritoneal/septic conditions of patients in their series. Most notably, 76% were older than 65 years, 84% were ASA IV/V, 63% had a >25 MPI and 22% had fecal peritonitis. Furthermore, 77% of all patients and 50% of patients with fecal peritonitis were discharged with their colon reconstructed. Although further evidence is clearly needed, this emergency option may be a valuable tool when dealing with older and frail patients at high risk of septic complications.

13.6 Diagnosis and Treatment of Diverticular Bleeding

Colonic diverticula are the most typical source of lower gastrointestinal bleeding accounting for more than 40% of episodes [123, 124]. Diverticular bleeding resolves spontaneously in up to 90% of episodes but has an overall recurrence rate from 22 to 38% [125–127]. Severe haemorrhage can arise in 3–5% of patients with diverticulosis [125, 126].

Early recurring or persistent or massive bleeding usually requires interventional treatment.

The following risk factors for recurring bleeding have been identified: old age, diverticulitis, peripheral vascular disease and chronic kidney disease [128]. Several other factors, such as blood pressure medications, tachycardia, low diastolic blood pressure, low haemoglobin and INR > 1.5, may help to predict severe diverticular haemorrhage at the time of presentation [129].

Female sex, warfarin use and chronic kidney disease were associated with significantly greater risk of transfusion need, while NSAID use was associated with significantly greater risk of further bleeding during hospitalization and subsequent prolonged stay [130].

Intuitively most of those conditions are associated with advanced age.

At the present time, diagnosis of diverticular bleeding is based on contrast-enhanced computed tomography and colonoscopy. In about 30% of patients, CT can identify the diverticular source of bleeding; hence, it should precede colonoscopy to guide haemostasis in these cases [131].

Though different algorithms have been suggested, the initial management is most commonly based on support and surveillance. Once it has been established that bleeding has not stopped spontaneously, interventional endoscopy is mandatory. Endoscopic haemostatic manoeuvres, by means of epinephrine injection, multipolar or heat probe coagulation, placement of endoclips, band ligation or combinations of the above, are successful in controlling most diverticular bleeding.

If colonoscopy is not available or if it fails to reveal or control the bleeding source, further intervention is required. Usually angiographic selective embolization or intraarterial infusion of vasopressin is performed, but the subsequent risk of bowel infarction must be considered.

Surgery may be required for massive bleeding with haemodynamic instability or failure of previous treatment attempts. Segmentary resection is appropriate when the bleeding source has been identified; otherwise a subtotal colectomy has to be performed. Urgent surgery is associated with high rates of post-operative complications and mortality (10–30%).

Elective resection might be considered in patients with comorbidity and two or more episodes of diverticular haemorrhage, but surgical decision is again on a case-by-case basis.

References

1. Kohler L, Sauerland S, Neugebauer E. Diagnosis and treatment of diverticular disease: result of a consensus development conference. The scientific Committee of the European Association for endoscopic surgery. Surg Endosc. 1999;13:430–6.
2. Liu CK, Hsu HH, Cheng SM. Colonic diverticulitis in the elderly. Int J Gerontol. 2009;3:9–15.
3. Petruzziello L, Iacopini F, Bulajic M, et al. Review article: uncomplicated diverticular disease of the colon. Aliment Pharmacol Ther. 2006;23:1379–91.
4. De Cecco CN, Ciolina M, Annibale B, Rengo M, Bellini D, Muscogiuri G, Maruotti A, Saba L, Iafrate F, Laghi A. Prevalence and distribution of colonic diverticula assessed with CT colonography (CTC). Eur Radiol. 2016;26:639–45.
5. Wheat CL, Strate LL. Trends in hospitalization for diverticulitis and diverticular bleeding in the United States from 2000 to 2010. Clin Gastroenterol Hepatol. 2016;14:96–103.
6. Bharucha AE, Parthasarathy G, Ditah I, Fletcher JG, Ewelukwa O, Pendlimari R, Yawn BP, Melton LJ, Schleck C, Zinsmeister AR. Temporal trends in the incidence and natural history of diverticulitis: a population-based study. Am J Gastroenterol. 2015;110:1589–96.
7. Cuomo R, Barbara G, Pace F, et al. Italian consensus conference for colonic diverticulosis and diverticular disease. United Eur Gastroenterol J. 2014;2:413–42.
8. Etzioni DA, Mack TM, Beart RWJ, et al. Diverticulitis in the United States: 1998–2005: changing patterns of dis- ease and treatment. Ann Surg. 2009;249:210–7.
9. Nguyen GC, Steinhart AH. Nationwide patterns of hospitalizations to centers with high volume of admissions for inflammatory bowel disease and their impact on mortality. Inflamm Bowel Dis. 2008;14:1688–94.
10. Monk BA, George SJ. The effect of ageing on vascular smooth muscle cell behaviour—a mini-review. Gerontology. 2015;61:416–26.
11. Reichert MC, Lammert F. The genetic epidemiology of diverticulosis and diverticular disease: emerging evidence. United European Gastroenterol J. 2015;3:409–18.
12. Isbit J. Why diverticulosis haunts the western world. Tech Coloproctol. 2016;20:267–8.
13. Humes DJ, Ludvigsson JF, Jarvholm B. Smoking and the risk of hospitalization for symptomatic diverticular disease: a population cohort study from Sweden. Dis Colon Rectum. 2016;59:110–4.
14. Aldoori WH, Giovannucci EL, Rimm EB, Ascherio A, Stampfer MJ, Colditz GA, Wing AL, Trichopoulos DV, Willett WC. Prospective study of physical activity and the risk of symptomatic diverticular disease in men. Gut. 1995;36:276–82.
15. Williams PT. Incident diverticular disease is inversely related to vigorous physical activity. Med Sci Sports Exerc. 2009;41:1042–7.
16. Strate LL, Liu YL, Aldoori WH, Syngal S, Giovannucci EL. Obesity increases the risks of diverticulitis and diverticular bleeding. Gastroenterology. 2009;136:115–22.
17. Rosemar A, Angerås U, Rosengren A. Body mass index and diverticular disease: a 28-year follow-up study in men. Dis Colon Rectum. 2008;51:450–5.
18. Cirocchi R, Grassi V, Cavaliere D, Renzi C, Tabola R, Poli G, Avenia S, Farinella E, Arezzo A, Vettoretto N, D'Andrea V, Binda GA, Fingerhut A. New trends in acute management of colonic diverticular bleeding: a systematic review. Medicine (Baltimore). 2015;94:e1710. https://doi.org/10.1097/MD.0000000000001710.
19. Kvasnovsky CL, Papagrigoriadis S, Bjarnason I. Increased diverticular complications with nonsteriodal anti-inflammatory drugs and other medications: a systematic review and meta-analysis. Color Dis. 2014;16:189–96.
20. Delvaux M. Diverticular disease of the colon in Europe: epidemiology, impact on citizen health and prevention. Aliment Pharmacol Ther. 2003;18(Suppl 3):71.

21. Jeyarajah S, Faiz O, Bottle A, Aylin P, Bjarnason I, Tekkis PP, Papagrigoriadis S. Diverticular disease hospital admissions are increasing, with poor outcomes in the elderly and emergency admissions. Aliment Pharmacol Ther. 2009;30:1171–82.
22. McGillicuddy EA, Schuster KM, Davis KA, Longo WA. Factors predicting morbidity and mortality in emergency colorectal procedures in elderly patients. Arch Surg. 2009;144:1157–62.
23. Modini C, Romagnoli F, De Milito R, Romeo V, Petroni R, La Torre F, Catani M. Octogenarians: an increasing challenge for acute care and colorectal surgeons. An outcomes analysis of emergency colorectal surgery in the elderly. Colorect Dis. 2012;14:e312–8.
24. Wong WD, Wexner SD, Lowry A, et al. Standards task force, American Society of Colon and Rectal Surgeons. Practice parameters for the treatment of sigmoid diverticulitis: supporting documentation. Dis Colon Rectum. 2000;43:290–7.
25. Anaya DA, et al. Risk of emergency colectomy and colostomy in patients with diverticular disease. Arch Surgery. 2005;140:681–5.
26. Ricciardi R, Baxter NN, Read TE, Marcello PW, Hall J, Roberts PL. Is the decline in the surgical treatment for diverticulitis associated with an increase in complicated diverticulitis? Dis Colon Rectum. 2009;52:1558–63.
27. Morris CR, Harvey IM, Stebbings WS, et al. Epidemiology of perforated colonic diverticular disease. Postgrad Med J. 2002;78:654–8.
28. Chapman J, Davies M, Wolff B, et al. Complicated diverticulitis: is it time to rethink the rules? Ann Surg. 2005;242:576–81.
29. Rafferty J, Shellito P, Hyman NH, et al. Practice parameters for sigmoid diverticulitis. Dis Colon Rectum. 2006;49:939–44.
30. Simianu VV, Fichera A, Bastawrous AL, Davidson GH, Florence MG, Thirlby RC, Flum DR. Number of diverticulitis episodes before resection and factors associated with earlier interventions. JAMA Surg. 2016;151:604–10.
31. Simianu VV, Strate LL, Billingham RP, et al. The impact of elective colon resection on rates of emergency surgery for diverticulitis. Ann Surg. 2016;263:123–9.
32. Feingold D, Steele SR, Lee S, et al. Practice parameters for the treatment of sigmoid diverticulitis. Dis Colon Rectum. 2014;57:284–94.
33. Fozard JBJ, Armitage NC, Schofield JB, Jones OM. ACPGBI position statement on elective resection for diverticulitis. Colorectal Dis. 2011;13(Suppl 3):1–11.
34. Binda GA, Cuomo R, Laghi A, Nascimbeni R, Serventi A, Bellini D, Gervaz P, Annibale B. Practice parameters for the treatment of colonic diverticular disease: Italian Society of Colon and Rectal Surgery (SICCR) guidelines. Tech Coloproctol. 2015;19:615–26.
35. Makela JT, Kiviniemi H, Laitinen S. Prognostic factors of perforated sigmoid diverticulitis in the elderly. Dig Surg. 2005;22:100–6.
36. Kwon S, Billingham R, Farrokhi E, et al. Surgical care and outcomes assessment program (SCOAP) collaborative. Adoption of laparoscopy for elective colorectal resection: a report from the surgical care and outcomes assessment program. J Am Coll Surg. 2012;214:909–18.
37. Kehlet H, Büchler MW, Beart RW Jr, Billingham RP, Williamson R. Care after colonic operation: is it evidence-based? Results from a multinational survey in Europe and the United States. J Am Coll Surg. 2006;202:45–54.
38. Colorectal Writing Group for the SCOAP-CERTAIN Collaborative. The impact of delaying elective resection of diverticulitis on laparoscopic conversion rate. Am J Surg. 2015;209:913–8.
39. Lidor AO, Segal JB, Wu AW, Yu Q, Feinberg R, Schneider EB. Older patients with diverticulitis have low recurrence rates and rarely need surgery. Surgery. 2011;150:146–53.
40. Klarenbeek BR, Veenhof A, De Lange E, Bemelman WA, Bergamaschi R, Heres P, Lacy AM, Van den Broek WT, Van der Peet DL, Cuesta MA. The sigma-trial protocol: a prospective double-blind multi-centre comparison of laparoscopic versus open elective sigmoid resection in patients with symptomatic diverticulitis. BMC Surg. 2007;7:16.
41. Reissfelder C, Burh HJ, Ritz JP. What is the optimal time of surgical intervention after an acute attack of sigmoid diverticulitis: early or late elective laparoscopic resection? Dis Colon Rectum. 2006;49:1842–9.

42. Zingg U, Pasternak I, Guertler L, Dietrich M, Wohlwend K-A, Metzger U. Early vs, delayed elective laparoscopic-assisted colectomy in sigmoid diverticulitis: timing of surgery in relation to the acute attack. Dis Colon Rectum. 2007;50:1911–7.
43. Benn PL, Wolff BG, Ilstrup DM. Level of anastomosis and recurrent colonic diverticulitis. Am J Surg. 1986;151:269–71.
44. Lehmann RK, Brounts LR, Johnson EK, Rizzo JA, Steele SR. Does sacrifice of the inferior mesenteric artery or superior rectal artery affect anastomotic leak following sigmoidectomy for diverticulitis? A retrospective review. Am J Surg. 2011;201:623–7.
45. Cirocchi R, Trastulli S, Farinella E, Desiderio J, Listorti C, Parisi A, et al. Is inferior mesenteric artery ligation during sigmoid colectomy for diverticular disease associated with increased anastomotic leakage? A meta-analysis of randomized and non-randomized clinical trials. Color Dis. 2012;14:e521–9.
46. Masoni L, Mari FS, Nigri G, Favi F, Gasparrini M, Dall'Oglio A, et al. Preservation of the inferior mesenteric artery via laparoscopic sigmoid colectomy performed for diverticular disease: real benefit or technical challenge: a randomized controlled clinical trial. Surg Endosc. 2013;27:199–206.
47. Tocchi A, Mazzoni G, Fornasari V, Miccini M, Daddi G, Tagliacozzo S. Preservation of the inferior mesenteric artery in colorectal resection for complicated diverticular disease. Am J Surg. 2001;182:162–7.
48. Stevenson AR, Stitz RW, Lumley JW, Fielding GA. Laparoscopically assisted anterior resection for diverticular disease: follow-up of 100 consecutive patients. Ann Surg. 1998;227:335–42.
49. Klarenbeek BR, Veenhof AA, Bergamaschi R, van der Peet DL, van den Broek WT, de Lange ES, et al. Laparoscopic sigmoid resection for diverticulitis decreases major morbidity rates: a randomized control trial: short-term results of the sigma trial. Ann Surg. 2009;249:39–44.
50. Gervaz P, Inan I, Perneger T, Schiffer E, Morel P. A prospective, randomized, single-blind comparison of laparoscopic versus open sigmoid colectomy for diverticulitis. Ann Surg. 2010;252:3–8.
51. Siddiqui MR, Sajid MS, Qureshi S, Check E, Baig MK. Elective laparoscopic sigmoid resection for diverticular disease has fewer complications than conventional surgery: a meta-analysis. Am J Surg. 2010;200:144–61.
52. Jones OM, Stevenson AR, Clark D, Stitz RW, Lumley JW. Laparoscopic resection for diverticular disease: follow-up of 500 consecutive patients. Ann Surg. 2008;248:1092–7.
53. Cirocchi R, Farinella E, Trastulli S, Sciannameo F, Audisio RA. Elective sigmoid colectomy for diverticular disease. Laparoscopic vs open surgery: a systematic review. Color Dis. 2012;14:671–83.
54. Mbadiwe T, Obirieze AC, Cornwell EE 3rd, Turner P, Fullum TM. Surgical management of complicated diverticulitis: a comparison of the laparoscopic and open approaches. J Am Coll Surg. 2013;216:782–8.
55. Aalbers AG, Biere SS, van Berge Henegouwen MI, Bemelman WA. Hand-assisted or laparoscopic-assisted approach in colorectal surgery: a systematic review and meta-analysis. Surg Endosc. 2008;22:1769–80.
56. Lee SW, Yoo J, Dujovny N, Sonoda T, Milsom JW. Laparoscopic vs. hand-assisted laparoscopic sigmoidectomy for diverticulitis. Dis Colon Rectum. 2006;49:464–9.
57. Anderson J, Luchtefeld M, Dujovny N, Hoedema R, Kim D, Butcher J. A comparison of laparoscopic, hand-assist and open sigmoid resection in the treatment of diverticular disease. Am J Surg. 2007;193:400–3.
58. Kang JC, Chung MH, Chao PC, et al. Hand-assisted laparoscopic colectomy vs open colectomy: a prospective randomized study. Surg Endosc. 2004;18:577–81.
59. Champagne BJ, Lee EC, Leblanc F, Stein SL, Delaney CP. Single-incision vs straight laparoscopic segmental colectomy: a case-controlled study. Dis Colon Rectum. 2011;54:183–6.
60. Vestweber B, Alfes A, Paul C, Haaf F, Vestweber KH. Single-incision laparoscopic surgery: a promising approach to sigmoidectomy for diverticular disease. Surg Endosc. 2010;24:3225–8.

61. Ragupathi M, Ramos-Valdez DI. Robotic-assisted laparoscopic surgery for recurrent diverticulitis: experience in consecutive cases and review of literature. Surg Endosc. 2011;25:199–206.
62. Casillas S, Delaney CP, Senagore AJ, Brady K, Fazio VW. Does conversion of a laparoscopic colectomy adversely affect patient outcome? Dis Colon Rectum. 2004;47:1680–5.
63. Maciel V, Lujan HJ, Plasencia G, Zeichen M, Mata W, Jorge I, Lee D, Viamonte M 3rd, Hartmann RF. Diverticular disease complicated with colovesical fistula: laparoscopic versus robotic management. Int Surg. 2014;99:203–10.
64. Nguyen GC, Sam J, Anand N. Epidemiological trends and geographic variation in hospital admissions for diverticulitis in the United States. World J Gastroenterol. 2011;17:1600–5.
65. Alonso S, Pera M, Parés D, Pascual M, Gil MJ, Courtier R, et al. Outpatient treatment of patients with uncomplicated acute diverticulitis. Color Dis. 2009;12:278–82.
66. Comparato G, Pilotto A, Franzè A, Franceschi M, Di Mario F. Diverticular disease in the elderly. Dig Dis. 2007;25:151–9.
67. Rodríguez-Cerrillo M, Poza-Montoro A, Fernandez-Diaz A, Matesanz-David M, Iñurrieta Romero A. Treatment of elderly patients with uncomplicated diverticulitis, even with comorbidity, at home. Eur J Int Med. 2013;24:430–2.
68. van Randen A, Laméris W, van Es HW, van Heesewijk HP, van Ramshorst B, Ten Hove W, Bouma WH, van Leeuwen MS, van Keulen EM, Bossuyt PM, Stoker J, Boermeester MA, OPTIMA Study Group. A comparison of the accuracy of ultrasound and computed tomography in common diagnoses causing acute abdominal pain. Eur Radiol. 2011;21:1535–45.
69. Ambrosetti P, Becker C, Terrier F. Colonic diverticulitis: impact of imaging on surgical management – a prospective study of 542 patients. Eur Radiol. 2002;12:1145–9.
70. Ukkonen M, Karlsson S, Laukkarinen J, Rantanen T, Paajanen H, Finnsepsis Study Group. Severe sepsis in elderly patients undergoing gastrointestinal surgery-a prospective multicenter follow-up study of finish intensive care units. J Gastrointest Surg. 2016;20:1028–33.
71. Lamb MN, Kaiser AM. Elective resection versus observation after nonoperative management of complicated diverticulitis with abscess: a systematic review and meta-analysis. Dis Colon Rectum. 2014;57:1430–40.
72. Devaraj B, Liu W, Tatum J, Cologne K, Kaiser AM. Medically treated diverticular abscess associated with high risk of recurrence and disease complications. Dis Colon Rectum. 2016;59:208–15.
73. Brandt D, Gervaz P, Durmishi Y, et al. Percutaneous CT scan-guided drainage vs. antibiotherapy alone for Hinchey II diverticulitis: a case-control study. Dis Colon Rectum. 2006;49:1533–8.
74. Siewert B, Tye G, Kruskal J, et al. Impact of CT-guided drainage in the treatment of diverticular abscesses: size matters. Am J Roentgenol. 2006;186:680–4.
75. Kumar R, Kim JT, Haukoos JS, et al. Factors affecting the successful management of intra-abdominal abscesses with antibiotics and the need for percutaneous drainage. Dis Colon Rectum. 2006;49:183–9.
76. Ambrosetti P, Chautems R, Soravia C, Peiris-Waser N, Terrier F. Long-term outcome of mesocolic and pelvic diverticular abscesses of the left colon: a prospective study of 73 cases. Dis Colon Rectum. 2005;48:787–91.
77. Elagili F, Stocchi L, Ozuner G, Mody R, Baker ME, Kiran RP. Predictors of postoperative outcomes for patients with diverticular abscess initially treated with percutaneous drainage. Am J Surg. 2015;209:703–8.
78. Felder SI, Barmparas G, Lynn J, Murrell Z, Margulies DR, Fleshner P. Can the need for colectomy after computed tomography-guided percutaneous drainage for diverticular abscess be predicted? Am Surg. 2013;79:1013–6.
79. Subhas G, Rana G, Bhullar J, Essad K, Mohey L, Mittal VK. Percutaneous drainage of a diverticular abscess should be limited to two attempts for a resilient diverticular abscess. Am Surg. 2014;80:635–9.
80. Gaertner WB, Willis DJ, Madoff RD, Rothenberger DA, Kwaan MR, Belzer GE, Melton GB. Percutaneous drainage of colonic diverticular abscess: is colon resection necessary? Dis Colon Rectum. 2013;56:622–6.

81. Chautems RC, Ambrosetti P, Ludwig A, Mermillod B, Morel P, Soravia C. Long-term follow-up after first acute episode of sigmoid diverticulitis: is surgery mandatory?: a prospective study of 118 patients. Dis Colon Rectum. 2002;45:962–6.
82. Nagorney DM, Adson MA, Pemberton JH. Sigmoid diverticulitis with perforation and generalized peritonitis. Dis Colon Rectum. 1985;28:71–5.
83. Salem L, Anaya DA, Roberts KE, Flum DR. Hartmann's colectomy and reversal in diverticulitis: a population-level assessment. Dis Colon Rectum. 2005;48:988–95.
84. Jacobs DO. Clinical practice. Diverticulitis. N Engl J Med. 2007;357:2057–66.
85. Vermeulen J, Akkersdijk GP, Gosselink MP, Hop WC, Mannaerts GH, van der Harst E, Coene PP, Weidema WF, Lange JF. Outcome after emergency surgery for acute perforated diverticulitis in 200 cases. Dig Surg. 2007;24:361–6.
86. Janes SE, Meagher A, Frizelle F. Management of diverticulitis. BMJ. 2006;332:271–5.
87. Constantinides VA, Heriot A, Remzi F, Darzi A, Senapati A, Fazio VW, Tekkis PP. Operative strategies for diverticular peritonitis: a decision analysis between primary resection and anastomosis versus Hartmann's procedures. Ann Surg. 2007;245:94–103.
88. Oberkofler CE, Rickenbacher A, Raptis DA, Lehmann K, Villiger P, Buchli C, Grieder F, Gelpke H, Decurtins M, Tempia-Caliera AA, Demartines N, Hahnloser D, Clavien PA, Breitenstein S. A multicenter randomized clinical trial of primary anastomosis or Hartmann's procedure for perforated left colonic diverticulitis with purulent or Fecal peritonitis. Ann Surg. 2012;256:819–27.
89. Binda GA, Karas JR, Serventi A, Sokmen S, Amato A, Hydo L, Bergamaschi R, for the Study Group on Diverticulitis. Primary anastomosis vs nonrestorative resection for perforated diverticulitis with peritonitis: a prematurely terminated randomized controlled trial. Color Dis. 2012;14:1403–10.
90. Masoomi H, Stamos MJ, Carmichael JC, Nguyen B, Buchberg B, Mills S. Does primary anastomosis with diversion have any advantages over Hartmann's procedure in acute diverticulitis? Dig Surg. 2012;29:315–20.
91. Gawlick U, Nirula R. Resection and primary anastomosis with proximal diversion instead of Hartmann's: evolving the management of diverticulitis using NSQIP data. J Trauma Acute Care Surg. 2012;72:807–14.
92. Jiménez Fuertes M, Costa Navarro D. Resection and primary anastomosis without diverting ileostomy for left colon emergencies: is it a safe procedure? World J Surg. 2012;36:1148–53.
93. Trenti L, Biondo S, Golda T, Monica M, Kreisler E, Fraccalvieri D, Frago R, Jaurrieta E. Generalized peritonitis due to perforated diverticulitis: Hartmann's procedure or primary anastomosis? Int J Color Dis. 2011;26:377–84.
94. Zingg U, Pasternak I, Dietrich M, Seifert B, Oertli D, Metzger U. Primary anastomosis vs Hartmann's procedure in patients undergoing emergency left colectomy for perforated diverticulitis. Color Dis. 2010;12:54–60.
95. Vermeulen J, Coene PP, Van Hout NM, van der Harst E, Gosselink MP, Mannaerts GH, Weidema WF, Lange JF. Restoration of bowel continuity after surgery for acute perforated diverticulitis: should Hartmann's procedure be considered a one-stage procedure? Color Dis. 2009;11:619–24.
96. Richter S, Lindemann W, Kollmar O, Pistorius GA, Maurer CA, Schilling MK. One-stage sigmoid colon resection for perforated sigmoid diverticulitis (Hinchey stages III and IV). World J Surg. 2006;30:1027–32.
97. Regenet N, Pessaux P, Hennekinne S, Lermite E, Tuech JJ, Brehant O, Arnaud JP. Primary anastomosis after intraoperative colonic lavage vs. Hartmann's procedure in generalized peritonitis complicating diverticular disease of the colon. Int J. Color Dis. 2003;18:503–7.
98. Schilling MK, Maurer CA, Kollmar O, Büchler MW. Primary vs. secondary anastomosis after sigmoid colon resection for perforated diverticulitis (Hinchey stage III and IV): a prospective outcome and cost analysis. Dis Colon Rectum. 2001;44:699–703.
99. Gooszen AW, Gooszen HG, Veerman W, Van Dongen VM, Hermans J, Klien Kranenbarg E, Tollenaar RA. Operative treatment of acute complications of diverticular disease: primary or secondary anastomosis after sigmoid resection. Eur J Surg. 2001;167:35–9.
100. Constantinides VA, Tekkis PP, Athanasiou T, Aziz O, Purkayastha S, Remzi FH, Fazio VW, Aydin N, Darzi A, Senapati A. Primary resection with anastomosis vs. Hartmann's procedure

in nonelective surgery for acute colonic diverticulitis: a systematic review. Dis Colon Rectum. 2006;49:966–81.
101. Abbas S. Resection and primary anastomosis in acute complicated diverticulitis, a systematic review of the literature. Int J Color Dis. 2007;22:351–7.
102. Salem L, Flum DR. Primary anastomosis or Hartmann's procedure for patients with diverticular peritonitis? A systematic review. Dis Colon Rectum. 2004;47:1953–64.
103. Constantinides VA, Aydin HN, Tekkis PP, Fazio VW, Heriot AG, Remzi FH. Long-term, health-related, quality of life comparison in patients undergoing single stage vs staged resection for complicated diverticular disease. Color Dis. 2006;8:663–71.
104. de Korte N, Klarenbeek BR, Kuyvenhoven JP, Roumen RM, Cuesta MA, Stockmann HB. Management of diverticulitis: results of a survey among gastroenterologists and surgeons. Color Dis. 2011;13:e411–7.
105. Aydin HN, Tekkis PP, Remzi FH, Constantinides V, Fazio VW. Evaluation of the risk of a nonrestorative resection for the treatment of diverticular disease: the Cleveland Clinic diverticular disease propensity score. Dis Colon Rectum. 2006;49:629–39.
106. Jafferji MS, Hyman N. Surgeon, not disease severity, often determines the operation for acute complicated diverticulitis. J Am Coll Surg. 2014;218:1156–61.
107. O'Sullivan GC, Murphy D, O'Brien MG, Ireland A. Laparoscopic management of generalized peritonitis due to per- forated colonic diverticula. Am J Surg. 1996;171:432–4.
108. Myers E, Hurley M, O'Sullivan GC, Kavanagh D, Wilson I, Winter DC. Laparoscopic peritoneal lavage for generalized peritonitis due to perforated diverticulitis. Br J Surg. 2008;95:97–101.
109. Toorenvliet BR, Swank H, Schoones JW, Hamming JF, Bemelman WA. Laparoscopic peritoneal lavage for perforated colonic diverticulitis: a systematic review. Color Dis. 2010;12:862–7.
110. Vennix S, Musters GD, Mulder IM, et al. Laparoscopic peritoneal lavage or sigmoidectomy for perforated diverticulitis with purulent peritonitis: a multicentre, parallel-group, randomised, open-label trial. Lancet. 2015;386:1269–77.
111. Angenete E, Thornell A, Burcharth J, et al. Laparoscopic lavage is feasible and safe for the treatment of perforated diverticulitis with purulent peritonitis: the first results from the randomized controlled trial DILALA. Ann Surg. 2016;263:117–22.
112. Schultz JK, Yaqub S, Wallon C, et al. Laparoscopic lavage vs primary resection for acute perforated diverticulitis: the SCANDIV randomized clinical trial. JAMA. 2015;314:1364–75.
113. Slim K. Role of peritoneal lavage for sigmoid perforation peritonitis surgery: what do the meta-analyses tell us? J Visc Surg. 2016;154:139. https://doi.org/10.1016/j.jviscsurg.2016.09.009.
114. Ceresoli M, Coccolini F, Montori G, Catena F, Sartelli M, Ansaloni L. Laparoscopic lavage in perforated purulent diverticulitis-is it time for definitive conclusions? Int J Color Dis. 2016;32(1):159. https://doi.org/10.1007/s00384-016-2674-7.
115. Angenete E, Bock D, Rosenberg J, Haglind E. Laparoscopic lavage is superior to colon resection for perforated purulent diverticulitis-a meta-analysis. Int J Color Dis. 2016;32(2):163–9. https://doi.org/10.1007/s00384-016-2636-036.
116. Marshall JR, Buchwald PL, Gandhi J, et al. Laparoscopic lavage in the management of Hinchey grade III diverticulitis: a systematic review. Ann Surg. 2016;265(4):670–6. https://doi.org/10.1097/SLA.0000000000002005.
117. Cirocchi R, Di Saverio S, Weber DG, et al. Laparoscopic lavage versus surgical resection for acute diverticulitis with generalized peritonitis: a systematic review and meta-analysis. Tech Coloproctol. 2017;21(2):93–110. https://doi.org/10.1007/s10151-017-1585-0.
118. Tridente A, Clarke GM, Walden A, McKechnie S, Hutton P, Mills GH, Gordon AC, Holloway PA, Chiche JD, Bion J, Stuber F, Garrard C, Hinds CJ, GenOSept Investigators. Patients with faecal peritonitis admitted to European intensive care units: an epidemiological survey of the GenOSept cohort. Intensive Care Med. 2014;40:202–10.
119. Rosenthal G, Kaboli P, Barnett M. Age and the risk of in-hospital death: insights from a multihospital study of intensive care patients. J Am Geriatr Soc. 2002;50:1205–12.

120. Van Den Noortgate N, Vogelaers D, Afschrift M, Colardyn F. Intensive care for very elderly patients: outcome and risk factors for in-hospital mortality. Age Ageing. 1999;28:253–6.
121. Perathoner A, Klaus A, Muhlmann G, et al. Damage control with abdominal vacuum therapy (VAC) to manage perforated diverticulitis with advanced generalized peritonitis—a proof of concept. Int J Color Dis. 2010;25:767–74.
122. Kafka-Ritsch R, Birkfellner F, Perathoner A, et al. Damage control surgery with abdominal vacuum and delayed bowel reconstruction in patients with perforated diverticulitis Hinchey III/IV. J Gastrointest Surg. 2012;16:1915–22.
123. Peura DA, Lanza FL, Gostout CJ, Foutch PG. The American College of Gastroenterology bleeding registry: preliminary findings. Am J Gastroenterol. 1997;92:924–8.
124. Longstreth GF. Epidemiology and outcome of patients hospitalized with acute lower gastrointestinal hemorrhage: a population-based study. Am J Gastroenterol. 1997;92:419–24.
125. McGuire HH Jr, Haynes BW Jr. Massive hemorrhage for diverticulosis of the colon: guidelines for therapy based on bleeding patterns observed in fifty cases. Ann Surg. 1972;175:847–55.
126. Zuckerman GR, Prakash C. Acute lower intestinal bleeding. II. Etiology, therapy, and outcomes. Gastrointest Endosc. 1999;49:228–38.
127. McGuire HH Jr. Bleeding colonic diverticula: a reappraisal of natural history and management. Ann Surg. 1994;220:653–6.
128. Aytac E, Stocchi L, Gorgun E, Ozuner G. Risk of recurrence and long-term outcomes after colonic diverticular bleeding. Int J Color Dis. 2014;2:373–8.
129. Lee KK, Shah SM, Moser MA. Risk factors predictive of severe diverticular hemorrhage. Int J Surg. 2011;9:83–5.
130. Nagata N, Niikura R, Aoki T, Moriyasu S, Sakurai T, Shimbo T, Sekine K, Okubo H, Watanabe K, Yokoi C, Akiyama J, Yanase M, Mizokami M, Fujimoto K, Uemura N. Risk factors for adverse in-hospital outcomes in acute colonic diverticular hemorrhage. World J Gastroenterol. 2015;21:10697–703.
131. Nakatsu S, Yasuda H, Maehata T, Nomoto M, Ohinata N, Hosoya K, Ishigooka S, Ozawa S, Ikeda Y, Sato Y, Suzuki M, Kiyokawa H, Yamamoto H, Itoh F. Urgent computed tomography for determining the optimal timing of colonoscopy in patients with acute lower gastrointestinal bleeding. Intern Med. 2015;54:553–8.

Surgical Management of Colorectal Cancer in the Elderly Patient

14

Andrea Mazzari, Pasquina Tomaiuolo, Federico Perrone, Federico Sicoli, and Antonio Crucitti

14.1 Epidemiology

Colorectal cancer is the third most common cancer in men and the second most common in women with 1,360,000 newly diagnosed patients worldwide [1] and almost 694,000 estimated deaths in 2012. There is a higher incidence in older populations [2]; in fact, the highest risk of developing a colorectal cancer occurs around the age of 70 years, while it is infrequently diagnosed before the age of 40 years. Seventy-five percent of colorectal cancer diagnoses are in patients over 65 years. In both Europe and the United States, approximately 50% of colorectal cancer patients are older than 70 years of age, and, among these, colorectal cancer is the second leading cause of cancer death [3]. Moreover, life expectancy has lengthened in elderly patients. According to World Health Organization (WHO) reports, estimated life expectancy at age 60 years was 21.5 years in women and 18.5 years in men in 2012 [4]. Increasing life expectancy corresponds to a rapid increase of the elderly population. Thus, age could be considered as a major risk factor for the development of this cancer [5].

14.2 Who Is "Elderly?"

Elderly patients form a specific population due to comorbidities, disability, and organ-specific physiological changes that have impaired their enrollment in clinical trials and thus the transposition of current guidelines which have been established in younger patients. One of the most difficult problems in evaluating the outcomes of colorectal surgery in elderly patients is that there is no clear definition of an

A. Mazzari • P. Tomaiuolo • F. Perrone • F. Sicoli • A. Crucitti (✉)
Department of General and Mini-invasive Surgery, Cristo Re Hospital, Rome, Italy
e-mail: antonio.crucitti@unicatt.it

A. Crucitti (ed.), *Surgical Management of Elderly Patients*,
https://doi.org/10.1007/978-3-319-60861-7_14

elderly patient, with ages varying from 65 to 80 years in different publications [6]. "Elderly" is a very subjective definition that arises from the environmental culture of the patient: it has been defined as a chronological age of ≥65 years of age, which, in turn, has been divided into early and late elderly for those who are 65–74 years of age and over 75 years, respectively [7].

14.3 Histopathology

Adenocarcinoma occurs in more than 95% of colorectal cancer with lesions that can be infiltrative, ulcerated, or polypoid; histologically, it can be well differentiated, moderately differentiated, or poorly differentiated. Mucinous adenocarcinoma (5%) is diagnosed when mucosa occurs in more than 50% of the tumor tissue and usually has a worse prognosis. Other histotypes (<5%) are lymphomas, sarcomas, and carcinoid tumors. In accordance with the international literature data, the proportion of right-sided colon cancer is relatively high in patients aged under 40 years and over 80 years. Right-sided colon cancer is more likely to be detected at an advanced stage with severe symptoms. Polypoid-type early cancer is dominant in the left colon, while the proportion of flat-type early cancer is significantly higher in the right colon than in the left colon.

14.4 Risk Assessment

Elderly patients frequently have one or more comorbidities and are often "frail"; for these reasons, they have a very high risk of morbidity and mortality. While the cutoff for a definition of elderly patients varies from 65 to 70 years of age [8], as previously said, defining elderly patients based on functional status is more accurate than age itself. Aging, especially if associated with cancer, is commonly associated with a functional decline, cognitive disorders, frailty, comorbidities, malnutrition, falls, and polypharmacy, resulting in increased vulnerability and institutionalization as well as an increase in health system costs.

The International Society of Geriatric Oncology (SIOG) recommended that patients affected by colorectal diseases ≥65 years of age undergoing surgery should experience a preoperative whole-patient assessment of the most common physiological side effects of aging, physical and mental ability, and social support [9]. Many studies have shown that age alone is not a significant prognostic factor in survival after colonic surgery [10]. Several authors have tried to quantify the correlation between comorbidities and postoperative mortality or morbidity [11]. Physical frailty increases the risk of major complications following surgery [odds ratio (OR) 4.1 (1.4–11.6)] in patients ≥75 years (range 75–93) and is predictive for both complications and survival in patients ≥70 years following surgery [12].

It is mainly frail elderly patients who suffer postoperative complications such as cardiac problems, pneumonia, and deep vein thrombosis. Due to the high rate of postoperative complications in the elderly, geriatricians designed the comprehensive geriatric assessment (CGA) as a multidimensional tool that accurately predicts postoperative morbidity, in order to assess preoperative risks and physiological reserves of the elderly. The results of the CGA can lead to developing individualized geriatric intervention programs, and in many subfields of geriatrics, the CGA is used to evaluate geriatric conditions that are associated with frailty [13]. A preoperative CGA may be used to assess the condition of each patient's health within 6 months of surgery. In this protocol all patients related face-to-face with a geriatric team, composed of geriatricians, nurse specialists, dieticians, and pharmacists. The preoperative CGA had eight domains: burden of comorbidity (Charlson Comorbidity Index, CCI), polypharmacy, physical function according to activities of daily living (ADL), instrumental ADL (IADL), cognitive status (Mini-Mental State Examination), risk of postoperative delirium (Nursing Delirium Screening Scale), Geriatric Depression Scale, and nutritional status (Mini Nutritional Assessment). The definition of "deficit" in each domain is a score of 3 or more for comorbidities [14], the regular use of eight or more drugs [15], poor physical function assessed by using the ADL, poor physical function assessed by using the IADL [16], cognitive dysfunction assessed by using the Mini-Mental State Examination, severe depression, and malnutrition.

As seen in a recent Korean large study [17], a preoperative CGA indicating "high risk" (patient who had deficits in two or more domains) was associated with major postoperative complications (Clavien-Dindo grade II or higher within 30 days of surgery) in elderly patients who underwent surgery for colorectal cancer. Thus, using the CGA, we are able to identify elderly colorectal cancer patients who should be given greater attention during pre- and postoperative management in order to achieve a clinical benefit.

14.5 Diagnosis and Screening

Colorectal cancer in older patients is more often diagnosed at a later stage than in younger patients. As a result, older patients more frequently require emergency and palliative surgery, which increases the risk of perioperative morbi-mortality. Delays in colorectal cancer diagnosis are multifactorial: older people consult later, symptoms could be atypical or poorly recognized, and investigations and screening are generally organized up to the age of 74 years.

Colorectal cancer screening leads to detecting polyps, precancerous lesions, and early colorectal cancer with lower incidence of cancer (17–33%) and reduction of mortality from 11 to 53% [18]. At present many screening methods are available such as fecal occult blood test (FOBT), endoscopy, and CT colonography, but neither is universally accepted in elderly patients. Many consensus documents (3, 4, 5, 6) are recommended (Table 14.1).

Screening for colorectal cancer with the fecal occult blood test (FOBT) reduces colorectal cancer mortality [18]. Nevertheless, studies that have demonstrated the benefit of colorectal cancer screening with FOBT enrolled few or no elderly patients. The majority of other organized mass screening programs and the national

Table 14.1 Screening programs for colorectal cancer in the elderly

US Multi-Society Task Force and the American Cancer Society	Discontinuation of surveillance colonoscopy should be considered in persons with serious comorbidities and expectancy of life less than 10 years
American Gastroenterological Association	Individualized approach
American Geriatrics Society	Not recommended in points with high comorbidity and with expectancy of life <5 years
British Society of Gastroenterology	FOB every 2 years, ages 50–69, plan to extend to over 75 years

screening program for colorectal cancer are restricted to a population aged 50–74 years. The efficacy of colorectal cancer screening with FOBT has never been prospectively evaluated in elderly subjects.

Age is a critical factor in the occurrence of adverse events related to colonoscopy. Adequate bowel preparation is more difficult to achieve in very old patients. Thus, patient selection for colonoscopy is an important challenge. In the elderly population, the risk of colorectal surveillance may outweigh its benefit due to comorbidities and specific age-related risks. Most of the society agree that colorectal cancer screening in the elderly should be tailored. Older patients have a 30% higher risk of perforation during colonoscopy than younger patients [19] and a higher morbidity if the colonoscopy is performed under general anesthesia. Bowel preparation should be considered in elderly patients because adverse events have been observed with minor ones like abdominal pain, nausea, and fecal incontinence and major ones like electrolyte abnormalities, aspiration pneumonia, ischemic colitis, and acute kidney failure [20]. Many considerations relate to the compliance and the high incidence (5–60%) of poor bowel preparation. Poor bowel preparation plays a key role in the completion of colonoscopy with a high risk of being unsuccessful in very elderly patients (52–95%) [21]. It is still debated when to interrupt the surveillance in the elderly. Most authors agree with the decision to go through an individual assessment that considers the risks and the benefits and balances these with the patients' health, functional status, and expectancy of life.

14.6 Surgical Treatment

Age continues to be considered as one of the main factors of perioperative mortality after colorectal surgery. However, elderly patients are more susceptible to postoperative infectious complications, particularly chest complications. The resection of nonmetastatic tumors in operable elderly patients with long life expectancy is common sense; however, in patients with short life expectancy, a multidisciplinary meeting including, if possible, a geriatrician should decide on the treatment strategy. The survival benefit of liver metastatic surgery is maintained above 70 years in selected patients. There are, however, no consistent data regarding patients over 80 years.

Surgery is the gold standard for the treatment of colorectal cancer, and it is performed either with curative intent or for problem-solving when patients present with colon perforation or obstruction. In fact, colorectal cancer can particularly manifest as an acute abdomen characterized by occlusion (15–20% of cases) and perforation (3–8% of cases) [22]. These events are characteristic in geriatric age; in fact, the incidence of most surgical interventions as a matter of urgency is for patients aged over 70 years, while patients between 60 and 70 years most frequently undergo elective surgery [23]. Although in recent years, thanks to the use of staplers, the prognosis of colorectal carcinoma has significantly improved for elective operations, for those in an emergency it has remained poor [24]. The high mortality linked to emergency interventions [25] emphasizes the importance of careful preoperative assistance that aims to improve comorbidities and the special deficit conditions due to the colorectal cancer (state of anemia and malnutrition). Therefore, a close collaboration between surgical associations and geriatric societies is necessary in order to produce guidelines for the perioperative assessment and the management of postoperative geriatric events [26, 27].

14.7 Laparoscopic Colorectal Surgery in Elderly Patients

Over the past decade, many studies have widely demonstrated that a laparoscopic surgical approach to colon resections is not inferior to open colon resections. It has been proven to be a safe procedure, even in high-risk patients [28]. Most evidence suggests that laparoscopic colorectal surgery (LCS) can be performed safely for several pathologic conditions in elderly patients [29]. In addition, recent randomized controlled trials and a meta-analysis show, with Level 1 evidence, that laparoscopic colorectal surgery achieves good oncological results compared to the open method [30].

The short-term benefits of laparoscopic colorectal surgery compared to the open method are well known and include less pain, better pulmonary function, shorter postoperative small bowel obstruction, and shorter hospital stay [31]. Decreases in blood loss and postoperative pain reduce the stress of surgery and therefore reduce overall morbidity. The reduction in cardiovascular complications might also be due to decrease in blood loss. Bowel obstruction and ileus are also reduced in laparoscopic colorectal surgery. The exposure of intestines and major trauma to the abdominal wall might increase in incidence of bowel paralysis and adhesion in open colorectal surgery. A recent systematic review on the incidence of nonsurgical (cardiopulmonary) complications in randomized clinical trials addressing surgery for colorectal cancer found that laparoscopic colectomy reduces the incidence of postoperative cardiac complications [32]. Large-scale, randomized studies and reviews that compare long-term results between laparoscopic colorectal surgery and open colorectal surgery in all generations report no difference in colon cancer patients [33].

These outcomes are particularly important in elderly patients who are at a higher risk of postoperative morbidity and mortality than younger ones. It would seem natural then that laparoscopic colorectal surgery should be the ideal surgical approach for elderly patients. The only area where laparoscopic colorectal surgery did not show a benefit over open colorectal surgery was for operative time. Despite the fragility of elderly patients and the longer operative times needed to perform laparoscopy, many studies show that laparoscopy for colorectal surgery does not create a greater risk in elderly patients [34].

In conclusion, laparoscopic colorectal surgery is a safe and good option in elderly patients. Advanced age should not be a contraindication for laparoscopic colorectal surgery, even for complex procedures, such as laparoscopic rectal resection. Safer laparoscopic colorectal surgery can be provided to elderly patients with rectal cancer by selecting an appropriate operative procedure according to each individual patient's condition.

14.8 Robotic Colorectal Surgery in Elderly Patients

Robotic technology for colorectal surgery was introduced for the first time in 2002 by Weber et al. in order to improve the feasibility of a minimally invasive surgical approach, starting out with laparoscopy at least 20 years ago. As with all new techniques, robotic colorectal surgery started to be performed in selected patients, young people with low BMI and ASA scores and good performance status: at the beginning, patients older than 70 years were ruled out of robotic colorectal surgery. Some concerns were recognized with the use of robotics in the elderly population, especially when considering a longer operative time as reported by several studies; furthermore, some procedures require prolonged and steep Trendelenburg position (e.g., rectal and prostatic surgery), with possible consequences regarding pulmonary and cardiovascular implications. When robotic colorectal surgery was shown to be feasible and safe, with improved systemic outcomes for young patients, many authors started to use this robotic approach with elderly patients too. Their results assessed the feasibility of extending the benefits of this improved minimally invasive approach to elderly people as well [35].

Colorectal cancer is one of the most frequent malignancies worldwide, especially in elderly people. Over the last two decades, minimally invasive techniques have been extensively used for the surgical management of this disease, with better short-term outcomes and equivalent oncological results when compared to open surgery, including in the elderly. The robotic surgical approach has been shown to be a feasible, safe, and oncologically adequate treatment for colorectal disease. As many authors have already demonstrated, it offers satisfactory systemic outcomes in terms of short hospital stay, early first flatus, quick soft diet intake, good systemic procedure tolerance, low conversion, and postoperative complication rate. All these benefits have been demonstrated for elderly patients as well.

As is compatible with the reports of high-volume robotic centers, age alone cannot be considered an exclusion criteria to the robotic surgical approach; moreover, elderly people with comorbidities can benefit, even more than younger patients, from this technological improvement. The high conversion rate and long learning curve of laparoscopy may be overcome by robotic surgery that represents the natural evolution of minimal access surgery, with the addition of a computer interface between the surgeon and the patient.

At present, there is no evidence that robotic surgery should be considered better than conventional minimally invasive surgery, with only a few randomized clinical trials having been performed.

Nevertheless, considering the high direct costs, minimally invasive robot-assisted surgery should be done on a case-by-case basis, tailored to each patient with their specific histories and comorbidities.

14.9 Fast Track

Enhanced recovery after surgery (ERAS) is a multidisciplinary approach to obtain better results for patients after a surgical procedure. Fast-track protocol focuses on preoperative, intraoperative, and postoperative period, and the main goal is to reduce surgical stress to optimize perioperative management [36]. Many authors have demonstrated that ERAS in colorectal surgery is feasible and safe. Adhesion to protocol leads to minimizing morbidity and reducing the length of hospital stay [37]. Some studies in the literature have reported that elderly patients undergoing colorectal surgery could benefit from the ERAS protocol and that it improves postoperative outcomes when compared to traditional perioperative management [38].

The ERAS protocol includes the following statements:

- Preoperative phase: assessment with complete nutritional status, preadmission education and preoperative multidisciplinary counseling, no mechanical bowel preparation for colon resections, and carbohydrate-rich drinks 1 day prior to and 2 h before surgery
- Intraoperative phase: antibiotic prophylaxis, epidural analgesia, avoidance of opioid analgesia, no nasogastric tube and drains when possible, and no fluid overload
- Postoperative phase: oral fluids during the early postoperative period (meaning 6–8 h after surgery), soft-food diet by the second postoperative day, early mobilization and rehabilitation, removal of urinary catheter on postoperative day 1, and early termination of IV fluid

Results from the Perioperative Italian Society Registry demonstrate that elderly patients can be managed with the ERAS protocol with good reported outcomes in terms of reduction of hospital stay, compliance rates, morbidity, and readmission rates [39].

14.10 Outcomes After Colorectal Surgery in Elderly Patients

Elderly patients are often categorized as high-risk patients due to their having significant comorbidity with increasing postoperative morbidity and mortality. As a result of this, age has received increasing multidisciplinary attention as a prognostic factor for postoperative complications.

The impact of age on postoperative outcomes after major colorectal surgery remains controversial. Furthermore, curative surgery of colonic cancer in elderly patients is debatable, especially in very elderly patients who have limited prospects of survival.

Historically there has been a tendency to exclude very old patients from entering clinical trials (not just those within surgery), making evidence-based clinical decision-making more challenging [40]. The majority of randomized controlled trials evaluating the efficacy of chemotherapy and surgery as treatment for colorectal cancer do not include patients over the age of 75 years. It is difficult, therefore, to accurately guide this group of patients who have been assessed as being fit for surgery. Traditionally, patients over the age of 80 years undergoing segmental colonic resection have been less likely to receive adjuvant therapies or additional surgery (for recurrence or metastatic disease) following their diagnosis of colorectal cancer when compared to patients under the age of 80 years [41]. However, studies have supported the view that even very frail older people can be offered tailored colorectal chemotherapy regimens safely [42]. Some authors promote extensive surgery, including multistage procedures, as performed in younger patients [43]; others promote less aggressive surgery [44], withholding curative treatment with radical surgical procedures and opting for more "conservative" or palliative therapies in elderly patients. In a systematic review, published in the Lancet in 2000, it has been demonstrated that a resection of the tumor is performed less often in elderly patients than in younger patients [45].

Improved diagnostic procedures, intensive perioperative care, better anesthesia, and surgical techniques have made it possible to perform high-risk surgical procedures in older age patients. As a result of this, many recent publications have encouraged the same surgical approach as for younger patients [46]. Nowadays, many studies demonstrate that age alone is not a predictor of postoperative complications [47]. Elderly patients have similar rates of morbidity and mortality as younger patients of the same clinical status. Therefore, it is better to talk about biological age rather than chronological age when assessing risk factors for surgery, which focuses more on the overall condition of the patient.

A number of predictive tools, such as validated online risk calculators (e.g. www.riskcalculator.facs.org), are available in order to assess risk of morbidity and mortality after surgery based on the comorbid and general health status of elderly patients [48]. Any effect of age on systemic complications can be explained by other factors such as patient's American Society of Anesthesia (ASA) grading, performance status, and Charlson Comorbidity Index Scores. It would be beneficial to test these tools on local populations and use these rather than age alone as criteria to select surgical treatment.

Another specific problem related to evaluation of outcomes of colorectal surgery in elderly patients is the significantly higher number of emergency presentations. It is well documented that emergency surgery is related to a higher mortality rate than elective surgery [49]. However, for those patients presenting as acute surgical emergencies, often with physiological derangement, clinical decision-making is challenging and treatment options limited. There is little available evidence upon which to base a surgical opinion of when to operate and when not to operate. The latter of which is invariably more difficult. Surgical intervention for obstructing colonic tumors (segmental resection or proximal defunctioning stoma) has been the mainstay of treatment. However, colonic stenting, which was previously seen as a "bridge" to surgery, is becoming increasingly readily available for the definitive management of obstructing colonic tumors.

In conclusion, age itself is not a risk factor for the development of complications in patients undergoing surgery for colorectal cancer. Age alone should not be a reason to avoid therapeutic or palliative surgery in these patients; instead, patient selection should focus on clinical condition and assessment scores. The type and number of comorbidities influence postoperative mortality and morbidity. Treatment of these comorbidities prior to surgery may influence postoperative outcome.

References

1. Ferlay J, Soerjomataram I, Dikshit R, et al. Cancer incidence and mortality worldwide: sources, methods and major patterns in GLOBOCAN 2012. Int J Cancer. 2015;136(5):E359–86.
2. Kahn KL, Adams JL, Weeks JC, et al. Adjuvant chemotherapy use and adverse events among older patients with stage III colon cancer. JAMA. 2010;303(11):1037–45.
3. Folprecht G, Cunningham D, Ross P, Glimelius B, Di Costanzo F, Wils J, Scheithauer W, Rougier P, Aranda E, Hecker H, Köhne CH. Efficacy of 5-fluorouracil-based chemotherapy in elderly patients with metastatic colorectal cancer: a pooled analysis of clinical trials. Ann Oncol. 2004;15:1330–8.
4. Mathers CD, Stevens GA, Boerma T, White RA, Tobias MI. Causes of international increases in older age life expectancy. Lancet. 2015;385(9967):540–8.
5. de Rijke JM, Schouten LJ, Hillen HF, Kiemeney LA, Coebergh JW, van den Brandt PA. Cancer in the very elderly Dutch population. Cancer. 2000;89:1121–33.
6. Seishima R, Okabayashi K, Hasegawa H, Tsuruta M, Shigeta K, Matsui S, et al. Is laparoscopic colorectal surgery beneficial for elderly patients? A systematic review and meta-analysis. J Gastrointest Surg. 2015;19:756–65.
7. Bircan HY, Koc B, Ozcelik U, Adas G, Karahan S, Demirag A. Are there any differences between age groups regarding colorectal surgery in elderly patients? BMC Surg. 2014;14:44.
8. Uyar D, Frasure HE, Markman M, et al. Treatment patterns by decade of life in elderly women (C70 years of age) with ovarian cancer. Gynecol Oncol. 2005;98:403–8.
9. Papamichael D, Audisio R, Horiot JC, et al. Treatment of the elderly colorectal cancer patient: SIOG expert recommendations. Ann Oncol. 2009;20:5–16.
10. Hermans E, Van Schaik PM, Prins HA, et al. Outcome of colonic surgery in elderly patients with colon cancer. J Oncol. 2010;2010:1–5. https://doi.org/10.1155/2010/865908.
11. Kristjansson SR, Farinella E, Gaskell S, et al. Surgical risk and post-operative complications in older unfit cancer patients. Cancer Treat Rev. 2009;35:499–502.
12. Tan KY, Kawamura YJ, Tokomitsu A, et al. Assessment for frailty is useful for predicting morbidity in elderly patients undergoing colorectal cancer resection whose comorbidities are already optimized. Am J Surg. 2012;204:139–43.

13. Pal SK, Katheria V, Hurria A. Evaluating the older patient with cancer: understanding frailty and the geriatric assessment. CA Cancer J Clin. 2010;60:120–32.
14. Charlson ME, Pompei P, Ales KL, MacKenzie CR. A new method of classifying prognostic comorbidity in longitudinal studies: development and validation. J Chronic Dis. 1987;40:373–83.
15. Topinková E, Mádlová P, Fialová D, Klán J. New evidence-based criteria for evaluating the appropriateness of drug regimen in seniors. Criteria STOPP (screening tool of older person's prescriptions) and START (screening tool to alert doctors to right treatment). Vnitr Lek. 2008;54:1161–9.
16. Stone SP, Ali B, Auberleek I, Thompsell A, Young A. The Barthel index in clinical practice: use on a rehabilitation ward for elderly people. J R Coll Physicians Lond. 1994;28:419–23.
17. Lee YH, Oh H-K, Kim D-W, et al. Use of a comprehensive geriatric assessment to predict short-term postoperative outcome in elderly patients with colorectal cancer. Ann Coloproctol. 2016;32(5):161–9.
18. Lindholm E, Brevinge H, Haglind E. Survival benefit in a randomized clinical trial of faecal occult blood screening for colorectal cancer. Br J Surg. 2008;95:1029–36.
19. Day LW, Kwon A, Inadomi JM, Walter LC, Somsouk M. Adverse events in older patients undergoing colonoscopy: a systematic review and meta-analysis. Gastrointest Endosc. 2011;74:885–96.
20. Lukejohn W, Velayos F. Colorectal cancer screening and surveillance in the elderly: updates and controversies. Gut Liver. 2015;9(2):143–51.
21. Lee-Kong S, Lisle D. Surgical management of complicated colon cancer. Clin Colon Rectal Surg. 2015;28:228–33.
22. Darby CR, Berry AR, Mortensen N. Management variability in surgery for colo-rectal emergencies. Br J Surg. 1992;79:206–10.
23. Fukuda N, Wada J, Niki M, et al. Factors predicting mortality in emergency abdominal surgery in the elderly. World J Emerg Surg. 2012;7:1.
24. Van Gestel YR, Lemmens VE, De Hingh IH, et al. Influence of comorbidity and age on 1-, 2-, and 3-month postoperative mortality rates in gastrointestinal cancer patients. Ann Surg Oncol. 2013;20:371–80.
25. Kumar R, et al. A population-based study of metastatic colorectal cancer in individuals aged ≥ 80 years: findings from the South Australian Clinical Registry for metastatic colorectal cancer. Cancer. 2013;119:722–8.
26. Kang CY, Halabi WJ, Chaudhry OO, Nguyen V, et al. A nationwide analysis of laparoscopy in high-risk colorectal surgery patients. J Gastrointest Surg. 2013;17(2):382–91.
27. Schiphorst AHW, Verweij NM, Pronk A, Borel Rinkes IH, Hamaker ME. Non-surgical complications after laparoscopic and conventional surgery for colorectal cancer – a systematic review of randomized controlled trials. Eur J Surg Oncol. 2015;41:1118–27.
28. Senagore AJ, Madbouly KM, Fazio VW, Duepree HJ, Brady KM, Delaney CP, et al. Advantages of laparoscopic colectomy in older patients. Arch Surg. 2003;138:252–6.
29. Bonjer HJ, Hop WC, Nelson H, Sargent DJ, Lacy AM, Castells A, et al. Laparoscopically assisted vs open colectomy for colon cancer. A meta-analysis. Arch Surg. 2007;142:298–303.
30. Odermatt M, Flashman K, Khan J, Parvaiz A. Laparoscopic assisted abdominoperineal resection for low rectal cancer provides a shorter length of hospital stay while not affecting the recurrence or survival: a propensity score-matched analysis. Surg Today. 2016;46:798–806.
31. Fleshman J, Sargent DJ, Green E, et al. Laparoscopic colectomy for cancer is not inferior to open surgery based on 5-year data from the COST study group trial. Ann Surg. 2007;246:655–62.
32. Kuhry E, Schwenk WF, Gaupset R, Romild U, Bonjer HJ. Long term results of laparoscopic colorectal cancer resection. Cochrane Database Syst Rev. 2008;2:CD003432. https://doi.org/10.1002/14651858.
33. Yamamoto S, Watanabe M, Hasegawa H, et al. Short-term surgical outcomes of laparoscopic colonic surgery in octogenarians: a matched case-control study. Surg Laparosc Endosc Percutan Tech. 2003;13:95–100.

34. Buchs NC, Addeo P, Bianco FM, et al. Safety of robotic general surgery in elderly patients. J Robot Surg. 2010;4:91–8.
35. Zeng WG, Zhou ZX. Mini-invasive surgery for colorectal cancer. Chin J Cancer. 2014;33:277–84.
36. ERAS Compliance Group. The impact of enhanced recovery protocol compliance on elective colorectal cancer resection. Ann Surg. 2015;261(6):1153–9.
37. Adamina M, Kehlet H, Tomlison GA, Senagore AJ, Delaney CP. Enhanced Recovery pathways optimize health outcomes and resource utilization: a meta analysis of randomized controlled trials in colorectal surgery. Surgery. 2011;149:830–40.
38. Bagnall NM, Malietzis G, Kennedy RH, et al. A systematic review of enhanced recovery after colorectal surgery in elderly patients. Color Dis. 2014;16:947–56.
39. Braga M, Pecorelli N, Scatizzi M, Borghi F, Missana G, Radrizzani D, PeriOperative Italian Society. Enhanced recovery program in high-risk patients undergoing colorectal surgery: results from the Perioperative Italian Society Registry. World J Surg. 2016;41:860–7.
40. McMurdo ME, Roberts H, Parker S, Wyatt N, Helen May H, et al. Improving recruitment of older people to research through good practice. Age Ageing. 2011;40:659–65.
41. Smith JJ, Lee J, Burke C, Contractor KB, Dawson PM. Major colorectal cancer resection should not be denied to the elderly. Eur J Surg Oncol. 2002;28:661–6.
42. Seymour MT, Thompson LC, Wasan HS, Middleton G, Brewster AE, Shepherd SF, et al. Chemotherapy options in elderly and frail patients with metastatic colorectal cancer (MRC FOCUS2): an open-label, randomized factorial trial. Lancet. 2011;377:1749–59.
43. Wobbes T. Carcinoma of the colon and rectum in geriatric patients. Age Ageing. 1985;14(6):321–6.
44. Violi V, Pietra N, Grattarola M, et al. Curative surgery for colorectal cancer: long-term results and life expectancy in the elderly. Dis Colon Rectum. 1998;41(3):291–8.
45. Colorectal Cancer Collaberative Group. Surgery for colorectal patients in elderly patients: a systematic review. Lancet. 2000;356:968–74.
46. Basili G, Lorenzetti L, Biondi G, Preziuso E, Angrisano C, Carnesecchi P, Roberto E, Goletti O. Colorectal cancer in the elderly. Is there a role for safe and curative surgery? ANZ J Surg. 2008;78(6):466–70.
47. Paksoy M, Ipek T, Colak T, Cebeci H. Influence of age on prognosis and management of patients with colorectal carcinoma. Eur J Surg. 1999;165(1):55–9.
48. Kristjansson SR, Nesbakken A, Jordhoy MS, Skovlund E, Audisio RA, Johannessen HO, Bakka A, Wyller TB. Comprehensive geriatric assessment can predict complications in elderly patients after elective surgery for colorectal cancer: a prospective observational cohort study. Crit Rev Oncol Hematol. 2010;76(3):208–17.
49. Ugolini G, Rosati G, Montroni I, Zanotti S, Manaresi A, Giampaolo L, Blume JF, Taffurelli M. Can elderly patients with colorectal cancer tolerate planned surgical treatment? A practical approach to a common dilemma. Color Dis. 2009;11(7):750–5.

Surgical Management of Full-Thickness Rectal Prolapse in the Elderly Patient

15

Francesco Gabrielli, Angelo Guttadauro, Matteo Maternini, and Nicoletta Pecora

15.1 Epidemiology and Etiology

Though uncommon, full-thickness rectal prolapse (FTRP) is a debilitating condition that diminishes the quality of life. Its incidence in the general population is 0.2–0.4% and 1% in those aged over 65 years [1, 2], and it increases with advancing age: 21.7% in the seventh decade, 31.7% in the eighth decade, and 20% in the ninth decade, as observed by Keighley in 120 cases [3]. It is more prevalent among older women than older men [1].

Risk factors for the development of FTRP include multiparity by vaginal birth and a history of pelvic surgery, neurological or psychiatric disorders (stroke, spina bifida, dementia), and cystic fibrosis. Contributing factors are bowel dysfunction (IBS, chronic constipation, diarrhea) or bowel habits such as chronic excessive straining during defecation. In 30% of cases, it may be associated with rectal functional disorders (puborectal muscle syndrome, sphincter dyssynergia, descending perineum syndrome) or other perineal anomalies (genital or pelvic organ prolapse, enterocele, sigmoidocele).

The fact that over one hundred different procedures for rectal prolapse repair have been described to date reveals how little we actually know about the etiology [4, 5]. Factors predisposing to the development of rectal prolapse include sigmoid colon redundancy, abnormally deep pouch of Douglas, weakening and collapse of the anatomical structures derived from the pelvic fascia (lateral rectal ligaments), more obtuse anorectal angle at rest, and congenital or progressive weakening of the muscles of the pelvic diaphragm (levator ani muscle) [3]. A main causal role in its development has been attributed to intussusception [6]. A unifying explanation proposed for its pathogenesis is that the prolapse begins cranially as an internal or

F. Gabrielli (✉) • A. Guttadauro • M. Maternini • N. Pecora
Department of General Surgery, University of Milan Bicocca, Zucchi Hospital, Monza, Italy
e-mail: francesco.gabrielli4@tin.it; angelo.guttadauro@unimib.it; matteo.maternini@live.it; nicoletta.pecora@unimib.it

A. Crucitti (ed.), *Surgical Management of Elderly Patients*,
https://doi.org/10.1007/978-3-319-60861-7_15

occult sigmoidorectal or high rectorectal prolapse that then invaginates distally to form a rectoanal prolapse that eventually protrudes externally, becoming a FTRP, conventionally defined as rectal prolapse if the segment is up to 5–6 cm in length or sigmoidorectal if longer. As it continues to descend, an internal rectal prolapse can deform the anterior peritoneal wall, giving rise to rectocele: intussusception and rectocele thus contribute to dyschezia caused by obstructed defecation [5].

In 15–65% of cases, FTRP is associated with constipation; in 75% of patients, stretching of the nerve fibers and the anal sphincters leads to a variable degree of incontinence [3, 4, 7], which is more prevalent in patients over 60 years of age and especially in the multiparous (85% of cases) [3].

15.2 Surgical Therapy

Symptom severity and the risk of complications are indications for surgical treatment in elderly patients, too. Medical management is reserved for very frail patients, in which palliative treatment of functional symptoms is focused on correct diet, Kegel exercises to strengthen pelvic floor muscles, or biofeedback therapy to improve sphincter control [8].

15.3 Abdominal Procedures

15.3.1 Traditional Rectopexy

For nearly 30 years, traditional rectopexy procedures were the most widely used techniques and yielded good outcomes for prolapse repair [9–11]. In the Wells procedure (posterior sling rectopexy), a mesh is anchored to the sacrum and wrapped 270° posterolaterally around the rectum [12], while in the Orr-Loygue procedure, two prosthetic polytetrafluoroethylene (PTFE) strips are fixed to the anterolateral surface of the rectum and back to the sacral promontory [13]. The Ripstein procedure involved a mesh encircling the rectum entirely [14] but was subsequently abandoned because of the risk of occlusion from stenotic scarring. Simple rectopexy using nonabsorbable sutures instead of a mesh for fixation to the presacral fascia from 1–2 to 4–5 cm below the sacral promontory has been shown to be non-inferior to rectopexy with mesh [15]. Most commonly performed under general anesthesia, rectopexy can also be carried out under peridural anesthesia in selected patients.

In both male and female patients, the rectum is mobilized to the tip of the coccyx posteriorly and anteriorly to expose the plane of the levator muscles. Debate continues about whether or not to resect the lateral rectal ligaments, with some surgeons arguing that the ligaments are weakened in rectal prolapse [3] and the majority sustaining that ligament resection leads to parasympathetic denervation, resulting in the onset or worsening of constipation. On the other hand, while sparing the ligaments may reduce the risk of constipation, it increases the risk of prolapse recurrence [16, 17]. Furthermore, ligament resection may also affect colon transit time and increase the frequency of bowel movement, reducing rectal elasticity and capacity [18].

Rectopexy has been considered the gold standard of surgical treatment for rectal prolapse since it is associated with a recurrence rate of less than 5% (mean rate, 2–3%) [3, 4, 7, 9, 19–22]. The operative mortality rate ranges between 0 and 7% but remains acceptable on average. Morbidity ranges more widely (0–20%) [3, 7, 9, 10, 19–22]: the major complications are bleeding (even life-threatening in cases of sacral veins lesion), prosthesis infection producing pelvic abscess, stenotic scarring, and erosion fistulas. While prosthesis-related complications (infection, stenosis, erosion) are obviously absent in simple rectopexy, other complications are similar to those seen after rectopexy with the use of a mesh [3, 9, 10].

Incontinence after surgery is improved in about 60% of patients [3]. Since improvement may not be noted until at least 6 months after the operation, particularly in elderly patients, other therapeutic options for treating incontinence, especially further surgery, should be delayed accordingly. Studies seeking to identify predicting factors of functional improvement based on preoperative examinations have found that patients presenting with low basal pressure and maximum squeeze pressure have a higher probability of remaining incontinent after rectopexy [3]. Morphologic evaluation with CT and MR imaging of the perineal musculature has shown that impairment of sphincter and levator ani muscle function can be useful for diagnosis and prognosis [23].

Improvement in constipation after rectopexy ranges widely across studies, with some reporting improvement in 15–80% of patients and others noting new onset or worsening of constipation in 15–50% [4, 7, 9, 10, 22, 24–27]. Patients with preexisting constipation have a greater probability of not experiencing improvement or even worsening of the condition after surgery [3]. Other reasons for failed improvement are preexisting colonic inertia, complete rectal mobilization with resection of the lateral rectal ligaments, and kinking of a convoluted sigmoid. Hence, the real problem with traditional rectopexy is postoperative constipation, which has dampened the initial expectations driven by the lower recurrence rates associated with the procedure.

15.3.2 Combined Abdominal Rectopexy and Sigmoid Resection

The Frykman-Goldberg procedure [28] is primarily indicated in patients with preexisting constipation and in those having undergone rectopexy in which the sigmoid colon is so twisted that replacing it in the abdominal cavity would not only be difficult but also would arouse suspicion as to the cause of constipation. For technical reasons, rectopexy is performed after sigmoid resection and without the use of a mesh to minimize the risk of bacterial infection.

The few comparative trials that have been conducted to date (rectopexy alone vs. resection combined with rectopexy) [29–31] have found no meaningful difference in recurrence rates, a lower incidence of postoperative constipation after Frykman-Goldberg procedure (12 vs. 48%), and a statistically significant improvement of incontinence. Enlarging colon resection from sigmoidectomy to left hemicolectomy does not appear to provide additional improvement in bowel function, particularly as regards constipation [32].

Several studies have shown that colon resection with anastomosis increases both the rate of operative mortality (1–2%) and the risk of major complications (34 vs. 22%) [29–31].

15.3.3 Ventral Rectopexy

This procedure derives from the laparotomic technique Loygue originally devised in 1984 [13]. In 2004, D'Hoore et al. [33] proposed a simplified approach by laparoscopy, in which posterior dissection is limited to exposure of the sacral promontory, opening of the peritoneum to the right of the rectum without resecting the pouch of Douglas, and preparing the anterior rectal subperitoneal fascia as far as the levator muscles. The rectum is then suspended with a mesh (3 cm large) fixed cranially to the sacral promontory, and the mesh is then extraperitonealized.

In France, ventral rectopexy is also performed using a limited dissection, fixation with prosthetic strips, and excision of the lowest portion of the pouch of Douglas [25].

Following initial good outcomes published by D'Hoore's group in Belgium [34] and by others in Great Britain [35, 36], the technique quickly gained wider acceptance owing to its simplicity and effectiveness, becoming the abdominal suspension method of choice for prolapse repair. Its indication from FTRP repair was expanded to include rectal intussusception and rectocele, which cause obstructed defecation, and associated with gynecological suspension procedures for the repair of multi-compartment prolapses [37].

There is a growing body of evidence documenting good long-term outcomes after ventral rectopexy. Two recent meta-analyses [38, 39] examined the follow-up results in 574 and 789 patients, respectively. The conversion rate was 2.9%; no operative deaths occurred. The postoperative complication rate was lower than 20%, and serious complications were noted in 4.8% of patients. The recurrence rate at 2 years was 3.4% and 4.7%, respectively. A net improvement in incontinence was achieved in 30–40% and in up to 80–90% of cases.

Also of interest was the long-term improvement in constipation. Both meta-analyses substantiated the initial reports by D'Hoore et al. [40] and the Oxford group [35]. As compared with traditional rectopexy, a greater improvement in constipation and reduced risk postoperative constipation were associated with ventral rectopexy: improvement in constipation in 3–70% of patients and incidence of new onset constipation or worsening of constipation in 0–20% of patients [38, 39]. The improvement in constipation can be explained by the fact that the lateral rectal ligaments are spared, thus avoiding rectal inertia due to parasympathetic denervation.

Improvement in incontinence (improved in over 80% of patients) has also been reported in elderly patients [41]. Despite advanced age, the basal tone and squeeze pressure values were found to improve during the first 2 months following the operation and continued to improve at 1-year follow-up assessment, with a statistically significant increase in basal tone.

Taken together, these results show that ventral rectopexy is an effective and safe procedure. Although it entails minor and simpler rectal mobilization, it is not associated with a higher recurrence rate. Functional improvement in incontinence and constipation appears promising, making the technique particularly attractive for FTRP repair in older patients [36].

15.3.4 Mesh Selection in Rectopexy Procedures

Following reports of its oncogenicity in experimental studies, the use of the Ivalon sponge was abandoned [3]. Most surgeons opted for other types of mesh made from synthetic materials, mostly polypropylene, for traditional rectopexy. Though no significant difference in functional outcome or complication rates has been found for mesh made from absorbable material (polyglycolic acid), it appears to be burdened by a slightly higher rate of recurrence [42].

An emerging problem of synthetic mesh prostheses, sometimes causing severe erosion of rectal or contiguous visceral tissues after ventral rectopexy, has recently come to light. Initially estimated at 1% [43], the risk of erosion seems to be higher (2%) and far greater than that associated with biological prostheses (0.7–2.4 vs. 0–0.7%) [44]. Owing to their antigenic properties, polyester prostheses appear to be more erosive than mesh made from polypropylene or titanium-coated propylene prostheses.

Biological mesh made from porcine skin or submucosa, though safer, is more expensive. They are less durable, which is thought to be the reason for the higher number of recurrences found at long-term follow-up [45]. Their use in laparoscopic ventral rectopexy should be reserved for young males, women of reproductive age, and particularly for patients at higher risk for developing sepsis due to the presence of comorbid conditions such as diabetes or inflammatory bowel disease or a history of pelvic radiation therapy or rectal or vaginal surgery [46].

When selecting a synthetic mesh, the material of choice seems to be titanium-coated polypropylene because of its strength and greater resistance to infections [46]. Furthermore, suturing of the mesh to the sacral promontory appears to be safer with staples rather than with simple sutures [47].

15.3.5 Open and Minimally Invasive (Laparoscopy or Robot-Assisted) Procedures

The choice of technique depends on the surgeon's preference and experience. Minimally invasive procedures should be carried out at centers specialized in these techniques. Of note is that the recent ventral rectopexy is almost always performed in laparoscopy [33, 35, 36].

The wider acceptance of laparoscopic rectopexy has been driven in part by optimal long-term complications and recurrence rates [27, 38, 48]. Comparative trials evaluating open surgery and laparoscopy have not reported significant differences in recurrence rates or functional outcomes (improvement in constipation and incontinence) [49, 50]. Moreover, laparoscopy affords the advantages of better cosmesis, less pain, shorter duration of postoperative ileus, and shorter length of hospital stay. Its drawbacks are the longer operative time and limiting problems such as abdominal adhesions [10]. Though more expensive than open surgery, the greater cost is offset by shorter hospitalization and less morbidity [30, 49, 50].

Even recent meta-analyses have reported that, in trained hands, long-term recurrence rates and functional outcomes are similar for laparotomy and laparoscopy, while the latter seems to be associated with lower operative morbidity and complication rates [51, 52].

Robot-assisted surgery appears to combine the advantages of laparoscopy, with better 3D visualization [53, 54]; however, the technique is seldom used and is limited by its lengthy operating time and high costs [55].

15.4 Perineal Procedures

15.4.1 Rectosigmoidectomy (Altemeier Procedure)

Perineal resection of the sigmoid colon and rectum for prolapse repair was first described by Auffret in 1882 in France. Following reports by Mikulicz and St. Mark's Hospital in London, the procedure was gradually abandoned because of its high failure rates [56]. It gained renewed interest in the mid-twentieth century through refinements by Altemeier in the United States [57]. According to Altemeier, its combination with levatorplasty was the reason for the less than 3% long-term recurrence rate in his series [58]. The procedure subsequently gained wide acceptance, becoming the most commonly used technique in the United States, particularly in the treatment of high-risk geriatric patients [59]. Many colorectal surgeons now consider it an elective procedure in all patients, irrespective of age [56, 60].

The Altemeier procedure offers distinct advantages for the older patient subpopulation: it can be performed under spinal anesthesia, no scar formation, low postoperative complications, painless rapid course, and early hospital discharge [61].

Controversy surrounds its recurrence rates. In their literature review of studies involving a total of 1635 patients, Cirocco [56] observed a 37% recurrence rate for series treated before 1971 and a 10% rate for series treated after 1971. Specifically regarding geriatric surgery, Altomare et al. [61] examined case series of patients in which the mean age was 77 years (over 80 years in 40% and over 90 years in 7.5% of patients in their own case series) and found a mean recurrence rate of 18%, with a wide individual range (0–58%).

Various reasons have been proposed for the continuing improvement in recurrence rates. Foremost is enhanced awareness of the correct execution of the technique, which entails opening the pouch of Douglas to completely exteriorize the prolapse [56]. Combining the procedure with levatorplasty is also important, as originally suggested by Altemeier [57] and as underlined by some surgeons [62–64] but not accepted by all [56, 61]. Another explanation for the variability in outcome reported in single case series is the diverse length of follow-up periods, given that the recurrence rate will increase with advancing patient age and that prolonged follow-up of elderly patients is difficult to achieve [7, 56, 61]. Other factors (sex, age, length of operative specimen, preoperative incontinence) have not been demonstrated to have a predictive value [61].

The operative mortality rate is extremely low (0.6% of 1635 operations) [57] and the morbidity rate ranges between 3 and 14% [7, 56, 60]. Major early complications (6–7%) include pelvic hematoma, anastomotic dehiscence, sigmoid perforation, and pararectal abscess [61]. The percentage and severity of complications appear to be lower than those associated with abdominal procedures [7, 65, 66].

The use of new technologies (resection with ultrasound or radiofrequency devices and coloanal stapler anastomosis) does not appear to confer meaningful advantages over traditional techniques, except for a lower risk of recurrence (10 vs. 15%) [49].

In most of the patients with preexisting incontinence, the condition improved: 80–100% in large series [56] and in geriatric patients as well [61]. Particular importance has been given to combining the procedure with levatorplasty to improve post-operative incontinence rather than prevent prolapse recurrence [56, 63, 67].

On the other hand, new-onset incontinence was found to develop in 15% of patients who were continent before the operation [56]. This may be explained by the fact that part of the rectal ampulla is removed, resulting in loss of its reservoir function [61]. Comparison between perineal rectosigmoidectomy and an abdominal procedure (resection plus rectopexy) showed that the latter is associated with a significant improvement in continence and less postoperative defecation urgency [68]. For this reason, completing an Altemeier procedure with creation of a pouch has been recommended especially in elderly patients [69].

Postoperative constipation has been reported to improve in 50–60% of cases (range, 15–100%), without worsening of the condition [7, 56, 61]. Therefore, perineal procedures are not burdened by the most severe functional risk associated with rectopexy. The lower risk of postoperative constipation may be attributed to the reduced volume of the rectal ampulla and the consensual resection of the possible intussusception associated with external prolapse.

The good functional outcomes translate into improved quality of life, as measured with the EuroQol (EQ-5D) questionnaire for measuring generic health status and the Patient Assessment of Constipation Quality of Life (PAC-QoL). The improvement after perineal rectosigmoidectomy, unlike other surgical techniques, does not appear to be influenced by advanced age or comorbidities [70].

15.4.2 Perineal Stapled Prolapse Resection (PSPR)

Scherer [71] recently described a new abdominal perineal resection procedure that offers the advantages of rapidity and ease of execution, which make it of particular interest in geriatric surgery. Based on the variant described by Romano et al. [72], the procedure begins with division of the prolapse using a linear cutter (75 mm) at 3 and 9 o'clock approximately 2 cm above the dentate line. Then resection-suture of the prolapse is performed by a curved cutter stapler (Contour® CCS 30). After insertion, the head is rotated counterclockwise along the two hemi-conferences for complete removal of the prolapse and creation of a suture line cranial to and parallel with the dentate line.

The results are inferior to those obtained with the Altemeier technique, with a recurrence rate of 20–40% in the few cases operated on to date [73–75]. The reason for such high recurrence may derive from resection performed with traction applied only to the visible portion of the prolapse, resulting in a smaller amount of protruding rectal tissue that can be resected. Furthermore, controlled opening of the pouch of Douglas is not possible, which would allow complete mobilization and exteriorization of the prolapse, and the technique cannot be combined with levatorplasty [74].

Technical limitations may arise from excessive prolapse length (>5–6 cm) and especially excessive prolapse thickness (7–8 mm) owing to the risk of the staples failing to close. Moreover, the method entails performing several steps without visual control: resection-suture of the pouch of Douglas may inadvertently involve the intestinal loops or the vaginal vault in hysterectomized patients. Finally, effective hemostasis cannot be achieved in cases of resection-suturing of a thick mesorectum.

Another problem is the procedure's elevated costs, which may run to about US $1600 if multiple staples are used [74]. This leads to the question of whether the method is justifiable when the Altemeier procedure is less costly and safer in terms of recurrence [56].

Summarizing, PSPR should be reserved only for high-risk elderly patients (high ASA class) in which the duration of the operation should be as short as possible and, owing to technical limitations, for cases of prolapse repair neither too long nor too thick [76].

15.4.3 Other Perineal Procedures

Encircling holds only a historical interest because of its high failure rates [3].

The Delorme procedure continues to be used in Europe, mainly in France [3, 77]. It may be considered as an alternative to rectosigmoidectomy in cases of short prolapse (<5 cm in length). It is not always easy to perform, and it has been associated with recurrence rates of over 30% [78], but lower rates (5–22%) are reported by expert surgeons [77]. The only comparative trial carried out to date [31] found no significant differences in recurrence or functional outcome between the Delorme and the Altemeier procedures. When combined with levatorplasty, the procedure yields improvement in incontinence and recurrence rates, though the difference in recurrence rates was not statistically significant [79].

15.5 Management of Prolapse Recurrence

Most recurrences occur within 3 months of the operation, with the elderly and women at greater risk [80, 81]. The patient's general health condition permitting recurrent prolapse repair can be performed using the same surgical procedures [82]. While the same access as in the primary operation may be used, most surgeons feel it more prudent in cases of failed rectopexy to switch to a perineal approach. In recurrences after a perineal procedure, especially in elderly patients, the same procedure can be safely and effectively repeated even if laparoscopic ventral rectopexy could be employed if the patient is in good health.

A meta-analysis of studies comparing prolapse recurrence after an abdominal procedure (158 patients) and after a perineal procedure (144 patients) reported a mortality rate of 0% and 15%, respectively; those who had undergone a perineal procedure were evidently in poorer health. The morbidity rate ranged between 0 and 32% and the recurrence rate between 0 and 50% [83]. These results appear somewhat questionable. Undoubtedly, the risk of a new recurrence after repair for prolapse recurrence is higher [80–82, 84].

15.6 Selecting a Surgical Procedure

A long-standing principle that guided the selection of surgical treatment was that abdominal procedures were associated with lower recurrence but greater morbidity, whereas perineal procedures were associated with lower mortality and morbidity and faster postoperative recovery but burdened by higher recurrence. More recently, however, this principle has been revised following reports from trials comparing recurrence rates after abdominal procedures (resection combined with rectopexy) and those after perineal procedures (Altemeier procedure): there was no statistically significant difference [31, 68]. Moreover, case studies with a follow-up period of up to 4–5 years reported a similar range of recurrence rates, between 0 and 18% [85].

The major factors guiding the choice of treatment, especially in elderly patients, are that a perineal procedure can be carried out under spinal anesthesia with shorter operating time, is less demanding on the patient, and allows earlier recovery [10]. Accurate assessment of the patient's general health is essential, given that biological age is more important than chronological age in evaluating elderly patients. Based on the American Society of Anesthesiologists (ASA) risk classification system, low-risk elderly patients may be considered fit for an abdominal procedure, pending a more valid permanent definitive result, whereas a perineal procedure, because it is less demanding on the patient, should be considered for higher-risk patients.

Several other factors will also need to be considered when selecting a surgical procedure. An abdominal procedure may be the better choice (combined with a suspension procedure) when repair of multicompartment prolapse (genital or bladder) or coexisting conditions (enterocele or sigmoidocele) needs to be performed in a single stage. In cases of associated gynecological prolapse, priority should be given to repair of the genital prolapse since its treatment (anterior, lateral, posterior colpopexy) may resolve also the posterior problem, obviating the need to operate on the rectum.

On the other hand, because suspending a denervated rectum already weakened due to prolapse may not only be useless but also counterproductive, some surgeons have further expanded the indications for perineal resection which, in expert hands, appears to considerably reduce mortality, morbidity, and long-term recurrence [56].

Also, bowel function before surgery may influence the choice of surgical treatment, with the option of selecting between an abdominal and a perineal procedure in patients with normal bowel function. Differently, in patients with preexisting constipation, owing to the risk of persistent or worsening postoperative constipation, either abdominal rectopexy combined with sigmoid resection or perineal resection, which does not significantly worsen constipation, should be performed [10].

Patient sex is irrelevant in geriatric surgery, whereas in young patients, an abdominal procedure can be indicated to reduce the risk of pelvic organ denervation in young males, and mesh suspension in women of reproductive age should be critically considered to minimize the risk of infertility.

15.7 The Evolution of Geriatric Surgery

Historically, patient age has been a major factor in FTRP repair. Perineal procedures, because less demanding on the patient, are the preferred choice in the surgical treatment of elderly patients [85]. Up until 2010, perineal resection was the most commonly performed procedure in patients aged over 70 years in the United States, followed by laparotomy and laparoscopy [86]. In their study, Fang et al. [87] retrospectively examined the data from the American College of Surgeons National Surgical Quality Improvement Program (ACS NSQIP) database and found that the percentage of patients undergoing an abdominal procedure (by laparotomy or laparoscopy) decreased with advancing patient age. Furthermore, patients aged 80 years or older were twice as likely to undergo a perineal procedure, and those aged under 80 years and with an ASA status of 3 or 4 were 1.5 times more likely than those with an ASA score of 1 or 2. Finally, operative mortality was lower after an abdominal than after a perineal procedure (0.13 vs. 0.9%) and was 0 after a laparoscopic procedure.

As the situation continues to evolve, more and more studies are reporting favorably on the wider use of laparoscopic rectopexy in geriatric patients. In patients aged 80 years or older, ventral rectopexy has been associated with a long-term complication rate of 15 and a 3% recurrence rate [36]. A study comparing laparoscopic techniques (rectopexy with or without mesh combined with colon resection) in patients with a mean age of 70 years reported a morbidity rate of 28% and a 3.3% recurrence rate, both of which were similar to those reported for younger patients. Reports on outcomes after robotic surgery in patients aged over 75 years have also begun to appear [88].

In terms of acceptable morbidity rates and effective outcomes, there is a new emerging trend for minimally invasive abdominal suspension procedures in low-risk older patients [85, 86]. Nonetheless, evidence is still scarce and doubt remains about functional outcomes. To fill this gap in geriatric surgery, large-scale multi-center trials with longer follow-up are needed.

References

1. Kairaluoma MV, Kellokumpu IH. Epidemiologic aspects of complete rectal prolapse. Scand J Surg. 2005;94:207–10.
2. Stein EA, Stein DE. Rectal procidentia: diagnosis and management. Gastrointest Endosc Clin N Am. 2006;16:189–201.
3. MRB K, Williams NS. Rectal prolapse. In: Surgery of the anus rectum and colon, Saunders, vol. 23. London; 1999. p. 794–842.
4. Madoff RD, Mellgren A. One hundred years of rectal prolapse surgery. Dis Colon Rectum. 1999;42:441–50.
5. Jayne D, Stuto A. The evidence for stapled hemorrhoidopexy and STARR. In: Transanal stapling techniques for anorectal prolapse, vol. 7. London: Springer; 2009. p. 95–115.
6. Broden B, Snellman B. Procidentia of the rectum studied with cineradiography: a contribution to the discussion of the causative mechanism. Dis Colon Rectum. 1968;11:330–47.
7. Kim DS, Tsang CB, Wong WD, et al. Complete rectal prolapse: evolution of management and results. Dis Colon Rectum. 1999;42:460–6.
8. Khaikin M, Wexner SD. Treatment strategies in obstructed defecation and fecal incontinence. World J Gastroenterol. 2006;12:3168–73.
9. Madiba TE, Baig MK, Wexner SD. Surgical management of rectal prolapse. Arch Surg. 2005;140:63–73.
10. Tou S, Brown SR, Nelson RL. Surgery for complete (full-thickness) rectal prolapse in adults. Cochrane Database Syst Rev. 2015;11:CD001758. https://doi.org/10.1002/14651858.CD001758.pub3.
11. Karas JR, Uranues S, Altomare DF, et al. No rectopexy versus rectopexy following rectal mobilization for full-thickness rectal prolapse: a randomized controlled trial. Dis Colon Rectum. 2011;54:29–34.
12. Wells C. New operation for rectal prolapse. Proc R Soc Med. 1959;52:602–3.
13. Loygue J, Huguier M, Malafosse M, Biotois H. Complete prolapse of the rectum. A report on 140 cases treated by rectopexy. Br J Surg. 1971;58:847–8.
14. Ripstein CB. Procidentia: definitive corrective surgery. Dis Colon Rectum. 1972;15:334–6.
15. Novell JR, Osborne MJ, Winslet MC, Lewis AA. Prospective randomized trial of Ivalon sponge versus sutured rectopexy for full-thickness rectal prolapse. Br J Surg. 1994;81(6):904–6.
16. Speakman CTM, Madden MV, Nicholls RJ, Kamm MA. Lateral ligament division during rectopexy causes constipation but prevents recurrence: results of a prospective randomized study. Br J Surg. 1991;78(12):1431–3.
17. Selvaggi F, Scotto di Carlo E, Silvestri L, Festa L, Piegari V. Surgical treatment of rectal prolapse: a randomised study. Br J Surg. 1993;80(Suppl):S89.
18. Mollen RM, Kuijpers JH, van Hoek F. Effects of rectal mobilization and lateral ligaments division on colonic and anorectal function. Dis Colon Rectum. 2000;43:1283–7.
19. Watts JD, Rothenberger DA, Buls JG, et al. The management of procidentia. 30 years' experience. Dis Colon Rectum. 1985;28:96–102.
20. Madbouly KM, Senagore AJ, Delaney CP, et al. Clinically based management of rectal prolapse. Surg Endosc. 2003;17:99–103.
21. Raftopoulos Y, Senagore AJ, Di Giuro G, et al. Recurrence rates after abdominal surgery for complete rectal prolapse: a multicenter pooled analysis of 643 individual patient data. Dis Colon Rectum. 2005;48:1200–6.

22. Portier G, Iovino F, Lazorthes F. Surgery for rectal prolapse: Orr-Loygue ventral rectopexy with limited dissection prevents postoperative-induced constipation without increasing recurrence. Dis Colon Rectum. 2006;49:1136–40.
23. Gabrielli F, Campanelli GP, Leopaldi E, Poggi L, et al. Terapia chirurgica del prolasso rettale: vantaggi e limiti delle rettopessie per via addominale. Chirurgia. 1993;6:535–40.
24. Lechaux JP, Atienza P, Goasguen N, et al. Prosthetic rectopexy to the pelvic floor and sigmoidectomy for rectal prolapse. Am J Surg. 2001;182:465–9.
25. Laubert T, Kleemann M, Schorcht A, et al. Laparoscopic resection rectopexy for rectal prolapse: a single-center study during 16 years. Surg Endosc. 2010;24:2401–6.
26. Dulucq JL, Wintringer P, Mahajna A. Clinical and functional outcome of laparoscopic posterior rectopexy (Wells) for full-thickness rectal prolapse. A prospective study. Surg Endosc. 2007;21:2226–30.
27. Lechaux D, Trebuchet G, Siproudhis L, Campion JP. Laparoscopic rectopexy for full-thickness rectal prolapse: a single-institution retrospective study evaluating surgical outcome. Surg Endosc. 2005;19:514–8.
28. Frykman HM, Goldberg SM. The surgical treatment of rectal procidentia. Surg Gynecol Obstet. 1969;129:1225–30.
29. Luukkonen P, Mikkonen U, Jarvinen H. Abdominal rectopexy with sigmoidectomy versus rectopexy alone for rectal prolapse: a prospective, randomized study. Int J Color Dis. 1992;7(4):219–22.
30. Tjandra JJ, Fazio VW, Church JM, Milsom JW, Oakley JR, Lavery IC. Ripstein procedure is an effective treatment for rectal prolapse without constipation. Dis Colon Rectum. 1993;36:501–7.
31. Senapati A, Gray RG, Middleton LJ, Harding J, Hills RK, Armitage NCM, et al. PROSPER: a randomised comparison of surgical treatments for rectal prolapse. Color Dis. 2013;15(7):858–68.
32. Yoshioka K, Heyen F, Keighley MRB. Functional results after posterior abdominal rectopexy for rectal prolapse. Dis Colon Rectum. 1989;32:835–8.
33. D'Hoore A, Cadoni R, Penninckx F. Long-term outcome of laparoscopic ventral rectopexy for total rectal prolapse. Br J Surg. 2004;91:1500–5.
34. D'Hoore A, Penninckx F. Laparoscopic ventral recto(colpo)pexy for rectal prolapse: surgical technique and outcome for 109 patients. Surg Endosc. 2006;20:1919–23.
35. Boons P, Collinson R, Cunningham C, Lindsey I. Laparoscopic ventral rectopexy for external rectal prolapse improves constipation and avoids de novo constipation. Color Dis. 2010;12:526–32.
36. Wijffels N, Cunningham C, Dixon A, Greenslade G, Lindsey I. Laparoscopic ventral rectopexy for external rectal prolapse is safe and effective in the elderly. Does this make perineal procedures obsolete? Color Dis. 2011;13:561–6.
37. Gurland B. Ventral mesh rectopexy: is this the new standard for surgical treatment of pelvic organ prolapse? Dis Colon Rectum. 2014;57:1446–7.
38. Faucheron JL, Trilling B, Girard E, Sage P, Barbois S, Reche F. Anterior rectopexy for full-thickness rectal prolapse: technical and functional results. World J Gastroenterol. 2015;21:5049–55.
39. Samaranayake CB, Luo C, Plank AW, et al. Systematic review on ventral rectopexy for rectal prolapse and intussusception. Color Dis. 2010;12:504–12.
40. van Geluwe B, Wolthuis A, Penninckx F, D'Hoore A. Lessons learned after more than 400 laparoscopic ventral rectopexies. Acta Chir Belg. 2013;113:103–6.
41. Bjerke T, Mynster T. Laparoscopic ventral rectopexy in an elderly population with external rectal prolapse: clinical and anal manometric results. Int J Color Dis. 2014;29:1257–62.
42. Galili Y, Rabau M. Comparison of polyglycolic acid and polypropylene mesh for rectopexy in the treatment of rectal prolapse. Eur J Surg. 1997;163:445–8.
43. Smart NJ, Pathak S, Boorman P, Daniels IR. Synthetic or biological mesh use in laparoscopic ventral mesh rectopexy: a systematic review. Color Dis. 2013;15:650–4.
44. Evans C, Stevenson AR, Sileri P, et al. A multicenter collaboration to assess the safety of laparoscopic ventral rectopexy. Dis Colon Rectum. 2015;58:799–807.

45. Bhandarkar DS. Laparoscopic rectopexy for complete rectal prolapse: mesh, no mesh or a ventral mesh? J Minimal Access Surg. 2014;10:1–3.
46. Mercer-Jones MA, D'Hoore A, Dixon AR, et al. Consensus on ventral rectopexy: report of a panel of experts. Color Dis. 2014;16:82–8.
47. Darzi A, Henry MM, Guillou PJ, Shorvon P, Monson JR. Stapled laparoscopic rectopexy for rectal prolapse. Surg Endosc. 1995;9:301–3.
48. Kariv Y, Delaney CP, Casillas S, et al. Long-term outcome after laparoscopic and open surgery for rectal prolapse: a case-control study. Surg Endosc. 2006;20:35–42.
49. Boccasanta P, Venturi M, Barbieri S, Roviaro G. Impact of new technologies on the clinical and functional outcome of Altemeier's procedure: a randomized, controlled trial. Dis Colon Rectum. 2006;49:652–60.
50. Salkeld G, Bagia M, Solomon M. Economic impact of laparoscopic versus open abdominal rectopexy. Br J Surg. 2004;91:1188–91.
51. Purkayastha S, Tekkis P, Athanasiou T, et al. A comparison of open vs. laparoscopic abdominal rectopexy for full-thickness rectal prolapse: a meta-analysis. Dis Colon Rectum. 2005;48:1930–40.
52. Sajid MS, Siddiqui MRS, Baig MK. Open vs laparoscopic repair of full-thickness rectal prolapse: a re-meta-analysis. Color Dis. 2010;12:515–25.
53. Munz Y, Moorthy K, Kudchadkar R, et al. Robotic assisted rectopexy. Am J Surg. 2004;187:88–9.
54. Heemskerk J, de Hoog DE, van Gemert WG, et al. Robot-assisted vs. conventional laparoscopic rectopexy for rectal prolapse: a comparative study on costs and time. Dis Colon Rectum. 2007;50:1825–30.
55. Mäkelä-Kaikkonen J, Rautio T, Klintrup K, Takala H, Vierimaa M, Ohtonen P, Mäkelä J. Robotic-assisted and laparoscopic ventral rectopexy in the treatment of rectal prolapse: a matched-pairs study of operative details and complications. Tech Coloproctol. 2014;18:151–5.
56. Cirocco WC. The Altemeier procedure for rectal prolapse: an operation for all ages. Dis Colon Rectum. 2010;53:1618–23.
57. Altemeier WA, Giuseffi J, Hoxworth P. Treatment of extensive prolapse of the rectum in aged or debilitated patients. Arch Surg. 1952;65:72–80.
58. Altemeier WA, Culbertson WR, Schowengerdt C, Hunt J. Nineteen years' experience with the one-stage perineal repair of rectal prolapse. Ann Surg. 1971;173:993–1006.
59. Schoetz DJ Jr. Evolving practice patterns in colon and rectal surgery. J Am Coll Surg. 2006;203:322–7.
60. Glasgow SC, Birnbaum EH, Kodner IJ, Fleshman JW Jr, Dietz DW. Recurrence and quality of life following perineal proctectomy for rectal prolapse. J Gastrointest Surg. 2008;12:1446–51.
61. Altomare DF, Binda G, Ganio E, De Nardi P, Giamundo P, Pescatori M, Rectal Prolapse Study Group. Long-term outcome of Altemeier's procedure for rectal prolapse. Dis Colon Rectum. 2009;52:698–703.
62. Agachan F, Pfeiffer J, Joo JS, et al. Results of perineal procedures for the treatment of rectal prolapse. Am Surg. 1997;63:9–12.
63. Chun SW, Pikarsky AJ, You SY, et al. Perineal rectosigmoidectomy for rectal prolapse: role of levatorplasty. Tech Coloproctol. 2004;8:3–9.
64. Williams JG, Rothenberger DA, Madoff RD, Goldberg SM. Treatment of rectal prolapse in the elderly by perineal rectosigmoidectomy. Dis Colon Rectum. 1992;35:830–4.
65. Azimuddin K, Khubchandani IT, Rosen L, Stasik JJ, Riether RD, Reed JF. Rectal prolapse: a search for the "best" operation. Am Surg. 2001;67:622–7.
66. Habr-Gama A, Jacob CE, Jorge JM, et al. Rectal procidentia treatment by perineal rectosigmoidectomy combined with levator ani repair. Hepato-Gastroenterology. 2006;53:213–7.
67. Prasad ML, Pearl RK, Abcarian H, Orsay CP, Nelson RL. Perineal proctectomy, posterior rectopexy, and postanal levator repair for the treatment of rectal prolapse. Dis Colon Rectum. 1986;29:547–52.
68. Deen KI, Grant E, Billingham C, Keighley MRB. Abdominal resection rectopexy with pelvic floor repair versus perineal rectosigmoidectomy and pelvic floor repair for full-thickness rectal prolapse. Br J Surg. 1994;81:302–4.

69. Yoshioka K, Ogunbiyi OA, Keighley MRB. Pouch perineal rectosigmoidectomy gives better functional results than conventional rectosigmoidectomy in elderly patients with rectal prolapse. Br J Surg. 1998;85:1525–6.
70. Kim M, Reibetanz J, Schlegel N, Germer CT, Jayne D, Isbert C. Perineal rectosigmoidectomy: quality of life. Color Dis. 2013;15:1000–6.
71. Scherer R, Marti L, Hetzer F. Perineal stapled prolapse resection: a new procedure for external rectal prolapse. Dis Colon Rectum. 2008;51:1727–30.
72. Romano G, Bianco F, Caggiano L. Modified perineal stapled rectal resection with contour transtar for full-thickness rectal prolapse. Color Dis. 2009;11:878–81.
73. Tschuor C, Limani P, Nocito A, Dindo D, Clavien PA, Hahnloser D. Perineal stapled prolapse resection for external rectal prolapse: is it worthwhile in the long-term? Tech Coloproctol. 2013;17:537–40.
74. Ram E, Krissi H, Zbar A, Atar E, Joubran S, Rath-wolfson L. Perineal stapled prolapse resection (PSPR) in elderly patients for external rectal prolapse: early experience. Tech Coloproctol. 2014;18:1003–7.
75. Raahave D, Jensen AK, Dammegaard L, et al. Primary and repeated perineal stapled prolapse resection. Tech Coloproctol. 2016;20:853–7.
76. Maternini M, Guttadauro A, Pecora N, Gabrielli F. Perineal stapled prolapse resection (PSPR) for external rectal prolapse in high morbidity patients. Ann Ital Chir. 2016;87:476–80.
77. Tsunoda A, Yasuda N, Yokoyama N, et al. Delorme's procedure for rectal prolapse. Clinical and physiological analysis. Dis Colon Rectum. 2003;46:1260–5.
78. Senapati A, Nicholls RJ, Thomson JP, Phillips RK. Results of Delorme's procedure for rectal prolapse. Dis Colon Rectum. 1994;37:456–60.
79. Youssef M, Thabet W, El Nakeeb A, Magdy A, Alla EA, El Nabeey MA, et al. Comparative study between Delorme operation with or without postanal repair and levatorplasty in treatment of complete rectal prolapse. Int J Surg. 2013;11:52–8.
80. Hool GR, Hull TL, Fazio VW. Surgical treatment of recurrent complete rectal prolapse: a thirty-year experience. Dis Colon Rectum. 1997;40:270.
81. Pikarsky AJ, Joo JS, Wexner SD, et al. Recurrent rectal prolapse: what is the next good option? Dis Colon Rectum. 2000;43:1273–6.
82. Steele SR, Goetz LH, Minami S, et al. Management of recurrent rectal prolapse: surgical approach influences outcome. Dis Colon Rectum. 2006;49:440–5.
83. Hotouras A, Ribas Y, Zakeri S, et al. A systematic review of the literature on the surgical management of recurrent rectal prolapse. Color Dis. 2015;17:657–64.
84. Ding JH, Canedo J, Lee SH, et al. Perineal rectosigmoidectomy for primary and recurrent rectal prolapse: are the results comparable the second time? Dis Colon Rectum. 2012;55:666–70.
85. Hrabe J, Gurland B. Optimizing treatment for rectal prolapse. Clin Colon Rectal Surg. 2016;29:271–6.
86. Clark CE, Jupiter DC, Thomas JS, Papaconstantinou HT. Rectal prolapse in the elderly: trends in surgical management and outcomes from the American College of Surgeons National Surgical Quality Improvement Program database. J Am Coll Surg. 2012;215:709–14.
87. Fang SH, Cromwell JW, Wilkins KB, et al. Is the abdominal repair of rectal prolapse safer then perineal repair in the highest risk patients? An NSQIP analysis. Dis Colon Rectum. 2012;55:1167–72.
88. Germain A, Perrenot C, Scherrer ML, et al. Long-term outcome of robotic-assisted laparoscopic rectopexy for full-thickness rectal prolapse in elderly patients. Color Dis. 2014;16:198–202.

Part IV

Vascular Disorders

Cerebrovascular Disease and Critical Limb Ischaemia

16

Carlo Setacci, Maria Agnese Mele, Giuseppe Galzerano, Giuseppe de Donato, Domenico Benevento, Massimiliano Walter Guerrieri, Francesco Setacci, and Bruno Amato

16.1 Cerebrovascular Disease (Figs. 16.1, 16.2, 16.3, 16.4, and 16.5)

16.1.1 Introduction

Cerebrovascular disease is the second leading cause of death worldwide and accounts for approximately 9.5% of all deaths. The primary goal of treatment of cerebrovascular disease is the prevention of stroke, the third leading cause of death in the United States; those who survive the acute event have a markedly shortened life expectancy. Approximately 80% of strokes are ischaemic, and 20% are haemorrhagic, with haemorrhagic strokes approximately equally divided between subarachnoid and intracranial haemorrhage. As regards ischaemic strokes, carotid disease accounts for about two thirds, this as a consequence of embolization of carotid artery bifurcation plaque to the intracranial vessels, usually to the middle cerebral artery (MCA), in the anterior circulation, or as a consequence of low flow. These strokes can also result from lesions in the common carotid artery (CCA) or in the distal or intracranial portion of the internal carotid artery (ICA). Age, gender and race are clearly risk factors for stroke. Similarly, the well-established cardiovascular risk factors (i.e. atrial fibrillation), hypertension, diabetes, smoking and recognized cerebrovascular disease, seem to have ramifications for stroke risk.

C. Setacci (✉) • M.A. Mele • G. Galzerano • G. de Donato • D. Benevento • M.W. Guerrieri
F. Setacci
Department of Medicine, Surgery and Neurosciences, Vascular and Endovascular Unit, Siena University, Siena, Italy
e-mail: setacci@unisi.it

B. Amato
Dipartimento Medicina Clinica e Chirurgia, Università degli studi di Napoli Federico II, Naples, Italy

A. Crucitti (ed.), *Surgical Management of Elderly Patients*,
https://doi.org/10.1007/978-3-319-60861-7_16

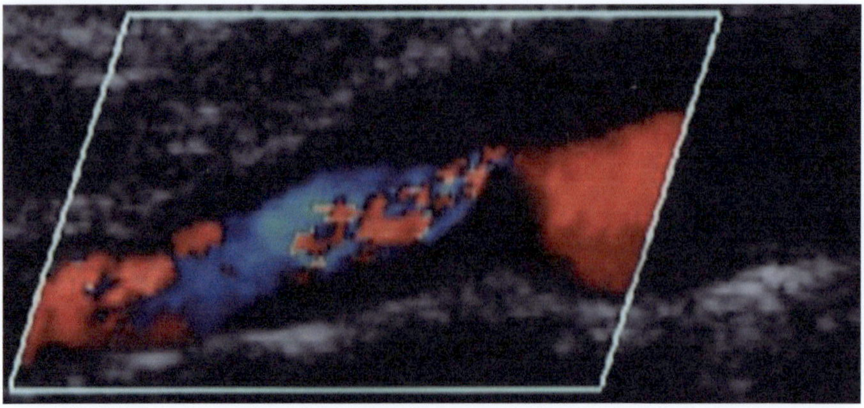

Fig. 16.1 Echocolordoppler US: soft plaque

The majority of carotid occlusive disease occurs at the carotid bifurcation. Since the area of the carotid bulb is wider than points proximal or distal, this change in calibre, along with the flow divider at the carotid bifurcation, creates a pattern of turbulent flow and areas of variable shear stress along the walls of the carotid vessels. Similar to atherosclerotic plaques that form in other vessels, the carotid plaque begins as fibrointimal thickening and progresses to become symptomatic in a variety of ways. Studies relating pathologic findings with symptoms have demonstrated that intraplaque haemorrhage, thrombus formation and ulceration are consistent with a vulnerable plaque that may cause symptoms. Most plaque ruptures occur at the midpoint of the plaque, rather than at the edges or shoulders. Embolic potential and symptomatic status have been correlated with hypoechogenic patterns on duplex ultrasonography.

Patients presenting with symptoms of carotid disease will typically have focal neurological dysfunction in the form of numbness, paraesthesias, slurred speech, weakness or monocular blindness (amaurosis fugax). If these symptoms resolve within 24 h without any permanent neurological deficit, the incident is termed a transient ischaemic attack (TIA). Symptoms lasting for longer than 24 h represent a completed stroke and can be classified according to the National Institutes of Health Stroke Scale. Patients who have multiple episodes of focal neurological deficit punctuated by failure to return to baseline are classified as having crescendo TIAs. Those patients whose symptoms progress and worsen over the course of hours to days are classified clinically as having a stroke-in-evolution. Patients with any of the symptoms described here should undergo bilateral carotid duplex ultrasound to determine whether carotid stenosis is a contributing factor to their symptoms. These symptomatic patients, however, represent a minority of patients who present with carotid disease. The majority of patients are asymptomatic.

The era of carotid surgery began in 1954 when Eastcott, Pickering and Rob published a case report documenting the first auspicious reconstruction of the carotid artery in the treatment of carotid occlusive disease in a woman with recurrent transient ischaemic attacks (TIAs). Her treatment included excision of the carotid bifurcation, ligation of the external carotid artery (ECA) and reconstruction with direct anastomosis of the CCA to the ICA. Over the years, much headway has been made in the field of carotid surgery, including the introduction of endovascular techniques for the treatment of carotid obstructive disease. In the 1970s, Mathias et al. reported successful outcomes with percutaneous angioplasty for carotid stenosis, employing techniques derived from peripheral arterial angioplasty which developed rapidly during the subsequent years. In the endovascular era, classical surgery still possesses a certain importance and dignity, remaining the gold standard for the treatment of primitive carotid lesions. The indication for surgery is atherosclerotic stenosis ≥70% (conforming to the European Carotid Surgery Trial, ECST), both in symptomatic and asymptomatic patients, and ≥50% when an ulcer is clearly evident in an asymptomatic patient or when the contralateral carotid was occluded. Colour Doppler ultrasound (DUS) constitutes the preferred first-line imaging modality for identifying patients with 70–99% ICA stenosis because of its low cost, its rapid availability, its robustness in sensitivity analysis and its capability of meeting the exigencies of contemporary surgery.

The most important considerations for decision-making regarding an endovascular versus open procedure for carotid bifurcation disease are the risks of complications associated with the respective approaches and their long-term effectiveness. The gravity of both early and late complications should be weighed. The patient's comorbid conditions, as well as predicted longevity, obviously impact on the importance of procedural perils versus longevity.

16.1.2 Surgical Anatomy and Anatomical Variations of the Carotid Artery Bifurcation

Arterial vascularization of the head and neck area derives from the CCA, the branches of the CCA, the ECA, the ICA and the vertebral arteries which comprise the circle of Willis. The CCA differs on the right and left sides with respect to their origins. On the right, the common carotid emerges from the brachiocephalic artery as it passes behind the sternoclavicular joint. On the left, the common carotid artery originates from the arch of the aorta in the superior mediastinum. Following a similar course on both sides, the common carotid artery ascends, diverging laterally from behind the sternoclavicular joint to the level of the upper border of the thyroid cartilage of the larynx (C3–C4 junction), where it bisects into the external and internal carotid arteries. The carotid bifurcation (CB), and, in particular, the height of the carotid bifurcation (HCB), is an anatomical and surgical landmark of special significance for the surgical approach to carotid artery disease. In fact, the extremes of the HCB ("high" and "low" CB) may alter the appropriate surgical techniques, including selection between carotid endarterectomy and carotid stenting (i.e. high CB is usually a contraindication for carotid endarterectomy). Anatomically, we speak of high bifurcation when the CCA bifurcates as high as C2 vertebra making a carotid endarterectomy (CEA) technically difficult. It is more common in Japanese, females, at the left side and in an Ethiopian population, indicating a genetic component. On the other hand, its counterpart, a low CB, is defined as a bifurcation under C4 vertebra, often at the level of C6–C7; in some rare cases, thoracic bifurcation of the CCA may be seen, which may be associated with the Klippel-Feil anomaly. It is a very rarely encountered anatomical variation. It has an incidence of 3.75 and 7.5% and traditionally does not represent a challenge for surgery [1].

16.1.3 Diagnosis

Carotid duplex ultrasound is the first-line imaging tool for patients with suspected carotid occlusive disease. Duplex criteria for diagnosis of carotid stenosis were standardized in 1987 by Dr. Strandness at the University of Washington. This first set of criteria, known as the University of Washington criteria, stratified carotid stenosis into six categories, using both duplex and B mode evaluation. The percentage of stenosis in the carotid artery could be reliably predicted as 0, 1–15%, 16–49%, 50–79%, 80–99% or complete occlusion based on duplex criteria. These methods had a sensitivity of 99% and a specificity of 84% when compared with angiography. In addition to being highly operator dependent, other limitations of duplex ultrasound are its inability to accurately determine velocities in the presence of heavily calcified plaque because of an artefact created by the shadowing and in the setting of contralateral carotid occlusion. Although many surgeons can safely rely on carotid duplex for preoperative imaging, there are certain cases in which more information is necessary before proceeding to surgery, such as with the aforementioned heavy calcifications, unexpectedly low velocities or atypical presentation. Digital subtraction angiography (DSA) was, for a number of years, the gold standard for diagnosis of carotid stenosis; however, CTA and MRA have now supplanted DSA as an anatomic imaging modality. In particular CTA and MRA should be reserved for patients in whom duplex results are unequivocal or for preoperative planning.

16.1.4 Medical and Surgical Treatment

The primary management of both symptomatic and asymptomatic carotid diseases is aggressive medical therapy including statin therapy, antiplatelet therapy and antihypertensive therapy with risk factor modification, and in particular cessation of smoking is strongly advised.

Evidence for the treatment of patients with symptomatic carotid stenosis higher than 70% with either CAS or CEA is compelling, and several trials demonstrate the benefit of carotid revascularization in the symptomatic patient population. Asymptomatic carotid stenosis is perhaps more controversial, with the largest trials [2] only demonstrating a 1% per year risk stroke reduction with CEA. Although there are sufficient data to advocate for aggressive medical therapy as the primary mode of treatment for asymptomatic carotid stenosis, there are data to suggest that

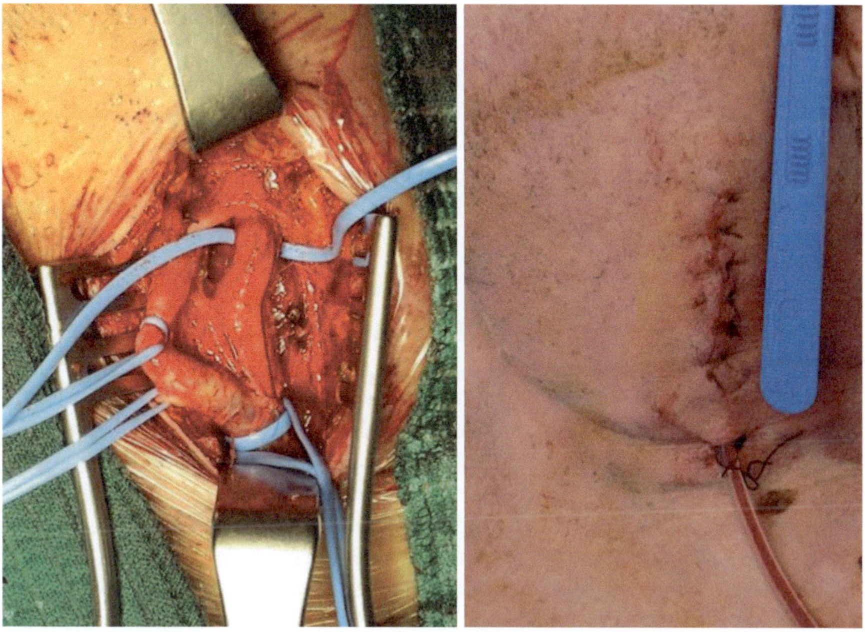

Fig. 16.2 and 3 CEA: Miniskin incision performed in our centre

certain patient populations will benefit from stroke risk reduction with carotid revascularization. The best available evidence with regard to CAS versus CEA demonstrates no difference between the two procedures in early perioperative stroke, MI or death and no difference in 4-year ipsilateral stroke risk. However, as a result of a higher perioperative risk of stroke in patients undergoing CAS, particularly in symptomatic, female or elderly patients, it is difficult to recommend CAS over CEA except in populations with prohibitive cardiac risk, previous carotid surgery or prior neck irradiation. In recent years, several studies have demonstrated low risk for CEA in women, octogenarians and patients undergoing CEA using local anaesthesia. Regarding randomized trials, ACAS and the early phase of NASCET excluded patients older than 79 years. ACST and ECST did not arbitrarily exclude older patients, although the number of patients of 80 years or older was small. Age is an inconsistent indicator of increased surgical risk, especially when associated comorbidity is accounted for. In symptomatic patients, over 75 years of age was associated with a higher risk for stroke with medical therapy than was under 65 years of age, comparable surgical risk, and thus overall greater benefit of CEA in older patients. This increased benefit should not necessarily be extrapolated to asymptomatic patients. The subset over 75 years in ACST did not show significant benefit with CEA versus medical therapy, and ACAS excluded patients older than 79 years. The long-time survival necessary to achieve a benefit of prophylactic CEA in asymptomatic patients would suggest conservatism in patients older than 80 years unless they are in good health.

Several papers have also favoured the eversion technique of CEA, reporting that it prevents carotid sinus denervation and low baroreflex sensitivity, an independent risk factor for cardiovascular disease. Likewise, several studies have identified factors predicting risk stratification for carotid disease, such as contralateral occlusion, chronic kidney disease, homocysteine levels and plaque quality based on advanced imaging modalities [3].

16.1.5 Operative Techniques: CEA Versus CAS

A fundamental consideration in the conduct of CEA is selection of the anaesthetic method. CEA may be performed under general anaesthesia (GA), under regional anaesthesia (RA) with deep or superficial cervical block and even under pure local anaesthesia (LA). Careful positioning of the patients is important to ensure patient comfort and adequate operative exposure. Positioning begins with placing a roll behind the scapulae to achieve some hyperextension of the neck. The patient is placed in the flexed position with the table rotated to expose the side of the neck to be operated on. The standard skin incision is a longitudinal incision parallel to the medial border of the sternocleidomastoid muscle. An alternative method is to place the incision in an appropriately located skin crease, usually 1–2 cm inferior to the angle of the jaw.

There are two basic surgical techniques for CEA: conventional and eversion. Regardless of which method is used, meticulous surgical technique is paramount for a successful operation. Manipulation of the carotid artery should be minimized because intraoperative embolization can result from careless handling. The conventional technique for CEA consists of a vertical arteriotomy and closure by patch angioplasty. In this case, a vertical arteriotomy is begun on the CCA and continued through the carotid bifurcation into the ICA. If a shunt is used, it is placed in the distal ICA and backbled before the proximal end is placed into the CCA.

The endarterectomy is begun in the CCA in the plane between the media and adventitia, and then it is continued into the orifice of ECA and up into the ICA. A technically perfect endpoint in the ICA is critical to avoid perioperative stroke and recurrent stenosis. After the endarterectomy, the arteriotomy is repaired with a patch angioplasty (autologous vein, PTFE, Dacron or bovine pericardium). The patch is sewn in with running non-absorbable suture.

Eversion endarterectomy is an excellent alternative technique that is practised successfully in many centres throughout the world. Two different versions of eversion endarterectomy are performed. DeBakey originally described eversion endarterectomy with partial transection of the anterior portion of the carotid bifurcation. Etheredge improved on DeBakey's technique with complete transection of the bifurcation, which allowed the origins of both the ICA and ECA to be everted for a longer distance. The endarterectomy is performed by mobilizing the entire circumference of the carotid adventitia off the plaque and then everting the adventitia and mobilizing it upward while gentle caudad traction is applied to the plaque. This

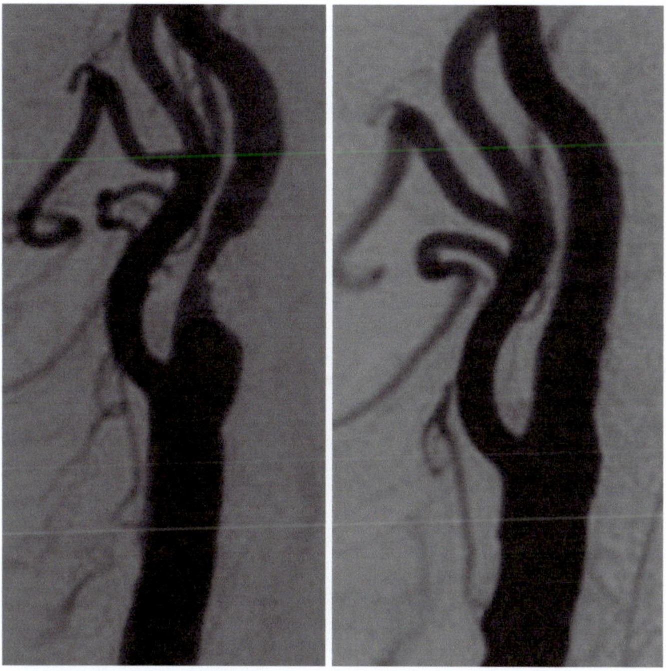

Fig. 16.4 Angiograms of Carotid artery stenosis before and after CAS

manoeuvre is performed distally into the orifices of the ICA and ECA and then proximally into the CCA. Once the endarterectomy is complete, the divided bifurcation is reunited with a simple end-to-end anastomosis. Advantages of this technique are that the anastomosis can be performed rapidly and it is not prone to restenosis, and therefore patching is not required.

CAS has emerged as an alternative to CEA in patient at high risk for complication from endarterectomy, such as those with contralateral occlusion, severe coronary artery disease, prior neck radiation or prior carotid endarterectomy. It involves placing a small, expandable stent in the narrowed artery using a transfemoral or radial approach with the position of a cerebral protection filter before the stent deployment.

Carotid artery stenting technologies are rapidly evolving. Options for endovascular surgeons and interventionist who treat occlusive carotid disease continue to expand. Carotid technologies addressed include the carotid stents themselves as well as adjunct neuroprotective devices. Aspects of stent technology include bare metal versus covered stents, stent tapering and free-cell area. Bare metal and covered stents provide unique advantages and disadvantages. Stent tapering may allow for a more fitted contour to the calibre decrement between the common carotid and internal carotid arteries but also introduces new technical challenges. Studies regarding free-cell area are conflicting with respect to benefits and associated risk; clinical relevance of associated adverse effects associated with either type is unclear.

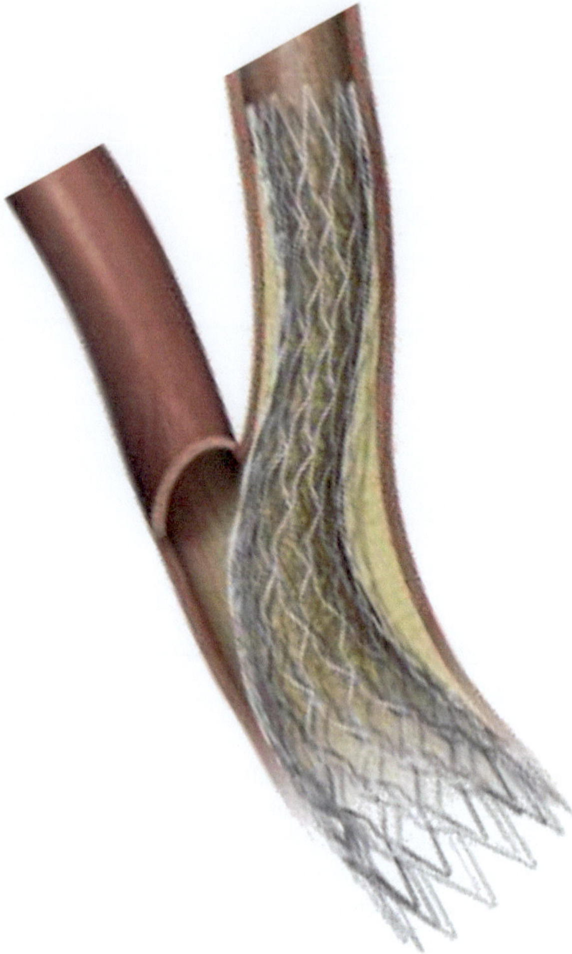

Fig. 16.5 Carotid artery stenting

Embolization protection strategies include distal filter protection and flow reversal (a proximal protection device in which a triple-lumen catheter with a double balloon was utilized to occlude the CCA and ECA; the reversed flow was then directed through the catheter to a filtered external femoral venous system). Though flow reversal was initially met with some scepticism, it has gained wider acceptance and may provide the advantage of not crossing the carotid lesion before protection is established. Carotid stenting is a new and exciting field with rapidly advancing technologies. Embolization protection, low-risk deployment and lesion assessment and stratification are active areas of research [4].

Although CAS has emerged as an attractive alternative to CEA in patients who are at high risk for surgical complications, conflicting data exist about the risks associated with carotid stenting in the very elderly (≥80 years old) population. Octogenarian patients are more likely to have baseline characteristics that predispose the patient to adverse outcome including: Type III aortic arch, decreased cerebral reserve, aortic arch calcification, excessive vessel tortuosity and severe lesion calcification. While these characteristics represent a challenge to operators performing CAS on octogenarian patients, they do not constitute absolute contraindications to the procedure. It is noteworthy that the outcomes in this patient population seem to correlate with operator experience [5].

16.2 Critical Limb Ischaemia (Figs. 16.6, 16.7, 16.8, and 16.9)

Critical limb ischaemia (CLI) is a manifestation of peripheral arterial disease (PAD) that describes patients with typical chronic ischaemic rest pain (Tables 16.1 and 16.2) or patients with ischaemic skin lesions, either ulcers or gangrene. The term CLI should only be used in relation to patients with chronic ischaemic disease, defined as the presence of symptoms for more than 2 weeks. The diagnosis of CLI should be confirmed by the ankle-brachial index (ABI), toe systolic pressure or transcutaneous oxygen tension. Ischaemic rest pain most commonly occurs below an ankle pressure of 50 mm Hg or a toe pressure < 30 mm Hg. Other causes of pain, a rest should, therefore, be considered in patients with an ankle pressure > 50 mm Hg, although CLI could be the cause. Some ulcers are entirely ischaemic in aetiology; others initially have other causes (e.g. traumatic, venous or neuropathic) but will not heal because of the severity of the underlying PAD. Healing requires an inflammatory response and additional perfusion above that required for supporting intact skin and underlying tissues. The ankle and toe pressure levels needed for healing are, therefore, higher than the pressures found in ischaemic rest pain. For patients with

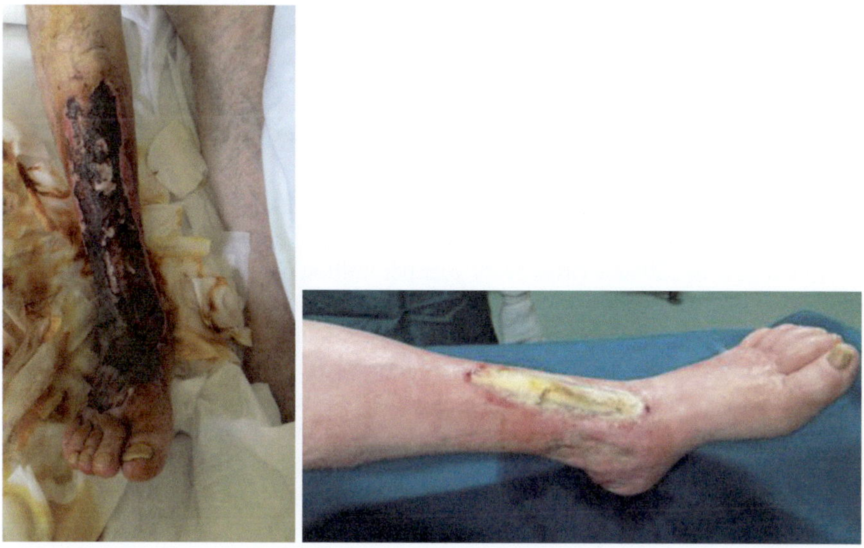

Fig. 16.6 and 7 Ulcers with tendon exposition

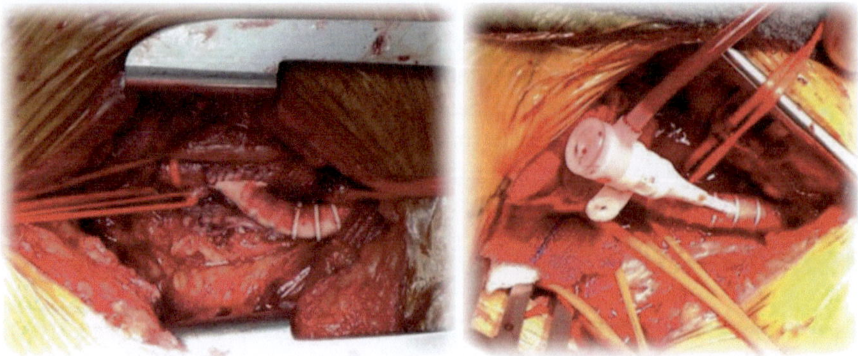

Fig. 16.8 and 9 Hybrid approach: F-P bypass + angiografic control and PTA tibial vessels

Table 16.1 Fontaine classification of peripheral arterial disease

Stage	Clinical
I	Asymptomatic
IIa	Mild claudication
IIb	Moderate to severe claudication
III	Ischaemic rest pain
IV	Ulceration or gangrene

Table 16.2 Rutherford classification of peripheral arterial disease

Grade	Stage	Clinical
0	0	Asymptomatic
I	1	Mild claudication
I	2	Moderate claudication
I	3	Severe claudication
II	4	Ischaemic rest pain
III	5	Minor tissue loss
III	6	Major tissue loss

ulcers or gangrene, the presence of CLI is suggested by an ankle pressure < 70 mm Hg or a toe systolic pressure > 50 mm Hg. CLI population are difficult to study, with large numbers of patients lost to follow-up or dying in longitudinal studies, leading to incomplete data sets. The incidence of CLI, based on large prospective population studies, is of 220 new cases every year per million population [6]. Although the diagnosis of arterial occlusive disease of the lower limb could be made on the basis of history and physical examination, imaging is mandatory for localization and quantification of the arterial lesions. Traditionally intraarterial digital subtraction arteriography (DSA) is considered the diagnostic standard to evaluate the lower extremity arterial tree. However, DSA is invasive and may be associated with well-documented limitations that make this method unsuitable for screening or follow-up examinations. Other limitations for the use of DSA as routine diagnostic technique include the need of catheterization, contrast allergic reactions, arterial injury, haemorrhage, atheroembolism, potential pseudoaneurysm formation at the puncture site and most importantly contrast-induced nephropathy despite the use of non-ionic contrast media. Furthermore, even with bi-planar views, arteriography can underestimate the severity of eccentric arterial stenosis. For these reasons, many forms of less invasive modalities include multidetector tomography angiography, magnetic resonance angiography (MRA) and duplex ultrasonography (DU) that have been devised for grading lower extremity arterial disease. In the last few years, several studies have raised the possibility of using DU arterial mapping as the sole investigation method to assess the most suitable treatment plan for CLI. In fact, this non-invasive method, with colour Doppler technology, if used appropriately, provides most of the essential anatomic information plus haemodynamic data for extensive peripheral arterial mapping and allows to distinguish between thigh stenosis and occlusion, to determine the grade of stenosis severity into multiple levels during pre-operatory study. Moreover, it can be used as a follow-up exam [7].

As regards the treatment, CLI has always been considered a primary indication for bypass surgery. Nevertheless, not all patients with CLI can undergo surgical revascularization because of prohibitive surgical risk or anatomical unfavourable conditions. The ideal treatment for CLI lesions has raised great amount of discussion and controversy among specialists. Aside from differing opinions regarding the preferred method of treatment, specialists suggest that many additional variables must be considered: lesion location, severity, degree of calcification and the patient's associated symptoms. Limb salvage rates >90% at 1 year are reported in recent series using bypass surgery. Unfortunately, an adequate vein is often unavailable, and long-term results of bypasses constructed with prosthetic materials are much less satisfactory. Nowadays the use of endovascular procedures as primary treatment for CLI has increased due to the continuous advances in imaging techniques, angioplasty equipment (i.e. low-profile balloons and new guidewires) and endovascular expertise. The clinical advantages of the endovascular approach in CLI are well established, especially for high-risk, elderly and vascular compromised patients: there is no need for general or spinal anaesthesia; there are few or no surgical wounds, especially risky in diabetic patients; the hospital stay is shorter; complication and mortality rates are low; and a failed angioplasty attempt does not preclude a subsequent bypass graft. Therefore, it's important (1) to identify the patient (comorbidities), (2) to identify the lesion location/extension and (3) to distinguish between haemodynamically significant and non-significant lesions in order to establish the optimal revascularization treatment for CLI. Treatment strategy is strongly determined not only by the type of lesion but also by the anatomical site, since there are large differences in approaches and outcomes for proximal lesions on large vessels (aortoiliac) and distal lesion on small vessels (tibial arteries). In 2000 and 2007, the TransAtlantic Inter-Society Consensus (TASC) allowed stratification by length and morphology of lesions (iliac occlusive disease and femoropopliteal and infrapopliteal lesions) and reinforced the concept of treating short, focal stenoses (TASC A lesions) via endovascular means and using surgical revascularization for long-segment occlusions (TASC D lesions). In cases of diffused aortoiliac occlusive disease although aortobifemoral bypass appears to have better long-term patency than endovascular treatment, the risks of surgery are significantly greater than the risk of an endovascular approach, in terms not only of mortality but also of major morbidity and delay in return to normal activities. As regards the femoropopliteal and infrapopliteal disease, PTA is the primary option for short and focal disease <3 cm in length; for lesions that are between 3 and 5 cm in length, there are too many variables to recommend a single treatment protocol. If a patient has vessels with a poor runoff, small vessels and calcified lesions that are 5–10 cm in length, the surgical option may be the optimal treatment. For patients with high comorbidities, the ideal treatment seems to be endovascular (bare metal stent or stent graft). Endovascular procedures below the popliteal artery are usually indicated for limb salvage, and there are no data comparing endovascular procedures to bypass surgery for intermittent claudication in this region. PTA seems to be feasible and effective in patients with CLI and infrapopliteal artery occlusion.

The techniques used are:

- Angioplasty: PTA of a short anterior or posterior tibial artery stenosis may be performed in conjunction with popliteal or femoral angioplasty. Treatment of longer lesions is often more complex and has a worse prognosis than treatment of short lesions.
- Stents: stent application in below-the-knee vessels remains highly controversial; the high risk of early thrombosis and luminal loss due to intimal hyperplasia formation leading to insufficient long-term patency rates can explain the reluctance on implanting stents in these small diameter vessels. Infrapopliteal stent implantation is generally reserved for cases with suboptimal outcome after PTA.
- Cutting balloon: this technique decreases vessel elastic recoil and perivascular injury by a focal concentration of dilatation force.
- Subintimal angioplasty: this technique, by passing a wire into the subintimal space and inflating a balloon to create a channel for blood flow, is largely employed for long-segment occlusion below the knee recanalization [8].

Several endovascular devices have been shown to be safe and feasible in the infrapopliteal segment but have failed to show superiority when compared with PTA. The development of self-expanding nitinol stent has improved the therapeutic outcome of femoropopliteal lesions compared with conventional angioplasty. However, restenosis remains a key unresolved issue. Restenosis usually occurs 6 months after the implantation of bare nitinol stents, with a peak onset at 12 months. In an effort to curb restenosis, manufacturers engineered stents to elute antiproliferative agents. Drug-eluting stents (DES) significantly reduced restenosis rates compared with bare stents [9].

However, the employment of DES did not give good results in infrapopliteal arteries where restenosis rates remain high. The favourable results of below-the-knee (BTK) DES treatment were limited to PTA of short lesions that are not representative of the diffuse BTK vessel disease typical of diabetic patients with CLI. The cause of these difficulties with regard to peripheral angioplasty and stenting in obtaining acceptable good long-term patency rate resides in the peculiar characteristics of the infrainguinal vessel physiology and disease: in patients with CLI, infrainguinal vessels have a multisegmental and diffuse disease which necessitate an extensive treatment, resulting in an extraordinary mean length of the treated PTA lesions (it is well known that restenosis is proportional to the length of the treated vessel); inferior limb arteries undergo intense mechanical stress due to hip, knee and ankle movements, muscle contraction and to the interaction of the limb with external bodies during daily activities (standing up, sitting, walking, lying, etc.); stents interfere with the original physical behaviour of the arteries, leading to chronic mechanical stress, fractures, inflammation and subsequent restenosis [10].

With this in mind, faced with the limits of peripheral angioplasty and stenting in infrainguinal vessels, the drug-eluting balloon (DEB) presents some advantages with respect to DES and seems able to prevent restenosis and to avoid, when possible, the metallic burden of stenting [11].

Given the evolving demographics and the increasing prevalence of CLI with age in Western countries, there has been an enhanced focus on developing safe and effective treatment. Related to endovascular and surgical options, in recent years the hybrid approach (the combination of the two techniques) is considered an interesting alternative approach to improve life expectancy of patients with CLI. This treatment is reserved for patients with a multilevel disease (involvement of more than two districts among the iliac, the femoral, the popliteal and the tibial areas) or a previous surgical intervention or an adequate length of the greater saphenous vein or leg ulcer prohibiting distal graft implantation. In the CA, the union of the endovascular and surgical techniques was used to complete the revascularization in different anatomical districts or to correct inadequate results of the first procedure (inadequate inflow or outflow) or to correct inadequate results due to iatrogenic complications of the first technique (arterial rupture or residual dissection) [12].

The treatment of CLI in the United States has been characterized as a pathway to amputation, as 67% of Medicare patients who underwent a major amputation did not have any other exploratory or therapeutic procedures prior to losing their limb. This finding was confirmed in a recent study of 20,464 Medicare patients with CLI who underwent amputations, which revealed that 71% had no revascularization and 54% did not even undergo angiography, underscoring the fact that revascularization procedures (endovascular and surgical) have largely been underutilized. This could be ascribed, at least in part, to the paucity of randomized control trials (RCTs) comparing both strategies, which have been difficult to implement. This represents an example of the existing gap between "real-world CLI practices" and the availability of evidence-based therapies [13].

In conclusion CLI continues to be a significant challenge to the vascular surgeon. Despite great advances in the treatment of CLI, a significant number of amputations are still performed. Limb salvage may represent the goal even if, unfortunately, some patients still require primary amputation due to many variables which are impossible to resolve.

References

1. Michalinos A, Chatzimarkos M, Arkadopoulos N, et al. Anatomical consideration on surgical anatomy of the carotid bifurcation. Anat Res Int. 2016;2016:1–8.
2. ACST-2 Collaborative Group. Status update and interim results from the Asymptomatic Carotid Surgery Trial-2 (ACST 2). Eur J Vasc Endovasc Surg. 2013;46(5):511–8.
3. O'Brien M, Chandra A. Carotid revascularization: risk and benefits. Vasc Health Risk Manag. 2014;10:103.
4. Morr S, Lin N, Siddqui AH. Carotid artery stenting: current and emerging options. Med Devices Evid Res. 2014;7:343.
5. Grant A, White C, Ansel G. Safety and efficacy of carotid stenting in the very elderly. Catheter Cardiovasc Interv. 2009;75(5):651–5.
6. De Donato G, Chisci E, Setacci F, et al. Critical limb ischemia: definition, epidemiology and economic impact. Chapter I. Critical limb ischemia. New developments and perspectives. 2010.
7. Benedetti-Valentini F, et al. Arterial mapping by duplex scanning in patients with CLI: Chapter IV. New developments and perspectives. 2010.
8. Brambilla D, Casalino A, Barbante M, et al. Decision chart for optimal endovascular treatment. Chapter 6. New developments and perspectives. 2010.
9. Soga Y. Can new drug-eluting stents put an end to the debate? J Endovasc Ther. 2016;23(5):708–9.
10. Schlager O, Dick P, Sabeti S, et al. Long-segment SFA stenting- the dark sides: in-stent restenosis, clinical deterioration and stent fractures. J Endovasc Ther. 2005;12:676–84.
11. Ferrares R, Aprigliano A, Palloshi A, et al. Drug-eluting balloon technologies and results. How drug eluting balloon going to chance our practice? Chapter XVI. Critical limb ischemia. New developments and perspectives. 2010.
12. Setacci C, Galzerano G, Sirignano P, et al. The role of hybrid procedures in the treatment of critical limb ischemia. J Cardiovasc Surg. 2013;54:729–36.
13. Diaz-Sandoval LJ, Mustapha JA, Saab F. Evidence-based CLI therapies in 2016. Endovasc Today Eur. 2016;4(4).

Acute Peripheral Arterial Disease

17

Francesco Speziale, Pasqualino Sirignano, Simone Cuozzo, Wassim Mansour, Chiara Pranteda, Martina Formiconi, Alessandro d'Adamo, and Laura Capoccia

17.1 Introduction

Acute limb ischemia (ALI) is a pathological condition resulting from a sudden blood interruption (or, at least, from an important reduction in flow) limiting tissues' survival [1]. ALI is always a serious event requiring immediate diagnosis and treatment, also considering the high associated amputation risk (from 10% to 25%). Unfortunately, ALI is not a rare occurrence, with an estimated incidence of about 1.5 new cases per 10,000 person/year [2].

The most frequent causes of acute limb ischemia are embolism, thrombosis, and trauma [3]. Symptoms include intermittent claudication, rest pain, paresthesia, muscle weakness, anesthesia, and paralysis. Physical examination could be characterized by the absence of pulses distally to the occlusion site, hypothermia, and pale or mottled skin.

Those clinical findings are grouped together in a series mnemonic note as "6P of Pratt": pain, pallor, pulselessness, poikilothermia, paresthesia, and paralysis.

All those data—in association with a duplex ultrasound scan (DUS)—allow classification of the syndrome into different classes of severity as reported by Rutherford in 1997 (Table 17.1) [4].

Considering the peculiarity of the symptoms and their frequent (if not constant) association, the diagnosis of ALI is mainly based on clinical features. The instrumental investigations, however, are indispensable to obtain a diagnosis of certainty, to recognize the causes, and to have correct treatment planning (open surgery, endovascular surgery, hybrid procedures, or fibrinolytic treatment) [5].

F. Speziale • P. Sirignano (✉) • S. Cuozzo • W. Mansour • C. Pranteda • M. Formiconi • A. d'Adamo • L. Capoccia
Vascular and Endovascular Surgery, Department of Surgery "Paride Stefanini", "Policlinico Umberto I", "Sapienza" Università di Roma, Viale del Policlinico, 155, 00161 Rome, Italy
e-mail: Francesco.speziale@uniroma1.it; pasqualino.sirignano@uniroma1.it; laura.capoccia@uniroma1.it

A. Crucitti (ed.), *Surgical Management of Elderly Patients*,
https://doi.org/10.1007/978-3-319-60861-7_17

Table 17.1 Clinical stages of acute limb ischemic syndrome (edited by the Society for Vascular Surgery standards [4])

Stage	Description and prognosis	Objectivity		Doppler signal	
		Sensory damage	Muscle weakness	Arterial	Venous
I	Limb vital, not immediately threatened	Absent	Absent	Present	Present
II	Limb threatened				
IIa	Limb marginally threatened that can be saved if treated promptly	Minimum (limited to the fingers) or absent	Absent	Often absent	Present
IIb	Limb immediately threatened, recoverable with immediate revascularization	Extended beyond the fingers, associated with pain	Medium or moderate	Often absent	Present
III	Limb irreversibly damaged, major tissue loss, or permanent damage to the inevitable nerves	Spread/anesthesia	Severe/paralysis	Absent	Absent

17.2 Physiopathology and Diagnostic Evaluation

DUS in concert with the clinical features assumes a primary and crucial role in diagnostic and preoperative evaluation of ALI patients. The bidimensional (B-Mode) ultrasound provides the typical image of endoluminal material, presenting variable echogenicity. In cases of embolic occlusions, generally, it is not possible to observe atherosclerotic lesions, while typical atherosclerotic lesions will be more frequently found in cases of thrombotic genesis of the syndrome. Moreover, DUS allows evaluation of the pathognomonic sign of *meniscus* and the absence of color signal downstream. DUS also evaluates the complete absence of flow signal at the level of the occlusion.

Upstream and downstream of the stretch of the acutely occluded vessel, it may be possible to highlight characteristic indirect signs of ALI: increased resistance and pulsatility of the blood flow (increases modulation of the curve with the amplitude reduction). In cases, with the absence of collateral circulation, there will not be any detectable DUS signal in downstream vessels; instead, in cases with a preexisting collateral circulation, DUS signal will be present with a curve characterized by a clear reduction in resistance indices and secondary pulsatility at the reduction of systolic-diastolic modulation. In most severe cases, the curve assumes a continuous form. Accuracy, sensitivity, and specificity of DUS are 86, 84, and 89%, respectively [6].

A fundamental aspect (unfortunately, not always easy to interpret) is the differential diagnosis between embolism and thrombosis, a crucial aspect in choosing different treatment options [7].

Indeed, in consideration of the difficulty in distinguishing embolic and thrombotic arterial occlusion, in recent years the vascular surgery team of Cairo published two articles with the aim of helping the vascular surgeon in this difficult differential diagnosis.

In 2010 Elmahdy et al. performed a study of 107 surgically treated ALI. To be able to make an accurate diagnosis of the etiology of ALI (embolic versus thrombotic) without the use of angiography (gold standard for this condition but not free of risk, with an overall complication rate of about 2%), they have examined several parameters such as risk factors, systemic vascular atherosclerosis, time of symptom onset, and clinical presentation. The presence of atherosclerotic vascular disease was defined based on the presence of one myointimal thickness > 0.1 mm. They also rated the arterial diameter (*intima-intima*) at the level of the occlusion (d_{occl}), compared to the diameter at the same artery level in the contralateral limb ($d_{control}$). The difference between these two diameters ($\Delta = d_{occl} - d_{control}$) was calculated. Patients were consequently divided into two groups: embolic ALI (Group E) and thrombotic ALI (Group T). No statistically significant differences were found between the two groups for any examined features (calcifications, collateral circulation, atrial fibrillation), except for Δ diameter. In Group E, the Δ diameter results were 0.95 ± 0.92 mm, while in Group T, results were −0.13 ± 1.02 mm (p: < 0.001). Their results show an increase in the diameter of vessels in embolic etiology of ALI and, even though minimal, an average reduction of the diameter of vessels in thrombotic etiology of this syndrome. Analyzing ROC curves, the authors stated that a change in diameter of ±0.5 mm between the occluded vessel and the contralateral one could be considered as a valid DUS cutoff to differentiate embolic from thrombotic ALI, with a sensitivity of 85% and a specificity of 76% (CI 0.72–0.90, $p < 0.007$) [8–10]. Otherwise, when emboli origin is macroscopically evident, such as in case of a popliteal aneurysm, it should be easier to recognize the embolic etiology of the syndrome. Up to 60% of popliteal aneurysm is presenting with ALI due to distal mobilization of aneurysmal intraluminal thrombus [11, 12]. DUS is considered the technique of choice in those situations, allowing evaluation of the localization and size of the aneurysm, amount and characteristics of the intraluminal thrombus, and patency of the aneurysms and the outflow vessels.

From a diagnostic point of view, another important problem to solve is represented by ALI resulting from a failure of previous recanalization surgery. Those failures usually present with acute symptom onset, with an incidence ranging between 10% (within 14 days after surgery, *early thrombosis*) and 30% (within 2 years of follow-up, *late thrombosis*) [13, 14]. DUS, the method of choice in lower limb revascularizations follow-up, showed a sensitivity of 95% and a specificity of 100% in diagnosis and localization of occlusion and stenosis >50% after bypass (either prosthetic or vein) and after endovascular revascularization (angioplasty, stenting, and endo-bypass). Occluded vessels may be characterized by complete absence of DUS signal, variously associated with intraluminal material [15] (Fig. 17.1).

Another important and relatively new cause of ALI is represented by thrombosis of the percutaneous access site after endovascular treatment. The underlying causes can be divided into distal embolization of atheromatous material, intimal flap, and

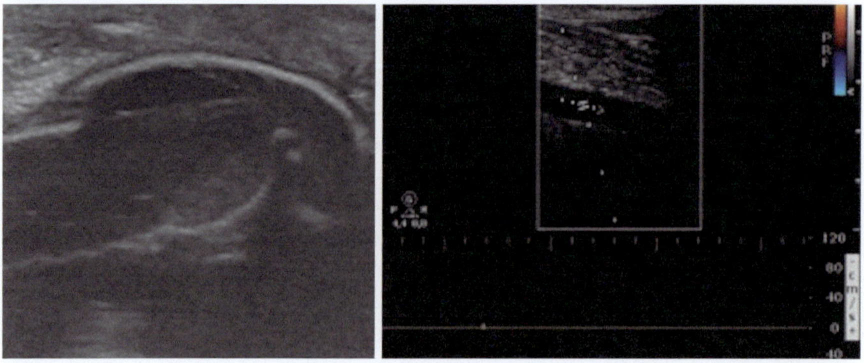

Fig. 17.1 Acute occlusion of prosthetic infra-inguinal bypass; the DUS can highlight the bypass whose lumen is occupied by intraluminal material, no flow detectable inside the prosthetic graft

delamination of an atherosclerotic plaque. From a clinical point of view, all those forms of ALI are not different from others previously described. The B-Mode ultrasound could directly display the endoluminal material in case of embolism, which appears with a variable echogenicity, also associated with preexisting parietal lesions. In secondary thrombosis, consequent to intimal flap, the latter will be easily recognizable within the lumen as hyperechoic and mobile flap. The outflow vessels are filled by hypoechoic material, with preserved diameter, and sometimes apparently pulsating (paradoxical pulse). ALI due to percutaneous hemostasis device malfunction are emerging as a new entity with a reported incidence ranging between 0.9 and 1.7% of treated cases [16, 17]. When devices based on the use of hemostatic material are at the origin of the occlusion, the material could be directly detectable at B-Mode as a foreign hyperechoic material inside the arterial lumen. Even in this case, as already described for the embolic and thrombotic occlusion, DUS could show the complete absence of signal at the level of the occlusion, associated with an increase of resistances and pulsatility of the blood flow upstream to the occlusion (increased modulation of the curve with amplitude reduction). In those cases, without collateral circulation, any detectable DUS signal in downstream vessels could be recognized, while in those cases with a preexisting collateral circulation, DUS shows a curve characterized by a clear reduction in resistance indices and secondary pulsatility at the reduction of systolic-diastolic modulation. In more severe cases, the curve assumes a continuous form, as previously described (Fig. 17.2).

A totally different situation is represented by ALI as consequence of a trauma. Clearly, in those situations, it is crucial to promptly recognize the lesion. Vascular lesion in the presence of an active bleeding wound is certainly more prone to be identified immediately, in comparison with lesions localized in depth tissue or in anatomically difficult places to investigate. DUS has a primary role both in open and closed trauma. In closed traumas, three different features should be distinguished:

- *Arterial spasm*: a result of contraction of the smooth muscle of the *tunica media* (medial layer), typical of medium-sized arteries. It can be observed in the affected artery or to all the downstream arterial tree.

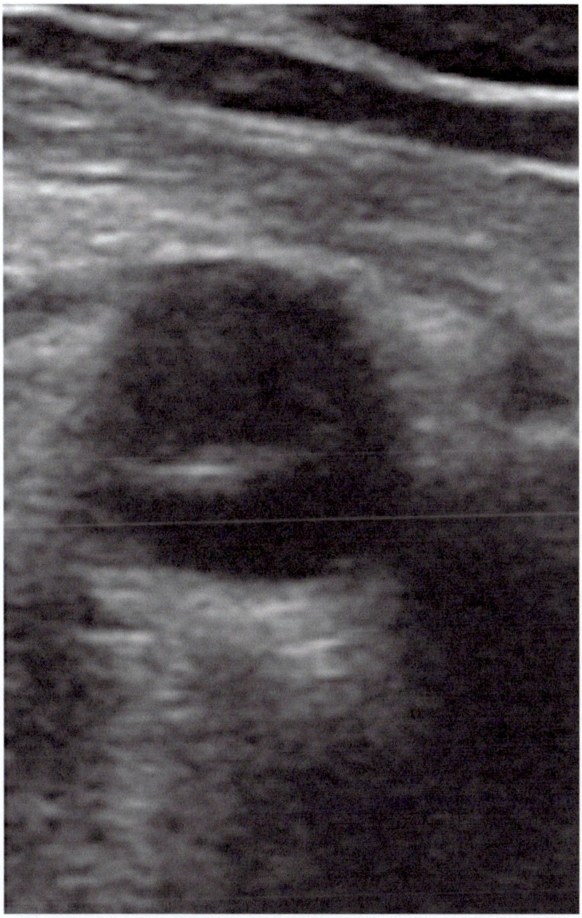

Fig. 17.2 Common femoral artery dissection after failure of percutaneous hemostasis system; inside the lumen a hyperechoic flap is clearly visible

- *Arterial contusion*: consists of a continuous solution of one or more layers of the arterial wall, in the absence of the full section of the vessel. It usually only affects the *adventitia* or the *intima*, with the integrity of the *media*. In those cases, DUS allows to highlight the exact anatomical localization of the lesion.
- *Arterial laceration*: consists of a continuous solution to the entire thickness of the vessel wall which involves all the three layers. The most important local consequences are ischemia of the downstream tissues, external bleeding, and/or hematoma; the pain is only present in 25% of cases [18]. Also in those situations, the sole DUS allows highlighting of the exact anatomical localization of the lesion.

In all those situations, DUS allows highlighting of the site of the trauma and, consequently, the site of the arterial lesion in more than 90% of cases, confirming the high sensitivity and specificity of this exam [16].

17.3 Therapeutic Management

Once the diagnosis of ALI has been established and its severity classified, a plethora of immediate interventions are critical to optimize patient outcomes.

Systemic anticoagulation with unfractionated heparin should be initiated to minimize the risk of further clot propagation and to prevent microvascular thrombosis of under perfused distal vessels.

Other measures that may be beneficial in patients with ALI include intravenous hydration, supplemental oxygen, and intravenous analgesia. Indeed, ALI patients are often relatively volume depleted, and careful fluid resuscitation is necessary in reducing myoglobinuria due to ischemia reperfusion and the potential risk of acute renal insufficiency.

Treatment for ALI largely depends on the clinical presentation according to the abovementioned Rutherford's classification [4].

Class I ALI patients may require only medical therapy, such as anticoagulation. Revascularization, if contemplated, can be performed electively and can consist of either thrombolytic or open surgical intervention, depending on the duration of ALI, its location, and the underlying cause of the occlusion, as well as the presence or absence of a preexistent atherosclerotic occlusive disease and the patient's overall medical condition.

All class II ALI patients require revascularization to preserve the functional integrity of the affected limb. However, because the ischemic insult in class IIa ALI is mild, therapy may be performed on an urgent, rather than emergency, basis. Either endovascular or surgical options may be adopted considering the duration of symptoms of prime importance in operative planning. Percutaneous endovascular options are more effective in patients with ischemia of less than 2 weeks' duration, whereas ischemic symptoms of more than 2 weeks' duration are better served by surgical revascularization [19]. For a duration of symptoms of less than 14 days, prospective studies comparing thrombolytic and surgical intervention favor the initial use of thrombolytic therapy, with surgical intervention reserved for those limbs that do not show response to lytic therapy.

Patients with more severe class IIb ALI, in which both sensory and motor deficits are present, require emergency revascularization. Historically, surgical revascularization has been preferred. However, advances in catheter-based thrombolytic delivery and percutaneous mechanical thrombectomy devices have convinced several physicians to use those techniques as first-line therapy.

Class III ALI manifests as a profound neurologic deficit (insensate, paretic limb), muscle rigidity, and absence of arterial and venous Doppler ultrasound signals in the affected vascular bed. In patients with class III ALI, revascularization is usually futile, and primary amputation should be considered.

17.3.1 Open Surgery

Balloon catheter thrombectomy, first introduced by Fogarty in 1963 [20], has been the cornerstone of therapy for the surgical management of ALI. Severe ALI (class IIb), manifested by both sensory and motor deficits, requires urgent intervention, and surgical therapy has remained the treatment of choice [21].

Balloon Catheter Thrombectomy or Embolectomy—Balloon thrombectomy is routinely used to deal with an embolic event or chronic graft thrombosis (Fig. 17.3). The technique involves direct cutdown over either the common femoral artery or the brachial artery with proximal and distal control of the major branches. A transverse arteriotomy is performed immediately proximal to the common femoral artery or brachial artery bifurcation to allow for direct visualization of the distal branches, with the ability to directly pass an appropriate-sized embolectomy catheter into those branches. A longitudinal arteriotomy is made when there is concern that end-arterectomy with patch angioplasty closure will be required. Balloon embolectomy catheters are passed proximally and distally until no visible thrombus is removed and a pulse or backflow is established. Completion angiography is important to evaluate the effectiveness of thrombus removal. Over-the-wire embolectomy catheters may also be used to direct the embolectomy catheter into the tibial branches [21].

Bypass Procedures—Bypass procedures are more commonly performed in patients with known peripheral arterial disease or after failed open balloon thrombectomy. The ideal graft is an ipsilateral saphenous vein of adequate caliber (>3 mm). Otherwise, contralateral saphenous vein, arm veins, or lesser saphenous vein is preferred if below-the-knee revascularization is performed; synthetic grafts can be used for above-the-knee revascularizations [22].

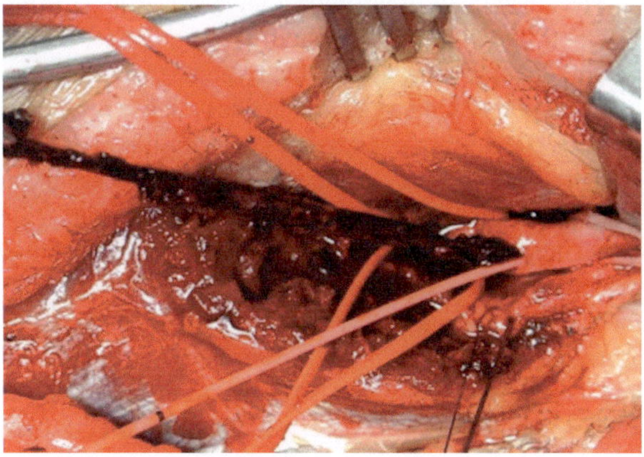

Fig. 17.3 Intraoperative findings of thrombus removal by Fogarty catheter

Although improvements in open surgical technique have diminished the rate of limb loss associated with ALI, the mortality rate remains unacceptably high, ranging from 10 to 25% mortality and 7 to 12% amputation rates. Moreover, despite the rate of amputation diminishing over the decades (mainly due to improvements in surgical techniques), mortality rate is unchanged over the years. A potential explanation could be that the ability to rapidly restore arterial flow to the extremity with an operative procedure represents a significant insult to a severe medically compromised patient, frequently culminating in the patient's death despite ALI resolution [23].

17.3.2 Endovascular Surgery

Catheter-based endovascular procedures offer potential advantages to ALI patients, less-invasive revascularization strategies for sick or elderly patients (theoretically decreasing surgical-related morbidity and mortality rates) and a direct way to clear the occluding thrombus from a periphery, restore blood flow to the extremity, and allow the identification of underlying atherosclerotic lesions (culprit lesions) responsible for the occlusive event. Culprit lesions could then be directly treated, directed by angioplasty, stenting, or atherectomy. Currently available percutaneous endovascular procedures include catheter-directed thrombolysis, pharmacomechanical thrombolysis, catheter-directed thrombus aspiration, and percutaneous mechanical thrombectomy [1, 2, 24, 25].

Intra-arterial thrombolytic infusion therapy, the first adopted endovascular solution for ALI patients, is often performed as a two-step procedure with a catheter-based infusion lasting >12 h. During the intra-arterial lysis, the patient is usually observed in a higher-care nursing unit. Thrombolytic infusion is time- and resource-consuming, and also associated with a not negligible bleeding risk.

The advantages of thrombectomy devices include the immediate reestablishment of blood flow without the use of thrombolytics, reducing the risk of bleeding and potentially reducing costs. Vacuum-assisted thrombectomy (VAT) is a catheter-based thrombectomy system that does not use intra-arterial thrombolytics. The VAT systems (Penumbra or Indigo, Penumbra Inc., Alameda, CA, USA) consist of four components: a catheter (tapered and not collapsible during suction), a separator wire, a reinforced tubing, and an aspiration pump.

Standard technique for using the VAT systems consists of contralateral 6F percutaneous arterial access, diagnostic angiography, systemic anticoagulation, and aspiration. The use of a separator wire is at the discretion of the operator. A catheter is advanced over a wire to the proximal aspect of the occlusion, the wire is removed, and the vacuum is initiated. The catheter is embedded in the proximal centimeter of the thrombus as long as there is no free-flowing blood into the vacuum device. When a clot is pulled through the device and flow reestablished, the device is advanced further into the lesion. If thrombus is not being removed, the catheter would be pulled back, with the vacuum still on, and removed through the sheath (removing the sheath valve) and flushed outside the patient. In this way, a thrombus that is too large to be removed through the catheter is suctioned on the end and

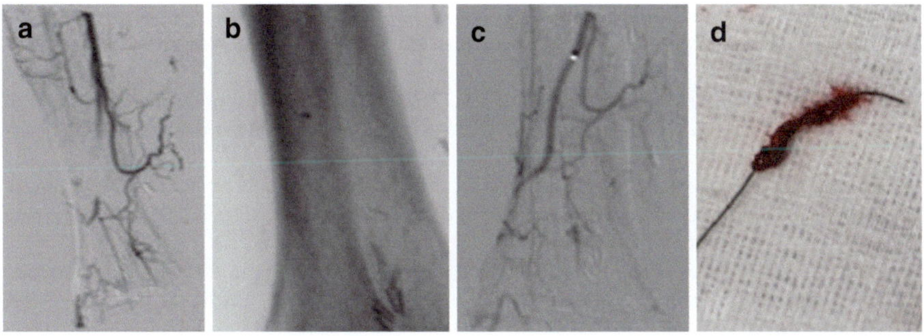

Fig. 17.4 Endovascular thrombectomy using VAT devices (**a**) preoperative angiography; (**b**) VAT catheter placement; (**c**) final result with complete flow restoration; (**d**) removed thrombus

removed. Intermittent angiographies and VAT are performed until blood flow is reestablished and the thrombus burden reduced (Fig. 17.4) [26].

17.3.3 Hybrid Surgery

Hybrid treatment of ALI syndrome, consisting of a selective angiography at the end of open surgical operative time, has become more and more frequently adopted in standard surgical practice.

The decision to perform an on-table angiography is mainly based on the absence of satisfactory back-bleeding from distal vessels, the demonstration of signals of poor revascularization by the DUS at the ankle, the poor clinical appearance of the foot after surgical procedure, and the impossibility of advancing the Fogarty catheter far enough distally.

Angiography is generally performed by direct puncture of the exposed artery or, in case of below-the-knee arterial vessel exposure, by puncture of the ipsilateral common femoral artery. When the angiography diagnoses an incomplete restoration of perfusion, all the abovementioned endovascular options could be adopted after careful evaluation of the residual clot extension and its location [5].

References

1. Norgren L, Hiatt WR, Dormandy JA, et al. Inter-society consensus for the management of peripheral arterial disease (TASC II). J Vasc Surg. 2007;45:5–67.
2. Creager MA, Kaufman JA, Conte MS. Clinical practice. Acute limb ischemia. N Engl J Med. 2012;366(23):2198–206.
3. Rajan DK, Patel NH, Valji K, et al. CIRSE and SIR standards of practice committees quality improvement guidelines for percutaneous management of acute limb ischemia. J Vasc Interv Radiol. 2009;20(7):208–18.
4. Rutherford RB, Baker JD, Ernst C, et al. Recommended standards for reports dealing with lower extremity ischemia: revised version. J Vasc Surg. 1997;26:517–38. [Erratum, J Vasc Surg 2001;33:805]

5. de Donato G, Setacci F, Sirignano P, et al. The combination of surgical embolectomy and endovascular techniques may improve outcomes of patients with acute lower limb ischemia. J Vasc Surg. 2014;59(3):729–36.
6. Löfberg AM, Karacagil S, Hellberg A, et al. The role of duplex scanning in the selection of patients with critical lower-limb ischemia for infrainguinal percutaneous transluminal angioplasty. Cardiovasc Intervent Radiol. 2001;24(4):229–32.
7. Katsamouris AN, Giannoukas AD, Tsetis D, et al. Can ultrasound replace arteriography in the management of chronic arterial occlusive disease of the lower limb? Eur J Vasc Endovasc Surg. 2001;21(2):155–9.
8. Elmahdy MF, Ghareeb Mahdy S, et al. Value of duplex scanning in differentiating embolic from thrombotic arterial occlusion in acute limb ischemia. Cardiovasc Revasc Med. 2010;11(4):223–6.
9. Egglin TK, O'Moore PV, Feinstein AR, et al. Complications of peripheral arteriography: a new system to identify patients at increased risk. J Vasc Surg. 1995;22(6):787–94.
10. El-Gengehe AT, Ammar WA, Baligh Ewiss E, et al. Acute limb ischemia: role of preoperative and postoperative duplex in differentiating acute embolic from thrombotic ischemia. Cardiovasc Revasc Med. 2013;14(4):197–202.
11. Speziale F, Sirignano P, Menna D, et al. Ten years' experience in endovascular repair of popliteal artery aneurysm using the viabahn endoprosthesis: a report from two Italian vascular centers. Ann Vasc Surg. 2015;29(5):941–9.
12. de Donato G, Setacci F, Galzerano G, et al. Endovascular treatment of popliteal aneurysm. J Cardiovasc Surg. 2015;56(4):587–97.
13. Foshager MC, Sane SS. Evaluation of lower extremity bypass grafts with use of color duplex sonography. Radiographics. 1996;16(1):9–25.
14. Willmann JK, Mayer D, Banyai M, et al. Evaluation of peripheral arterial bypass grafts with multi-detector row CT angiography: comparison with duplex US and digital subtraction angiography. Radiology. 2003;229(2):465–74.
15. Polak JF, Donaldson MC, Dobkin GR, et al. Early detection of saphenous vein arterial bypass graft stenosis by color-assisted duplex sonography: a prospective study. Am J Roentgenol. 1990;154(4):857–61.
16. Toursarkissian B, Mejia A, Smilanich RP, et al. Changing patterns of access site complications with the use of percutaneous closure devices. Vasc Surg. 2001;35(3):203–6.
17. Meyerson SL, Feldman T, Desai TR, et al. Angiographic access site complications in the era of arterial closure devices. Vasc Endovasc Surg. 2002;36(2):137–44.
18. Cihan HB, Gülcan O, Hazar A, et al. Peripheral vascular injuries. Ulus Travma Derg. 2001;7(2):113–6.
19. Ouriel K, Shortell CK, DeWeese JA, et al. A comparison of thrombolytic therapy with operative revascularization in the initial treatment of acute peripheral arterial ischemia. J Vasc Surg. 1994;19:1021–30.
20. Fogarty TJ, Cranley JJ, Krause RJ, et al. A method for extraction of arterial emboli and thrombi. Surg Gynecol Obstet. 1963;116:241–4.
21. Kasirajan K, Ouriel K. Management of acute lower extremity ischemia: treatment strategies and outcomes. Curr Intervent Cardiol Rep. 2000;2:119–29.
22. Baril DT, Patel VI, Judelson DR, et al. Outcomes of lower extremity bypass performed for acute limb ischemia. J Vasc Surg. 2013;58(4):949–56.
23. Eliason JL, Wainess RM, Proctor MC, et al. A national and single institutional experience in the contemporary treatment of acute lower extremity ischemia. Ann Surg. 2003;238(3):382–9. Discussion 389-390
24. Oklu R, Ghasemi-Rad M, Irani Z, et al. Aspiration thrombectomy using the Penumbra catheter. J Vasc Interv Radiol. 2015;26:454–5.
25. Schernthaner MB, Samuels S, Biegler P, et al. Ultra-sound-accelerated versus standard catheter-directed thrombolysis in 102 patients with acute and subacute limb ischemia. J Vasc Interv Radiol. 2014;25:1149–56.
26. Baumann F, Sharpe E 3rd, Peña C, et al. Technical results of vacuum-assisted thrombectomy for arterial clot removal in patients with acute limb ischemia. J Vasc Interv Radiol. 2016;27(3):330–5.

Aortic Aneurysm in Elderly Patients

18

Andrea Stella, Erico Gallitto, Chiara Mascoli, Rodolfo Pini, and Alessia Sonetto

18.1 Introduction

In industrialized countries, elderly represent an increasing group among the entire population [1]. In the United States, the number of people over 85 years will reach 21 million within 2050, representing the 5% of the overall population [2]. Also in Europe, similar data are expected, estimating a triplication from 21.8 billion people to 61.4 billion in 2060 [3].

The incidence of abdominal aortic aneurysm (AAA) increases with the ageing of the population. Given the increasing of median age in the population, a rapid increase of AAA that will need to be treated during the next decades is expected.

At the same time, considering all their comorbidities, elderly patients are usually considered unfit for a traditional open repair (OR). Endovascular aneurysm repair (EVAR) is a safe and effective mini-invasive therapeutics option for elderly [4–7].

18.2 EVAR Literature Review

During the last 10 years, randomized controlled trials (RCTs) reported EVAR outcomes compared with OR [4–7].

The main RCTs (EVAR-1, DREAM, OVER and FACE) have been analysed and summarized in a recent Cochrane review [8]. These studies included AAA that matched the morphological inclusion criteria of EVAR and that could be suitable for both procedures (open and EVAR).

A. Stella • E. Gallitto (✉) • C. Mascoli • R. Pini • A. Sonetto
Vascular Surgery - Bologna University, Bologna, Italy
e-mail: andrea.stella2@unibo.it

A. Crucitti (ed.), *Surgical Management of Elderly Patients*,
https://doi.org/10.1007/978-3-319-60861-7_18

Patients who underwent EVAR had significantly lower 30-day (1.4% vs 4.2% in EVAR and open, respectively) and intra-hospitalization (1:4 proportion in EVAR vs OR) mortality [8].

EVAR-1 and DREAM reported shorter procedural time, intensive care unit (ICU) stay and hospitalization, less blood loss/transfusion, reduced pain, faster mobilization and reduced gastrointestinal, pulmonary, cardiac and nephrological complications in EVAR if compared with OR [8]. These results were related with the lower EVAR invasiveness compared with OR. EVAR was associated with better 30-day results probably due to the lower cardiac stress during the procedure.

DREAM and FACE underlined a correlation between a patient who underwent OR and has a higher risk of intra-procedural mortality and the onset of moderate to severe perioperative complications, especially respiratory complications.

DREAM, EVAR-1 and OVER trials reported also the long-term results [8–11]. The mean follow-up was 6 years (5–10 years) [8]. Despite initial benefits of EVAR vs open repair, patient survival in the follow-up was similar for both techniques [8–11].

DREAM reported a mean survival of 69.9% at 6 years for OR and of 68.9% for EVAR group [8]. EVAR-1 trial reports an overall survival of 54% for both groups, and OVER study presents similar results [8–11]. The higher peri-procedural mortality of OR is balanced by higher rates of complications during long-term follow-up in EVAR patients. EVAR complications seem to increase in a period between 6 and 4 years from the procedure. The RCTs [4–7] also reported a higher rate of re-intervention in EVAR group. Patients who underwent EVAR had a significantly higher re-intervention rate (23.4%) than open surgery group (13.1%) [8]. Moreover, the DREAM study showed that re-interventions in open group were related mostly to the onset of laparocele, while in the EVAR group, re-interventions were more related to endograft complications such as endoleaks, migration and/or thrombosis. As regards long-term complications, all the RCTs reported homogeneous data between EVAR and open procedures [8].

In conclusion, the Cochrane review showed that EVAR has an advantage in terms of early/midterm mortality and cardiac morbidity, while OR showed better results in terms of freedom from re-intervention.

The two techniques didn't show significant differences in long-term survival, so that different parameters should be considered in order to decide which treatment, OR or EVAR, is better for each patient.

Due to the lower invasiveness and cardiac morbidity, EVAR has extended the possibility of treatment to patients at high surgical risk. Thanks to EVAR, risks and benefits in the treatment of AAA have changed, and also patients affected by a relevant number of comorbidities can now be treated.

Even if EVAR is associated with lower morbidity and short-term complications compared with OR, procedure-related complications and re-interventions remain an open issue.

Re-intervention rate of EVAR is around 1–2% per year. Octogenarian patients have a life expectancy of 6.1 years, and they are likely to die for other disease, not related to the AAA.

It is also remarkable that the reduced period of hospitalization has defined EVAR as the most indicated technique for the treatment of octogenarians. In fact open surgery requires long time of complete recovery (between 3 and 6 months), and 36% of patients did not completely recovered.

Some comorbidities have been defined as relevant in determining the success of a surgical procedure: high grade of ASA (American Society of Anesthesiologists) score; cardiac, pulmonary, nephrological, neurologic and hematologic issues; elevated body mass index; impaired renal function; reduced haematocrit and low levels of albumin.

According to these factors, a new score based on ASA score and on a system suggested by Ad Hoc Committee for Standardized Reporting Practices in Vascular Surgery by SVS has been proposed [12]. This score considers the presence of cardiac, pulmonary and renal comorbidities and allows stratifying patients in low, medium and high risk.

18.3 Literature Review in Patients Under and Over 80s

Previous studies showed a higher 30-day mortality in octogenarians versus younger patients [13, 14]. In particular, Lange et al. [15] reported a 30-day mortality rate of 5%. In a more recent paper, Geisbusch et al. [16] showed that 30-day mortality of patients who underwent EVAR was higher in octogenarians (2.8% vs 1%). However, in this study, age did not influence survival in high-risk patients. Tsilimparis et al. [17] reported a 30-day mortality rate stratified on the basis of age: 13, 7 and 4% in nonagenarian, octogenarians and younger patients, respectively. Cardiac and pulmonary complications were the main complications related to 30-day mortality. These complications were not related with the procedure but with the clinical conditions.

As regards long-term outcomes, Geisbuch et al. [16] reported a survival of 64% in octogenarians at 4 years of follow-up. A lower survival has been reported in over 80s patients at 1, 2 and 5 years. Death was aneurysm related in only 1.1% of cases, while 40% is related to comorbidities, and in 58% the cause of death was unknown. A higher mortality rate has been found in patients classified as ASA 4.

Elderly patients seem to have lower rate of re-interventions during follow-up. Visser et al. [18] reported 8.2 and 19.8% of re-interventions at 3 years in elderly and in young patients, respectively. This result could be related with a stricter follow-up of octogenarians. Other authors reported a re-intervention rate in octogenarian about 10–15% [19, 20].

18.4 Our Experience

In our experience, among 1135 consecutive EVAR performed in an 8-year period (2006–2015), 201 (15.9%) were octogenarian.

Due to the increment of mean life duration, the number of patients that need a treatment has increased (from 8 cases in 2006 to 26 cases in 2014). The mean age was 84 ± 2 years (range 81–100 years), 84% were male, and the mean AAA diameter was 61 ± 8 mm. Thirty-four patients (16%) had ASA score of 4.

Loco-regional anaesthesia was the preferable method and was performed in 84% of patients.

Short-term results were encouraging, both regarding the technical success (96.7%) and the absence of 30-day conversions and re-interventions. Technical success was not reached in case of type Ia endoleak that has not influenced a 30-day mortality.

The 30-day mortality was 2.5%, and it was lower if compared to literature 30-day mortality in elderly patients (2.8, 5 and 7.2%, respectively, by Geibusch et al. [16], Lange et al. [15] and Tsilimparis et al. [17]) but higher if compared to younger patients (1.4% Paravastu et al. [8]). Mortality was significantly higher in ASA 4 patients compared with ASA < 4 patients (9.4% vs 0.6%).

In our experience, perioperative morbidity was 23.5%, similar to morbidity rate reported from Tsilimparis et al. [17] (24.7%). Geibusch et al. [16] reported a lower morbidity rate (11.5%) without considering nephrological complications. If we consider only cardiopulmonary complications, our morbidity rate is 9.9%.

The mean follow-up was 36 ± 18 months, and the overall survival at 1, 2, 3 and 5 years was 88 ± 2%, 84 ± 3%, 79 ± 3% and 56 ± 5%, respectively.

Among elderly, we divided and compared the population into two groups on the basis of the age: survival of patients over 85 years was 66.8% vs 64.5% of patients between 80 and 85 years at a mean follow-up of 35 months (p:ns). Long-term mortality related to AAA was 3.1% vs 33.3% of total deaths.

Re-interventions rate at 35 months of follow-up was 6.2%, slightly lower if compared to the current literature (8.2% Visser et al. [18] and 12.6% Biebl et al. [14]). Re-intervention rate in elderly was significantly lower than in patients under 80s (23.4%). This could be related to the stricter attention offered to elderly.

In our experience, we evaluated other possible variables that can influence survival (COPD, CKF, PAOD and ASA 3 or ASA > 3. At multivariate analysis, PAOD was one of the variables that affects more midterm survival (2 years), together with ASA > 3 score (signal of higher systemic comorbidities). Only patients with one or no risk factors reached the 5-year follow-up.

Conclusions

Octogenarians are affected by a higher risk of peri-procedural mortality compared to patients under 80s, but this risk is sufficiently low to allow EVAR treatment in these patients.

Obviously the decision to treat this group of patients remains controversial and has to be valued case by case, considering comorbidities, aneurysm dimension and life expectancy of each patient.

With a life expectancy of 6.1 years, octogenarians with anatomical and clinical features fit for EVAR seem to benefit from a preventive AAA treatment. EVAR in >80-year-old patients is associated with an overall low early mortality rate of 2% especially in ASA < 4 (0.6%).

According to the literature, we can state that age should not be considered first as an exclusion criteria for these patients, not even if over 85 years.

Exclusion criteria should be clinical conditions of patient, because the survival of patients with none or only one risk factor justifies the treatment for AAA; however, patients with ASA 4 and PAOD had a significantly higher mortality rate and reduction of life expectancy; therefore, the EVAR treatment could be justified only in particular cases of AAA with impending rupture.

References

1. Bennett JE, Li G, Foreman K, Best N, Kontis V, Pearson C, Hambly P, Ezzati M. The future of life expectancy and life expectancy inequalities in England and Wales: Bayesian spatiotemporal forecasting. Lancet. 2015;386(9989):163–70.
2. U.S. Census Bureau. U.S. interim projections by age, sex, race, and hispanic origin: 2000–2050. http://www.census.gov/population/www/projections/usinterimproj/.
3. Eurostat. Population projections. http://epp.eurostat.ec.europa.eu/statistics_explained/index.php/Population_projections/.
4. EVAR trial participants. Endovascular aneurysm repair versus open repair in patients with abdominal aortic aneurysm (EVAR trial 1): randomised controlled trial. Lancet. 2005;365(9478):2179–86.
5. Greenhalgh RM, Brown LC, Kwong GP, Powell JT, Thompson SG. EVAR trial participants. Comparison of endovascular aneurysm repair with open repair in patients with abdominal aortic aneurysm (EVAR trial 1), 30-day operative mortality results: randomised controlled trial. Lancet. 2004;364(9437):843–8.
6. Prinssen M, Verhoeven EL, Buth J, Cuypers PW, Van Sambeek MR, Balm R, et al. A randomized trial comparing conventional and endovascular repair of abdominal aortic aneurysms. N Engl J Med. 2004;351(16):1607–18.
7. Lederle FA, Freischlag JA, Kyriakides TC, Padberg FT Jr, Matsumura JS, Kohler TR, et al. Outcomes following endovascular vs open repair of abdominal aortic aneurysm: a randomized trial. JAMA. 2009;302(14):1535–42.
8. Paravastu SC, Jayarajasingam R, Cottam R, Palfreyman SJ, Michaels JA, Thomas SM. Endovascular repair of abdominal aortic aneurysm. Cochrane Database Syst Rev. 2014;1:CD004178.
9. United Kingdom EVAR Trial Investigators, Greenhalgh RM, Brown LC, Powell JT, Thompson SG, Epstein D, Sculpher MJ. Endovascular versus open repair of abdominal aortic aneurysm. N Engl J Med. 2010;362:1863–71.
10. De Bruin JL, Baas AF, Buth J, Prinssen M, Verhoeven EL, Cuypers PW, van Sambeek MR, Balm R, Grobbee DE, Blankensteijn JD, DREAM Study Group. Long-term outcome of open or endovascular repair of abdominal aortic aneurysm. N Engl J Med. 2010;362(20):1881–9.
11. Schermerhorn ML, Buck DB, O'Malley AJ, Curran T, McCallum JC, Darling J, Landon BE. Long-term outcomes of abdominal aortic aneurysm in the Medicare population. N Engl J Med. 2015;373(4):328–38.
12. Chaikof EL, Fillinger MF, Matsumura JS, Rutherford RB, White GH, Blankensteijn JD, Bernhard VM, Harris PL, Kent KC, May J, Veith FJ, Zarins CK. Identifying and grading factors that modify the outcome of endovascular aortic aneurysm repair. J Vasc Surg. 2002;35:1061–6.
13. Pol RA, Zeebregts CJ, van Sterkenburg SM, Reijnen MM, ENGAGE Investigators. Thirty-day outcome and quality of life after endovascular abdominal aortic aneurysm repair in octogenarians based on the endurant stent graft natural selection global postmarket registry (ENGAGE). J Vasc Surg. 2012;56(1):27–35.
14. Biebl M, Lau LL, Hakaim AG, Oldenburg WA, Klocker J, Neuhauser B, McKinney JM, Paz-Fumagalli R. Midterm outcome of endovascular aortic aneurysm repair in octogenarians: a single institution's experience. J Vasc Surg. 2004;40(3):435–42.

15. Lange C, Leurs LJ, Buth J, Myhre HO, EUROSTAR collaborators. Endovascular repair of abdominal aortic aneurysm in octogenarians: an analysis based on EUROSTAR data. J Vasc Surg. 2005;42(4):624–30.
16. Geisbüsch P, Katzen BT, Tsoukas AI, Arango D, Peña CS, Benenati JF. Endovascular repair of infrarenal aortic aneurysms in octogenarians and nonagenarians. J Vasc Surg. 2011;54(6):1605–13.
17. Tsilimparis N, Perez S, Dayama A, Ricotta JJ 2nd. Age-stratified results from 20,095 aortoiliac aneurysm repairs: should we approach octogenarians and nonagenarians differently? J Am Coll Surg. 2012;215(5):690–701.
18. Visser L, Pol RA, Tielliu IF, van den Dungen JJ, Zeebregts CJ. A limited and customized follow-up seems justified after endovascular abdominal aneurysm repair in octogenarians. J Vasc Surg. 2014;59(5):1232–40.
19. Pol RA, Zeebregts CJ, van Sterkenburg SM, Ferreira LM, Goktay Y, Reijnen MM, Endurant Stent Graft Natural Selection Global Postmarket Registry (ENGAGE) Investigators. Outcome and quality of life after endovascular abdominal aortic aneurysm repair in octogenarians. J Vasc Surg. 2014;60(2):308–17.
20. Prenner SB, Turnbull IC, Serrao GW, Fishman E, Ellozy SH, Vouyouka AG, Marin ML, Faries PL. Outcome of elective endovascular abdominal aortic aneurysm repair in nonagenarians. J Vasc Surg. 2011;54(2):287–94.

Venous Disorders of the Leg

19

Stefano de Franciscis and Raffaele Serra

Abbreviations

ASVAL	Ablation sélective des varices sous anésthesie locale
CDT	Catheter-directed thrombolysis
CEAP	Clinical-etiology-anatomy-pathophysiology
CHIVA	Cure Hémodynamique de l'insuffisance veineuse en ambulatoire
CT	Compression therapy
CVD	Chronic venous disease
CVI	Chronic venous insufficiency
CVLU	Chronic venous leg ulceration
DVT	Deep vein thrombosis
ECM	Extracellular matrix
EVLA	Endovascular laser therapy
GAG	Glycosaminoglycan
LMWH	Low molecular weight heparin
PAPS	Percutaneous ablation of perforators
PAT	Percutaneous aspiration thrombectomy
PCDT	Pharmacomechanical catheter-directed thrombolysis
PTS	Post-thrombotic syndrome
RFA	Radiofrequency ablation
SEPS	Subfascial endoscopic perforator vein surgery
VAD	Venoactive drug

S. de Franciscis • R. Serra (✉)
Department of Medical and Surgical Sciences, Interuniversity Center of Phlebolymphology (CIFL), International Research and Educational, Program in Clinical and Experimental Biotechnology, University Magna Graecia of Catanzaro, Catanzaro, Italy
e-mail: defranci@unicz.it; rserra@unicz.it

A. Crucitti (ed.), *Surgical Management of Elderly Patients*,
https://doi.org/10.1007/978-3-319-60861-7_19

19.1 Introduction

Venous disorders of the leg refer to either chronic or acute conditions related to or caused by veins that become diseased or abnormal. These problems can include chronic venous disease (CVD) which involves primarily the superficial venous system and deep vein thrombosis (DVT) which affects primarily the deep venous system.

CVD and DVT may occur at any age; nevertheless, most of the complications of venous disorders are more prevalent in the elderly [1].

19.2 Chronic Venous Disease

The prevalence of chronic venous disease (CVD) is <10% for men and for women younger than 30 years and goes up to 57 and 77% in men and women aged >70 years, respectively. The spectrum of CVD can be described using the clinical-etiology-anatomy-pathophysiology (CEAP) classification, and according to the "C" (clinical classes) of this classification, it ranges from the mild manifestations such as telangiectases/reticular veins (C1) and truncal varicose veins (C2) to the more advanced signs represented by leg edema (C3) and the serious dermal manifestations

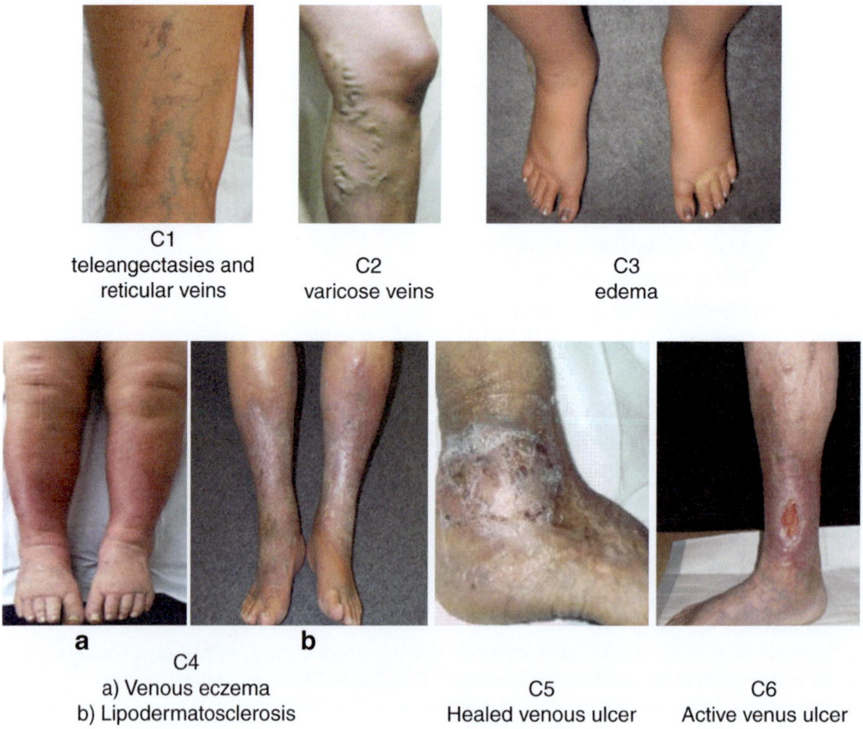

Fig. 19.1 Clinical classes (C) of the CEAP classification

consisting of hyperpigmentation, eczema, lipodermatosclerosis (C4), and chronic venous leg ulceration (CVLU) (C5–C6) (Fig. 19.1).

Clinical manifestations from C3 to C6 pertain to the condition called chronic venous insufficiency (CVI).

Each clinical class is further characterized by a subscript for the presence of symptoms (S, symptomatic) or absence of symptoms (A, asymptomatic). Symptoms include aching, pain, tightness, itching, heaviness, and muscle cramps. A particular subgroup of patients are defined C0s, which means that these patients have no evident sign or instrumental abnormalities, but they complain of venous symptoms.

Loss of calf muscle pump and poor mobility in elderly patients more often lead to important increase of venous hypertension, with subsequent skin changes formation and, thus, with the risk of venous ulceration becoming even higher. In fact, venous ulcers occur more commonly in the elderly, the peak prevalence occurring between ages 60 and 80 years. Venous ulceration is a condition that often requires long-term care. Nonhealing ulcers can be complicated by infection that may require hospitalization. Furthermore, venous ulcer recurrences are common with rates ranging from 54 to 78%. In the western world, the treatment cost of venous ulcers has been estimated to require up to 2% of the annual health-care budget.

Mixed arterial and venous disease may also coexist in elderly patients. In fact, in several clinical studies, the reported incidence of arterial insufficiency in patients with venous ulceration has reached up to 30%, especially in the elderly. This condition is responsible for chronic delayed healing among lower extremity wounds.

From a clinical point of view, venous ulcers are typically superficial and irregularly shaped. Granulation tissue is often present along with the aforementioned signs of CVI, such as edema and skin changes. These wounds traditionally present in the lower third of the leg, especially around the gaiter region. Usually, there is no pain unless the ulcer becomes infected.

On the other side, arterial ulcers can have a punched out appearance with distinct borders and may involve the foot and/or the toes, and at the end stage, gangrene may be present. Furthermore, patients with arterial ulcers may complain of more leg pain compared to patients with venous ulcers alone.

In patients suffering from an ulcer of mixed arterial and venous origin, features of both ulcer types may be present (Fig. 19.2).

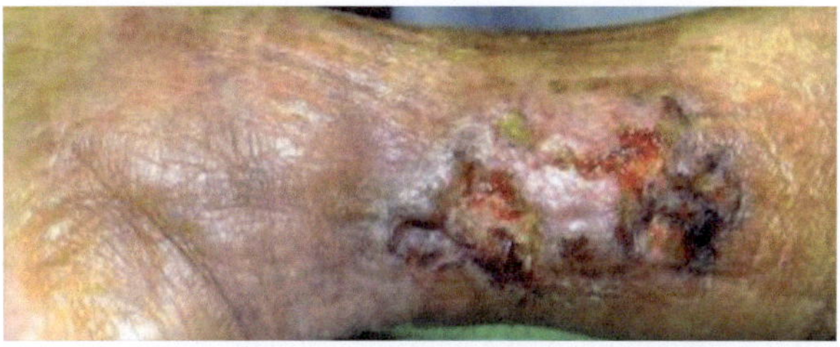

Fig. 19.2 Mixed arterial and venous ulcer

Although many elderly patients have associated diseases or particular medical conditions that make them less suitable for a general anesthetic, the full range of interventions dedicated for the superficial venous disease can be performed safely under tumescent local anesthetic, often as an outpatient, with considerable advantage for the elderly.

There is no evidence that surgical treatment of CVD in the elderly is less safe or less effective than in younger people. Conversely, elderly patients with CVD, being more likely to have complications for their condition, have the most gain from active treatment.

Apart from classic operations such as saphenectomy, surgery has made important progress in the last 25 years. Operations are now more limited, considering the extension of the segments to treat, and they intend to correct the hemodynamic alterations, preserving the competent venous segments (hemodynamic surgery).

Furthermore the treatment of varicose veins has also undergone dramatic changes with the introduction of percutaneous endovenous ablation techniques, including endovascular laser therapy (EVLA), radiofrequency ablation (RFA), and liquid or foam sclerotherapy [1–11].

19.2.1 Operating Techniques

The basic indication for the treatment of varicose veins in the elderly is the prevention of possible secondary complications and sequels which are particularly frequent in these patients. Therefore, for these patients, varicose vein surgery is basically a preventive surgery [7–18].

19.2.1.1 Saphenous Stripping

This surgery involves making incisions (usually the groin and medial thigh, for the short vein stripping, or the lower part of the leg, for the long vein stripping) followed by insertion of a special metal or plastic wire into the vein. The vein is attached to the wire and then pulled out from the body. The incisions are stitched up, and a pressure bandage followed by elastic stockings is a common recovery prescription. This procedure may be performed under general or locoregional anesthetic and more frequently under local or tumescent anesthetic. For this reason and for the risk of saphenous nerve injury, more frequently in the elderly, the reasons explained below are not routinely considered for elderly people.

Saphenous nerve injury is known for a long time to be a potential complication of the saphenous vein long stripping. The proximity of the vein and nerve, especially at the level of shank, results in injuries during the vein resection, especially in the patients, such as the elderly, with advanced varicose veins in this area caused by a large number of insufficient perforators. Additionally, in the elderly patients suffering from long-lasting varicose veins, it can lead to an accretion of the widened vein, resulting in the saphenous nerve neuropraxy. This pathology also facilitates in injury of the nerve fibers during the operation [9–12].

19.2.1.2 Local Phlebectomy and Hemodynamic Correction

Surgical treatment for varicose veins had a great and creative improvement with Muller's invention of the local stab avulsion method, developing some specific and useful hooks. Soon after, Franceschi developed a minimally invasive surgical approach, the cure hémodynamique de l'insuffisance veineuse en ambulatoire (CHIVA), meaning a therapy (cure) which preserves veins and restores the hemodynamics for insufficient veins on an outpatient basis. In fact, CHIVA strategy aims to perform a hemodynamic correction, more than to a radical avulsion of the varicose bed, based upon a meticulous preoperative duplex ultrasound examination. CHIVA treatment corrects the blood flow by using ligatures of specific blood vessels. In fact, the duplex ultrasound examination allows the physician to create a precise map of the patient's venous anatomy and blood flow and, therefore, determine how to correct it. This technique may preserve the saphenous veins, and most of all, by suppressing the hemodynamic overload, it normalizes the venous flow and make varicose vein disappear. Generally the result is an efficient, cheap, and ambulatory minimally invasive surgery.

Recently the ablation sélective des varices sous anésthesie locale (ASVAL), based on the ascending theory, describing the disease process as developing in the lower most part of the leg and propagating cranially, aims to eliminate collateral varicose veins, considered at the origin of the disease, under local anesthesia and by means of multiple micro-incisions, and without treating the saphenous trunk [10,12,13–16].

19.2.1.3 Endovenous Thermal Ablation Surgery

The advantages of endovascular ablation are lower incidence of complications, shorter post-intervention hospital stays, less postoperative pain, and earlier return to normal physical activities and, therefore, are particular adequate in the elderly.

The main techniques are represented by endovenous laser ablation (EVLA) and radiofrequency ablation (RFA) which are performed ultrasonographically guided and under tumescent local anesthetic.

EVLA is performed by introducing a laser fiber into the lumen of the vein to treat. The heat generated and transferred by the laser energy causes a direct thermal injury to the vein wall, resulting in the destruction of the endothelial wall, collagen denaturation of the media, and then followed by fibrosis. EVLA can be used to treat both axial veins and collaterals.

RFA is performed by inserting a special radiofrequency catheter into the targeted saphenous vessel under ultrasound guidance from the knee to the groin, usually up to the level of the epigastric vein or 1–2 cm away from the saphenofemoral junction. The initial thermal injury is then followed by fibrosis of the treated vein. This procedure appears to be safe and efficacious, shortening the operation time and preventing patient procedural discomfort. RFA has been initially proposed for the treatment of axial reflux (saphenous veins) but seems to have also a role in the treatment of tributary varices.

The introduction of ultrasonographically guided thermal ablations has also revolutionized the techniques of perforator vein ablation. Percutaneous ablation of perforators (PAPS) consists in the application of an ablative technique (RF, EVLA, or even sclerotherapy) within the lumen of the target veins through an ultrasound-guided percutaneous intraluminal port. These techniques seem to get advantages over the most traditional ablative treatments (Linton and Cockett procedures) and even over the less invasive subfascial endoscopic perforator vein surgery (SEPS) for the necessity of simple local anesthesia and for the possibility to be performed ambulatorially because no dissections and incisions are needed [1,11,17].

19.2.1.4 Skin Grafts

One of the most important surgical procedures for the treatment of CVLUs is skin grafting, especially when lesions are large and refractory to standard treatments.

Autografts, allografts, or human skin equivalents can be used, with a resulting healing rate of 73%. Overall, all patients suffering with CVLUs and being considered for skin graft should undergo surgery for venous insufficiency in order to correct the underlying venous abnormalities causing the ulcerations and avoid surgical breakdown. Skin grafting for CVLUs can also be followed by additional treatment to try to speed up the healing such as long-term LMWH therapy. Also the use of platelet gel after skin grafting appears to be effective and a safe tool in order to increase the healing rate of difficult-to-treat ulcers, reaching a healing rate up to 90% at 5 years [1, 18].

19.2.1.5 Nonsurgical Treatments

Nonsurgical approaches are mainly represented by compression therapy, medical treatment, and sclerotherapy that will be briefly resumed here for completeness, as they are not included within the aim and the scope of this surgical chapter, but they may be used as adjuvant treatments to surgery.

Currently, compression therapy represents the basic and most frequently used treatment of CVD and its complications. This treatment has been extensively validated. Compression therapy (CT) must overcome the abnormal hemodynamics of venous hypertension; it is important to achieve the optimal pressure according to the clinical class of the patient. Therefore, CT has been designed as the primary therapeutic modality for healing venous ulcers and as adjuvant device to superficial vein surgery and skin grafting in order to avoid also ulcer recurrence. CT may be executed by compression stockings and compression bandages. Depending on the clinical situations, generally the grade of compression may range 10–40 mmHg or even more.

Difficulties regarding putting on and removing of the compression stockings remain significant in the elderly population, and this may affect the compliance of this category of patients to these important and useful devices.

Venoactive drugs (VADs) have been employed, along the years, in case of all the clinical classes of CVD. The most used are flavonoids which seem to reduce endothelial alterations and improve the property of smooth muscle cells within the media of the vein, with phlebotonic effect. Glycosaminoglycan (GAG) drugs seem to reduce inflammation and extracellular matrix (ECM) imbalance which is one of the major components of CVD.

Sclerotherapy has become a very popular treatment for varicose veins in Europe. It consists of the injection of a sclerosing substance into the refluxing vessels. The sclerosant substance, in the liquid form or in the foam form if it has been mixed with a gas, such as air, is able to determine chemical endothelial damage and vessel fibrosis [1, 19].

19.3 Deep Vein Thrombosis

One of the most recent understood aspects of venous deep vein thrombosis (DVT) risk is advancing age. Incidence rates of DVT increase dramatically at about age 55 and by age 80 are nearly 1 in 100 per year, approximately 1000-fold higher than for those aged 45 or younger. Furthermore, rates of its life-threatening complication pulmonary embolism (PE) rise faster than DVT in the elderly so that the disease has greater fatal impact in this population. For DVT (Fig. 19.3), prompt, effective, and sustained anticoagulation is pivotal because of the risk of recurrent events, including PE, and also complications such as post-thrombotic syndrome (PTS) and chronic thromboembolic pulmonary hypertension, which may greatly affect a patient's quality of life, especially in the elderly.

PTS is the consequence of venous valvular incompetence, venous outflow obstruction, and calf muscle pump dysfunction following an acute episode of DVT. Signs and symptoms of PTS may include lower extremity pain, edema, hyperpigmentation, and CVLU. For PTS, proximal DVT and recurrent ipsilateral DVT are the two principal established risk factors for PTS, and the best way to prevent it is to provide optimal anticoagulation for the acute phase of DVT once it occurs. From this, it follows that most of the treatment of DVT pertains to medicine rather than surgery.

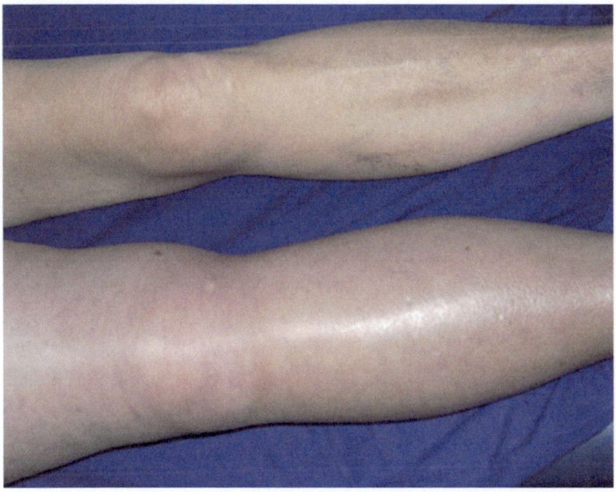

Fig. 19.3 Deep vein thrombosis

For the subgroup of patients with acute iliofemoral DVT and recently formed thrombus (<10–14 days), endovascular treatment options may also be considered such as catheter-directed thrombolysis (CDT), pharmacomechanical catheter-directed thrombolysis (PCDT), percutaneous aspiration thrombectomy (PAT), vena cava filter protection, venous balloon dilatation, and venous stent implantation. Current practice shows strong clinical tendency for the use of PCDT with or without other endovascular methods and an individualized approach for each DVT patient. PCDT seems also to be the most promising interventional modality for prevention of PTS. PCDT aims to improve early mechanical thrombus removal and promote lysis of remaining clot.

Current guidelines from the American College of Chest Physicians suggest that directed thrombolysis should be used in those with life expectancy >1 year, good functional status, extensive iliofemoral thrombosis, and presenting soon after the onset of symptoms (fewer than 14 days) (level 2B evidence) [20–25].

Acknowledgments The authors have no conflict of interests to declare.
This chapter received no funding.

Authors' Contribution SdF and RS contributed equally to this work.
They both conceived the chapter, participated in its design, drafted, and revised it critically.

References

1. Serra R, Grande R, Butrico L, Fugetto F, de Franciscis S. Epidemiology, diagnosis and treatment of chronic venous disease: a systematic review. Chirurgia. 2016;29(2):34–45.
2. Serra R, Buffone G, de Franciscis A, Mastrangelo D, Molinari V, Montemurro R, et al. A genetic study of chronic venous insufficiency. Ann Vasc Surg. 2012;26:636–42.
3. Robertson L, Evans C, Fowkes FG. Epidemiology of chronic venous disease. Phlebology. 2008;23:103–11.
4. Beebe-Dimmer JL, Pfeifer JR, Engle JS, Schottenfeld D. The epidemiology of chronic venous insufficiency and varicose veins. Ann Epidemiol. 2005;15:175–84.
5. Eklöf B, Rutherford RB, Bergan JJ, Carpentier PH, Gloviczki P, Kistner RL, et al. Revision of the CEAP classification for chronic venous disorders: consensus statement. J Vasc Surg. 2004;40:1248–52.
6. Serra R, Andreucci M, De Caridi G, Massara M, Mastroroberto P, de Franciscis S. Functional chronic venous disease: a systematic review. Phlebology. 2017;1:268355516686451. https://doi.org/10.1177/0268355516686451. [Epub ahead of print].
7. O'Hare JL, Earnshaw JJ. Practical advice for the treatment of venous disease in the elderly. Phlebology. 2008;23(3):101–2.
8. Etufugh CN, Phillips TJ. Venous ulcers. Clin Dermatol. 2007;25(1):121–30.
9. Canonico S, Campitiello F, Pacifico F, Sepe D, Lauletta V. Day care surgery of varicose veins in elderly patients. Vasc Surg. 1996;30(5):387–92.
10. de Franciscis S, Gasbarro V, Amato B, Buffone G, Grande R, Serra R. Hemodynamic surgery versus conventional surgery in chronic venous disease: a multicenter retrospective study. Acta Phlebologica. 2013;14:109–14.
11. Serra R, Gasbarro V, Barbetta A, De Caridi G, Massara M, Perri P, Ciranni S, Torcia G, Abatucci G, Andreucci M, Buffone G, de Franciscis S. Endovenous radiofrequency ablation of tributary veins reflux. Acta Phlebologica. 2016;17:61–3.
12. Müller R. Traitement des varices par la phlebéctomie ambulatoire. Bull Soc Fr Phléb. 1966;19:277–9.

13. Francheschi C. Thèorie et pratique de la cure conservatrice de l'insufisance veineuse en ambulatoire. Précy-sous- Thil: Editions de l'Armancon; 1988.
14. Solis JV, Ribè L, Portero JL, Rio J. Stripping saphenectomy, CHIVA and laser ablation for the treatment of the saphenous vein insufficiency. Ambul Surg. 2009;15:11–4.
15. Onida S, Davies AH. CHIVA, ASVAL and related techniques—concepts and evidence. Phlebology. 2015;30(2 Suppl):42–5.
16. Jaworucka-Kaczorowska A, Oszkinis G, Huber J, Wiertel-Krawczuk A, Gabor E, Kaczorowski P. Saphenous vein stripping surgical technique and frequency of saphenous nerve injury. Phlebology. 2015;30(3):210–6.
17. Lam H, Chao L. Endovascular ablation therapies for varicose veins in elderly patients. Int J Gerontol. 2014;8:219–22.
18. Serra R, Rizzuto A, Rossi A, Perri P, Barbetta A, Abdalla K, Caroleo S, Longo C, Amantea B, Sammarco G, de Franciscis S. Skin grafting for the treatment of chronic leg ulcers – a systematic review in evidence-based medicine. Int Wound J. 2017;14:149–57.
19. Carpentier PH, Becker F, Thiney G, Poensin D, Satger B. Acceptability and practicability of elastic compression stockings in the elderly: a randomized controlled evaluation. Phlebology. 2011;26(3):107–13.
20. Silverstein RL, Bauer KA, Cushman M, Esmon CT, Ershler WB, Tracy RP. Venous thrombosis in the elderly: more questions than answers. Blood. 2007;110(9):3097–101.
21. Prandoni P. Treatment of patients with acute deep vein thrombosis and/or pulmonary embolism: efficacy and safety of non-VKA oral anticoagulants in selected populations. Thromb Res. 2014;134(2):227–33.
22. Rabinovich A, Kahn SR. The postthrombotic syndrome: current evidence and future challenges. J Thromb Haemost. 2017;15(2):230–41. https://doi.org/10.1111/jth.13569. [Epub ahead of print].
23. Goktay AY, Senturk C. Endovascular treatment of thrombosis and embolism. Adv Exp Med Biol. 2017;906:195–213.
24. Kuo TT, Huang CY, Hsu CP, Lee CY. Catheter-directed thrombolysis and pharmacomechanical thrombectomy improve midterm outcome in acute iliofemoral deep vein thrombosis. J Chin Med Assoc. 2017;80(2):72–9.
25. Patterson BO, Hinchliffe R, Loftus IM, Thompson MM, Holt PJ. Indications for catheter-directed thrombolysis in the management of acute proximal deep venous thrombosis. Arterioscler Thromb Vasc Biol. 2010;30(4):669–74.

Part V

Hepato-Biliary System

Cholecystectomy in Elderly: Challenge and Critical Analysis of Available Evidence

20

Alessandro Puzziello, Domenico Landi, Fernando Vicinanza, Giulia Pacella, Giulio Orlando, and Ileana Maria Luppino

20.1 Introduction

The incidence of gallstone disease in the elderly population ranges from 14 to 27%. The prevalence of gallstones increases with age. It ranges from 20 to 30% in patients aged ≥60 years [1, 2], and according to several potentially high severity studies, especially with patients presenting with complications, the prevalence increases to 80% in institutionalized individuals aged ≥90 years [3]. One such complication is acute cholecystitis, which is a frequent reason for an emergency presentation to hospital. Surgery for cholelithiasis is more common in elderly patients since the incidence of gallstones increases with age (13–50%). It is the higher frequency of associated pathologies in patients older than 60 years of age that can influence the type and effectiveness of treatment. In elderly patients, the optimal treatment of acute cholecystitis remains controversial. Laparoscopic cholecystectomy (LC) is the gold standard for the treatment of gallbladder stone disease. Even though laparoscopic cholecystectomy has become the gold standard for the treatment of gallbladder stones, its safety in elderly patients is still questioned [4–6]. In comparison with the open approach, the advantages of this procedure include better cosmetic results, less postoperative pain, shorter operative time, less intraoperative and postoperative complications and shorter postoperative hospital stay both in younger and older people.

A. Puzziello (✉) • D. Landi • F. Vicinanza • G. Pacella
General and Day Surgery Unit, AOU San Giovanni di Dio e Ruggi d'Aragona, Department of Medicine Surgery and Dentistry, University of Salerno, Salerno, Italy
e-mail: apuzziello@unisa.it

G. Orlando
University Magna Graecia of Catanzaro, Catanzaro, Italy

I.M. Luppino
Gastroenterology and Endoscopy Unit, AO Annunziata, Cosenza, Italy

A. Crucitti (ed.), *Surgical Management of Elderly Patients*,
https://doi.org/10.1007/978-3-319-60861-7_20

This chapter considers the question of whether to recommend laparoscopic or open cholecystectomy in elderly patients of over 70 years of age. The most important points of the discussion are addressed.

20.2 Discussion Points

The literature contains many criteria, none of which have led to the defining of an agreed single cutoff age. The National Institute on Aging and the National Institute of Health identify three age classes: "young old" (65–74 years), "older (middle) old" (75–85 years) and "oldest old" (>85 years). Census predictions indicate that from 1995 to 2020, the percentage of the population aged 65 years or older will increase from 12.8 to 15%, those aged 75 years or older will increase from 5.6 to 6.8% and those aged 85 years or older will increase from 1.4 to 2% [7]. Cholecystectomy is a common operation in ageing patients, due to the increasing prevalence of gallstones in an increasingly older population [8, 9].

The laparoscopic approach to a cholecystectomy is standard. Their only opportunity to perform an open procedure is a simultaneous cholecystectomy, such as in a total gastrectomy, a pancreatoduodenectomy, or major liver resections.

The only a priori indications for an open procedure are in the case of a suspected malignant disease, gallbladder cancer or major anaesthesia restrictions, mostly related to respiratory function during pneumoperitoneum.

20.3 Biliary Lithiasis

Biliary tract disorders are amongst the most common reasons for surgery in older patients. Fifty percent of women and 16% of men in young old have been shown to have gallbladder disease [10]. When bile duct stones are suspected, an MRCP (magnetic resonance cholangiopancreatography) is performed, which is a sensitive noninvasive and rather sensitive method. Once the biliary stones have been identified, the use of Endoscopic Retrograde Cholangio Pancreatography (ERCP) allows the clearance of the principal bile duct. In the study carried out by Charfare et al., a preoperative ERCP was performed, and postoperatively retained stones were present in 1.2% of these patients [11]. In another study by Collins et al. amongst 997 laparoscopic cholecystectomy patients, clinically silent choledocholithiasis was present in 3.4%, one-third of which were passed spontaneously within 6 weeks of the operation [12]. The extremely elderly frequently present with several biliary diagnoses and complicated gallstone disease, which explains the higher rate of complications and mortality usually seen in this age group [11–15].

The incidence of choledocholithiasis ranges from 5 to 10% in patients undergoing laparoscopic cholecystectomy for symptomatic cholelithiasis and from 18 to 33% of patients with acute biliary pancreatitis. The clinical presentation of choledocholithiasis may vary widely, as up to half the cases of common bile duct stones (CBDS) may be asymptomatic or associated with various symptoms and conditions [16].

Over the last 30 years, the diagnosis and management of CBDS have radically changed following the dramatic diffusion of imaging, including endoscopic ultrasound (EUS) and magnetic resonance cholangiography (MRC), endoscopy and laparoscopy. During the 2000s, a critical appraisal of management options [17, 18] and the diffusion of new diagnostic examinations led to a more cautious, patient-tailored preoperative workup, based on patient risk of carrying CBDS, and management based on the perception that CBDS [19, 20] may be treated in a multidisciplinary way.

The 2006 European Society for Endoscopic Surgery (EAES) guideline update justified an expectant attitude in elderly patients [21]. In 2008, the British Society of Gastroenterology guidelines [22] recommended that whenever patients have symptoms and investigations suggest ductal stones, possible extraction should be performed; the American Society for Gastrointestinal Endoscopy (ASGE) guidelines [23] incorporated those recommendations and proposes a stratification of patients according to the risk for choledocholithiasis, thus influencing subsequent management [23].

According to ASGE guidelines, cholangitis, total bilirubin >4 mg/dL and common bile duct stone (CBDS) on US were considered very strong predictors. Total bilirubin 1.8–4 mg/dL and dilated CBD on US were considered strong predictors. Abnormal liver biochemical tests, patients aged >55 years and gallstone pancreatitis were considered moderate predictors (Fig. 20.1) [23].

A retrospective study confirms that the combination of choledocolithiasis predictors may improve risk estimation of choledocholithiasis and should be considered to optimize patient selection for ERCP. However, even in the "high-risk group", the specificity was low (56.2%), meaning that a significant proportion of patients will still have an unnecessary ERCP [24].

There are two main approaches for patients with an intermediate to high risk of carrying CBDS: on one hand, the "laparoscopy-first" approach and on the other hand, the "endoscopy-first" approach [25].

Since no consensus has been achieved, CBDS diagnosis and management seem to be more conditioned by availability of instrumentation, personnel and skills than cost-effectiveness [19, 23].

The optimal timing for therapeutic ERC in the management of choledocholithiasis is variable and depends on the specific clinical scenario. In elderly patients, it is better to bring forward the therapeutic time to prevent cascades of pathological events linked to associated pathologies [25].

The ageing population of Western countries together with the increasingly less invasive nature of CBDS management is rekindling the debate concerning the most appropriate treatment not only for the "young old" and "older old" but also for oldest old, where procedure-related complications may become severe or fatal [25]. Operative ERCP is proposed for CBDS retrieval in the very elderly [16, 26]. In oldest old patients and those with serious comorbidities, where other endoscopic or surgical procedures may confer unacceptably high risks, endoscopic biliary stenting is a useful alternative [27, 28].

In general, although results of mini-invasive CBDS management in very elderly patients seem to be worse than in younger patients, they mostly consist of longer operating times and hospital stays. Since clinical impact and morbidity appear lower than those of traditional surgery, age should not contraindicate per se CBDS

Predictors of choledocholithiasis

"Very strong"

- CBD stone on transabdominal US
- Clinical ascending cholangitis
- Bilirubin > 4 mg/dL

"strong"

- Dilated CBD on US (> 6 mm with gallbladder *in situ*)
- Bilirubin level 1.8-4 mg/dL

"Moderate"

- Abnormal liver biochemical test other than bilirubin
- Age older than 55 years
- Clinical gallstone pancreatitis

Assigning a likelihood of choledcholithiasis based on clinical predictors	
Presence of any very strong predictor	High
Presence of both strong predictors	High
No predictors Present	Low
All other patients	Intermediate

Fig. 20.1 Taken from Maple JT, Ikenberry SO, Anderson MA, Appalaneni V, Decker GA, et al. The role of endoscopy in the management of choledocholithiasis. Gastrointest Endosc. 2011; 74: 731–744

management. Biliary stent placement is a possible alternative in elderly patients but is likely to put the patients at risk for cholangitis as a result of stent clogging. To avoid this adverse event, a periodic (e.g. every 3 months) exchange of biliary stents is needed [24]. An emerging dilemma is whether to proceed with cholecystectomy after successful CBD clearance in patients of 80 years or over [25, 29].

The goal of treatment for the elderly is to provide them with the best possible quality of life with the lowest physiological cost.

20.4 Postoperative Course: Hospital Stay

Laparoscopic cholecystectomy has been shown to provide a shorter hospital stay, less postoperative physiological dysfunction and an earlier return to daily activities than open cholecystectomy. The attainment of such goals is particularly desirable in the elderly patient [30]. Advanced age is frequently associated with significant comorbidity and limited functional reserve, which may complicate a postoperative course. Preoperative assessment of cardiovascular risk factors and adequate monitoring of the patient is necessary for detection and treatment of possible complications [31]. In the Yetkin et al. study [32], the length of hospitalization was significantly longer in the elderly group compared with that in the younger group. These results indicated that elderly patients also benefited from the shorter hospital stay offered by the laparoscopic technique.

20.5 Morbidity and Mortality

The reported incidence of morbidity and mortality with open cholecystectomy in the geriatric population is approximately 23–28% and 1.5–2% respectively [33, 34]. In the elderly who underwent laparoscopic cholecystectomy, complication rates of 5–15% and an overall mortality rate of 0–1% have been observed [4, 13, 14]. Higher complication rates observed in oldest old patients seem to result from more difficult cholecystectomies. The best surrogate markers of biological age are the functional reserves of the organism. The functional reserves represent the difference between basal and maximum function of the organ/system and are a measure of the capability of the organism to cope with conditions of increased stress or disease [58].

Kuy et al. [36] have shown that the oldest old are ≥3 times more likely to need blood transfusions and to require continuous mechanical ventilation and ≥5 times more likely to develop aspiration pneumonitis. Other studies have proven that age > 65 years, male gender, acute cholecystitis, thickened gallbladder wall, diabetes mellitus, ASA 3 and previous upper abdominal surgery were significantly associated with an increased risk of conversion to the open technique [37, 38]. In oldest old patients, the rates of acute cholecystitis, conversion to open surgery and postoperative complications were significantly higher than in other groups (Tables 20.1 and 20.2) [32]. On the other hand, the enhanced recovery offered by laparoscopy, with reduced postoperative pain, improved mobilization, a shorter length of hospital stay and fewer complications may be most advantageous in this group with a prevalent comorbidity and reduced physiologic reserve [31, 39]. The extremely elderly frequently present with complicated gallstone disease, which explains the higher rate of

Table 20.1 Significantly higher incidence of postoperative complications compared to their fit counterparts

	Postoperative complication			
	Present *N* (%)	Absent *N* (%)	OR (95% CI)	*P*
CGA assessment				
Fit	2 (15.4)	23 (52.3)	1.0	0.026
Frail	11 (84.6)	21 (47.7)	6.0 (1.2–30.4)	
Age				
<75	8 (61.5)	28 (65.1)	1.0	1.000
≥75	5 (38.5)	15 (34.9)	1.2 (0.3–4.2)	
ASA				
<3	3 (23.1)	2 (4.5)	1.0	0.072
≥3	10 (76.9)	42 (95.5)	6.3 (0.9–42.8)	

Table 20.2 Post-operative stay as outcome in elderly group

	Postoperative stay			
	≤2 days *N* (%)	>2 days *N* (%)	OR (95% CI)	*P*
CGA assessment				
Fit	13 (65.0)	11 (30.6)	1.0	0.023
Frail	7 (35.0)	25 (69.4)	4.2 (1.3–13.5)	
Age				
<75	14 (70.0)	22 (61.1)	1.0	0.571
≥75	6 (30.0)	14 (38.9)	0.7 (0.2–2.2)	
ASA score				
<3	0 (0)	5 (13.9)	1.0	0.148
≥3	20 (100)	31 (86.1)	5.6 (0.8–35.8)	

Taken from Lasithiotakis K, Petrakis J, Venianaki M, Georgiades G, Koutsomanolis D, Andreou A, Zoras O, Chalkiadakis G. Frailty predicts outcome of elective laparoscopic cholecystectomy in geriatric patients. Surg Endosc. 2013;27(4):1144–50

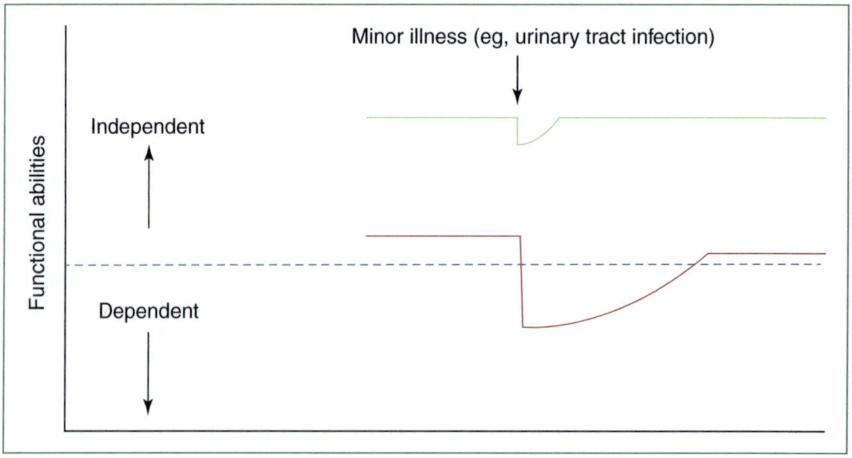

Fig. 20.2 Vulnerability of frail elderly people to a sudden change in health status after a minor illness. The *green line* represents a fit elderly individual who after a minor stressor event has a small deterioration in function and then returns to homeostasis. The *red line* represents a frail elderly individual who after a similar stressor event undergoes a larger deterioration and does not return to baseline homeostasis. Taken from Clegg A. Frailty in elderly people. Lancet. 2013; 381:752–62

complications and mortality usually seen in this group [5, 30]. It is estimated that the 30% residue of the functional reserve may represent the minimum threshold for the functionality of the system itself. Therefore, it is possible to lose 70% of a function without any symptomatic manifestation, especially if such reduction occurs over time (Fig. 20.2) [58].

20.6 Pneumoperitoneum

In laparoscopic cholecystectomy, CO2 pneumoperitoneum has potentially harmful intraoperative circulatory and ventilatory effects because of absorbed carbon dioxide and elevated intraabdominal pressure. Pneumoperitoneum decreases functional residual capacity, lung compliance and peak airway pressures, and absorbed intraperitoneal CO2 causes hypercarbia and acidemia. Both increased intra-abdominal pressure and reduced cardiac function and renal and hepatic hypoperfusion resulting in oliguria and transient hepatocellular injury [40, 41, 57]. Cardiac output decreases by up to 30% during laparoscopic surgery, due to a decrease in stroke volume. Pneumoperitoneum also causes an increase in systemic vascular resistance [42, 43]. Findings from the Koivusola et al. [15] report show that during laparoscopic cholecystectomy, the pneumoperitoneum induced with 10–12 mm Hg pressure in patients with ASA scores 3 or 4 did not pose additional risks in elderly patients.

20.7 Acute Cholecystitis

Applying strict criteria to select patients who might benefit from early cholecystectomy as treatment for acute cholecystitis (AC) may contribute to a better perioperative outcome. Fuks et al. [44] assessed the perioperative outcome of early cholecystectomy in elderly patients. It included only patients with grades I and II acute cholecystitis based on the severity assessment criteria from the Tokyo Guidelines [45]. To reduce the risk of perioperative morbidity and mortality, a severity assessment of pre-existing comorbid conditions should be performed. This review showed that patients who died had been suffering from severe pre-existent comorbidities or a poor clinical preoperative condition [44, 46, 47].

Previous studies have shown that the incidence of acute cholecystitis is higher in elderly patients [10, 13]. The Yetkin study in older old patients revealed that the rate of acute cholecystitis was 45.5%, and in oldest old patients, it was significantly higher than that of other groups (*P* 0.029) [32]. This finding seems to explain the higher complication rate in oldest old patients [39, 48]. Even though elderly patients are more likely to present with several comorbidities in advanced stages, early laparoscopic cholecystectomy for elderly patients with acute gallbladder disease proved to be safe and effective. It should be regarded as the standard of care in conjunction with an appropriate selection of cases [13, 49]. Loozen demonstrated that early cholecystectomy for acute cholecystitis in patients aged ≥70 years is associated with a perioperative morbidity of 24% and a mortality of 3.5% [50].

20.8 Conversion

In many surgical teams, conversion is mandatory in cases of anatomic difficulties or complications. A conversion does not make the operation easier or safer. The conversion rate depends on the surgical team's experience and work volume. The correlation between age and conversion has been previously reported in elective surgery for cholelithiasis [32, 51] as well as in AC [30]. Conversion to open surgery is more frequent in elderly patients and ranges between 5 and 25% [10, 47, 52]. Yetkin et al. [32] report a conversion rate of 8% in the younger age group. Although the conversion rates were higher in the elderly group of "young old", this did not reach statistical significance (*P* 0.765) [32]. However, subgroup analysis of group of "young old" and "older old" revealed that patients aged 80 or over had a significantly higher conversion rate than that of other subgroups (*P* 0.01), a finding which is also in agreement with the literature. Increased age has been noted in the literature as a preoperative risk factor for conversion, perhaps due to a longer history of gallstones and increased number of cholecystitis attacks [53, 54].

Conclusion

The evaluation of a new technology and/or innovative surgical technique has many problems, which are related in part to a cultural attitude towards evidence-based surgery [55]. In addition, some factors can also bias the best randomized trials with random sampling. Moreover, the success of an intervention is not only related to the surgeon's skills and experience but also to the patient's characteristics. Diffusion of new techniques in surgery is also related to sociological factors. Whatever the quality of innovation, these factors affect its adoption on a large scale, thus making any attempt at objective analysis useless: "It is always too early (for rigorous evaluation) until, unfortunately, it's suddenly too late" (Buxton's law) [56].

In elderly patient, the laparoscopic approach was initially reserved for low-risk patients, although age has never been a contraindication [47]. It is therefore important to consider the impact that this procedure has had on the fastest growing segment of our population, ageing patients, who are at high risk for surgery [5]. LC can be performed safely in extremely elderly patients. However, the presence of inflammation is the main factor that influences the adverse outcome in the elderly.

References

1. Lirussi F, Nassuato G, Passera D, Toso S, Zalunardo B, Monica F, et al. Gallstone disease in an elderly population: the Silea study. Eur J Gastroenterol Hepatol. 1999;11:485–91.
2. Festi D, Dormi A, Capodicasa S, Staniscia T, Attili AF, Loria P, et al. Incidence of gallstone disease in Italy: results from a multicenter, population-based Italian study (the MICOL project). World J Gastroenterol. 2008;14:5282–9.
3. Ratner J, Lisbona A, Rosenbloom M, Palayew M, Szabolcsi S, Tupaz T. The prevalence of gallstone disease in very old institutionalized persons. JAMA. 1991;265:902–3.

4. Tagle FM, Lavergne J, Barkin JS, Unger SW. Laparoscopic cholecystectomy in the elderly. Surg Endosc. 1997;11(6):636–8.
5. Brunt LM, Quasebarth MA, Dunnegan DL, Soper NJ. Outcomes analysis of laparoscopic cholecystectomy in the extremely elderly. Surg Endosc. 2001;15(7):700–5.
6. McMahon AJ, Fischbacher CM, Frame SH, MacLeod MC. Impact of laparoscopic cholecystectomy: a population-based study. Lancet. 2000;356(9242):1632–7.
7. U.S. Bureau of the Census Current population reports, series P-25, N. 952. Projections of the population of the United States by age, sex, and race: 1983–2080. Washington: U.S. Government Printing Office; 1975.
8. Kurbanov FS, Abbasova SF, Aliev IG, Sushko AN, Dobrovol'skii SR. The laparoscopic cholecystectomy in elderly patients. Khirurgiia. 2012;9:38–41.
9. Elwood DR. Cholecystitis. Surg Clin North Am. 2008;88:1241–52.
10. Bingener J, Richards ML, Schwesinger WH, Strodel WE, Sirinek KR. Laparoscopic cholecystectomy for elderly patients: gold standard for golden years? Arch Surg. 2003;138(5):531–5.
11. Charfare H, Cheslyn-Curtis S. Selective cholangiography in 600 patients undergoing cholecystectomy with 5-year follow-up for residual bile duct stones. Ann R Coll Surg Engl. 2003;85(3):167–73.
12. Collins C, Maguire D, Ireland A, Fitzgerald E, O'Sullivan GC. A prospective study of common bile duct calculi in patients undergoing laparoscopic cholecystectomy: natural history of choledocholithiasis revisited. Ann Surg. 2004;239(1):28–33.
13. Polychronidis A, Botaitis S, Tsaroucha A, et al. Laparoscopic cholecystectomy in elderly patients. J Gastrointestin Liver Dis. 2008;17(3):309–13.
14. Annamaneni RK, Moraitis D, Cayten CG. Laparoscopic cholecystectomy in the elderly. J Soc Laparoendosc Surg. 2005;9(4):408–10.
15. Koivusalo AM, Pere P, Valjus M, Scheinin T. Laparoscopic cholecystectomy with carbon dioxide pneumoperitoneum is safe even for high-risk patients. Surg Endosc. 2008;22(1):61–7.
16. Magalhaes J, Rosa B, Cotter J. Endoscopic retrograde cholangiopancreatography for suspected choledocholithiasis: from guidelines to clinical practice. World J Gastrointest Endosc. 2015;7(2):128–34.
17. Ong TZ, Khor JL, Selamat DS, Yeoh KG, Ho KY. Complications of endoscopic retrograde cholangiography in the postMRCP era: a tertiary center experience. World J Gastroenterol. 2005;11:5209–12.
18. Machi J, Oishi AJ, Tajiri T, Murayama KM, Furumoto NL, Oishi RH. Routine laparoscopic ultrasound can significantly reduce the need for selective intraoperative cholangiography during cholecystectomy. Surg Endosc. 2007;21:270–4.
19. ASGE Standards of Practice Committee, Maple JT, Ben-Menachem T, Anderson MA, Appalaneni V, Banerjee S, Cash BD, Fisher L, Harrison ME, Fanelli RD, Fukami N, Ikenberry SO, Jain R, Khan K, Krinsky ML, Strohmeyer L, Dominitz JA. The role of endoscopy in the evaluation of suspected choledocholithiasis. Gastrointest Endosc. 2010;71:1–9.
20. Gurusamy KS, Giljaca V, Takwoingi Y, Higgie D, Poropat G, Štimac D, Davidson BR. Endoscopic retrograde cholangiopancreatography versus intraoperative cholangiography for diagnosis of common bile duct stones. Cochrane Database Syst Rev. 2015;Issue 2.
21. Treckmann J, Sauerland S, Frilling A, Paul A. Common bile duct stones - update 2006. In: Neugebauer EAM, Sauerland S, Fingerhut A, Millat B, Buess G, editors. EAES guidelines for endoscopic surgery. Berlin: Springer; 2006. p. 329–33.
22. Williams EJ, Green J, Beckingham I, Parks R, Martin D, Lombard M. Guidelines on the management of common bile duct stones (CBDS). Gut. 2008;57:1004–21.
23. Maple JT, Ikenberry SO, Anderson MA, Appalaneni V, Decker GA, Early D, Evans JA, Fanelli RD, Fisher D, Fisher L, Fukami N, Hwang JH, Jain R, Jue T, Khan K, Krinsky ML, Malpas P, Ben-Menachem T, Sharaf RN, Dominitz JA. The role of endoscopy in the management of choledocholithiasis. Gastrointest Endosc. 2011;74:731–44.
24. He H, Tan C, Wu J, Dai N, Hu W, Zhang Y, Laine L, Scheiman J, Kim JJ. Accuracy of ASGE high-risk criteria in evaluation of patients with suspected common bile duct stones. Gastrointest Endosc. 2017.

25. Costi R, Gnocchi A, Di Mario F, Sarli L. Diagnosis and management of choledocholithiasis in the golden age of imaging, endoscopy and laparoscopy. World J Gastroenterol. 2014;20(37):13382–401.
26. Sugiyama M, Atomi Y. Endoscopic sphincterotomy for bile duct stones in patients 90 years of age and older. Gastrointest Endosc. 2000;52:187–91.
27. Bergman JJ, Rauws EA, Tijssen JG, Tytgat GN, Huibregtse K. Biliary endoprostheses in elderly patients with endoscopically irretrievable common bile duct stones: report on 117 patients. Gastrointest Endosc. 1995;42:195–201.
28. De Palma GD, Catanzano C. Stenting or surgery for treatment of irretrievable common bile duct calculi in elderly patients? Am J Surg. 1999;178:390–3.
29. Costi R, DiMauro D, Mazzeo A, Boselli AS, Contini S, Violi V, Roncoroni L, Sarli L. Routine laparoscopic cholecystectomy after endoscopic sphincterotomy for choledocholithiasis in octogenarians: is it worth the risk? Surg Endosc. 2007;21:41–7.
30. Tambyraja AL, Kumar S, Nixon SJ. Outcome of laparoscopic cholecystectomy in patients 80 years and older. World J Surg. 2004;28(8):745–8.
31. Kirshtein B, Bayme M, Bolotin A, Mizrahi S, Lantsberg L. Laparoscopic cholecystectomy for acute cholecystitis in the elderly: is it safe? Surg Laparosc Endosc Percutan Tech. 2008;18(4):334–9.
32. Yetkin G, Uludag M, Oba S, Citgez B, Paksoy I. Laparoscopic cholecystectomy in elderly patients. J Soc Laparoendosc Surg. 2009;13:587–91.
33. Lujan JA, Sanchez-Bueno F, Parrilla P, Robles R, Torralba JA, Gonzalez-Costea R. Laparoscopic vs. open cholecystectomy in patients aged 65 and older. Surg Laparosc Endosc. 1998;8(3):208–10.
34. Feldman MG, Russell JC, Lynch JT, Mattie A. Comparison of mortality rates for open and closed cholecystectomy in the elderly: Connecticut statewide survey. J Laparoendosc Surg. 1994;4(3):165–72.
35. Lasithiotakis K, Petrakis J, Venianaki M, Georgiades G, Koutsomanolis D, Andreou A, Zoras O, Chalkiadakis G. Frailty predicts outcome of elective laparoscopic cholecystectomy in geriatric patients. Surg Endosc. 2013;27(4):1144–50.
36. Kuy S, Sosa JA, Roman SA, Desai R, Rosenthal RA. Age matters: a study of clinical and economic outcomes following cholecystectomy in elderly Americans. Am J Surg. 2011;201:789–96.
37. Yang TF, Guo L, Wang Q. Evaluation of preoperative risk factor for converting 15. Laparoscopic to open cholecystectomy: a meta-analysis. Hepato-Gastroenterology. 2014;61(132):958–65.
38. Chang WT, Yu FJ, Hsieh MY, Huang MC, Lee KT, Chen JS, et al. Laparoscopic cholecystectomy in aged patients. Hepato-Gastroenterology. 2009;56(93):950–5.
39. Kwon AH, Matsui Y. Laparoscopic cholecystectomy in patients aged 80 years and over. World J Surg. 2006;30(7):1204–10.
40. Chesney T, Acuna A. Do elderly patients have the most to gain from laparoscopic surgery? Ann Med Surg. 2015;4(3):321–3.
41. Clergue F, Morel P, Pastor C. Perioperative management of patients 10. With increased risk of laparoscopy- induced hepatic hypoperfusion. Swiss Med Wkly. 2004;134(3–4):39–43.
42. O'Leary E, Hubbard K, Tormey W, Cunningham AJ. Laparoscopic cholecystectomy: haemodynamic and neuroendocrine responses after pneumoperitoneum and changes in position. Br J Anaesth. 1996;76(5):640–4.
43. Struthers AD, Cuschieri A. Cardiovascular consequences of laparoscopic surgery. Lancet. 1998;352(9127):568–70.
44. Fuks D, Duhaut P, Mauvais F, Pocard M, Haccart V, Paquet JC, et al. A retrospective comparison of older and younger adults undergoing early laparoscopic cholecystectomy for mild to moderate calculous cholecystitis. J Am Geriatr Soc. 2015;63:1010–6.
45. Yokoe M, Takada T, Strasberg SM, Solomkin JS, Mayumi T, Gomi H, et al. TG13 diagnostic criteria and severity grading of acute cholecystitis. J Hepatobiliary Pancreat Sci. 2013;20:35–46.
46. Fukami Y, Kurumiya Y, Mizuno K, Sekoguchi E, Kobayashi S. Cholecystectomy in octogenarians: be careful. Updat Surg. 2014;66:265–8.

47. Pessaux P, Regenet N, Tuech JJ, Rouge C, Bergamaschi R, Arnaud JP. Laparoscopic versus open cholecystectomy: a prospective comparative study in the elderly with acute cholecystitis. Surg Laparosc Endosc Percutan Tech. 2001;11(4):252–5.
48. Hazzan D, Geron N, Golijanin D, Reissman P, Shiloni E. Laparoscopic cholecystectomy in octogenarians. Surg Endosc. 2003;17(5):773–6.
49. Antoniou SA, Antoniou GA, Koch OO, Pointner R, Granderath FA. Meta- analysis of laparoscopic vs open cholecystectomy in elderly patients. World J Gastroenterol. 2014;20(46):17626–34.
50. Loozen CS, van Ramshorst B, van Santvoort HC, Boerma D. Early cholecystectomy for acute cholecystitis in the elderly population: a systematic review and meta-analysis. Dig Surg. 2017. https://doi.org/10.1159/000455241.
51. Kim KH, Sung CK, Park BK, Kim WK, Oh CW, Kim KS. Percutaneous gallbladder drainage for delayed laparoscopic cholecystectomy in patients with acute cholecystitis. Am J Surg. 2000;179:111–3.
52. Fried GM, Clas D, Meakins JL. Minimally invasive surgery in the elderly patient. Surg Clin North Am. 1994;74(2):375–87.
53. Simopoulos C, Botaitis S, Polychronidis A, Tripsianis G, Karayiannakis AJ. Risk factors for conversion of laparoscopic cholecystectomy to open cholecystectomy. Surg Endosc. 2005;19(7):905–9.
54. Lim KR, Ibrahim S, Tan NC, Lim SH, Tay KH. Risk factors for conversion to open surgery in patients with acute cholecystitis undergoing interval laparoscopic cholecystectomy. Ann Acad Med Singap. 2007;36(8):631–5.
55. Puzziello A, Orlando G, Siani C, Gervasi R, Lerose MA, Lucisano AM, Vescio G, Sacco R. From 3-port to new laparoendoscopic single-site (LESS) cholecystectomy: a critical analysis of available evidence.
56. Barkun JS, Aronson JK, Feldman LS, et al. Evaluation and stages of surgical innovations. Lancet. 2009;374:1089–96.
57. Joris JL, Chiche JD, Canivet JL, Jacquet NJ, Legros JJ, Lamy ML. Hemodynamic changes induced by laparoscopy and their endocrine correlates: effects of clonidine. J Am Coll Cardiol. 1998;32:1389–96.
58. Clegg A. Frailty in elderly people. Lancet. 2013;381:752–62.

Cancer of the Gallbladder and Biliary Tree

21

Marco Filauro, Giulio Angelini, Federico Fazio, and Andrea Barberis

21.1 Introduction

Cancer of the gallbladder and biliary tree are still stimulating challenges of modern surgery; the incidence of such diseases is not decreasing, and surgeons have become more aggressive in the last few years with the aim of radically removing neoplasms of this district. Studies from around the world demonstrate improvement of results in terms of long-term survival and quality of life, in elderly people as well. The purpose of this chapter is to review biliary diseases with emphasis on management in the older adult populations: until recently, age per se was considered the most important factor in the surgical decision-making process. However, efforts have been made to better understand the surgical risk and predict life expectancy of older cancer patients.

21.2 Gallbladder Cancer

Gallbladder cancer (GBC) is a form of malignant neoplasia equally rare and aggressive; because of its tendency to quickly spread by blood and in the lymphatic and in the intraperitoneal cavity, it's commonly found in its late presentation, often with disseminated disease. Similarly, gallbladder cancer is often found incidentally after cholecystectomy for benign disease such as cholelithiasis, and this may lead to the necessity of additional surgery. Radical surgery is the only potentially curative treatment.

M. Filauro (✉) • G. Angelini • F. Fazio • A. Barberis
E.O. Ospedali Galliera, Mura delle Cappuccine 14, 16128 Genova, Italy
e-mail: marco.filauro@galliera.it

A. Crucitti (ed.), *Surgical Management of Elderly Patients*,
https://doi.org/10.1007/978-3-319-60861-7_21

21.2.1 Epidemiology, Risk Factor, and Pathology

Worldwide the incidence of GBCs correlates with a prevalence of cholelithiasis; countries such as South America and those of Far East Asia have particularly high rates of GBC; in Europe GBC has elevated higher incidence mostly in eastern countries; the incidence data range from 1.5 to 3/100,000 of Northern Europe to 21.5/100,000 of Delhi, India [1]. The pathophysiologic factor underlying GBC is chronic gallbladder inflammation. Predisposing pathologic conditions are gallstone disease, porcelain gallbladder, gallbladder polyps, primary sclerosing cholangitis, abnormal pancreaticobiliary duct junction, and chronic infections such as salmonellosis or helicobacter colonization. The main associated risk factor identified so far is cholelithiasis (especially untreated chronic symptomatic gallstones) [2]; gallstone disease results typically from oversaturation of cholesterol in bile, even on a genetic background [3]; not only does it demonstrated a higher prevalence of GBC among people with cholelithiasis but also most patients with GBC have gallstone disease [4].

Porcelain gallbladder is characterized by the presence of calcification in the wall of the gallbladder, probably from a chronic inflammatory response, and is a risk factor for GBC as well, particularly in those cases where gallbladder wall calcification is not complete where the risk of malignancy rises to 41% [5].

Gallbladder polyps are also a risk factor for GBC, and size >1 cm is an independent factor for malignancy; risk of malignancy is 60–62% for polyps <1 cm but reaches 46–70% for polyps >1.5 cm [6].

Histologically most GBC are adenocarcinoma (about 90%); other kinds of malignancies are represented by squamous cell carcinoma (4%), neuroendocrine (3%), or sarcoma/others unspecified (3%) [7].

GBC spreads directly to the liver, via lymphatic vessels or by hematogenous means; the extreme facility of its spread is also due, on the side of the liver, to the absence of a serous layer with barrier functions, and, on peritoneal surface, there is only a very thin wall. Commonly it initially invades the liver or porta hepatis structures directly and other adjacent organs; the most common sites of lymphatic metastasis are locoregional lymph nodes. Hematogenous drainage leads to metastasize to the liver (typically IV and V segments) and to other extra-abdominal organs such as lungs [8].

21.2.2 Diagnosis

GBC can be diagnosed preoperatively, intraoperatively, or postoperatively, incidentally at pathological examination following routine cholecystectomy; over two thirds of affected by GBC are diagnosed intra- or postoperatively [9]. Symptoms are nonspecific, such as upper right abdominal quadrant pain, sometimes jaundice, nausea, anorexia, and/or weight loss, similar to those of a cholelithiasis or cholecystitis; unfortunately, only 25% of patients who present with symptoms are operable [10]. The most common situation is the discovery of the cancer at the time of pathological examination, which accounts for 30% of cases diagnosed with GBC. In three-large series combined, GBC was found in 0.33% of patients undergoing laparoscopic cholecystectomy [11–13].

When there is a diagnosis or a clinical suspicion of a GBC, it's important to make a correct preoperative imaging in order to reduce the number of unnecessary surgical attempts.

After blood tests with liver function, US imaging is recommended, followed by contrast-enhanced CT and/or MRI of the chest and abdomen, to evaluate the tumor extension and distant metastases. Endoscopic ultrasound is for some authors very helpful, allowing for good imaging with possible fine needle aspiration biopsy [14]. PET may be a useful method to detect distant or locoregional lymphonodal metastases, particularly in the follow-up, but it is not yet inserted in routine diagnostic work-up of GBC.

21.2.3 Surgical Management

Radical surgical resection, with negative margins, is the only potentially curative treatment; it consists in cholecystectomy, unless the patient has already undergone cholecystectomy with occasional finding at pathologic review, associated to liver resection of segments IVb and V and locoregional lymphadenectomy, including cystic node (Mascagni's node) and those of hepatic hilum; common bile duct resection is not recommended tout court but only to achieve radical resection with margins free of disease [15]; it can be useful to obtain an intraoperative frozen section of cystic duct stump to decide the need for further resections. Diagnostic laparoscopy avoids a nontherapeutic laparotomy in about 56% with unrespectable disease, and it demonstrates a higher yield primarily in locally advanced tumors than in early-stage tumors where disseminated peritoneal disease is quite rare [16]. A debated issue was the indication to remove the port site after laparoscopic cholecystectomy with successive incidental finding of GBG; this has not been shown to change outcomes, since these types of spreads were found in patients with advanced disease and correlates with peritoneal metastasis [17].

21.2.4 Treatment of Unresectable Disease

Patients with advanced GCA often have a short survival and need palliation for present or future symptoms such as jaundice, dyspepsia, or duodenal occlusion; the main techniques are based on the interventional or endoscopic approach; surgical bypass was in the past described with bilio-enteric anastomosis or with a segment III bypass when hepatic hilum is involved by tumor [18].

21.3 Cholangiocarcinoma

Cholangiocarcinoma (CCA) is a tumor arising from the epithelium of the biliary tree; it can be anatomically divided into intrahepatic (or peripheral) and extrahepatic CCA, depending on where it arises from: within the liver in the first case and within the extrahepatic bile ducts in the second; extrahepatic CCA are divided into perihilar or distal tumors: perihilar CCA, a more common type, arises from main bile duct confluence and distal CCA is localized between the confluence and the Vater's ampulla. This disease has a bad prognosis, also due to its late diagnosis.

21.3.1 Epidemiology, Risk Factor, and Pathology

First described in 1840 by Durand-Fardel [19], CCA is a rare malignancy and its incidence in autopsies is about 0.01–0.46%; in the USA; the reported incidence is about 1–2 cases per 100,000 population [20]. It is difficult to interpret data from the American Cancer Society: in fact, intrahepatic and extrahepatic CCA are classified, respectively, with primary liver cancer and in a separate subgroup that includes gallbladder cancer; the number of primary liver tumors diagnosed annually in the USA is about 39,000 [21], and about 15% are intrahepatic CCA; 15,500 extrahepatic biliary tumors are estimated to be one third of non-gallbladder neoplasms. Overall incidence of intrahepatic CCA has been rising; this aspect probably is related to new diagnostic methods but may also be due to the concomitant increase in risk factors. Extrahepatic CCA incidence, on the contrary, is decreasing and is substantially unexplained [22].

There are several risk factors for CCA, associated with chronic inflammation of the biliary epithelium.

Primary sclerosing cholangitis is a chronic inflammatory disease of the biliary tree that leads to fibrosis of bile ducts; sometimes it is associated with bowel inflammatory diseases, especially ulcerative colitis [23]; CCA rates of 8–40% have been reported in patients with primary sclerosing cholangitis [22].

Intrahepatic biliary stones are more common in Asia as opposed to the West, and are associated particularly with intrahepatic CCA; about 1/10 of patients with hepatolithiasis develop CCA [24]; the pathophysiological mechanism is thought to be the bile stasis and the recurrent biliary infections and epithelial inflammation.

Several chemical agents have been associated with CCA: rubber industry exposure to nitrosamines and dioxins which are considered risk factors [25]; thorotrast, a radiological contrast agent, seems to be an important risk factor as it has shown to increase the general population's risk by 300 times [26].

Liver cirrhosis has been also linked with CCA, with a tenfold risk compared to the otherwise healthy population [27]; moreover, hepatitis B and C viruses were associated with CCA [28]; in a study of patients with cirrhosis with hepatitis C virus, there were 3.5% risk of developing CCA at 10 years, which was about 1000 times higher than the estimated incidence of this cancer in the general population [29].

In Asia, a well-known risk factor is parasitic infection with liver flukes of the genera *Opisthorchis* and *Clonorchis* [30]; the infection is contracted via eating un- or undercooked fish; inoculated worms lay their eggs in the biliary tree; these parasites induce a chronic inflammation that presumably leads to malignant transformation.

Other abnormalities of biliary tree anatomy that are considered a risk factor include choledochal cysts and Caroli's disease (a congenital condition associated with biliary and renal cysts) [31]; the malignant transformation mechanism is not completely understood but seems to correlate to biliary stasis, pancreatic juice reflux causing activation of bile acids, and chronic inflammation [32].

Traditionally CCA are divided in intrahepatic CCA, arising from small biliary ductules present in liver parenchyma and extrahepatic CCA; the latter can be further divided according to their location along the biliary tree. It is possible to identify perihilar CCA (also called Klatskin tumors) that arise near/at the biliary confluence of the main left and right hepatic ducts and distal CCA originating from the common bile duct although they are mostly periampullary tumors; generally, perihilar CCA represents 50% of the total, distal CCA 40%, and intrahepatic CCA about 10% of the total [33]. Perihilar CCA has been further classified following the Bismuth-Corlette classification: type I, tumors below the confluence of the left and right hepatic ducts; type II, reaching the confluence but not involving left or right hepatic ducts; type III, occluding the common hepatic duct and either the right (IIIa) or the left (IIIb) hepatic duct; and type IV, multicentric or involving both right and left hepatic ducts (Fig. 21.1) [34].

Most of CCA (more than 90%) are well- or moderate-differentiated adenocarcinomas. Other carcinomas which is possible to find in the biliary tree are intestinal-type adenocarcinomas; signet cell carcinomas, with intracellular mucin, mucinous adenocarcinomas, adenosquamous carcinomas, clear-cell carcinoma (with similar morphology to renal cell carcinoma), and sarcomatoid/undifferentiated.

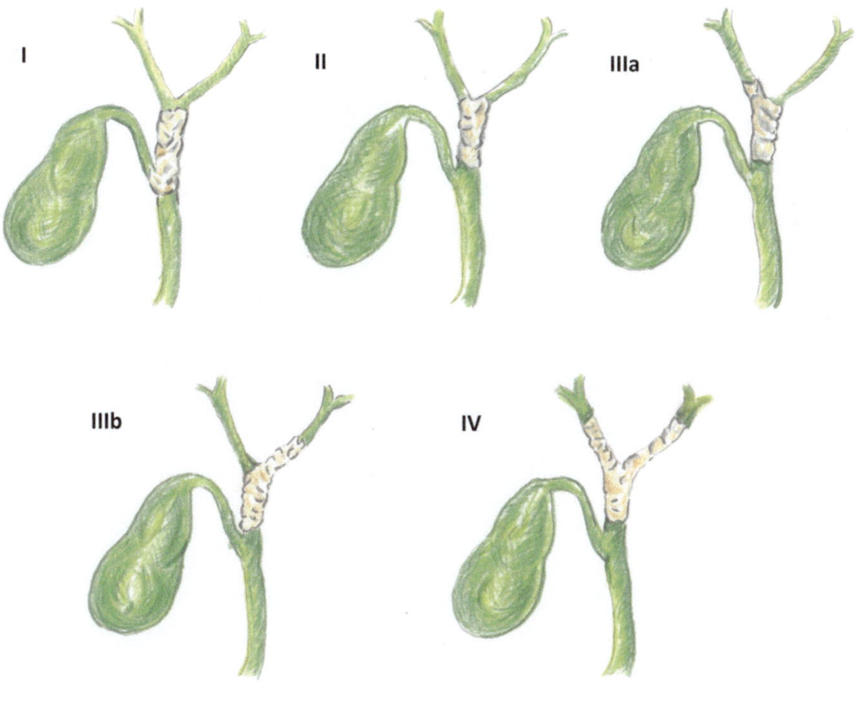

Fig. 21.1 Bismuth-Corlette classification of biliary tract cancers

Adenocarcinomas are divided in other subgroups: sclerosing (or periductal), nodular (mass-forming), mixed type (sclerosing and mass-forming), or polypoid (intraductal).

21.3.2 Diagnosis

Clinical diagnosis of CCA has to be distinguished from extrahepatic CCA and intrahepatic type. Extrahepatic CCA typically cause obstruction of biliary system; symptoms include jaundice, pruritus, pale stools, and dark urine; some patients can present abdominal pain (typically in right-upper quadrant), weight loss, and fever; sometimes it's possible to observe fatigue, night sweats, and malaise [35]. Intrahepatic CCA gives less frequently jaundice; more probably patients will present with right-upper quadrant pain, weight loss, and elevated alkaline phosphatase; sometimes instead intrahepatic CCA is diagnosed incidentally in the course of clinical investigations for other disease.

Blood tests are organized to assess liver function and tumor markers; CEA and CA19.9 can be considered for baseline assessment, bearing in mind that CA 19.9 is elevated in the presence of jaundice [36], and AFP can be utilized to distinguish CCA from hepatocellular carcinoma. After abdominal US, CT, and/or MRI is used to assess tumor stage and resectability (Fig. 21.2), the goal of such cross-sectional

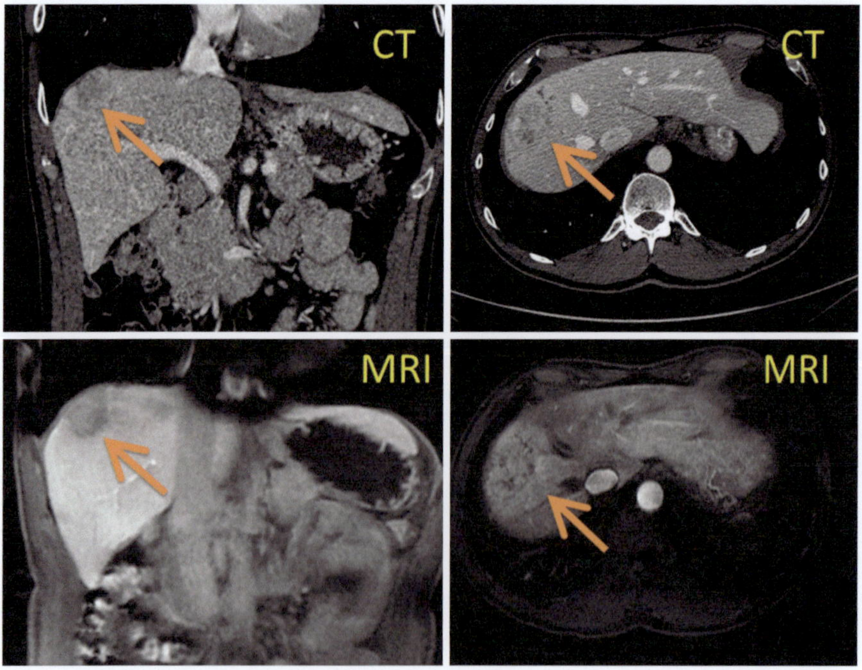

Fig. 21.2 CT and MRI imaging of intrahepatic (S8) CCA

imaging is to assess tumor dimensions, the relationship with vascular structures, lymph node involvement and the presence of metastases in the liver or other sites. Endoscopic ultrasound is also useful especially in distal CCA, and it allows endoscopic biopsy as well as the assessment of small lesions, which are not always directly visualized with radiographic imaging, and sometimes it is only possible to detect biliary tree dilatation [37]. Magnetic resonance cholangiopancreatography (MRCP) is an imaging modality useful in the preoperative assessment of CCA [38, 39] employed for its non-invasiveness and for the superiority of diagnostic accuracy when compared to endoscopic retrograde cholangiopancreatography (ERCP) and percutaneous transhepatic cholangiography (PTC) [40]. Direct cholangiography (ERCP and PTC) should be reserved for those patients considered for palliative strategies and also be used to collect brush cytology for pathologic evaluation. PET is equivocal to CT and MRI for the diagnosis of CCA but is superior in differentiating benign and malignant strictures [41], as well as being most accurate in terms of tumor staging and localization of metastases, resulting in management changes up to 17–30% [42].

21.3.3 Surgical Management

The first step in approaching elderly patients with CCA is to perform an accurate global evaluation, with the goal of assessing not only disease extent but also respiratory function, cardiac risk factors, and renal function as radical resection with histologically negative margins (R0 resection) remains the only potential cure for CCA, particularly in the elderly [43]. Unfortunately, even in patients undergoing radical resection, there remains a certain proportion of patients with as always a large part of resections with histology results demonstrating micro- or macroscopic positive margins which affects prognosis along with lymph node status, perineural invasion, TNM stage, microvascular invasion, and tumor grading [44]. Contraindications to resection include multifocal bilateral disease, the presence of distant metastases and comorbidities that increase perioperative risk [45], as well as encasement of the contralateral portal vein or hepatic artery, underlying liver parenchymal disease or insufficient future liver remnant (FLR 20–30%) and no or poor response to portal vein occlusion [46]. Liver transplant for CCA continues to be debated: several authors describe it as a potential therapeutic option, mainly for patients with unresectable perihilar CCA undergoing neoadjuvant chemoradiotherapy. In contrast to those patients with intrahepatic CCA, transplant should only be offered under the auspices of clinical studies, particularly in those patients with cirrhosis and/or primary sclerosing cholangitis [47, 48]; however, until survival for such cancers can be improved, perhaps in some subgroups of elderly liver transplant recipients, suitability for transplant should be seriously questioned [49].

21.3.3.1 Intrahepatic Cholangiocarcinoma

Radical surgical resection is the only potential strategy with curative intent in patients with intrahepatic CCA (Fig. 21.3); however, most patients with CCA,

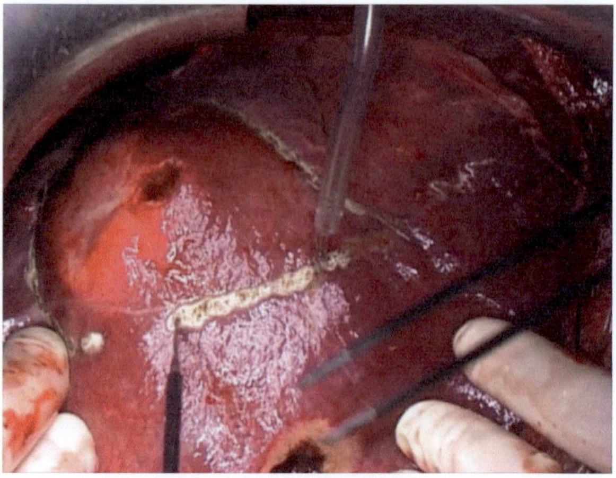

Fig. 21.3 Intraoperative view of intrahepatic (S8) CCA

particularly if elderly, are unfit for surgery at the time of presentation due to the presence of advanced disease or poor global clinical condition. Staging laparoscopy is useful to avoid unnecessary laparotomy, allowing the diagnosis of previously unrecognized peritoneal and liver metastases in one third of patients [50]. Life expectancy is influenced most strongly by margin-negative resection [51], the requirement for which often mandates the performance of major or extended liver resection; however, wedge and segmental resection remains possible if oncologically safe. Depending on tumor characteristics, any subsequent resection may involve the biliary tree, vena cava, or diaphragm, but the extent of resection must take in to account the patient's age and general clinical condition [52]. The role of routine lymphadenectomy has been debated as evidence suggests that it does not affect survival [53]; however, since the presence of nodal metastases has been demonstrated to affect prognosis, some authors continue to advocate regional lymphadenectomy for accurate classification and risk stratification [15, 54]. Recent literature shows that surgery for intrahepatic CCA should not be refused to elderly patients; indeed, even if the older patient has a higher perioperative morbidity, long-term survival appears to be determined more by cancer characteristics than age [55]. In fact, in the last two decades, there has been an increase in liver resections for intrahepatic CCA, even in elderly patients and octogenarians, with significantly longer median survival for resected patients in all age groups [56].

21.3.3.2 Perihilar Cholangiocarcinoma

Perihilar CCA arises at the biliary confluence, above the insertion of the cystic duct. The majority of such patients require a major hepatic resection, sometimes involving vascular structures, thus underlining the high postoperative morbidity and mortality seen with this disease which has been reported to be as high as 47.6 and 10% in some papers [57]. Upon consideration of resection or perihilar CCA, some crucial anatomical issues, important in surgical strategy planning, must be borne in mind. The biliary confluence is located to the right side of the hepatoduodenal

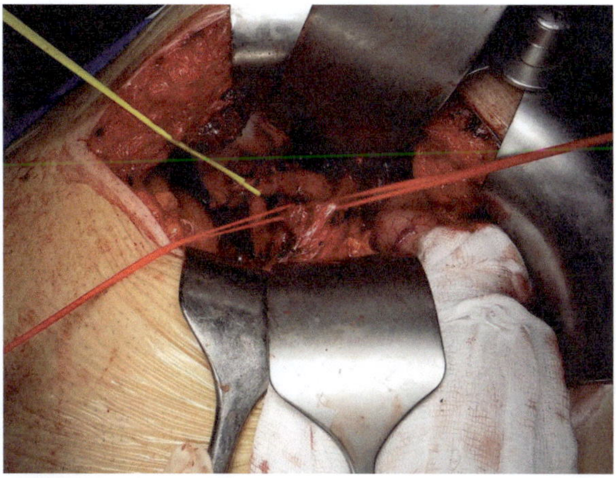

Fig. 21.4 Surgical preparation for perihilar CCA: right and left hepatic arteries on the *red* tapes, hepatic duct on the *yellow* tap

ligament; thus, the right hepatic artery and portal vein have a higher risk of neoplastic involvement. The right hepatic artery and portal vein have a shorter extrahepatic course before branching into second-order ducts, whereas, segment I bile ducts are also often involved by tumor spread because they enter the main bile duct near the confluence. Moreover, the operating surgeon should always remember this region has a high anatomic variability (Fig. 21.4) [58]. The exact surgical resection to be undertaken depends upon the tumor's anatomical location; however, major hepatic resection such as hepatectomy or trisectionectomy is usually extended to the caudate lobe, according to Brisbane terminology for liver resection [59] and always with the main goal of achieving negative margins (Fig. 21.5).

Biliary drainage, either endoscopic or percutaneous, positively affects the function and regeneration of the FLR, reducing the incidence of postoperative hepatic failure; however, cholangitis caused by drain position and enteric fluid contamination might, on the contralateral side, increase infectious complications and mortality [60]. In summary, even in light of the most recent available guidelines, there is consensus that preoperative drainage of the FLR should be undertaken even if it is anticipated to be of low volume, such as following extended hepatectomy [15, 61, 62].

Portal vein embolization (PVE) is useful to prevent postoperative hepatic failure resulting in enlargement of the FLR in cases of major hepatectomy. Some authors also suggest that the use of PVE can result in patient previously described as inoperable due to low anticipated FLR becoming resectable [63] and recent review also demonstrates a benefit of PVE when the FLR is expected <40% [64].

A last issue to be mentioned is the association of vascular resection with hepatic resection for perihilar cholangiocarcinoma: portal vein resection, when performed with the aim of achieving a negative margin resection appears to improve survival rate [65]. Some authors advocate a "hilar en bloc resection" with a no-touch technique, avoiding surgical preparation of vascular structures, with combined liver, biliary, and vascular resection to improve survival after surgery for perihilar CCA

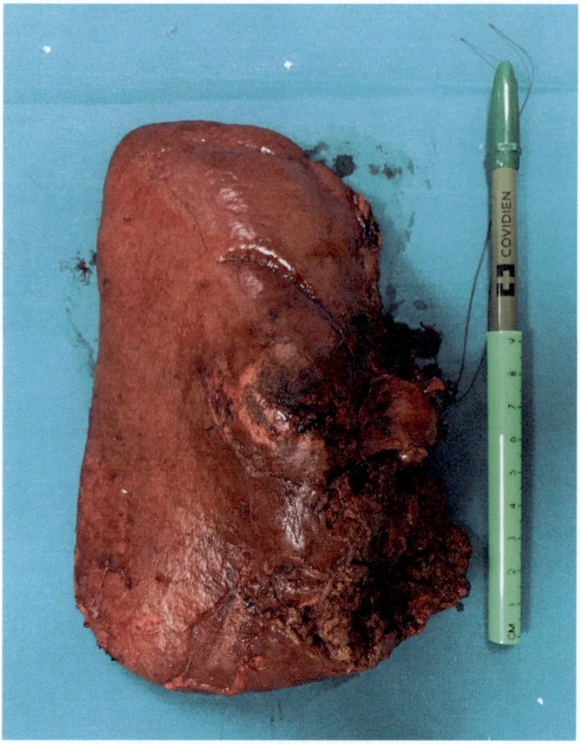

Fig. 21.5 Surgical specimen of right hepatectomy for perihilar CCA

[66]. At present, there is less evidence available regarding the benefits of combined arterial resection for patients with arterial involvement.

Regional lymphadenectomy is recommended for accurate staging even if it does not appear to affect prognosis, with a recent review suggesting that a lymph node count greater than or equal to seven is adequate for prognostic staging [67].

With regard to minimally invasive surgery, there are very few articles about laparoscopic or robotic procedures, demonstrating that these techniques are feasible but should be reserved for selected cases [68, 69].

Recent literature seems to demonstrate that such surgery is feasible in elderly people too; although geriatric patients have several comorbidities and less physiological reserve, an accurate preoperative selection aids in identification of patients that will benefit most from surgery, with similar outcomes to younger patients [70].

21.3.3.3 Distal Cholangiocarcinoma

Pancreatoduodenectomy is the first choice for most distal bile duct cancers; whereas, a more limited resection is only possible in selected mid-bile duct cancers [71]. Pancreatoduodenectomy is a surgical procedure associated with high morbidity and mortality; however, recent studies show that it is not the patient's age but the type of pathology that mainly determines the outcomes. However, some complications, particularly infectious sequelae, are found more commonly in the elderly [72]; thus, octogenarians too can undergo major surgical procedure with outcomes similar to younger patients, and patients should not be denied a potentially curative surgical option for distal bile duct or pancreatic head malignancy based on advanced age alone [73]. According to a recent paper investigating pancreatic cancer outcomes, most elderly adults undergoing pancreatoduodenectomy survive more than 1 year, whereas over one third of patients survive longer than 2 years. Such individuals benefit from an aggressive procedure and are likely to have acceptable long-term morbidity and overall good quality of life, representative of their age [74].

21.3.4 Treatment of Unresectable Disease

Previously, the majority of patients are unresectable at diagnosis, due to advanced disease or poor performance status, particularly in the elderly; however, palliation of pain and obstructive symptoms remains as important issues in the management of such patients. CCA palliation is particularly crucial in those cancers arising from the biliary confluence where it aids in the resolution of impaired liver function and permits progression to treatment modalities such as chemotherapy.

The main strategy available for the treatment of jaundice is the insertion of biliary stents, via either an endoscopic or percutaneous route.

Bare self-expandable metallic stents (SEMS) are widely used in the treatment of unresectable biliary neoplasms; they have a larger caliber than plastic stents, and they have a tendency to embed into the bile duct (for this reason, they are not indicated in patients scheduled for surgery), reducing the risk of migrations. However, the main problem associated with their use is the fact that neoplastic tissue can grow through the mesh usually within approximately 6 months, mandating the placement of a new stent.

Covered biliary stents are coated by a thin membrane of silicone (most common), polyurethane or PTFE, reducing the risk of the cancer growing through the wall of the stent; however, there is the risk of stent migration.

Endobiliary radio-frequency (RF) ablation utilizes radio frequency directly inside the bile duct, causing coagulative necrosis of malignant tissue. RF probes may be introduced with a percutaneous approach or endoscopic approach. Main complications include the disseminating of the RF energy into nearby structures, causing vascular or gastrointestinal wall lesions or thermal injury (e.g., skin burning at the grounding pad site) [75].

Photodynamic therapy is an alternate palliative strategy and is a local ablative method that uses a systemic photosensitizing agent that accumulates preferentially in malignant cells and is subsequently activated by a nonthermal light leading to tumor cells death through a process mediated by oxygen-free radicals. This procedure requires general anesthesia and involves intravenous infusion of agents, usually hematoporphyrin-derivate, followed by laser light directly to the tumor via endoscopic or percutaneous access [76].

Conclusions

In the last few decades, significant progress has been made in the surgical management of biliary tract cancer, and more articles have been published regarding strategies more relevant to the elderly patient. Robust diagnostic work-up is essential to reduce inappropriate or incomplete surgical procedures and to select those patients that will benefit from palliative treatments which continue to develop and evolve.

Wide resection margins are often required, together with locoregional lymphadenectomy, a strategy that is feasible in patients with good performance status. However, increasing evidence now shows that such a strategy is feasible in elderly patients too, without significant comorbidities with outcomes comparable to those of younger patients.

The delivery of such surgery requires dedicated technology and specific skills; therefore, it is important that the patient is referred to and managed in a tertiary hepatopancreatobiliary center where experienced multidisciplinary staff, including surgical, radiation and medical oncology, and interventional radiology, have high-volume experience in the management of such type of disease. Furthermore, patients can present in an idiosyncratic fashion, and it is important to individualize the specific type of treatment, taking into account family and social context of the patients themselves.

References

1. Randi G, Franceschi S, La Vecchia C. Gallbladder cancer worldwide: geographical distribution and risk factors. Int J Cancer. 2006;118:1591–602. https://doi.org/10.1002/ijc.21683.
2. Lazcano-Ponce EC, Miquel JF, Muñoz N, Herrero R, Ferrecio C, Alonso de Ruiz P, et al. Epidemiology and molecular pathology of gallbladder cancer. CA Cancer J Clin. 2001;51:349–64.
3. Xu HL, Cheng JR, Andreotti G, Gao YT, Rashid A. Cholesterol metabolism gene polymorphisms and the risk of biliary tract cancers and stones: a population-based case-control study in Shanghai, China. Carcinogenesis. 2011;32:58–62. https://doi.org/10.1093/carcin/bgq194.
4. Sheth S, Bedford A, Chopra S. Primary gallbladder cancer: recognition of risk factors and the role of prophylactic cholecystectomy. Am J Gastroenterol. 2000;95:1402–10. https://doi.org/10.1111/j.1572-0241.2000.02070.x.
5. Shimizu M, Miura J, Tanaka T, Itoh H, Saitoh Y. Porcelain gallbladder. Relation between its type by ultrasound and incidence of cancer. J Clin Gastroenterol. 1989;11:471–6.
6. Babu BI, Dennison AR, Garcea G. Management and diagnosis of gallbladder polyps: a systematic review. Langenbeck's Arch Surg. 2015;400:455–62. https://doi.org/10.1007/s00423-015-1302-2.
7. Duffy A, Capanu M, Abou-Alfa GK, Huitzil D, Jarnagin W, Fong Y, et al. Gallbladder cancer (GBC): 10-year experience at Memorial Sloan-Kettering Cancer Centre (MSKCC). J Surg Oncol. 2008;98:485–9. https://doi.org/10.1002/jso.21141.
8. Boerma EJ. Towards an oncological resection of gall bladder cancer. Eur J Surg Oncol. 1994;20:537–44.
9. Jin K, Lan H, Zhu T, He K, Teng L. Gallbladder carcinoma incidentally encountered during laparoscopic cholecystectomy: how to deal with it. Clin Transl Oncol. 2011;13:25–33. https://doi.org/10.1007/s12094-011-0613-1.

10. Miller G, Jarnagin WR. Gallbladder carcinoma. Eur J Surg Oncol. 2008;34:306–12. https://doi.org/10.1016/j.ejso.2007.07.206.
11. Konstantinidis IT, Deshpande V, Genevay M, Berger D, Fernandez-del Castillo C, Tanabe KK, Zheng H, et al. Trends in presentation and survival for gallbladder cancer during a period of more than 4 decades: a single-institution experience. Arch Surg. 2009;144:441–7. https://doi.org/10.1001/archsurg.2009.46.
12. Yamaguchi K, Chijiiwa K, Ichimiya H, Sada M, Kawakami K, Nishikata F, et al. Gallbladder carcinoma in the era of laparoscopic cholecystectomy. Arch Surg. 1996;131:981–4.
13. A prospective analysis of 1518 laparoscopic cholecystectomies. The Southern Surgeons Club. N Engl J Med. 1991;324:1073–8. https://doi.org/10.1056/nejm199104183241601.
14. Kanthan R, Senger JL, Ahmed S, Kanthan SC. Gallbladder cancer in the 21st century. J Oncol. 2015;2015:967472. https://doi.org/10.1155/2015/967472.
15. National Comprehensive Cancer Network. Hepatobiliary Cancer (Version 2.2016). https://www.nccn.org/professionals/physician_gls/pdf/hepatobiliary.pdf. Accessed December 20, 2016.
16. Agarwal AK, Kalayarasan R, Javed A, Gupta N, Nag HH. The role of staging laparoscopy in primary gall bladder cancer—an analysis of 409 patients: a prospective study to evaluate the role of staging laparoscopy in the management of gallbladder cancer. Ann Surg. 2013;258:318–23. https://doi.org/10.1097/SLA.0b013e318271497e.
17. Maker AV, Butte JM, Oxenberg J, Kuk D, Gonen M, Fong Y, et al. Is port site resection necessary in the surgical management of gallbladder cancer? Ann Surg Oncol. 2012;19:409–17. https://doi.org/10.1245/s10434-011-1850-9.
18. Soupault R, Couinaud C. New procedure for intrahepatic biliary shunt: left cholangiojejunostomy without hepatic sacrifice. Presse Med. 1957;65:1157–9.
19. Renshaw K. Malignant neoplasms of the extrahepatic biliary ducts. Ann Surg. 1922;76:205–21.
20. Pitt HA, Dooley WC, Yeo CJ, Cameron JL. Malignancies of the biliary tree. Curr Probl Surg. 1995;32:1–90.
21. Siegel RL, Miller KD, Jemal A. Cancer statistics, 2016. CA Cancer J Clin. 2016;66:7–30. https://doi.org/10.3322/caac.21332.
22. Shaib Y, El-Serag HB. The epidemiology of cholangiocarcinoma. Semin Liver Dis. 2004;24:115–25. https://doi.org/10.1055/s-2004-828889.
23. Broomé U, Olsson R, Lööf L, Bodemar G, Hultcrantz R, Danielsson A, et al. Natural history and prognostic factors in 305 Swedish patients with primary sclerosing cholangitis. Gut. 1996;38:610–5.
24. Kubo S, Kinoshita H, Hirohashi K, Hamba H. Hepatolithiasis associated with cholangiocarcinoma. World J Surg. 1995;19:637–41.
25. Hardell L, Bengtsson NO, Jonsson U, Eriksson S, Larsson LG. Aetiological aspects on primary liver cancer with special regard to alcohol, organic solvents and acute intermittent porphyria—an epidemiological investigation. Br J Cancer. 1984;50:389–97.
26. Sahani D, Prasad SR, Tannabe KK, Hahn PF, Mueller PR, Saini S. Thorotrast-induced cholangiocarcinoma: case report. Abdom Imaging. 2003;28:72–4. https://doi.org/10.1007/s00261-001-0148-y.
27. Sorensen HT, Friis S, Olsen JH, Thulstrup AM, Mellemkjaer L, Linet M, et al. Risk of liver and other types of cancer in patients with cirrhosis: a nationwide cohort study in Denmark. Hepatology. 1998;28:921–5. https://doi.org/10.1002/hep.510280404.
28. Shin HR, Lee CU, Park HJ, Seol SY, Chung JM, Choi HC, et al. Hepatitis B and C virus, Clonorchis Sinensis for the risk of liver cancer: a case-control study in Pusan, Korea. Int J Epidemiol. 1996;25:933–40.
29. Kobayashi M, Ikeda K, Saitoh S, Suzuki F, Tsubota A, Suzuki Y, et al. Incidence of primary cholangiocellular carcinoma of the liver in japanese patients with hepatitis C virus-related cirrhosis. Cancer. 2000;88:2471–7.
30. Watanapa P, Watanapa WB. Liver fluke-associated cholangiocarcinoma. Br J Surg. 2002;89:962–70. https://doi.org/10.1046/j.1365-2168.2002.02143.x.

31. Rustagi T, Dasanu CA. Risk factors for gallbladder cancer and cholangiocarcinoma: similarities, differences and updates. J Gastrointest Cancer. 2012;43:137–47. https://doi.org/10.1007/s12029-011-9284-y.
32. Ohtsuka T, Inoue K, Ohuchida J, Nabae T, Takahata S, Niiyama H, et al. Carcinoma arising in choledochocele. Endoscopy. 2001;33:614–9. https://doi.org/10.1055/s-2001-15324.
33. DeOliveira ML, Cunningham SC, Cameron JL, Kamangar F, Winter JM, Lillemoe KD. Cholangiocarcinoma: thirty-one-year experience with 564 patients at a single institution. Ann Surg. 2007;245:755–62. https://doi.org/10.1097/01.sla.0000251366.62632.d3.
34. Bismuth H, Nakache R, Diamond T. Management strategies in resection for hilar cholangiocarcinoma. Ann Surg. 1992;215:31–8.
35. Blechacz B, Komuta M, Roskams T, Gores GJ. Clinical diagnosis and staging of cholangiocarcinoma. Nat Rev Gastroenterol Hepatol. 2011;8:512–22. https://doi.org/10.1038/nrgastro.2011.131.
36. Mann DV, Edwards R, Ho S, Lau WY, Glazer G. Elevated tumour marker CA19-9: clinical interpretation and influence of obstructive jaundice. Eur J Surg Oncol. 2000;26:474–9. https://doi.org/10.1053/ejso.1999.0925.
37. Saini S. Imaging of the hepatobiliary tract. N Engl J Med. 1997;336:1889–94. https://doi.org/10.1056/NEJM199706263362607.
38. Halefoglu AM. Magnetic resonance cholangiopancreatography: a useful tool in the evaluation of pancreatic and biliary disorders. World J Gastroenterol. 2007;13:2529–34.
39. Hekimoglu K, Ustundag Y, Dusak A, Erdem Z, Karademir B, Aydemir S, et al. MRCP vs. ERCP in the evaluation of biliary pathologies: review of current literature. J Dig Dis. 2008;9:162–9.
40. Hyodo T, Kumano S, Kushihata F, Okada M, Hirata M, Tsuda T, et al. CT and MR cholangiography: advantages and pitfalls in perioperative evaluation of biliary tree. Br J Radiol. 2012;85:887–96. https://doi.org/10.1259/bjr/21209407.
41. Banks KP, Song WS. Role of positron emission tomography-computed tomography in gastrointestinal malignancies. Radiol Clin N Am. 2013;51:799–831. https://doi.org/10.1016/j.rcl.2013.05.003.
42. Sacks A, Peller PJ, Surasi DS, Chatburn L, Mercier G, Subramaniam RM. Value of PET/CT in the management of primary hepatobiliary tumors, part 2. Am J Roentgenol. 2011;197:W260–5. https://doi.org/10.2214/AJR.11.6995.
43. Murakami Y, Uemura K, Sudo T, Hashimoto Y, Nakashima A, Kondo N, et al. Prognostic factors after surgical resection for intrahepatic, hilar, and distal cholangiocarcinoma. Ann Surg Oncol. 2011;18:651–8. https://doi.org/10.1245/s10434-010-1325-4.
44. Ercolani G, Dazzi A, Giovinazzo F, Ruzzenente A, Bassi C, Guglielmi A, et al. Intrahepatic, peri-hilar and distal cholangiocarcinoma: three different locations of the same tumor or three different tumors? Eur J Surg Oncol. 2015;41:1162–9. https://doi.org/10.1016/j.ejso.2015.05.013.
45. Blechacz B. Cholangiocarcinoma: current knowledge and new developments. Gut Liver. 2017;11:13–26. https://doi.org/10.5009/gnl15568.
46. Ghouri YA, Mian I, Blechacz B. Cancer review: cholangiocarcinoma. J Carcinog. 2015;14:1. https://doi.org/10.4103/1477-3163.151940.
47. DeOliveira ML. Liver transplantation for cholangiocarcinoma: current best practice. Curr Opin Organ Transplant. 2014;19:245–52. https://doi.org/10.1097/MOT.0000000000000087.
48. Sapisochín G, Fernández de Sevilla E, Echeverri J, Charco R. Liver transplantation for cholangiocarcinoma: current status and new insights. World J Hepatol. 2015;7:2396–403. https://doi.org/10.4254/wjh.v7.i22.2396.
49. Levy MF, Somasundar PS, Jennings LW, Jung GJ, Molmenti EP, Fasola CG, et al. The elderly liver transplant recipient: a call for caution. Ann Surg. 2001;233:107–13.
50. Goere D, Wagholikar GD, Pessaux P, Carrère N, Sibert A, Vilgrain V. Utility of staging laparoscopy in subsets of biliary cancers: laparoscopy is a powerful diagnostic tool in patients with intrahepatic and gallbladder carcinoma. Surg Endosc. 2006;20:721–5. https://doi.org/10.1007/s00464-005-0583-x.
51. Ribero D, Pinna AD, Guglielmi A, Ponti A, Nuzzo G, Giulini SM. Surgical approach for long-term survival of patients with intrahepatic cholangiocarcinoma: a multi-institutional analysis of 434 patients. Arch Surg. 2012;147:1107–13. https://doi.org/10.1001/archsurg.2012.1962.

52. Poultsides GA, Zhu AX, Choti MA, Pawlik TM. Intrahepatic cholangiocarcinoma. Surg Clin North Am. 2010;90:817–37. https://doi.org/10.1016/j.suc.2010.04.011.
53. Choi SB, Kim KS, Choi JY, Park SW, Choi JS, Lee WJ, et al. The prognosis and survival outcome of intrahepatic cholangiocarcinoma following surgical resection: association of lymph node metastasis and lymph node dissection with survival. Ann Surg Oncol. 2009;16:3048–56. https://doi.org/10.1245/s10434-009-0631-1.
54. De Jong MC, Nathan H, Sotiropoulos GC, Paul A, Alexandrescu S, Marques H. Intrahepatic cholangiocarcinoma: an international multi-institutional analysis of prognostic factors and lymph node assessment. J Clin Oncol. 2011;29:3140–5. https://doi.org/10.1200/JCO.2011.35.6519.
55. Vitale A, Spolverato G, Bagante F, Gani F, Popescu I, Marques HP. A multi-institutional analysis of elderly patients undergoing a liver resection for intrahepatic cholangiocarcinoma. J Surg Oncol. 2016;113:420–6. https://doi.org/10.1002/jso.24148.
56. Cholankeril G, Sahai T, Ahmad A, Somasundar P. Intrahepatic cholangiocarcinoma: improved survival in the elderly with surgical intervention. Abstracts of the 12th World Congress of the International Hepato-Pancreato-Biliary Association, 20-23 April 2016, São Paulo, Brazil. J Hepatobiliary Pancreat Sci. 2016;18(Suppl 1):e1–e384.
57. Nuzzo G, Giuliante F, Ardito F, Giovannini I, Aldrighetti L, Belli G, et al. Improvement in perioperative and long-term outcome after surgical treatment of hilar cholangiocarcinoma: results of an Italian multicenter analysis of 440 patients. Arch Surg. 2012;147:26–34. https://doi.org/10.1001/archsurg.2011.771.
58. Hartog H, Ijzermans JN, van Gulik TM, Koerkamp BG. Resection of perihilar cholangiocarcinoma. Surg Clin North Am. 2016;96:247–67. https://doi.org/10.1016/j.suc.2015.12.008.
59. Belghiti J, Clavien P, Gadzijev E, Garden JO, Lau W, Makuuchi M. The Brisbane 2000 terminology of liver anatomy and resections. HPB. 2000;2:333–9.
60. Wiggers JK, Groot Koerkamp B, Cieslak KP, Doussot A, van Klaveren D, Allen PJ, et al. Postoperative mortality after liver resection for perihilar cholangiocarcinoma: development of a risk score and importance of biliary drainage of the future liver remnant. J Am Coll Surg. 2016;223:321–31. https://doi.org/10.1016/j.jamcollsurg.2016.03.035.
61. Moole H, Bechtold M, Puli SR. Efficacy of preoperative biliary drainage in malignant obstructive jaundice: a meta-analysis and systematic review. World J Surg Oncol. 2016;14:182. https://doi.org/10.1186/s12957-016-0933-2.
62. Miyazaki M, Yoshitomi H, Miyakawa S, Uesaka K, Unno M, Endo I, et al. Clinical practice guidelines for the management of biliary tract cancers 2015: the 2nd English edition. J Hepatobiliary Pancreat Sci. 2015;22:249–73. https://doi.org/10.1002/jhbp.233.
63. Abdalla EK, Barnett CC, Doherty D, Curley SA, Vauthey JN. Extended hepatectomy in patients with hepatobiliary malignancies with and without preoperative portal vein embolization. Arch Surg. 2002;137:675–80.
64. Glantzounis GK, Tokidis E, Basourakos SP, Ntzani EE, Lianos GD, Pentheroudakis G. The role of portal vein embolization in the surgical management of primary hepatobiliary cancers. A systematic review. Eur J Surg Oncol. 2017;43:32–41. https://doi.org/10.1016/j.ejso.2016.05.026.
65. Wang ST, Shen SL, Peng BG, Hua YP, Chen B, Kuang M. Combined vascular resection and analysis of prognostic factors for hilar cholangiocarcinoma. Hepatobiliary Pancreat Dis Int. 2015;14:626–32.
66. Neuhaus P, Thelen A, Jonas S, Puhl G, Denecke T, Veltzke-Schlieker W. Oncological superiority of hilar en bloc resection for the treatment of hilar cholangiocarcinoma. Ann Surg Oncol. 2012;19:1602–8. https://doi.org/10.1245/s10434-011-2077-5.
67. Kambakamba P, Linecker M, Slankamenac K, DeOliveira ML. Am J Surg. 2015;210:694–701. https://doi.org/10.1016/j.amjsurg.2015.05.015.
68. Lee W, Han HS, Yoon YS, Cho JY, Choi Y, Shin HK, et al. Laparoscopic resection of hilar cholangiocarcinoma. Ann Surg Treat Res. 2015;89:228–32. https://doi.org/10.4174/astr.2015.89.4.228.
69. Xu Y, Wang H, Ji W, Tang M, Li H, Leng J, et al. Robotic radical resection for hilar cholangiocarcinoma: perioperative and long-term outcomes of an initial series. Surg Endosc. 2016;30:3060–70. https://doi.org/10.1007/s00464-016-4925-7.

70. Takahashi Y, Ebata T, Yokoyama Y, Igami T, Sugawara G, Nagino M. Surgical treatment of perihilar cholangiocarcinoma in octogenarians: a single center experience. J Hepatobiliary Pancreat Sci. 2013;20:324–31. https://doi.org/10.1007/s00534-012-0529-3.
71. Akamatsu N, Sugawara Y, Hashimoto D. Surgical strategy for bile duct cancer: advances and current limitations. World J Clin Oncol. 2011;2:94–107. https://doi.org/10.5306/wjco.v2.i2.94.
72. Bergquist JR, Shubert CR, Ubl DS, Thiels CA, Kendrick ML, Truty MJ, et al. Risk by indication for pancreaticoduodenectomy in patients 80 years and older: a study from the American College of Surgeons National Surgical Quality Improvement Program. HPB (Oxford). 2016;18:900–7. https://doi.org/10.1016/j.hpb.2016.07.012.
73. Liang DH, Shirkey BA, Rosenberg WR, Martinez S. Clinical outcomes of pancreaticoduodenectomy in octogenarians: a surgeon's experience from 2007 to 2015. J Gastrointest Oncol. 2016;7:540–6. 10.21037/jgo.2016.03.04.
74. Gerstenhaber F, Grossman J, Lubezky N, Itzkowitz E, Nachmany I, Sever R, et al. Pancreaticoduodenectomy in elderly adults: is it justified in terms of mortality, long-term morbidity, and quality of life? J Am Geriatr Soc. 2013;61:1351–7. https://doi.org/10.1111/jgs.12360.
75. Alvarez-Sánchez MV, Napoléon B. Review of endoscopic radiofrequency in biliopancreatic tumours with emphasis on clinical benefits, controversies and safety. World J Gastroenterol. 2016;22:8257–70. https://doi.org/10.3748/wjg.v22.i37.8257.
76. Smith I, Kahaleh M. Biliary tumor ablation with photodynamic therapy and radiofrequency ablation. Gastrointest Endosc Clin N Am. 2015;25:793–804. https://doi.org/10.1016/j.giec.2015.06.013.

Pancreatitis

22

Francesco Basile, Antonio Biondi, Guido Basile,
and Marcello Donati

22.1 Introduction

The pancreatic parenchyma as well known is prone to a progressive atrophy during the time, being reduced to less than its original weight overcoming 80 years of age [1]. Also a progressive increase of Wirsung's duct over 8°years is to be observed [2]. So that in aged pancreas, a Wirsung's width till 1 cm can be occasionally observed without any evidence of obstruction; also calcification of splenic and mesenteric vessels can be registered without pathologic significance; even a progressive perilobular fibrosis is very often present in the elderly [3]. Not only the exocrine function but even the endocrine one was found to be progressively deteriorated with age; clinical significance of both remains not clear [4].

Anyway pancreatitis in the elderly represents a well-defined spectrum of diseases that we could first divide, relating to clinical evolution in acute pancreatitis and chronic pancreatitis. Those diseases represent completely different clinical conditions with different implications, early and long-term complications, and therefore must be separately considered.

If acute pancreatitis in the elderly can present a dramatic clinical evolution, with complications, requiring sometimes a multidisciplinary approach and sometimes also intensive care support, chronic pancreatitis shows usually an indolent clinical evolution starting often when patients are young and showing "effects" in the elderly.

F. Basile (✉) • A. Biondi • M. Donati
Department of Surgery and Medical-Surgical Specialties, Surgical Clinic, Vittorio-Emanuele University Hospital of Catania, Catania, Italy
e-mail: fbasile@unict.it

G. Basile
Department of Surgery and Medical-Surgical Specialties, Emergency Abdominal Surgery Unit, University Hospital of Catania, University of Catania, Catania, Italy

A. Crucitti (ed.), *Surgical Management of Elderly Patients*,
https://doi.org/10.1007/978-3-319-60861-7_22

22.2 Acute Pancreatitis

22.2.1 Etiology

The main cause of acute pancreatitis also in the elderly is the cholelithiasis amounting for round 60% of cases. In 20–25% of cases, a history of alcoholic abuses can be found in the anamnestic data of those patients [5] even in combination white smoke [6]. While other causes like medicament adverse reaction, neoplastic disease, trauma, and infections account for 5–10% of acute pancreatitis, it remains unclear the cause of about 10–15% that are defined idiopathic [7]. It's nowadays generally accepted that a big percentage of patients (round 70%) with an idiopathic acute pancreatitis is affected by microlithiasis in duodenal juice, and this aspect shows obviously also therapeutic implications [8]. The most important traumatic cause of traumatic pancreatitis seems to be surgical or endoscopic procedures in the elderly, instead of accident or violent trauma. Of course endoscopic procedures amount for the most important cause of pancreatitis even if most of them are not gaining clinical significance [9]. Diuretics, steroids, and tetracycline are those medicaments able to induce an acute pancreatitis generally; in the elderly the use of many different drugs for coexisting disease seems to be a rising problem for causing acute pancreatitis [10]. Etodolac, simvastatin, and isoniazid are medicaments more recently associated with acute pancreatitis induction; diffusion of this side effect in the elderly population is unknown.

A double binding exists between acute pancreatitis and pancreatic cancer, while round 10% of patients affected by pancreatic cancer are showing an acute pancreatitis, and on the other hand, in patients affected by pseudocyst as a consequence of acute pancreatitis rarely, a coexisting pancreatic cancer is to be observed (over 60 years round 8%).

There are some other minor causes of pancreatitis that should be mentioned; infectious disease like tuberculosis and fungal infections can be rarely responsible in the elderly of pancreatitis so like hypecalcemia, hypertriglyceridemia, and peptic ulcer.

22.3 Clinical Aspects, Diagnosis, and Complications

In the elderly like for young patients, the main symptom related to an acute pancreatitis is the epigastric pain, with typical belt-like irradiation. In a cholelithiasis-induced pancreatitis, also a right upper quadrant pain can be referred. A discrepancy between the referred high grade of spontaneous abdominal pain and the clinical objectivity of the abdomen are typical clinical aspects of pancreatitis. A rare clinical sign of severe pancreatitis is the Cullen's sign (periumbilical ecchymosis Fig. 22.1). In the elderly the clinical presentation can be attenuated, also because pancreatitis can often appear in patients in postoperatory recovery, under sedation or being intubated. Therefore the clinical course can be not so evident in a consistent proportion of patients (till 40%). Even laboratory tests considering serum amylase and serum

Fig. 22.1 Cullen sign: periumbilical ecchymosis due to retroperitoneal hemorrhagic lateral abdominal extension till subcutaneous area of a necrotich hemorrhagic acute pancreatitis

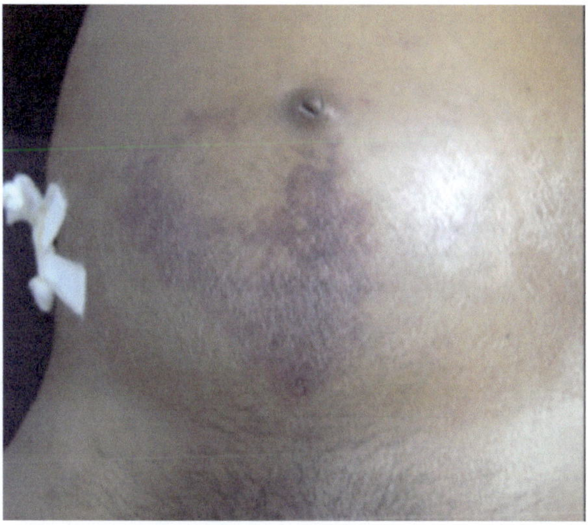

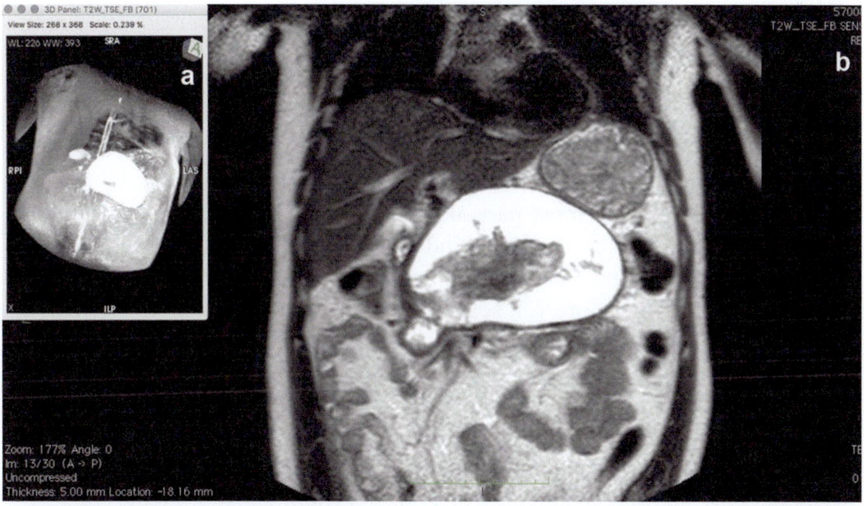

Fig. 22.2 Giant pancreatic pseudocyst as a complication of massive acute pancreatitis; 3D reconstruction (**a**). On MRI it shows as a transverse diameter of 17 cm (**b**)

lipase, and a threshold of 50 ng/mL for urinary trypsinogen-2, can fail to demonstrate an acute pancreatitis in one every ten patients, delaying correct diagnosis and treatment [11]. Interestingly the mortality of pancreatitis is similar in young as in the elderly patients but in the young patients is more due to local complication like necrosis (Fig. 22.3) or pseudocysts (Fig. 22.2), while in the elderly, septic and systemic complications are mainly responsible of death. In fact while in young patients, abscess, necrotizing pancreatitis, and pseudocyst are more frequent complications; in the elderly pulmonary or renal failure and gastrointestinal bleeding and septic

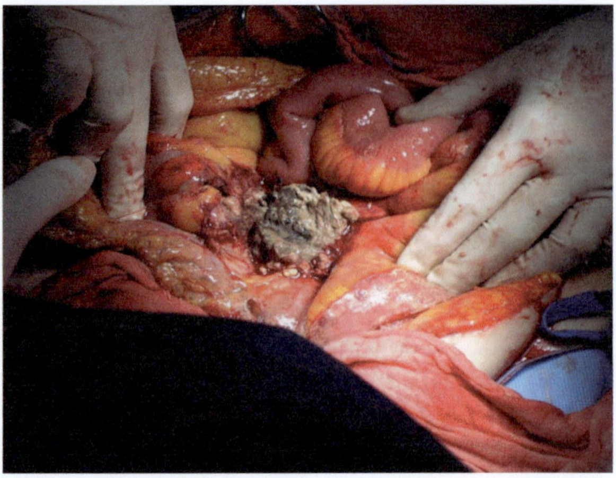

Fig. 22.3 Pancreatic head necrosis: intraoperative finding during a necrosectomy

shock are the most important and frequent complications. The mortality rate in the elderly can gain 20%, while in the young remains round 5–6%. This correlates well with the fact that age is intended to be a worse prognosis factor already in Ranson's criteria.

Diagnostic and evolution of acute pancreatitis out of labor tests is based on US and CT scan, even MRI is very useful to define retroperitoneal extension of disease, better identify choledocolitiasis or other coexistent diseases, and monitor complications' evolution. Ultrasound is usually intended to be the first-line imaging modality in the most part of first aid centers in order to confirm the diagnosis and/or to rule out other kind of acute abdomen. Unfortunately US examination considering the acute clinical settings shows a lot of limitations (Turkvatan 2015); therefore CT scan is very often the very first-line imaging technique to assess severity of involvement of peripancreatic structures and to check evolution of acute presentations. Rising interests in order to stage the severity of the disease were gained by magnetic resonance imaging. (It is especially useful for imaging of patients with iodine allergies, characterizing collections, and assessment of an abnormal or disconnected pancreatic duct.)

Not only age showed an influence on clinical evolution, but even the etiology is related to hospital stay. Idiopathic pancreatitis has shown a worse clinical evolution in front of biliary and alcohol-based pancreatitis; those patients are showing a longer hospital stay and a more severe clinical evolution [12].

One of most diffused complications of surgical interest is represented by pancreatic pseudocyst (Fig. 22.3). The risk of developing a pancreatic pseudocyst is in recent studies (estimated around 7%), most of them are symptomatic, and no specific studies are published for the elderly. Fluid collection becomes an emergency when infected leading in the elderly to a high mortality risk (Tables 22.1 and 22.2).

Table 22.1 Severity score of acute pancreatitis (an overview)

Score (year)	Factors	Sensitivity	Specificity
SOFA (1996/98) (sequential multiorgan failure assessment)	Arterial oxygen saturation, fraction of inspired oxygen, serum creatinine, total bilirubin, platelet count, itemized Glasgow Coma Scale score, mean arterial pressure, and use of vasopressors such as dopamine, dobutamine, adrenaline and noradrenaline	80%	79%
JSS (2009) (Japanese severity criteria for acute pancreatitis)	5 clinical items 10 blood test items CT findings SIRS signs Age	90%	79.8%
BISAP score (2009)	Blood urea nitrogen >25 mg/dl, impaired mental status, systemic inflammatory response syndrome (SIRS), age > 60 years, and pleural effusions	56%	91%
APACHE-II (1985) (Acute Physiology and Chronic Health Evaluation)	Age, Glasgow Coma score. Vital parameters, oxygenation, chemistry, hematology	90%	86.8%
Balthazar-CTSI (1990) (CT severity index)	Based on CT scan findings	66.7	67.1
Ranson (1974)	Age, leucocitosis, glucose blood levels, LDH, SGOT, azotemy, Ca++ blood levels, hematocrite reduction, PO_2, basis lost, seizure of liquids	70–80%	44.3

Table 22.2 Complications after acute pancreatitis

	Type of complications	Mortality
Young	Necrotizing pancreatitis, fluid collection, abscess, pseudocyst	3–4%
Elderly	Pneumonitis (respiratory failure), renal failure, septic shock	5–10%

22.4 Therapy

The treatment of an acute pancreatitis doesn't differ significantly from the same pathologic condition in the younger patients. Severe forms can require an intensive care setting. Out of clinical symptoms and evolution, CT scan and US scan are necessary to check evolution of diseases even when paucisymptomatic. Acute pancreatitis shows a variability of clinical presentation grades, ranging from light symptomatic to acute violent painful variants in which severe and extended necrosis of the parenchyma induces even a peritoneal involvement and can cause severe complications. Therapeutic options are surgical and endoscopic, or interventional radiologic methods are reserved to severe and complicated forms. Of course a biliary stone-based pancreatitis can be approached with ERCP, instead of early treating those patients; MRI and perendoscopic US of the biliary tract can avoid unnecessary early endoscopic exploration of biliary tract, due to the fact that most of the stones are passing spontaneously in the duodenum [13, 14]. Laparoscopic cholecystectomy is also in the elderly the necessary approach after reliefs of pancreatitis symptoms and laboratory signs in order to avoid recurrences; the mandatory delay of 4–5 weeks is able to reduce conversions to open cholecystectomy due to periportal inflammation making hard sometimes the identification of CBD (common bile duct) [15].

Fluids collection can be nowadays safely routinely drained by interventional radiology techniques [16] so that the high success rates of those methods are reducing surgical indications. Surgical exploration remains necessary in case of multilocular septic involvement and extended necrosis making surgical necrosectomy, abdominal cavity lavage and drainage, and sometimes laparotomy mandatory.

Also a conservative approach especially in the elderly can be in selected patients considered. The surgical exploration should be selectively considered also in the treatment of complications like pseudocyst. Although the transgastric drainage of pseudocyst becomes a standard of care, following some morphological features of pseudocyst is driving the surgeon in the choice of the kind of treatment. In fact the pseudocyst should be contiguous to gastric wall, not in an inferior position in order to avoid complications. MRI and transendoscopic US can clarify which kind of treatment should be adopted, underlying the importance of a multidisciplinary setting in the management of pancreatic pseudocysts.

22.5 Chronic Pancreatitis

22.5.1 Etiology and Epidemiology

Chronic pancreatitis in the elderly can be caused by many different factors such as:

- Alcohol abuses
- Autoimmune disease
- Pancreatic anatomical anomalies (pancreas divisum, etc.) [17]

There is also the idiopathic form that collects all other chronic pancreatitis in which an etiology cannot be identified.

Recent studies [18] have shown the role of autoimmune mechanism in the chronic pancreatitis classifying also this disease in two histological subgroups (types 1 and 2).

The autoimmune pancreatitis should also be mentioned correlated to high levels of IgG4-positive plasma cells infiltration of the pancreas and sensible to steroids treatment; this kind of acute pancreatitis was also associated to other clinical conditions like sclerosing cholangitis (50%), hilar lymphadenopathy (30%), and salivary gland involvement (20%) [19]. The idiopathic form seems to show to peaks of incidence: till 20 years and in the elderly after 65.

22.6 Symptoms and Therapy

Chronic pain especially postprandial pain and slow evidence of jaundice coming in an indolent way are the first clinical signs and symptoms of a chronic pancreatitis. During the years it appears also some progressive symptoms of pancreatic insufficiency. Instead of pancreatitis in the young patients, in the elderly the clinical course is oligosymptomatic and pain is rarely present. Also signs of exocrine insufficiency are slowly clinically evident and in most cases don't require a surgical approach. The clinical problem can be sometimes the differential diagnosis with pancreatic cancer due to gland atrophy and parenchymal changes to be differentiated from pancreatic cancer. Exocrine pancreas substitution and compensation of diabetes are therapeutical approach with medicaments. The surgical treatment of pain through Frey's procedure [20] (resection of pancreatic head for decompression of the Wirsung's duct) or Partington-Rochelle operation (longitudinal jejunum derivation of Wirsung's duct) [21] that are together with the alcoholization of celiac plexus for the pain control, the most adopted surgical options in the young patients, for this disease is rarely indicated in the elderly. Nowadays endotherapy [22] is the main therapeutical approach for symptoms relief of chronic pancreatitis under US control endoscopic sphincterotomy, and Wirsung's incannulation is able to obtain clinical resolution of pain. Even plastic ore metallic stent positioning is nowadays more adopted and diffused. Surgery in the elderly was quite completely replaced by endoscopic procedures [23].

References

1. Lillemoe KD. Pancreatic disease in the elderly patient. Surg Clin North Am. 1994;74(2):317–44.
2. Millbourn E. Calibre and appearance of the pancreatic ducts and relevant clinical problems. A roentgenographic and anatomical study. Acta Chir Scand. 1960;118:286–303.
3. Schmitz-Moormann P, Himmelmann GW, Brandes JW, Fölsch UR, Lorenz-Meyer H, Malchow H, Soehendra LN, Wienbeck M. Comparative radiological and morphological study of human pancreas. Pancreatitis like changes in postmortem ductograms and their morphological pattern. Possible implication for ERCP. Gut. 1985;26(4):406–14.
4. Chen G, Shi L, Cai L, Lin W, Huang H, Liang J, Li L, Lin L, Tang K, Chen L, Lu J, Bi Y, Wang W, Ning G, Wen J. Comparison of insulin resistance and β-cell dysfunction between the young and the elderly in normal glucose tolerance and prediabetes population: a prospective study. Horm Metab Res. 2017;49(2):135–41. https://doi.org/10.1055/s-0042-111325. Epub 2016 Jul 26
5. Browder W, Patterson MD, Thompson JL, Walters DN. Acute pancreatitis of unknown etiology in the elderly. Ann Surg. 1993;217(5):469–74. discussion 474–5
6. Sun X, Huang X, Zhao R, Chen B, Xie Q. Meta-analysis: Tobacco smoking may enhance the risk of acute pancreatitis. Pancreatology. 2015;15(3):286–94. https://doi.org/10.1016/j.pan.2015.03.001.
7. Portelli M, Jones CD. Severe acute pancreatitis: pathogenesis, diagnosis and surgical management. Hepatobiliary Pancreat Dis Int. 2017;16(2):155–9.
8. Saraswat VA, Sharma BC, Agarwal DK, Kumar R, Negi TS, Tandon RK. Biliary microlithiasis in patients with idiopathic acute pancreatitis and unexplained biliary pain: response to therapy. J Gastroenterol Hepatol. 2004;19(10):1206–11.

9. Ito K, Fujita N, Kanno A, Matsubayashi H, Okaniwa S, Nakahara K, Suzuki K, Enohara R, Post-ERCP Pancreatitis Prevention by Pancreatic Duct Stenting Research Group (PEP Study Group), Japan. Risk factors for post-ERCP pancreatitis in high risk patients who have undergone prophylactic pancreatic duct stenting: a multicenter retrospective study. Intern Med. 2011;50(24):2927–32. Epub 2011 Dec 15
10. Razavi D, Lindblad M, Bexelius T, Oskarsson V, Sadr-Azodi O, Ljung R. Polypharmacy and risk of acute pancreatitis. Pharmacoepidemiol Drug Saf. 2016;25(11):1337–41. https://doi.org/10.1002/pds.4109. Epub 2016 Sep 21
11. Türkvatan A, Erden A, Türkoğlu MA, Seçil M, Yener Ö. Imaging of acute pancreatitis and its complications. Part 1: acute pancreatitis. Diagn Interv Imaging. 2015;96(2):151–60. https://doi.org/10.1016/j.diii.2013.12.017.
12. Zhu Y, Pan X, Zeng H, He W, Xia L, Liu P, Zhu Y, Chen Y, Lv N. A study on the etiology, severity, and mortality of 3260 patients with acute pancreatitis according to the revised Atlanta classification in Jiangxi, China over an 8-year period. Pancreas. 2017;46(4):504–9. https://doi.org/10.1097/MPA.0000000000000776.
13. Rompianesi G, Hann A, Komolafe O, Pereira SP, Davidson BR, Gurusamy KS. Serum amylase and lipase and urinary trypsinogen and amylase for diagnosis of acute pancreatitis. Cochrane Database Syst Rev. 2017;4:CD012010. https://doi.org/10.1002/14651858.CD012010.pub2.
14. Cavdar F, Yildar M, Tellioğlu G, Kara M, Tilki M, Titiz Mİ. Controversial issues in biliary pancreatitis: when should we perform MRCP and ERCP? Pancreatology. 2014;14(5):411–4. https://doi.org/10.1016/j.pan.2014.08.002. Epub 2014 Aug 23
15. Şurlin V, Săftoiu A, Dumitrescu D. Imaging tests for accurate diagnosis of acute biliary pancreatitis. World J Gastroenterol. 2014;20(44):16544–9. https://doi.org/10.3748/wjg.v20.i44.16544.
16. Young SH, Peng YL, Lin XH, Chen YT, Luo JC, Wang YP, Hou MC, Lee FY. Cholecystectomy reduces recurrent pancreatitis and improves survival after endoscopic sphincterotomy. J Gastrointest Surg. 2017;21(2):294–301. https://doi.org/10.1007/s11605-016.
17. Gonoi W, Akai H, Hagiwara K, Akahane M, Hayashi N, Maeda E, Yoshikawa T, Tada M, Uno K, Ohtsu H, Koike K, Ohtomo K. Pancreas divisum as a predisposing factor for chronic and recurrent idiopathic pancreatitis: initial in vivo survey. Gut. 2011;60(8):1103–8.
18. Deshpande V, Gupta R, Sainani N, Sahani DV, Virk R, Ferrone C, Khosroshahi A, Stone JH, Lauwers GY. Subclassification of autoimmune pancreatitis: a histologic classification with clinical significance. Am J Surg Pathol. 2011;35(1):26–35.
19. Fernandez M, Arvanitakis M, Musala C, Devière J, Van Steenbergen W, Putzeys V, Ausloos F, Bastens B, Gast P, Roeyen G, Berrevoet F, Scheers I, Delhaye M, Deprez PH. The Belgian national registry on chronic pancreatitis: a prospective multi-centre study covering more than 800 patients in one year. Pancreatology. 2017;17(4):572–9. https://doi.org/10.1016/j.pan.2017.05.387. [Epub ahead of print]
20. Suzumura K, Hatano E, Okada T, Asano Y, Uyama N, Nakamura I, Hai S, Fujimoto J. Short- and long-term outcomes of the Frey procedure for chronic pancreatitis: a single-center experience and summary of outcomes in Japan. Surg Today. 2017;48(1):58–65. https://doi.org/10.1007/s00595-017-1548-0
21. Prochorov AV, Oldhafer KJ, Tretyak SI, Rashchynski SM, Donati M, Rashchinskaya NT, Audzevich DA. Surgical treatment of pain in patients with chronic pancreatitis. Hepatogastroenterology. 2012;59(116):1265–9.
22. Tandan M, Nageshwar Reddy D. Endotherapy in chronic pancreatitis. World J Gastroenterol. 2013;19(37):6156–64.
23. Costamagna G, Bulajic M, Tringali A, Pandol M, Gabbrielli A, Spada C, Petruzziello L, Familiari P, Mutignani M. Multiple stenting of refractory pancreatic duct strictures in severe chronic pancreatitis: long-term results. Endoscopy. 2006;38(3):254–9.

Benign and Malignant Lesions of the Liver

23

Francesca Romana Ponziani, Giulia Gibiino, and Antonio Gasbarrini

23.1 Introduction

Primary liver cancer represents approximately 4% of all new cancer diagnosed worldwide and is the third most common cause of cancer-related deaths among men and the sixth among women, respectively [1].

Hepatic tumors may derive from hepatocytes, bile duct epithelium, or mesenchymal tissue or spread to the liver from primary tumors in remote or adjacent organs.

In adults, hepatic metastases are more common than primary malignant tumors of the liver, whereas in children, primary malignant tumors outnumber both metastases and benign lesions. Except for cavernous hemangiomas, benign hepatic tumors are rare in all geographic regions and in all age groups. It is widely accepted that the risk of developing hepatocellular carcinoma (HCC) is age dependent [2]; hence, in Western countries, the diagnosis of HCC is more frequent in patients aged 70 or more, and being faced with elderly cirrhotic patients with HCC has become frequent in clinical practice [2–4].

23.2 Primary Malignant Tumors

23.2.1 Hepatocellular Carcinoma

Hepatocellular carcinoma is the most common primary malignant tumor of the liver, accounting for 85–90% of all primary liver cancers. It is the fifth most common cancer in men and the eighth most common in women, ranking fourth in annual cancer mortality rates [5]. The global age distribution of HCC varies by region,

F.R. Ponziani (✉) • G. Gibiino • A. Gasbarrini
Internal Medicine, Gastroenterology and Hepatology, Agostino Gemelli Hospital, Rome, Italy
e-mail: Antonio.Gasbarrini@unicatt.it

A. Crucitti (ed.), *Surgical Management of Elderly Patients*,
https://doi.org/10.1007/978-3-319-60861-7_23

incidence rate, gender, and etiology. In Western low-risk populations, men are generally more susceptible to HCC, and the highest rates occur among persons aged 75 and older [6, 7].

The mechanisms of HCC pathogenesis are complex and usually involve liver injury followed by inflammation, necrosis, and hepatocytes proliferation. The perpetuation of this destructive- regenerative process results in the development of liver cirrhosis, which is characterized by regenerating nodules that progress to dysplastic nodules and ultimately to HCC [8]. Indeed, cirrhosis is present in about 80–90% of patients with HCC being, therefore, the most frequent risk factor. Other risk factors are hepatitis B virus (HBV) and hepatitis C virus (HCV) infections, aflatoxin, alcohol intake, obesity, and diabetes.

Worldwide, around 400 million people are estimated to be chronically infected by HBV [9]. The HBV appears to be directly and indirectly carcinogenic, and HCC develops in as many as 25% of them [10].

HBV continues to be the major HCC risk factor worldwide, being the main leading factor to date compared to HCV, although its importance is expected to decrease during the coming decades due to the widespread diffusion of HBV vaccination in the newborns [5]. Approximately 170 million people in the world are chronically infected with HCV and are at increased risk of HCC development.

In Japan, Italy, and Spain, HCV is the cause of about 75% of HCCs, and, in other industrialized countries, chronic HCV infection, often in combination with alcohol abuse, is emerging as a major cause of this tumor. Patients with HCV-induced HCC are generally older than those with HBV-related tumors, and HCV infection was usually acquired in adult life [11].

Together, HBV and/or HCV chronic infections account for 80–90% of all HCC worldwide [12]. The variable age-specific patterns in different countries are related to differences in the dominant hepatitis virus in the population, the age at viral infection ,and the existence of other risk factors. According to EASL recommendations, in patients with chronic hepatitis, antiviral therapies leading to maintained HBV suppression in chronic hepatitis B and to sustained viral response in hepatitis C are recommended, since they have been shown to prevent progression to cirrhosis and hence HCC development [10].

Heavy alcohol intake, defined as ingestion of >50–70 g/day for prolonged periods, is a well-established risk factor for HCC, and there is also evidence of a synergistic effect of heavy alcohol intake with HCV or HBV chronic infection [13].

Nonalcoholic fatty liver disease (NAFLD) and nonalcoholic steatohepatitis (NASH), often associated with metabolic syndrome, are other well-known risk factors for HCC.

The relationship between cigarette smoking and HCC has been widely examined in both low- and high-risk areas, and discordant findings have been reported [5].

Although the typical clinical features of HCC (including abdominal pain and weight loss in patients with cirrhosis) are not always present and difficult to be recognized in patients with liver cirrhosis, nowadays more patients are being diagnosed at an early tumor stage, when they have no specific symptoms or signs. This is probably the result of the surveillance programs adopted among patients with cirrhosis,

[10] consisting in a semiannual abdominal ultrasound (US) all at-risk populations (cirrhotic patients, Child-Pugh stage A and B; cirrhotic patients, Child-Pugh stage C awaiting liver transplantation; non-cirrhotic HBV carriers with active hepatitis or family history of HCC; non-cirrhotic patients with chronic hepatitis C and advanced liver fibrosis). Paraneoplastic manifestations are rarely associated with HCC and include hypoglycemia (type A and B), polycythemia, hypercalcemia, and pityriasis rotunda.

The diagnosis of HCC in cirrhotic patients is made according to the "recall policy," which is based on the diameter of the nodule.

In cirrhotic patients, nodules <1 cm in diameter detected by ultrasound should be followed every 4 months in the first year and with regular checking every 6 months thereafter.

In cirrhotic patients, diagnosis of HCC for nodules of 1–2 cm in diameter should be based on imaging (computed tomography (CT) or magnetic resonance imaging) or biopsy-proven pathological confirmation.

In cirrhotic patients, nodules more than 2 cm in diameter can be diagnosed for HCC on one imaging technique or on the combination of CT scan and MRI techniques and/or liver biopsy as needed.

HCC diagnosis is therefore based on imaging or pathology. However, in the elderly, this may raise some concerns, especially regarding the risks associated with liver biopsy [1] and to the presence of contraindications to second-level radiologic imaging, due to chronic kidney disease with reduced creatinine clearance below 30 mL/min [14]. This is even truer in non-cirrhotic patients with HCC, because liver biopsy is recommended to ascertain the nature of the liver lesion independently of imaging behavior [15, 16]. Although great efforts of studies focused on molecular pathways and on the classification of HCC according to gene signatures or molecular abnormalities, they are not currently used for clinical application [17, 18].

The BCLC staging system has been recently recommended for prognostic prediction and treatment allocation of patients with HCC (Fig. 23.1) [19]. The severity of liver function impairment represents one of the most important prognostic parameters included in the BCLC algorithm, together with tumor stage and cancer-related symptoms. Based on these characteristics, in the BCLC system, patients are stratified in five categories (0, A–D), each one corresponding to specific therapeutic approaches and the patients' outcome.

Resection is the first-line treatment option for patients with a solitary tumor and very well-preserved liver function, defined as normal bilirubin with either hepatic venous pressure gradient $\leq$10 mmHg or platelet count $\geq$100,000. Perioperative mortality is expected to be 2–3% [20, 21]. Neoadjuvant or adjuvant therapies do not improve the outcome of patients treated with resection [22, 23].

Liver transplantation is considered to be the first-line treatment option for patients with single tumors less than 5 cm in size or with $\leq$3 nodules $\leq$3 cm in size (Milan criteria) who are not suitable for resection [24, 25]. A modest expansion of Milan criteria applying the "up-to-seven" criteria in patients without microvascular invasion undergoing liver transplantation seems also to achieve competitive

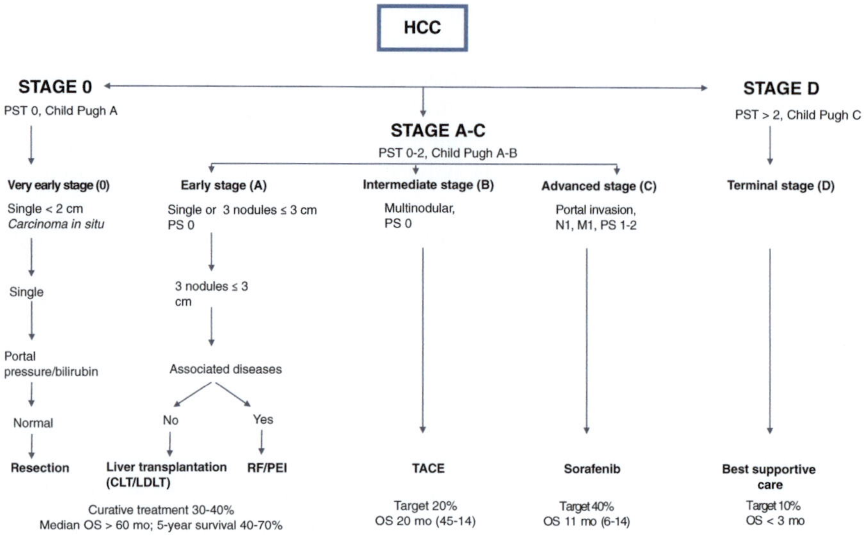

Fig. 23.1 Adapted from EASL- EORTC guidelines (2012)

outcomes [26]. However, most of the liver transplant centers have settled a cutoff for the age of liver transplant candidates, which usually does not exceed 65 years.

Local ablation with radiofrequency or percutaneous ethanol injection is considered the standard of care for patients with BCLC 0–A tumors not suitable for surgery. Studies reporting outcomes after radiofrequency ablation (RFA) in elderly patients showed that old age is not an independent predictor of reduced survival after RFA. However, the good safety profile of RFA is maintained in the elderly, and the rate of major complications was found to be similar in elderly and in younger cirrhotic patients [27–29].

Transarterial chemoembolization (TACE) is recommended for BCLC stage B patients, with multinodular asymptomatic tumors in the absence of vascular invasion or extrahepatic spread. It is instead discouraged in patients with decompensated liver disease, advanced liver dysfunction, macroscopic vascular invasion, or extrahepatic spread. There are only few studies addressing the use of TACE in the elderly, and its use in this setting is still debated. A prospective cohort study performed on 102 patients with HCC who underwent TACE showed similar survival and safety profile irrespective of age [30, 31]. In a large retrospective study from Korea, the authors found that TACE was associated with even better results in elderly than in younger patients, with respect to median OS and disease-specific survival; moreover, there was no significant difference in terms of TACE-related mortality [32]. These data suggest that in the elderly, TACE is an effective therapeutic option for HCC with a satisfactory safety profile.

Sorafenib is the only approved systemic therapy for HCC. It is indicated for patients with well-preserved liver function (Child-Pugh A) and with advanced tumors (BCLC C) or those tumors progressing upon locoregional therapies. The efficacy of sorafenib in elderly patients is supported by several studies, showing similar, or even a trend to longer, overall survival and time to progression in elderly patients compared with younger subjects [33, 34]. Overall, evidence collected to date shows that the efficacy and safety profile of sorafenib is not influenced by age. However, a stricter monitoring should be considered in the elderly because of the potential risk of developing and the reduced tolerability of adverse events.

23.2.2 Intrahepatic Cholangiocarcinoma

Intrahepatic cholangiocarcinoma (ICC) is a malignant tumor arising from the intrahepatic biliary tract. It is responsible for 10–20% of primary liver cancers worldwide and is the second most common primary liver malignancy [35]. ICC can be classified anatomically as perihilar or peripheral [36].

The incidence of ICC varies worldwide, with the highest rates in northeast Thailand (>80 per 100,000 population) and lower rates in the Western world (0.3–2.1 per 100,000 population) [37]. Hispanic females, American Indian/Alaskan Native, and Asian Pacific groups seem the most affected ethnic groups. Despite the significant geographical and ethnic variations, recent studies have reported a global increase in incidence of ICC over the last few decades [38] as well as an increasing mortality. Similar trends are observed in both sexes with an overall slight male predominance (M: F 1.2–1.5:1) [39].

Cholangiocarcinogenesis is a complex multistep process. It may occur in a healthy liver or in patients with underlying liver disease. Several risk factors for chronic inflammatory damage and increased cellular turnover have been established, such as hepatobiliary flukes (*Opisthorchis viverrini* and *Clonorchis sinensis*, classified as group 1 carcinogens in WHO classification 2009), primary sclerosing cholangitis (PSC), cysts of the biliary tract, hepatolithiasis, and toxins [40]. Cirrhosis, chronic hepatitis B and C, obesity, diabetes, and alcoholic liver disease, although recognized as risk factors for HCC, are also emerging as warning conditions for ICC. Mixed histotypes of hepatocellular-cholangiocarcinoma rather than the traditional adenocarcinoma can be also observed [41].

ICC early diagnosis is still a major clinical challenge, because patients with early-stage disease are often asymptomatic [42]. Weight loss, abdominal discomfort, biliary tract obstruction with jaundice, and hepatomegaly or palpable abdominal mass are usually observed at more advanced stages. The only potentially curative treatment option for patients who have resectable disease is surgery. Unfortunately, even the clinical outcomes of patients undergoing liver resection are disappointing, with a 5-year survival rate of 20–35% [43]. Furthermore, the role of adjuvant therapies, including systemic chemotherapy and radiotherapy, remains poorly defined and of scarce effect.

Many studies have investigated the mechanisms involved in the carcinogenetic process in ICC at different levels of cell biology, from single gene mutations to protein aberrations. In this perspective, there are many candidates for targeted therapies such as MET, EGFR and ERBB2, FGFR2, JAK/STAT, RAS/RAF/MAPK, and

PI3K/AKT/mTOR pathways and even IDH mutations, although no therapeutic approach has been currently introduced in clinical practice [44].

23.2.3 Hemangiosarcoma, Epithelioid Hemangioendothelioma, and Other Primary Malignant Tumors

Although rare, angiosarcoma is the most common malignant mesenchymal tumor of the liver [45]. It occurs almost exclusively in adults and is most prevalent in the sixth and seventh decades of life. Men are affected four times as often as women. The most common presenting symptom is upper abdominal pain. Other frequent complaints are abdominal swelling, rapidly progressing liver failure, malaise, weight loss, poor appetite, and nausea [46]. The duration of symptoms generally ranges from 1 week to 6 months, but a few patients have had symptoms for as long as 2 years before seeking medical attention. A rising serum bilirubin level and other evidence of progressive hepatic dysfunction may be present, especially in case of the later stages of the tumor.

Hepatic arteriography reveals a characteristic appearance. The hepatic arteries are displaced by the tumor, which shows a blush and "puddling" in the middle of the arterial phase that persist for many seconds, except in the central area, which may be hypovascular.

Hepatic angiosarcomas grow rapidly, and the prognosis is poor; death ensues within 6 months. Patients may have thrombocytopenia resulting from entrapment of platelets within the tumor (Kasabach-Merritt syndrome), disseminated intravascular coagulation with secondary fibrinolysis, or microangiopathic hemolytic anemia as a result of fragmentation of erythrocytes within the tumor circulation. Operative treatment is usually precluded by the advanced stage of the tumor, while chemo- and radiotherapy showed poor results [47].

Epithelioid hemangioendothelioma is a rare tumor, described in females at all ages in adulthood [48]. No specific symptoms are usually referred, and imaging studies show a characteristically highly vascular mass, which may infiltrate throughout the liver. Case reports indicate that the tumor can be visualized on PET. Correct diagnosis requires histologic examination of tissue obtained by biopsy. It is important to distinguish this tumor with low-grade malignant potential from hemangiosarcoma, as a better prognosis can be reached, if treated appropriately and aggressively. The first treatment modality for epithelioid hemangioendothelioma is surgery, including resection or liver transplantation [49].

Other rare sarcomas arising in the liver include liposarcoma, lymphoma, and rhabdomyosarcoma.

23.3 Benign Tumors

Benign liver tumors are frequently found incidentally, as a consequence of the widespread use of imaging tests, and often have a favorable course. Several types of benign liver tumors have been identified (Table 23.1); EASL guidelines [50]

Table 23.1 Histological classification of benign liver tumors, adapted from Coelho et al. indication and treatment of benign hepatic tumors

Epithelial origin	Type of tumor
Hepatocyte	Hepatocellular carcinoma
	Multiple adenomatosis
	Focal nodular hyperplasia
	Nodular rigenerative hyperplasia
Bile cells	Bile duct adenoma
	Biliary hamartomas (von Meyenburg complex)

Non-epithelial origin	Type of tumor
Mesenchymal	Hemangioma
	Angiomyolipoma
	Lipoma, myelolipoma
Others	Inflammatory pseudotumors

provide a contemporary aid for the practical diagnosis and management of the more common ones: hemangiomas, focal nodular hyperplasia (FNH), and hepatocellular adenoma (HCA). In association with an unremarkable baseline history, physical examination, blood tests, and imaging are usually sufficient to establish a diagnosis of a benign liver tumor and informed decisions on patients' management [50].

23.3.1 Hepatic Hemangiomas

Hepatic hemangiomas are the most common benign primary liver tumors, belonging to the group of non-epithelial lesions. Hemangiomas are present in 0.4–20% of the general population and are typically discovered incidentally during evaluation for non-specific abdominal complaints, most frequently diagnosed in women between 30 and 50 years [51]. Lesions measuring 10 cm are called "giant hemangiomas" and may be symptomatic, including pain and the Kasabach-Merritt syndrome [52].

Hemangiomas are most often asymptomatic as they are incidentally discovered and may change in size during long-term follow-up. There is no relationship between the size of hemangiomas and complications, while there is little relationship between symptoms and characteristics of the lesion. When observed at abdominal ultrasound (US), hemangiomas have a classic appearance as a homogeneous hypoechoic mass usually measuring less than 3 cm in diameter with acoustic enhancement and sharp margins [53]. Contrast enhancement (CE) study allows the definition of peripheral and globular enhancement of the lesion followed by a central enhancement on delayed phases [53]. MRI is the key imaging modality for the diagnosis of these lesions [54].

Surgical management is still debated in terms of advantages even in large lesions or lesions with mild symptoms. Symptomatic or giant hemangiomas are not common, and surgical resection is rarely indicated, except in the presence of KMS [52].

23.3.2 Focal Nodular Hyperplasia (FNH)

Focal nodular hyperplasia is the second most frequent benign tumor of the liver. The average age at presentation ranges between 35 and 50 years [55]. In most cases, it is solitary and smaller than 5 cm. It is widely thought that this lesion arises as a proliferative cell response to an aberrant dystrophic artery and may be associated with other conditions characterized by arterial damage [56].

On US, FNH is usually slightly hypo- or isoechoic and very rarely hyperechoic. Typically, Doppler US reveals central arteries with a spoke-wheel pattern.

MRI has the highest diagnostic performance for the diagnosis of FNH. CEUS achieves a high accuracy in FNH less than 3 cm.

Regardless of the specific imaging technique used, typical general findings are (1) homogeneity of the lesion except for the central scar, (2) slight difference from the adjacent liver on pre-contrast imaging, (3) strong and homogeneous enhancement on the arterial phase with a central vascular supply, (4) the lesion becomes similar to the adjacent liver on portal and delayed phases, (5) the central scar can be best seen on MRI, and (6) a lack of capsule and often lobulated contours [57].

In the absence of symptoms and given the rarity of complications, a conservative approach is recommended. For a lesion typical for FNH, the follow-up is unnecessary unless in the presence of an underlying vascular disease [58].

23.3.3 Hepatocellular Adenoma (HCA)

Hepatocellular adenoma is approximately ten times less common than FNH and is typically diagnosed in women 30–40 years old. Several studies have supported the potential role of sex hormones in the development of HCA. In particular, the link between oral contraceptive pills and increased risk of HCA in women was strengthened by the demonstration of occasional tumor regression upon drug withdrawal. Notably, the incidence of HCA has increased in males due to the increased use of anabolic-androgen steroids in body builders and gym activities. The recent increase in the HCA prevalence has been also associated with obesity and metabolic syndrome.

A molecular classification of HCA has been proposed showing two main types, respectively, observed in women and men. Indeed, the course of HCA diagnosed in women is more often benign, the content of fat is increased, and the hallmark is the absence of expression in tumor hepatocytes of genes controlled by HNF-1a, among them, liver fatty acid binding protein (LFABP), which is in contrast highly expressed in non-tumor hepatocyte.

The second subtype "inflammatory HCA" is characterized by the activation of the JACK/STAT pathway, a molecular key present in several malignancies. "Beta-catenin-activated HCA" is another subtype, highly associated with risk of malignant transformation [59].

MRI is superior to all other imaging modalities in the diagnosis of HCA and is useful to distinguish the different subtypes. Biopsy should be considered within a benign liver tumor to exclude malignancy. In the case of tissue availability obtained for diagnostic purpose, curative intervention is advised for the activated b-catenin-mutated HCA, irrespective of size [60].

Treatment decisions are usually based on gender, size, and patterns of progression. Upon HCA diagnosis, lifestyle changes such as weight loss and discontinuation of contraceptives should be recommended. HCA resection is recommended irrespective of size in men and in any instance of proven beta-catenin mutation; in women, a period of 6 months observation after lifestyle change is advised, and resection is indicated in the case of nodules ≥5 cm and for those continuing to grow. In case of lesions <5 cm in women, a reassessment at 1 year and annual imaging thereafter are recommended. A sure indication for embolization and subsequent resection is a bleeding HCA with hemodynamic instability [61].

References

1. Stewart BW, Kleihues P, editors. World cancer report. Lyon: IARC Press; 2003.
2. Borzio M, Dionigi E, Parisi G, Raguzzi I, Sacco R. Management of hepatocellular carcinoma in the elderly. World J Hepatol. 2015;7(11):1521–9.
3. Asahina Y, Tsuchiya K, Tamaki N, Hirayama I, Tanaka T, Sato M, Yasui Y, Hosokawa T, Ueda K, Kuzuya T, Nakanishi H, Itakura J, Takahashi Y, Kurosaki M, Enomoto N, Izumi N. Effect of aging on risk for hepatocellular carcinoma in chronic hepatitis C virus infection. Hepatology. 2010;52:518–27. https://doi.org/10.1002/hep.23691.
4. Borzio M, Fornari F, De Sio I, Andriulli A, Terracciano F, Parisi G, Francica G, Salvagnini M, Marignani M, Salmi A, Farinati F, Carella A, Pedicino C, Dionigi E, Fanigliulo L, Cazzaniga M, Ginanni B, Sacco R. Adherence to American Association for the Study of Liver Diseases guidelines for the management of hepatocellular carcinoma: results of an Italian field practice multicenter study. Future Oncol. 2013;9:283–94.
5. Nordenstedt H, White DL, El-Serag H. The changing pattern of epidemiology in hepatocellular carcinoma. Dig Liver Dis. 2010;42(Suppl):S206–14.
6. Kim YJ, Jang BK, Kim ES, Chung WJ, Park KS, Cho KB, Hwang JS. Hepatocellular carcinoma in the elderly: clinical characteristics, treatment, survival analysis in Korean patients older than 70 years. J Korean Med Sci. 2012;27:1147–54. https://doi.org/10.3346/jkms.2012.27.10.1147.
7. Pignata S, Gallo C, Daniele B, Elba S, Giorgio A, Capuano G, Adinolfi LE, De Sio I, Izzo F, Farinati F, Del Naja C, Stanzione M, Castiglione F, Marone G, Cuomo O, Felder M, Gaeta GB, De Maio E, Di Maio M, Signoriello G, Perrone F. Characteristics at presentation and outcome of hepatocellular carcinoma (HCC) in the elderly. A study of the Cancer of the Liver Italian Program (CLIP). Crit Rev Oncol Hematol. 2006;59:243–9. https://doi.org/10.1016/j.critrevonc.2006.01.002.
8. Sia D, Villanueva A, Friedman S, Llovet MJ. Liver cancer cell of origin, molecular class, and effects on patient prognosis. Gastroenterology. 2017;152:745–61.
9. Parkin DM, Bray F, Ferlay J, Pisani P. Global cancer statistics, 2002. CA Cancer J Clin. 2005;55:74–108.
10. European Association for the Study of the Liver. EASL-EORTC clinical practice guidelines: management of hepatocellular carcinoma. J Hepatol. 2012;56:908–43.
11. Nguyen VT, Law MG, Dore GJ. Hepatitis B-related hepatocellular carcinoma: epidemiological characteristics and disease burden. J Viral Hepat. 2009;16(7):453–63.
12. Bosetti C, Boffetta P, Lucchini F, Negri E, La Vecchia C. Trends in mortality from hepatocellular carcinoma in Europe 1980–2004. Hepatology. 2008;48:137–45.
13. Donato F, Tagger A, Gelatti U, et al. Alcohol and hepatocellular carcinoma: the effect of lifetime intake and hepatitis virus infection in men and women. Am J Epidemiol. 2002;155(4):323–31.

14. Forner A, Vilana R, Ayuso C, Bianchi L, Solé M, Ayuso JR, et al. Diagnosis of hepatic nodules 20 mm or smaller in cirrhosis: prospective validation of the noninvasive diagnostic criteria for hepatocellular carcinoma. Hepatology. 2008;47:97–104.
15. Stigliano R, Marelli L, Yu D, Davies N, Patch D, Burroughs AK. Seeding following percutaneous diagnostic and therapeutic approaches for hepatocellular carcinoma. What is the risk and the outcome? Seeding risk for percutaneous approach of HCC. Cancer Treat Rev. 2007;33:437–47.
16. Sersté T, Barrau V, Ozenne V, Vullierme MP, Bedossa P, Farges O, et al. Accuracy and disagreement of CT and MRI for the diagnosis of small hepatocellular carcinoma and dysplastic nodules: role of biopsy. Hepatology. 2011;55(3):800–6. https://doi.org/10.1002/hep.24746. [Epub ahead of print].
17. Boyault S, Rickman DS, de Reyniès A, Balabaud C, Rebouissou S, Jeannot E, et al. Transcriptome classification of HCC is related to gene alterations and to new therapeutic targets. Hepatology. 2007;45:42–52.
18. Chiang DY, Villanueva A, Hoshida Y, Peix J, Newell P, Minguez B, et al. Focal gains of VEGFA and molecular classification of hepatocellular carcinoma. Cancer Res. 2008;68:6779–88.
19. Llovet JM, Fuster J, Bruix J, Barcelona-Clinic Liver Cancer Group. The Barcelona approach: diagnosis, staging, and treatment of hepatocellular carcinoma. Liver Transpl. 2004;10(2, Suppl 1):S115–20.
20. Roayaie S, Llovet JM, Obeidat K, Labow D, Sposito C, Pellegrinelli A, et al. Hepatic resection for hepatocellular carcinoma <2 cm in diameter. Hepatology. 2012;49(44):518–23.
21. Llovet JM, Schwartz M, Mazzaferro V. Resection and liver transplantation for hepatocellular carcinoma. Semin Liver Dis. 2005;25:181–200.
22. Vitale A, Volk ML, Pastorelli D, Lonardi S, Farinati F, Burra P, et al. Use of sorafenib in patients with hepatocellular carcinoma before liver transplantation: a cost–benefit analysis while awaiting data on sorafenib safety. Hepatology. 2010;51:165–73.
23. Truesdale AE, Caldwell SH, Shah NL, Argo CK, Al-Osaimi AM, Schmitt TM, et al. Sorafenib therapy for hepatocellular carcinoma prior to liver transplant is associated with increased complications after transplant. Transpl Int. 2011;24:991–8.
24. Mazzaferro V, Bhoori S, Sposito C, Bongini M, Langer M, Miceli R, et al. Milan criteria in liver transplantation for HCC: an evidence-based analysis on 15 years of experience. Liver Transpl. 2011;17:S44–57.
25. Bruix J, Sherman M, AASLD Practice Guideline. Management of hepatocellular carcinoma: an update. Hepatology. 2011;53(3):1020–2.
26. Clavien PA, Lesurtel M, Bossuyt PM, Gores GJ, Langer B, Perrier A, et al. Recommendations for liver transplantation for hepatocellular carcinoma: an international consensus conference report. Lancet Oncol. 2012;13:e11–22.
27. Massarweh NN, Park JO, Farjah F, Yeung RS, Symons RG, Vaughan TL, Baldwin LM, Flum DR. Trends in the utilization and impact of radiofrequency ablation for hepatocellular carcinoma. J Am Coll Surg. 2010;210:441–8. https://doi.org/10.1016/j.jamcollsurg.2009.12.026.
28. Shiina S, Tateishi R, Arano T, Uchino K, Enooku K, Nakagawa H, Asaoka Y, Sato T, Masuzaki R, Kondo Y, Goto T, Yoshida H, Omata M, Koike K. Radiofrequency ablation for hepatocellular carcinoma: 10-year outcome and prognostic factors. Am J Gastroenterol. 2012;107:569–77. https://doi.org/10.1038/ajg.2011.425.
29. Tateishi R, Shiina S, Teratani T, Obi S, Sato S, Koike Y, Fujishima T, Yoshida H, Kawabe T, Omata M. Percutaneous radiofrequency ablation for hepatocellular carcinoma. An analysis of 1000 cases. Cancer. 2005;103:1201–9. https://doi.org/10.1002/cncr.20892.
30. Cohen MJ, Bloom AI, Barak O, Klimov A, Nesher T, Shouval D, Levi I, Shibolet O. Trans-arterial chemo-embolization is safe and effective for very elderly patients with hepatocellular carcinoma. World J Gastroenterol. 2013;19:2521–8. https://doi.org/10.3748/wjg.v19.i16.2521.
31. Cohen MJ, Levy I, Barak O, Bloom AI, Fernández-Ruiz M, Di Maio M, Perrone F, Poon RT, Shouval D, Yau T, Shibolet O. Trans-arterial chemo-embolization is safe and effective for

elderly advanced hepatocellular carcinoma patients: results from an international database. Liver Int. 2014;34:1109–17. https://doi.org/10.1111/liv.12486.
32. Yau T, Yao TJ, Chan P, Epstein RJ, Ng KK, Chok SH, Cheung TT, Fan ST, Poon RT. The outcomes of elderly patients with hepatocellular carcinoma treated with transarterial chemoembolization. Cancer. 2009;115:5507–15. https://doi.org/10.1002/cncr.24636.
33. Cabibbo G, Maida M, Cammà C, Craxì A. Is the efficacy of sorafenib treatment in patients with hepatocellular carcinoma affected by age? Expert Rev Anticancer Ther. 2013;13:1355–61. https://doi.org/10.1586/14737140.2013.859989.
34. Dufour JF. Hepatocellular carcinoma: sorafenib: for once age is not an issue. Nat Rev Gastroenterol Hepatol. 2014;11:273–4. https://doi.org/10.1038/nrgastro.2014.48.
35. Bridgewater J, Galle PR, Khan SA, Llovet JM, Park J, Patel T, Pawlik TM, Gores GJ. Guidelines for the diagnosis and management of intrahepatic cholangiocarcinoma. J Hepatol. 2014;60(6):1268–89.
36. Aishima S, Oda Y. Pathogenesis and classification of intrahepatic cholangiocarcinoma: different characters of perihilar large duct type versus peripheral small duct type. J Hepatobiliary Pancreat Sci. 2015;22:94–100.
37. Khan SA, Toledano MB, Taylor-Robinson SD. Epidemiology, risk factors, and pathogenesis of cholangiocarcinoma. HPB (Oxford). 2008;10:77–82.
38. Shaib Y, El-Serag HB. The epidemiology of cholangiocarcinoma. Semin Liver Dis. 2004;24:115–25.
39. Shaib YH, Davila JA, McGlynn K, El-Serag HB. Rising incidence of intrahepatic cholangiocarcinoma in the United States: a true increase? J Hepatol. 2004;40:472–7.
40. Khan SA, Thomas HC, Davidson BR, Taylor-Robinson SD. Cholangiocarcinoma. Lancet. 2005;366:1303–14.
41. Palmer WC, Patel T. Are common factors involved in the pathogenesis of primary liver cancers? A meta-analysis of risk factors for intrahepatic cholangiocarcinoma. J Hepatol. 2012;57:69–76.
42. Blechacz B, Gores GJ. Cholangiocarcinoma: advances in pathogenesis, diagnosis, and treatment. Hepatology. 2008;48:308–21.
43. Ruzzenente A, Conci S, Valdegamberi A, Pedrazzani C, Guglielmi A. Role of surgery in the treatment of intrahepatic cholangiocarcinoma. Eur Rev Med Pharmacol Sci. 2015;19(15):2892–900.
44. Andersen JB, Spee B, Blechacz BR, Avital I, Komuta M, Barbour A, Conner EA, Gillen MC, Roskams T, Roberts LR, Factor VM, Thorgeirsson SS. Genomic and genetic characterization of cholangiocarcinoma identifies therapeutic targets for tyrosine kinase inhibitors. Gastroenterology. 2012;142:1021–31.
45. Wu CH, Chiu NC, Yeh YC, Kuo Y, Yu SS, Weng CY, Liu CA, Chou YH, Chiou YY. Uncommon liver tumours: case report and literature review. Medicine (Baltimore). 2016;95(39):e4952. https://doi.org/10.1097/MD.0000000000004952. Review.
46. Lahat G, Dhuka AR, Hallevi H, et al. Angiosarcoma: clinical and molecular insights. Ann Surg. 2010;251:1098–106.
47. Maluf D, Cotterel A, Clark B, et al. Hepatic angiosarcoma and liver transplantation: case report and literature review. Transplant Proc. 2005;37:2195–9.
48. Miller WJ, Dodd GD, Federle MP, et al. Epithelioid hemangioendothelioma of the liver: imaging findings with pathologic correlation. AJR Am J Roentgenol. 1992;159:53–7.
49. Darras T, Moisse R, Colette JM. Epithelioid hemangioendothelioma of the liver. J Belg Radiol. 1988;71:722–33.
50. European Association for the Study of the Liver (EASL). EASL clinical practice guidelines on the management of benign liver tumours. J Hepatol. 2016;65:386–98.
51. Gandolfi L, Leo P, Solmi L, Vitelli E, Verros G, Colecchia A. Natural history of hepatic haemangiomas: clinical and ultrasound study. Gut. 1991;32:677–80.
52. O'Rafferty C, O'Regan GM, Irvine AD, Smith OP. Recent advances in the pathobiology and management of Kasabach-Merritt phenomenon. Br J Haematol. 2015;171:38–51.

53. Quaia E, Bertolotto M, Dalla Palma L. Characterization of liver hemangiomas with pulse inversion harmonic imaging. Eur Radiol. 2002;12:537–44.
54. Semelka RC, Brown ED, Ascher SM, Patt RH, Bagley AS, Li W, et al. Hepatic hemangiomas: a multi-institutional study of appearance on T2-weighted and serial gadolinium-enhanced gradient-echo MR images. Radiology. 1994;192:401–6.
55. Marrero JA, Ahn J, Rajender Reddy K, Americal College of Gastroenterology. ACG clinical guideline: the diagnosis and management of focal liver lesions. Am J Gastroenterol. 2014;109:1328–47. quiz 1348.
56. D'Halluin V, Vilgrain V, Pelletier G, Rocher L, Belghiti J, Erlinger S, et al. Natural history of focal nodular hyperplasia. A retrospective study of 44 cases. Gastroenterol Clin Biol. 2001;25:1008–10.
57. Buetow PC, Pantongrag-Brown L, Buck JL, Ros PR, Goodman ZD. Focal nodular hyperplasia of the liver: radiologic-pathologic correlation. Radiographics. 1996;16:369–88.
58. Birn J, Williams TR, Croteau D, Schwartz S, Sturza S, Getzen T. Transarterial embolization of symptomatic focal nodular hyperplasia. J Vasc Interv Radiol. 2013;24:1647–55.
59. Zucman-Rossi J, Jeannot E, Nhieu JT, Scoazec JY, Guettier C, Rebouissou S, et al. Genotype-phenotype correlation in hepatocellular adenoma: new classification and relationship with HCC. Hepatology. 2006;43:515–24.
60. Laumonier H, Bioulac-Sage P, Laurent C, Zucman-Rossi J, Balabaud C, Trillaud H. Hepatocellular adenomas: magnetic resonance imaging features as a function of molecular pathological classification. Hepatology. 2008;48:808–18.
61. Chun YS, Parker RJ, Inampudi S, Ehrenwald E, Batts KP, Burgart LJ, et al. Imaging surveillance of hypervascular liver lesions in non-cirrhotic patients. J Gastrointest Surg. 2015;20:564–7.

Pancreatic Tumors

24

Sergio Alfieri, Fausto Rosa, Dario Di Miceli,
and Giovanni Battista Doglietto

24.1 Introduction

The elderly population has been increasing rapidly in Western countries because of improvements in public health, nutrition, prevention, early detection of diseases, and continued medical progress. In 2008, in the United States, the elderly numbered 38.9 million or 12.8% of the population. They are projected to account for nearly 20% of the population by the year 2030 [1]. By 2050, over 85-year-old people are projected to account for 24% of the elderly population and 5% of the population overall [1, 2]. In 2050, there will be nearly six times as many octogenarians as in 2000 [3]. Moreover, in 2003, the average life expectancy of 75-year-old individuals in the United States was 11.8 years [4]. In 2004, the probability of survival for an 80-year-old person in Germany was 7.9 years [5]. For other Western countries and Japan, the estimations are comparable.

The incidence of pancreatic cancer is strongly related to a mean age of 72 years at the time of diagnosis. Approximately 29% of patients with this disease are 75–84 years of age, and 13% are 85 years of age [6, 7]. Recent improvements in surgical techniques and perioperative care in high-volume centers have allowed better results following pancreatic resection [8]. In fact, currently pancreatic surgeons are seeing more patients of 80 years or over with pancreatic cancer or periampullary neoplasms where they must make a decision as to whether to recommend a pancreatectomy. The decision to recommend a pancreatic resection for pancreatic cancer or other periampullary neoplasms in an elderly patient is complicated by the frailty of the patient, the strong surgical trauma, and the poor prognosis of the disease. The process of weighing up the risks and indications for surgical resection is made even more difficult by the lack of clinical data regarding major intra-abdominal surgery in the elderly.

S. Alfieri (✉) • F. Rosa • D. Di Miceli • G.B. Doglietto
Department of Digestive Surgery, Catholic University, "A. Gemelli" Hospital, Rome, Italy
e-mail: sergio.alfieri@unicatt.it

A. Crucitti (ed.), *Surgical Management of Elderly Patients*,
https://doi.org/10.1007/978-3-319-60861-7_24

In fact, although there is a large series of very elderly patients undergoing cardiothoracic [9–11] and vascular [12] procedures, few studies have analyzed the outcomes of very elderly patients following major intra-abdominal surgery.

Taking into consideration all the above factors and the likelihood that more very elderly people will present for surgery in the future, it is imperative to ask whether a pancreatic resection should be recommended for adenocarcinoma in patients of 80 years or over, especially when the 5-year survival rate is 25–30% after an R0 resection.

24.2 Clinicopathological Characteristics

The population of Western countries is aging, and because the incidence of cancer increases with age, the population of patients with cancer is growing. More than 50% of all newly diagnosed patients with cancer are over 60 years of age, and more than one third are over the age of 70 [13]. By 2030, 70% of all malignancies and 85% of all cancer-related deaths are expected to occur in individuals aged 65 years or over. Therefore, it is likely that older people will represent the prototypical cancer patient in the future [14]. Age is an important risk factor for the development of pancreatic cancer. Whereas the overall incidence rate of pancreatic cancer for all ages is 11.7%, the incidence rate among individuals older than 65 years is 66.4% and up to 91.1% for those over 80 years of age [15].

The association between aging and cancer is well established. Carcinogenesis is a time-consuming process with a final outcome (cancer) that is more likely to occur late in life. Older tissues are more vulnerable to environmental carcinogens. Changes in the environment of the body (such as chronic inflammation, immunosenescence) may favor the development of cancer [16, 17]. Furthermore, the immune system plays an important role in the progression of pancreatic cancer [18–20]. Very little data are available regarding pancreatic cancer in the elderly. Kamisawa et al. [21] compared the pathologic features of pancreatic cancer in older vs younger patients and found no differences in the grade, location, or incidence of the local spread, although elderly patients developed fewer hematogenous metastases. Other reports have indicated that older patients present more diploid tumors or p53 mutations, which are associated with a worse prognosis [22].

Several studies have shown that older cancer patients are often undertreated and have poorer outcomes compared with younger individuals [23, 24]. This may be due to the less aggressive treatment of elderly patients. Some studies focusing on pancreatic cancer have shown that nearly half of all elderly patients did not receive any treatment for locoregional pancreatic cancer. What's more, only 11% received a multimodal therapy (surgery ± chemoradiotherapy) [25].

Despite the rapidly growing oncogeriatric population, older cancer patients are underrepresented in clinical trials [26]. Talarico et al. [27] analyzed the age-related enrollment of cancer patients in clinical trials and found that the proportion of the overall patient population aged ≥65, ≥70, and ≥75 years was 36%, 20%, and 9% in clinical trials compared with 60%, 46%, and 31% in the US cancer population, respectively. This underrepresentation generates challenges because the results from clinical trials in younger patients cannot be extrapolated to the treatment of the elderly. The diverse effects of aging on organ function and the variety of potential comorbid diseases result in a heterogeneous elderly population. For example, pharmacokinetic and pharmacodynamic differences between younger and older patients, and indeed among elderly patients themselves, could result in considerable variability in the efficacy and safety of cancer treatments. Pharmacodynamic changes may cause resistance to cytotoxic drugs in older individuals due to resistance to apoptosis and poorer oxygenation in these neoplasms [28, 29]. Specifically, in patients aged 75 or older with advanced pancreatic adenocarcinoma and who were treated with gemcitabine, the median survival time was approximately 6–8 weeks shorter than that in trial patients [30]. Another important question concerns the effects of toxicity on older people. While grade 2 adverse events are not important in younger people and, in fact, are often not reported, the same level of toxicity may result in a considerable deterioration of functionality in older patients.

Several studies have shown that older patients are less likely to be staged than younger patients [31, 32]. Among those who are staged, it appears that older patients present with earlier-stage disease. Despite this, older patients have a worse overall 5-year survival compared to younger patients. This may be due to the less aggressive treatment of elderly patients and also deaths due to comorbid conditions. However, no studies are available that adequately address this issue.

Kamisawa et al. examined the pathologic features of pancreatic cancer in 89 elderly patients (>70 years) and compared them to 184 younger patients [21]. With advancing age, proportionally more women were diagnosed. There were no differences in the grade or location (head/body/tail) of tumors in younger vs older patients, and there was no difference in the incidence of local spread. Elderly patients, however, did have fewer hematogenous metastases than younger patients.

In another study, it appeared that older patients had more diploid tumors, and younger patients had more aneuploid tumors (which may help explain the difference in hematogenous spread) [33].

24.3 Surgery for Pancreatic Cancer in the Elderly

Despite a tendency toward worse surgical outcomes in the elderly, surgical resection for pancreatic cancer remains the only treatment modality that offers a complete cure. Surgeons have been compelled to push the age boundary in the hope of curing patients of over 60 years of age. A PubMed search was performed using the keywords "pancreatic cancer," "elderly," "resection," and "pancreaticoduodenectomy." All publications with original data of the surgical treatment of pancreatic cancer in the elderly within the last 15 years are included in Table 24.1.

Surgical resection is the only potentially curative treatment for pancreatic cancer. Unfortunately, only 15–20% of patients are candidates for pancreatectomy due to the late presentation of symptoms and/or detection of the disease [34–36]. Furthermore, the rate of resectability diminishes with age. Similarly, some authors

Table 24.1 Outcomes after pancreatic resection in the elderly patient

Study	Total No.	Age	Summary of findings	Median survival	Long-term survival
Bathe et al. [44]	70	75	No difference in 30-day mortality (8.5%), significant increase in morbidity in elderly (31 vs 63%). Measured endpoints for morbidity: gastric atony, pancreatic fistula, intra-abdominal abscess, biliary fistula, wound infection, line sepsis, urinary tract infection, gastrointestinal bleeding, bladder injury, pneumothorax, suppurative thrombophlebitis, pylephlebitis, chylous ascites, respiratory insufficiency, pneumonia, cardiovascular, multiple organ failure, hyperglycemia, pulmonary embolism, renal insufficiency, seizure, delirium, gout	24 months for patients less than 75 years old and 9 months in those over 75	5-year survival: 23% in patients less than 75 years old and 31% in those over 75
Hodul et al. [42]	122	70	No difference in 30-day mortality (only one death in the younger cohort) or morbidity. Measured endpoints for morbidity: wound infection, abscess, anastomotic leak, cardiac, urinary tract infection	Not reported	Not reported
Brozetti et al. [80]	166	70	Significant increase in 30-day mortality (4 vs 11%) and significant increase in morbidity (46 vs 49%) in the elderly. Measured endpoints for morbidity: pancreatic fistula, pancreatitis, biliary fistula, delayed gastric emptying, postoperative bleeding, sepsis, wound infection, urinary tract infection, pneumonia, cardiac, renal, or cerebrovascular disease	Not reported	Not reported
Makary et al. [39]	2698	80/90	Significant increase in 30-day mortality and morbidity for patients aged 80–90 compared to those less than 80 but not significant for those greater than 90. Measured endpoints for morbidity: reoperation, small bowel obstruction, ulcer, delayed gastric emptying, pancreatic fistula, pancreatitis, cardiac, pneumonia, sepsis, intra-abdominal abscess, lymph leak, cholangitis, bile leak, wound infection	40 months for patients less than 80 years old, 19 months for patients 80–90, and 15 months for patients over 90	5-year survival: 43.1% for patients less than 80 years old, 24.4% in those 80–90, and 0% in those over 90

Table 24.1 (continued)

Study	Total No.	Age	Summary of findings	Median survival	Long-term survival
Scurtu et al. [81]	70	75	No difference in 30-day mortality (0 vs 6.2%) or morbidity. Measured endpoints for morbidity: pancreatic fistula, delayed gastric emptying, bleeding, intestinal occlusion, intra-abdominal collection, abdominal wall sepsis, ulcer, biliary stenosis, sepsis, urinary infection, pneumopathy and pleural effusion, neurologic, pulmonary, diarrhea, thrombophlebitis	20 months for all patients	3-year survival: 33.1% in patients less than 75 years old and 27.7% in those over than 75
Finlayson et al. [41]	23,518	70/80	Significant increase in 30-day mortality with increased age for all groups (7 vs 9 vs 16%). Morbidity not reviewed	Not reported	5-year survival: 16% in patients less than 80 years old, 11% in those over 80
Riall et al. [36]	3736	60/70/80	Significant increase in 30-day mortality with increased age for all groups (2 vs 6 vs 7 vs 11%). Morbidity not reviewed	Not reported	Not reported
Ito et al. [43]	98	75	No difference in 30-day mortality (0 vs 3.2%) or morbidity. Measured endpoints for morbidity: pancreatic fistula, delayed gastric emptying, liver abscess, wound infection, intra-abdominal bleeding, respiratory insufficiency, intra-abdominal collection, sepsis, bile leakage, or gastrointestinal bleeding	Not reported	3-year survival: 65.9% for patients less than 75 years old and 50.5% for those over 75
Oguro et al. [22]	561	80	Significant increase in morbidity and significant decrease in median survival. Measured endpoints for morbidity: pancreatic fistula, delayed gastric emptying, abscess, hemorrhage, pneumonia, ascites	65 months in patients less than 80 years old and 43 months in those over 80	5-year survival: 51% in patients less than 80 years old and 46% in those over 80

(continued)

Table 24.1 (continued)

Study	Total No.	Age	Summary of findings	Median survival	Long-term survival
Frakes et al. [23]	193	70	No difference in mortality or morbidity. Measured endpoints for morbidity: Pancreatic leak, gastrojejunostomy leak, atrial fibrillation, pulmonary embolus, abscess, wound infection, wound dehiscence, anastomotic bleed, stricture, pancreatic fistula, enterocutaneous fistula, peritonitis	23 months in patients less than 70 years old, 23.4 months in those 70–75, 16.1 months those 76–80, and 18.7 months in those over 80	5-year survival: 26.7% in patients less than 70 years old, 23% in those 70–75, 0% in those 76–80, and 15.4% in those over 80
Zhang et al. [24]	216	70	No difference in mortality or morbidity. Measured endpoints for morbidity: delayed gastric emptying, pancreatic fistula, abscess, pleural effusion, cardiac, pulmonary, neurologic, urinary infections	14 months in those less than 70 and 20 months in those over 70	5-year survival: 14.8% in those less than 70 and 21.6% in those over 70

have reported that 40% of patients between the ages of 66 and 70 years are candidates for a pancreatectomy, but by the age of 85 years, only 7% are eligible candidates [37, 38].

Resection of the pancreas, either by pancreaticoduodenectomy (PD) (the Whipple procedure) or by total or partial pancreatectomy, is a complex surgical procedure with a high rate of morbidity and mortality.

Mortality rates after pancreatic surgery have dropped to less than 2–5% at experienced centers, but complication rates are high, reaching at least 30% in many centers [36]. Mortality also increases proportionally with age: 6.7% of patients aged 65–69 years, 9.3% of patients aged 70–79 years, and 15.5% of patients aged 80 years or older. Moreover, hospitals with a low pancreatic surgery volume (<11 resections per year) have higher mortality rates than high-volume hospitals (7.3 vs 3.2%, $P < 0.0001$) [39, 40]. These differences were accentuated with each increasing age group.

The Hopkins study showed that 33% of patients older than 80 years presented delayed gastric emptying compared with 18.6% of the patients younger than 80 years ($P = 0.03$) [41]. Other studies reported a similar trend in the occurrence of delayed gastric emptying but without statistical significance [42]. Ito et al. [43] showed a higher incidence of pancreatic fistulas in the elderly, but the results were not significant (45.1% vs 29.9%, respectively, $P = 0.14$). In the study by Hodul et al. [42], the rate of neurologic complications was 9.4% in the older group and 0% in the younger group.

The length of hospital stays increased proportionally with age [36]. The number of patients requiring ongoing inpatient nursing care at the time of discharge increased significantly with age. The proportion of patients who could not be discharged home was 10.6%, 19.2%, and 36.7% for ages 65–69, 70–79, and 80 years or older, respectively ($P < 0.0001$) [41].

The Memorial Sloan Kettering group showed a significant difference in 5-year survival between patients aged 70 years or older (21%, median = 18 mo) and <70 years (29%, median = 24 mo, $P = 0.03$) [44]. Finlayson et al. [41] evaluated the 5-year survival of patients following surgery for pancreatic cancer and demonstrated a decrease from 16.4% in patients aged 65–69 years to 15.6% in patients aged 70–79 years and 11.3% in patients aged 80 years or older, but this difference did not achieve statistical significance. Patients with more than two comorbidities undergoing pancreatectomy for pancreatic cancer had a 5-year survival rate of 10% compared with 14% in patients with fewer than two comorbidities (P = NS).

An accurate preanesthesia and cardiovascular risk assessment is needed to reduce the rates of morbidity and mortality in elderly patients undergoing pancreatic surgery. The perioperative management should also be standardized. Patients should be routinely admitted to the intensive care unit (ICU) or to recovery for the first 48–72 h postsurgery. All patients should receive broad-spectrum antibiotics for 2–3 days and an H2 blocker during the entire postoperative hospital stay [45].

Interestingly, minimally invasive surgery is associated with a lower rate of cardiorespiratory complications, diminished postoperative pain, shorter hospital stays, and a faster reincorporation into daily activities. Therefore, it is a very good option for elderly patients.

In summary, surgery is the only curative treatment in patients with pancreatic cancer. The benefits of surgery do not diminish with age, and therefore, elderly patients should not be denied the surgery a priori based on their age [46]. Although the elderly have a higher surgical mortality rate, this depends, among other factors, on the presence of comorbidities and the experience of the surgeon. Consequently, a proper preoperative assessment must be performed, as well as strict postoperative monitoring. Furthermore, this surgery must be conducted in a center with a high volume of pancreatic surgery patients. Under these conditions, surgical resection can be safely performed in older patients as well.

24.4 Locally Advanced Pancreatic Cancer in the Elderly

Locally advanced pancreatic cancer is defined as a tumor that encases a vascular structure, such as the superior mesenteric artery, celiac axis, or superior or mesenteric vein-portal confluence [47]. It represents approximately 20–25% of all newly diagnosed pancreatic cancers. In the strictest sense, in locally advanced pancreatic carcinoma, resection is not an option. In cases of locally non-resectable disease, the results of previous randomized trials indicated that concurrent external beam radiation therapy (EBRT) and 5-fluorouracil (5-FU) therapy resulted in significantly improved survival compared with EBRT alone or chemotherapy alone [48]. Thus, for locally advanced pancreatic cancer, chemoradiation is the standard of care [49, 50].

In elderly patients with locally advanced pancreatic adenocarcinoma, oncologists are hesitant to indicate chemoradiotherapy because of the associated poor prognosis and high risk of severe toxicities. In fact, in a retrospective cohort study in the United States conducted by Kryzanowska, only 21–27% of elderly patients with locally advanced pancreatic adenocarcinoma received chemoradiation therapy [51].

In the elderly, the tolerability, efficacy, and long-term outcomes associated with chemoradiotherapy remain unclear. Morizane et al. [52] reported the efficacy and tolerability of chemoradiotherapy (fluorouracil infusion 200 mg/m^2/day) plus concurrent radiotherapy (50.4 Gy in 28 fractions over 5.5 weeks) in older (>70 years) vs younger patients (<70 years) with locally advanced pancreatic cancer. The median survival time was longer in the older patients (11.3 vs 9.5 months), and there were no significant differences in the frequency of severe toxicity [52].

Similarly, Miyamoto et al. [53] analyzed a subset of elderly patients (median age of 78 years) receiving definitive chemoradiation therapy. The median overall survival time was 8.6 months, which is comparable to the survival time of younger historic controls. The authors also concluded that chemoradiation therapy in selected elderly patients with locally advanced pancreatic cancer can be considered an appropriate treatment and that further research is needed to reduce the high toxicity associated with this treatment approach [53].

Stereotactic body radiation therapy (SBRT) has been an important recent advance in RT for pancreatic cancer. Pioneered in the locally advance setting, much of the literature has shown that SBRT is well tolerated and effective, providing excellent local control and minimal toxicity [54]. Therefore, SBRT is a promising alternative modality as a definitive treatment for elderly patients with unresectable tumors. Several small studies have evaluated the efficacy and tolerability of SBRT in the locally advanced setting. Chang et al. [55] evaluated 77 patients with unresectable pancreatic adenocarcinoma who received 25 Gy in 1 fraction. In their study, the local free progression rates at 6 and 12 months were 91% and 84%, respectively, and the rate of grade >2 toxicity was 9% [56]. Another interesting recently reported study investigated 26 patients aged 80 years or over who were treated with SBRT (24 Gy in one fraction) alone or in conjunction with chemotherapy [57]. The median OS from SBRT was 7.6 months. More interestingly, there were no acute or late grade ≥3 toxicities, and the treatment was very effective for achieving symptom relief, particularly abdominal and back pain.

Chemotherapy alone without radiotherapy remains an option in the elderly subgroup of patients. Recent phase III studies comparing chemoradiotherapy with chemotherapy alone in patients with locally advanced non-resectable pancreatic cancer have shown that chemotherapy alone is more beneficial in terms of survival outcomes and is better tolerated than combined chemoradiation therapy [58, 59].

With the development of more sophisticated imaging tools, a greater number of patients have been included in a new subgroup: borderline resectable pancreatic cancer [60]. Several criteria have been proposed to define this group. MDACC criteria define borderline resectable pancreatic cancer following possible tumor-vessel relationships as follows: a tumor abutment of the superior mesenteric artery or celiac axis measuring ≤180°, encasement of the hepatic artery amenable to resection and reconstruction, or short-segment reconstructable occlusion of the superior mesenteric vein, portal vein, or superior mesenteric-portal vein confluence [61].

In this scenario, neoadjuvant therapies have been proposed as an alternative option with the aim of downstaging tumors in order to improve microscopic resection rates [62]. This approach could be interesting for elderly patients with borderline or resectable pancreatic cancer where the initiation of adjuvant chemotherapy is frequently delayed or is even discarded, due to surgical complications or comorbidities. Preoperative therapies also provide a time window in which patients who progress or develop distant metastases during treatment, or have a significant functional impairment, can be identified to avoid unnecessary surgery [55]. Few studies have explored the role of neoadjuvant therapy in elderly patients. At the 2014 ASCO Gastrointestinal Cancer Symposium, Miura et al. [63] reported the outcomes associated with neoadjuvant therapy (chemotherapy or chemoradiotherapy) in older patients with resectable or borderline resectable pancreatic cancer. They showed that the older group (aged 75 years or older) compared with the younger group (aged below 75 years) had more hospitalizations during neoadjuvant therapy (50% vs 28%, respectively) and was also less likely to complete the therapy (72.4% vs 89.5%, respectively). Among the patients who completed the therapy, there were no significant differences in complication rates or median overall survival between the two groups.

In conclusion, the neoadjuvant approach is an effective treatment option in elderly patients with borderline resectable pancreatic cancer and could be included in the treatment selection process for older patients who are not candidates for surgery.

24.5 Supportive and Palliative Care for Pancreatic Cancer in the Elderly

Pancreatic cancer is characterized by a high symptom burden at the time of diagnosis and a short survival expectancy because most patients present with incurable locally advanced or metastatic disease. Hence, palliative care plays a key role in the management of these patients.

The most common complications associated with pancreatic cancer are due to tumor growth and infiltration of adjacent structures (biliary obstruction, duodenal obstruction, pancreatic insufficiency, pain) and systemic phenomena (cachexia, thromboembolic events).

More than 75% of patients with pancreatic cancer experience pain due to pancreatic and celiac plexus infiltration [64]. In general, elderly patients with cancer pain are undertreated, and many of them underreport their pain [65]. Adequate treatment for pain is essential to avoid a decrease in quality of life, depression, and deterioration of performance status [66]. Pain should be treated according to the WHO analgesic recommendations. Major opioids are effective in the elderly, but some precautions must be considered because these patients often receive multiple medications [67]. Another treatment option that is available for pain control is a celiac plexus block [68]. This invasive technique achieves adequate pain control in 70–90% of cases and significantly reduces the consumption of narcotics [69]. However, the duration of the analgesic effect does not exceed 2–3 months.

Biliary obstruction is observed in up to 70% of pancreatic cancer patients. Most of these patients are treated successfully with an endoscopically placed stent, with resolution of the obstruction in 90% of cases [70]. When a plastic stent was used, older age was found to be an unfavorable prognostic factor for stent patency [71]. Surgical biliary bypass is usually the last option for patients when stent placement is ineffective. Duodenal obstruction occurs in approximately 20% of patients, and metal stents and palliative surgery are feasible therapeutic approaches [72]. Therefore, elderly patients with a reasonable life expectancy should be offered these palliative procedures which may improve the patient's quality of life.

Cachexia is closely related to pancreatic cancer. It is a multifactorial syndrome that is defined by an ongoing loss of skeletal muscle mass (with or without a loss of fat mass) that cannot be fully reversed via conventional nutritional support and leads to progressive functional impairments. Its physiopathology is characterized by a negative protein and energy balance that is driven by a variable combination of reduced food intake and abnormal metabolism [73]. There is currently no single or combined treatment strategy that has been shown to be successful in all patients [74]. Glucocorticoids and megestrol acetate are effective for improvement of cachexia in 30–50% of cases. Thus, the improved management of cancer cachexia may require a multimodal approach by a multidisciplinary team [75].

24.6 Other Pancreatic Tumors

24.6.1 Serous Cystic Tumor

Serous cystic tumors represent about 30% of cystic pancreatic tumors, more prevalent in the female population (65%) and with a mean age of 62 years (age range 35–84 years). In more than 50% of cephalic-based cases, dimensions vary greatly from a few centimeters up to 20–25 cm (average 6–10 cm).

Serous cystic tumors are considered benign and with a very low tendency to malignant degeneration; thus, the therapeutic strategy is careful clinical monitoring especially of asymptomatic forms in cephalic sites.

During follow-up, if serous cystic tumors become symptomatic in elderly patients being a benign lesion [76], endoscopic biliary stenting or gastrojejunal bypass should be considered instead of surgical resection.

24.6.2 Mucinous Cystic Tumor

Mucinous cystic tumors account for 44–49% of pancreatic cystic neoplasms affecting mainly females (>95%) with a greater incidence between the fifth and sixth decade of life. Despite their being increasing adopted at the level of the pancreatic body tail (75%), cephalic localization is not uncommon (25%).

Given the focal lesions and ultimately malignancy (despite the negativity of a biopsy), the recommended therapy is a radical surgical resection in order to prevent disease progression to more malignant forms, metastasis, and recurrence. For mucinous cystic tumors seated in the cephalopancreatic region, the procedure of choice is pancreaticoduodenectomy, while for the body tail, it is a left pancreatectomy.

Cystadenomas, moderate dysplasia, and noninvasive cystadenocarcinomas treated with radical surgery have a prognosis as high as 100% in 10 years. It should be stressed that in the literature, there are cases of tumor recurrence and metastasis after complete resection even in mucinous cystic tumor without atypia. The situation for invasive cystoadenocarcinomas is quite different, where the prognosis is drastically reduced to 15–33% at 5 years [77].

24.6.3 Intraductal Papillary Mucinous Neoplasm

The IPMN represents 5% of all pancreatic tumors, 11.5% of cystic tumors, and 16.3% of resected pancreatic cancer. They are most frequently localized in the cephalopancreatic region (~70%), predominantly affecting males (65–70%) more than females (30–35%) in around the sixth to seventh decade of life. These tumors are characterized by cystic dilatation of Wirsung and/or its subbranches with the presence of mucin and hairy intraductal proliferations. Originating in the ductal epithelium, in the context of the same lesion, they can simultaneously present different degrees of dysplasia, from simple adenoma to invasive carcinoma. Even though recent progress in imaging has allowed an increase in diagnosis, clinical features and borderline shape may vary in the benign form and in the malignant form, which are both noninvasive and invasive. Therefore, the most appropriate treatment is still subject to discussion. Being a slow-growing malignancy with a good prognosis, its management ranges from simple observation over time to surgical resection. However, distinguishing a benign form from a malignant form, based solely on preoperative imaging, is sometimes very difficult. In an advanced form of IPMN with infiltration of the pancreatic parenchyma, however, the prognosis is poor, and surgical resection of malignant IPMN is therefore crucial [78].

The IPMN can be divided into histological subtypes based on the degree of abnormality: adenoma, borderline, carcinoma in situ which are considered noninvasive forms and invasive carcinoma. It is estimated that approximately 25–48% of these tumors "hides" an invasive carcinoma. With regard to colorectal cancer, there are increasingly growing evidence and discussions which support the adenoma-carcinoma progression model for the intraductal papillary mucinous neoplasm, although the molecular mechanisms of this sequence have yet to be described. Today there is agreement on slow tumor progression, but neither the time required for neoplastic degeneration nor the slow tumor progression is known with any degree of precision. Some authors have calculated that it is on average 3–6 years, if all forms of noninvasive IPMN are potentially malignant. In relation to the extent of involvement of the IPMN ductal system, it can be divided into three subtypes: IPMN main pancreatic duct type (main duct type), IPMN secondary branches type (branch type), and IPMN mixed type (mixed type). The classification is not merely of descriptive and morphological interest but also has important prognostic implications. In fact, the main pancreatic duct type and the secondary branches type have a significant difference of malignancy, oscillating, according to the authors, from 57% to 92% and from 6% to 46%, respectively [79].

24.6.4 Main Pancreatic Duct Type

This is characterized by a partial or diffuse dilatation of the main pancreatic duct. The lumen may present large amounts of mucin, multiple polypoid lesions, and hairy papillary projection. It occurs mainly at the cephalopancreatic level and only occasionally in the tail. Intermittent obstructive episodes, but long-term Wirsung caused by papillary proliferations and precipitated mucin, may lead to chronic pancreatitis making the entire pancreas markedly fibrotic. The finding of a dilatation of the main pancreatic duct >1 cm and intraductal papillary nodules >1 cm in size is often poor prognostic signs as they indicate the presence of a malignant IPMN.

24.6.5 Side Branches Type

The side branches type involves one or more side branches of the main pancreatic duct which are dilated with solitary papillary formations or multiple plugs and intraluminal mucin. The presence of large papillae is indicative of an increased likelihood of the malignant nature of the lesion. The Wirsung is not dilated and contains papillae projecting into the lumen. However, it can make an occlusion of the lumen from which follows a chronic obstructive pancreatitis caused indirectly by the size of the tumor. This type of IPMN is less frequently associated to invasive cancer than the main pancreatic duct type, but no significant difference in prognosis has yet been demonstrated.

24.6.6 Mixed Type

The neoplasm involving both the Wirsung and its secondary branches can be considered as an advanced form of one of the two previous subtypes. In addition to the features found in the secondary branches type, in the mixed type, the main pancreatic duct presents with mucin plugs and buds in the lumen with different degrees of dysplasia. Therefore, if the Wirsung is only dilated as a result of mucin plugs but papillae are absent, it would be a mistake to include it in the mixed type.

Conclusion

In summary, the increasing incidence of pancreatic cancer in the elderly, in conjunction with the special features of this patient population and the poor information available from clinical trials regarding the management of older patients, has resulted in challenges in treatment. However, age should not be the determining factor in decisions regarding the best approach. An integral evaluation of the patient in accordance with appropriate tools should be conducted. Some clinical trials targeting the elderly population are currently underway to gain a better understanding of this disease in older patients.

References

1. Dimick JB, Diener-West M, Lipsett PA. Negative results of randomized clinical trials published in the surgical literature: equivalency or error? Arch Surg. 2001;136:796–800.
2. Rabeneck L, Davila JA, Thompson M, et al. Outcomes in elderly patients following surgery for colorectal cancer in the veterans affairs health care system. R Aliment Pharmacol Ther. 2004;5:1115–24.
3. World population ageing. United Nations: Department of Economic and Social Affairs Population Division. http://www.un.org/esa/population. Accessed 10 Sept 2013.
4. National Centre for Health Statistics. Health, United States. With chartbook on trends in the Health of Americans. Hyattsville: National Centre for Health Statistics; 2006. p. 176.
5. Federal Statistical Office. Germany's Population by 2050. Results of the 11th Coordinated Population Projection. Wiesbaden: Federal Statistical Office; 2006. p. 37.
6. Vladychenko A. Recent demographic developments in Europe. Strasbourg: Council of Europe Publishing; 2005. http://www.coe.int/t/e/social_cohesion/population/Demo2004EN.pdf. Accessed 10 Sept 2013.
7. Howlader N, Noone AM, Krapcho M, et al. SEER Cancer Statistics Review, 1975–2008. Bethesda, MD: National Cancer Institute. Based on November 2010 SEER data submission, posted to the SEERWeb site, 2011. http://seer.cancer.gov/csr/1975_2008/. Accessed 10 Sept 2013.
8. Gooiker GA, van Gijn W, Wouters MWJM, et al. Systematic review and meta-analysis of the volume-outcome relationship in pancreatic surgery. Br J Surg. 2011;98:485–94.
9. Williams DB, Carrillo RG, Traad EA, et al. Determinants of operative mortality in octogenarians undergoing coronary bypass. Ann Thorac Surg. 1995;60:1038–43.
10. Katz NM, Chase GA. Risks of cardiac operations for elderly patients: reduction of the age factor. Ann Thorac Surg. 1997;63:1309–14.
11. Sollano JA, Rose EA, Williams DL, et al. Cost-effectiveness of coronary artery bypass surgery in octogenarians. Ann Surg. 1998;228:297–306.
12. Nehler MR, Taylor LM, Moneta GL, et al. Indications for operation for infrarenal abdominal aortic aneurysms: current guidelines. Semin Vasc Surg. 1995;8:108–14.
13. Siegel RL, Miller KD, Jemal A. Cancer statistics, 2015. CA Cancer J Clin. 2015;65:5–29. https://doi.org/10.3322/caac.21254.
14. Yancik R, Ries LA. Cancer in older persons: an international issue in an aging world. Semin Oncol. 2004;31:128–36. https://doi.org/10.1053/j.seminoncol.2003.12.024.
15. Altekruse SF, Kosary CL, Krapcho M, Neyman N, Aminou R, Waldron W, Ruhl J, Howlader N, Tatalovich Z, Cho H, Mariotto A, Eisner MP, Lewis DR, Cronin K, Chen HS, Feuer EJ, Stinchcomb DG, Edwards BK. SEER cancer statistics review, 1975–2007. Bethesda: National Cancer Institute; 2010. http://seer.cancer.gov/csr/1975_2007/
16. Lasry A, Ben-Neriah Y. Senescence-associated inflammatory responses: aging and cancer perspectives. Trends Immunol. 2015;36:217–28. https://doi.org/10.1016/j.it.2015.02.009.
17. Grimes A, Chandra SB. Significance of cellular senescence in aging and cancer. Cancer Res Treat. 2009;41:187–95. https://doi.org/10.4143/crt.2009.41.4.187.
18. Amedei A, Niccolai E, Benagiano M, Della Bella C, Cianchi F, Bechi P, Taddei A, Bencini L, Farsi M, Cappello P, Prisco D, Novelli F, D'Elios MM. Ex vivo analysis of pancreatic

cancer-infiltrating T lymphocytes reveals that ENO-specific Tregs accumulate in tumor tissue and inhibit Th1/Th17 effector cell functions. Cancer Immunol Immunother. 2013;62:1249–60. https://doi.org/10.1007/s00262-013-1429-3.
19. Amedei A, Niccolai E, Prisco D. Pancreatic cancer: role of the immune system in cancer progression and vaccine-based immunotherapy. Hum Vaccin Immunother. 2014;10:3354–68. https://doi.org/10.4161/hv.34392.
20. Bazhin AV, Shevchenko I, Umansky V, Werner J, Karakhanova S. Two immune faces of pancreatic adenocarcinoma: possible implication for immunotherapy. Cancer Immunol Immunother. 2014;63:59–65. https://doi.org/10.1007/s00262-013-1485-8.
21. Kamisawa T, Yuyang T, Egawa N, Ishiwata J, Tsuruta K, Okamoto A, Koike M. Characteristics of pancreatic carcinoma in the elderly. Int J Pancreatol. 1998;24:31–4.
22. Sato Y, Nio Y, Song MM, Sumi S, Hirahara N, Minari Y, Tamura K. p53 protein expression as prognostic factor in human pancreatic cancer. Anticancer Res. 1997;17:2779–88.
23. Bouchardy C, Rapiti E, Blagojevic S, Vlastos AT, Vlastos G. Older female cancer patients: importance, causes, and consequences of undertreatment. J Clin Oncol. 2007;25:1858–69. https://doi.org/10.1200/JCO.2006.10.4208.
24. Quaglia A, Tavilla A, Shack L, Brenner H, Janssen-Heijnen M, Allemani C, Colonna M, Grande E, Grosclaude P, Vercelli M. The cancer survival gap between elderly and middle-aged patients in Europe is widening. Eur J Cancer. 2009;45:1006–16. https://doi.org/10.1016/j.ejca.2008.11.028.
25. Parmar AD, Vargas GM, Tamirisa NP, Sheffield KM, Riall TS. Trajectory of care and use of multimodality therapy in older patients with pancreatic adenocarcinoma. Surgery. 2014;156:280–9. https://doi.org/10.1016/j.surg.2014.03.001.
26. Hutchins LF, Unger JM, Crowley JJ, Coltman CA, Albain KS. Underrepresentation of patients 65 years of age or older in cancer treatment trials. N Engl J Med. 1999;341:2061–7. https://doi.org/10.1056/NEJM199912303412706.
27. Talarico L, Chen G, Pazdur R. Enrollment of elderly patients in clinical trials for cancer drug registration: a 7-year experience by the US Food and Drug Administration. J Clin Oncol. 2004;22:4626–31. https://doi.org/10.1200/JCO.2004.02.175.
28. Balducci L, Extermann M. Management of cancer in the older person: a practical approach. Oncologist. 2000;5:224–37. https://doi.org/10.1634/theoncologist.5-3-224.
29. Balducci L, Extermann M. Cancer and aging. An evolving panorama. Hematol Oncol Clin North Am. 2000;14:1–16. https://doi.org/10.1016/S0889-8588(05)70274-4.
30. Lamont EB, Schilsky RL, He Y, Muss H, Cohen HJ, Hurria A, Meilleur A, Kindler HL, Venook A, Lilenbaum R, Niell H, Goldberg RM, Joffe S. Generalizability of trial results to elderly medicare patients with advanced solid tumors (Alliance 70802). J Natl Cancer Inst. 2015;107:336. https://doi.org/10.1093/jnci/dju336.
31. Sener SF, Fremgen A, Menck HR, et al. Pancreatic cancer: a report of treatment and survival trends for 100,313 patients diagnosed from 1985–1995, using the National Cancer Database. J Am Coll Surg. 1999;189:1–7.
32. Niederhuber JE, Brennan MF, Menck HR. The National Cancer Database report on pancreatic cancer. Cancer. 1995;76:1671–6.
33. Hatori T. A clinicopathologic study of ductal adenocarcinoma of the head of the pancreas in aged patients 70 years and older. J Jpn Panc Soc. 1993;8:506–15.
34. Riall TS, Reddy DM, Nealon WH, Goodwin JS. The effect of age on short-term outcomes after pancreatic resection: a population-based study. Ann Surg. 2008;248(3):459–67. https://doi.org/10.1097/SLA.0b013e318185e1b3.
35. Ferfuson G. Pancreatico-duodenectomy: operation on two elderly patients. Br Med J. 1954. Riall TS. What is the effect of age on pancreatic resection? Adv Surg. 2009;43:233–49. https://doi.org/10.1016/j.yasu.2009.02.004.
36. Riall TS, Sheffield KM, Kuo YF, Townsend CM, Goodwin JS. Resection benefits older adults with locoregional pancreatic cancer despite greater short-term morbidity and mortality. J Am Geriatr Soc. 2011;59:647–54. https://doi.org/10.1111/j.1532-5415.2011.03353.x.
37. Sohn TA, Yeo CJ, Cameron JL, Lillemoe KD, Talamini MA, Hruban RH, Sauter PK, Coleman J, Ord SE, Grochow LB, Abrams RA, Pitt HA. Should pancreaticoduodenectomy

be performed in octogenarians? J Gastrointest Surg. 1998;2:207–16. https://doi.org/10.1016/S1091-255X(98)80014-0.
38. Meguid RA, Ahuja N, Chang DC. What constitutes a "high volume" hospital for pancreatic resection? J Am Coll Surg. 2008;206:622.e1–9. https://doi.org/10.1016/j.jamcollsurg.2007.11.011.
39. Makary MA, Winter JM, Cameron JL, et al. Pancreaticoduodenectomy in the very elderly. J Gastrointest Surg. 2006;10(3):347–56. https://doi.org/10.1016/j.gassur.2005.12.014.
40. Lieberman MD, Kilburn H, Lindsey M, Brennan MF. Relation of perioperative deaths to hospital volume among patients undergoing pancreatic resection for malignancy. Ann Surg. 1995;222:638–45. https://doi.org/10.1097/00000658-199511000-00006.
41. Finlayson E, Fan Z, Birkmeyer JD. Outcomes in octogenarians undergoing high-risk cancer operation: a national study. J Am Coll Surg. 2007;205(6):729–34. https://doi.org/10.1016/j.jamcollsurg.2007.06.307.
42. Hodul P, Tansey J, Golts E, et al. Age is not a contraindication to pancreaticoduodenectomy. Am Surg. 2001;67(3):270–5.
43. Ito Y, Kenmochi T, Irino T, et al. The impact of surgical outcome after pancreaticoduodenectomy in elderly patients. World J Surg Oncol. 2011;9:102. https://doi.org/10.1186/1477-7819-9-102.
44. Bathe OF, Levi D, Caldera H, et al. Radical resection of periampullary tumors in the elderly: evaluation of long-term results. World J Surg. 2000;24(3):353–8. https://doi.org/10.1007/s002689910056.
45. Aloia TA, Lee JE, Vauthey JN, Abdalla EK, Wolff RA, Varadhachary GR, Abbruzzese JL, Crane CH, Evans DB, Pisters PW. Delayed recovery after pancreaticoduodenectomy: a major factor impairing the delivery of adjuvant therapy? J Am Coll Surg. 2007;204:347–55. https://doi.org/10.1016/j.jamcollsurg.2006.12.011.
46. Targarona J, Callacondo D, Pino C, Rodriguez C, Coayla G, Garatea R, Barreda C, Barreda L. Impact of duodenopancreatectomy in elder patients. Rev Gastroenterol Peru. 2013;33:217–22.
47. Li D, Xie K, Wolff R, Abbruzzese JL. Pancreatic cancer. Lancet. 2004;363:1049–57. https://doi.org/10.1016/S0140-6736(04)15841-8.
48. Shinchi H, Takao S, Noma H, Matsuo Y, Mataki Y, Mori S, Aikou T. Length and quality of survival after external-beam radiotherapy with concurrent continuous 5-fluorouracil infusion for locally unresectable pancreatic cancer. Int J Radiat Oncol Biol Phys. 2002;53:146–50. https://doi.org/10.1016/S0360-3016(01)02806-1.
49. Sultana A, Tudur Smith C, Cunningham D, Starling N, Tait D, Neoptolemos JP, Ghaneh P. Systematic review, including metaanalyses, on the management of locally advanced pancreatic cancer using radiation/combined modality therapy. Br J Cancer. 2007;96:1183–90. https://doi.org/10.1038/sj.bjc.6603719.
50. Moertel CG, Frytak S, Hahn RG, O'Connell MJ, Reitemeier RJ, Rubin J, Schutt AJ, Weiland LH, Childs DS, Holbrook MA, Lavin PT, Livstone E, Spiro H, Knowlton A, Kalser M, Barkin J, Lessner H, Mann-Kaplan R, Ramming K, Douglas HO, Thomas P, Nave H, Bateman J, Lokich J, Brooks J, Chaffey J, Corson JM, Zamcheck N, Novak JW. Therapy of locally unresectable pancreatic carcinoma: a randomized comparison of high dose (6000 rads) radiation alone, moderate dose radiation (4000 rads + 5-fluorouracil), and high dose radiation + 5-fluorouracil: The Gastrointestinal Tumor Study Group. Cancer. 1981;48:1705–10. https://doi.org/10.1002/1097-0142(19811015)48:8<1705.
51. Krzyzanowska MK, Weeks JC, Earle CC. Treatment of locally advanced pancreatic cancer in the real world: population-based practices and effectiveness. J Clin Oncol. 2003;21:3409–14. https://doi.org/10.1200/JCO.2003.03.007.
52. Morizane C, Okusaka T, Ito Y, Ueno H, Ikeda M, Takezako Y, Kagami Y, Ikeda H. Chemoradiotherapy for locally advanced pancreatic carcinoma in elderly patients. Oncology. 2005;68:432–7. https://doi.org/10.1159/000086985.
53. Miyamoto DT, Mamon HJ, Ryan DP, Willett CG, Ancukiewicz M, Kobayashi WK, Blaszkowsky L, Fernandez-del Castillo C, Hong TS. Outcomes and tolerability of chemoradiation therapy for pancreatic cancer patients aged 75 years or older. Int J Radiat Oncol Biol Phys. 2010;77:1171–7. https://doi.org/10.1016/j.ijrobp.2009.06.020.

54. Rwigema JC, Parikh SD, Heron DE, Howell M, Zeh H, Moser AJ, Bahary N, Quinn A, Burton SA. Stereotactic body radiotherapy in the treatment of advanced adenocarcinoma of the pancreas. Am J Clin Oncol. 2011;34:63–9. https://doi.org/10.1097/COC.0b013e3181d270b4.
55. Chang DT, Schellenberg D, Shen J, Kim J, Goodman KA, Fisher GA, Ford JM, Desser T, Quon A, Koong AC. Stereotactic radiotherapy for unresectable adenocarcinoma of the pancreas. Cancer. 2009;115:665–72. https://doi.org/10.1002/cncr.24059.
56. Kim CH, Ling DC, Wegner RE, Flickinger JC, Heron DE, Zeh H, Moser AJ, Burton SA. Stereotactic body radiotherapy in the treatment of pancreatic adenocarcinoma in elderly patients. Radiat Oncol. 2013;8:240. https://doi.org/10.1186/1748-717X-8-240.
57. Chauffert B, Mornex F, Bonnetain F, Rougier P, Mariette C, Bouché O, Bosset JF, Aparicio T, Mineur L, Azzedine A, Hammel P, Butel J, Stremsdoerfer N, Maingon P, Bedenne L. Phase III trial comparing intensive induction chemoradiotherapy (60 Gy, infusional 5-FU and intermittent cisplatin) followed by maintenance gemcitabine with gemcitabine alone for locally advanced unresectable pancreatic cancer. Definitive results of the 2000-01 FFCD/SFRO study. Ann Oncol. 2008;19:1592–9. https://doi.org/10.1093/annonc/mdn281.
58. Loehrer PJ, Feng Y, Cardenes H, Wagner L, Brell JM, Cella D, Flynn P, Ramanathan RK, Crane CH, Alberts SR, Benson AB. Gemcitabine alone versus gemcitabine plus radiotherapy in patients with locally advanced pancreatic cancer: an Eastern Cooperative Oncology Group trial. J Clin Oncol. 2011;29:4105–12. https://doi.org/10.1200/JCO.2011.34.8904.
59. Varadhachary GR, Tamm EP, Abbruzzese JL, Xiong HQ, Crane CH, Wang H, Lee JE, Pisters PW, Evans DB, Wolff RA. Borderline resectable pancreatic cancer: definitions, management, and role of preoperative therapy. Ann Surg Oncol. 2006;13:1035–46. https://doi.org/10.1245/ASO.2006.08.011.
60. Katz MH, Pisters PW, Evans DB, Sun CC, Lee JE, Fleming JB, Vauthey JN, Abdalla EK, Crane CH, Wolff RA, Varadhachary GR, Hwang RF. Borderline resectable pancreatic cancer: the importance of this emerging stage of disease. J Am Coll Surg. 2008;206:833–846.; discussion 846–8. https://doi.org/10.1016/j.jamcollsurg.2007.12.020.
61. Lim KH, Chung E, Khan A, Cao D, Linehan D, Ben-Josef E, Wang-Gillam A. Neoadjuvant therapy of pancreatic cancer: the emerging paradigm? Oncologist. 2012;17:192–200. https://doi.org/10.1634/theoncologist.2011-0268.
62. Liao WC, Chien KL, Lin YL, Wu MS, Lin JT, Wang HP, Tu YK. Adjuvant treatments for resected pancreatic adenocarcinoma: a systematic review and network meta-analysis. Lancet Oncol. 2013;14:1095–103. https://doi.org/10.1016/S1470-2045(13)70388-7.
63. Miura JT, Krepline AN, Duelge KD, George B, Ritch PS, Erickson B, Thomas JP, Mahmoud A, Quebbeman EJ, Turaga K, Johnston FM, Christians KK, Gamblin TC, Evans DB, Tsai S. Neoadjuvant therapy for pancreatic cancer in patients older than age 75. J Clin Oncol. 2014;32(Suppl 3):287.
64. Wyse JM, Chen YI, Sahai AV. Celiac plexus neurolysis in the management of unresectable pancreatic cancer: when and how? World J Gastroenterol. 2014;20:2186–92. https://doi.org/10.3748/wjg.v20.i9.2186.
65. Ferrell BA, Ferrell BR, Osterweil D. Pain in the nursing home. J Am Geriatr Soc. 1990;38:409–14. https://doi.org/10.1111/j.1532-5415.1990.tb03538.x.
66. Torgerson S, Wiebe LA. Supportive care of the patient with advanced pancreatic cancer. Oncology. 2013;27:183–90.
67. Caraceni A, Hanks G, Kaasa S, Bennett MI, Brunelli C, Cherny N, Dale O, De Conno F, Fallon M, Hanna M, Haugen DF, Juhl G, King S, Klepstad P, Laugsand EA, Maltoni M, Mercadante S, Nabal M, Pigni A, Radbruch L, Reid C, Sjogren P, Stone PC, Tassinari D, Zeppetella G. Use of opioid analgesics in the treatment of cancer pain: evidence-based recommendations from the EAPC. Lancet Oncol. 2012;13:e58–68. https://doi.org/10.1016/S1470-2045(12)70040-2.
68. Seicean A. Celiac plexus neurolysis in pancreatic cancer: the endoscopic ultrasound approach. World J Gastroenterol. 2014;20:110–7. https://doi.org/10.3748/wjg.v20.i1.110.
69. McGreevy K, Hurley RW, Erdek MA, Aner MM, Li S, Cohen SP. The effectiveness of repeat celiac plexus neurolysis for pancreatic cancer: a pilot study. Pain Pract. 2013;13:89–95. https://doi.org/10.1111/j.1533-2500.2012.00557.x.

70. Maire F, Hammel P, Ponsot P, Aubert A, O'Toole D, Hentic O, Levy P, Ruszniewski P. Long-term outcome of biliary and duodenal stents in palliative treatment of patients with unresectable adenocarcinoma of the head of pancreas. Am J Gastroenterol. 2006;101:735–42. https://doi.org/10.1111/j.1572-0241.2006.00559.x.
71. Matsuda Y, Shimakura K, Akamatsu T. Factors affecting the patency of stents in malignant biliary obstructive disease: univariate and multivariate analysis. Am J Gastroenterol. 1991;86:843–9.
72. Jeurnink SM, van Eijck CH, Steyerberg EW, Kuipers EJ, Siersema PD. Stent versus gastrojejunostomy for the palliation of gastric outlet obstruction: a systematic review. BMC Gastroenterol. 2007;7:18. https://doi.org/10.1186/1471-230X-7-18.
73. Fearon KC, Voss AC, Hustead DS. Definition of cancer cachexia: effect of weight loss, reduced food intake, and systemic inflammation on functional status and prognosis. Am J Clin Nutr. 2006;83:1345–50.
74. Fearon KC. Cancer cachexia: developing multimodal therapy for a multidimensional problem. Eur J Cancer. 2008;44:1124–32. https://doi.org/10.1016/j.ejca.2008.02.033.
75. Tuca A, Jimenez-Fonseca P, Gascón P. Clinical evaluation and optimal management of cancer cachexia. Crit Rev Oncol Hematol. 2013;88:625–36. https://doi.org/10.1016/j.critrevonc.2013.07.015.
76. Sarr MG, Kendrick ML, Nagorney DM, Thompson GB, Farley DR, Farnell MB. Cystic neoplasms of the pancreas; benign to malignant epithelial neoplasms. Surg Clin North Am. 2001;81:497–509.
77. Wilentz RE, Albores-Saavedra J, Hruban RH. Mucinous cystic neoplasms of the pancreas. Semin Diagn Pathol. 2000;17:31–42.
78. Tanaka M, Chari S, Adsay V, Fernandez-del Castello C, Falconi M, Shimuzu M, Yamaguchi K, Yamao K, Matsuno S. International consensus guidelines for management of intraductal mucinous neoplasm and mucinous cystic neoplasm of the pancreas. Pancreatology. 2006;6:17–32.
79. Terris B, Ponsot P, Paye F, Hammel P, Sauvanet A, Molas G, Bernades P, Belghiti J, Ruszniewski P, Flejou JF. Intraductal papillary mucinous tumors of the pancreas confined to secondary ducts show less aggressive pathologic features as compared with those involving the main pancreatic duct. Am J Surg Pathol. 2000;24:1372–7.
80. Brozzetti S, Mazzoni G, Miccini M, et al. Surgical treatment of pancreatic head carcinoma in elderly patients. Arch Surg. 2006;141(2):137–42. https://doi.org/10.1001/archsurg.141.2.137.
81. Scurtu R, Bachellier P, Oussoultzoglou E, Rosso E, Maroni R, Jaeck D. Outcome after pancreaticoduodenectomy for cancer in elderly patients. Gastrointest Surg. 2006;10(6):813–22. https://doi.org/10.1016/j.gassur.2005.12.010.
82. Oguro S, Shimada K, Kishi Y, et al. Perioperative and longterm outcomes after pancreaticoduodenectomy in elderly patients 80 years of age and older. Langenbeck's Arch Surg. 2013;398(4):531–8. https://doi.org/10.1007/s00423-013-1072-7.
83. Frakes JM, Strom T, Springett GM, et al. Resected pancreatic cancer outcomes in the elderly. J Geriatr Oncol. 2015;6(2):127–32. https://doi.org/10.1016/j.jgo.2014.11.005.
84. Zhang D, Gao J, Li S, et al. Outcome after pancreaticoduodenectomy for malignancy in elderly patients. Hepato-Gastroenterology. 2015;62(138):451–4.

Part VI

Abdominal Wall Defect and Soft Tissue Sarcoma

Primitive Groin Hernias

25

Bruno Martella, Renata Lorenzetti, and Anna Claudia Colangelo

25.1 Introduction

Over the last decades, there have been several doubts about age limits in surgery, but now we can finally assert that there are none. This statement can be considered as a dogma especially with regard to hernia surgery: any hernia in the inguino-femoral region cannot be operated on, because the patient is considered too old. On the other hand, how often must we perform controversial or dangerous procedures (e.g. how often are we requested to perform PEG in terminal patients, whose life expectancy is only about a few weeks), whereas an accurate and non-traumatic (we do not aim to minimise) hernia surgery can provide an elderly patient with a good quality of life? Some observational studies have proven that follow-up delays but seldom prevents surgery [1, 2].

Based on this background knowledge, modern surgical techniques with mesh employment, anaesthesiology improvement, and the possibility to adjust drug administration to individual patients, as well as a positive attitude to a faster recover of everyday activities, allow achievement of similar outcomes with young adult patients.

We should bear in mind that, if a different approach from the above-mentioned one is adopted, a high operation incidence for complication persists, with a higher mortality and morbidity rate than in the elective surgery [3].

B. Martella (✉) • R. Lorenzetti
Geriatric Surgery Unit, University of Padua, Padua, Italy
e-mail: bruno.martella@unipd.it

A.C. Colangelo
General Surgery Residency Program of the University of Padua, Padua, Italy

A. Crucitti (ed.), *Surgical Management of Elderly Patients*,
https://doi.org/10.1007/978-3-319-60861-7_25

25.2 Elderly and Groin Hernias

Approximately 700,000 groin hernia repairs are performed annually in the United States: more than 30% of these operations are carried on an outpatient basis in patients who are 75 years old or over [4]. The incidences of hernia are common in elderly patients, many of whom are unaware of their diagnosis and are not waiting for surgical care. Strangulation is the most important complication and the main cause of postoperative morbidity and mortality.

Literature reports that inguinal hernia prevalence is 1.7% in the general population, whereas in people over 45 years, it is 4%. Inguinal hernia has an incidence of 200/10,000 patients in men over 75 years [5]. It is demonstrated that older patients with long-stay and non-reducible hernia have a high risk of complications, which is higher for femoral hernia. Asymptomatic patients have a high risk of developing pain which is the reason for surgery, as we can assume from previous observational studies [1, 2]. Truss use is never recommended as an ultimate treatment [5]. Elective surgery mortality is very low and is the same as in young adult. Moreover, it is higher in elderly patients who had had emergency surgery with ASA three or more. A Scottish study shows that mortality only relates to people older than 79 years old in emergency surgery (133 deaths out of 31, 525; 0.42%) [6]. Mortality was highest among femoral hernia operations in women (37 deaths/1184 operations; 3.1%); in the same study, it is recommended to perform elective surgery, not outside of normal working hours [6].

In the experience of the Geriatric Surgical Unit of Padua University, 12% of >75-year-old patients were affected by groin hernias vs 1.5% of the general population. Elective surgery mortality rate was zero, whereas complicated hernia treated as emergency had 5% mortality rate (2/5 of over 90-year-old patients died after surgical complications for emergency hernia surgery, on average). Patients 80 years old or older were operated on in an emergency setting in 8% of the cases. In 57% of the cases, the pathological pattern was femoral hernia [7].

25.3 Pre-surgical Assessment

Pre-surgical assessment plays a key role in elderly patients. For general principles, please refer to another chapter of this book. Anaesthesiology assessment for hernia surgical repair in elderly patients does not differ from young patients. Blood tests and radiological examinations are the same for every age. We should bear in mind that elderly patients quite often are already taking complex pharmacological therapies. In this situation, antiplatelet and anticoagulant drugs play an important role. For this reason, an accurate clinical history is needed, avoiding general information, and not minimising important issues, especially with regard to the aforementioned therapies [8].

25.4 Local Anaesthesia

Every kind of anaesthesia can be performed in elderly people. Local anaesthesia plays a fundamental role in elderly patients thanks to its feasibility and efficacy. It is safe, and respiratory and thrombotic complications are minimised because of immediate resumption of deambulation. Patients never suffer sore throat or acute urine retention, seldom nausea or vomiting. In the last few years, local anaesthesia has been associated with laryngeal mask airway ventilation technique. This is very useful, especially for those patients with low adaptation to surgical settings. Loco-regional techniques and general anaesthesia remain very important, especially in an urgent setting, when the chance of a laparotomy increases. Patients undergoing to surgical hernia repair are often obese, whereby these techniques can appear more indicated [9].

Regional anatomy and nerve distribution knowledge is crucial. First of all, an accurate infiltration of the skin and subcutaneous tissue is performed, and then a small dose of anaesthetic is injected under the aponeurosis of the external oblique muscle along the next incision line. So ilio-hypogastric and ilio-inguinal nerves are exposed, and about 0.5 mL of anaesthetic into the more proximal part is enough to obtain an adequate and durable analgesic control. Some millilitres injected near the pubic tubercle and along the inguinal ligament facilitate the isolation of the spermatic cord and then detection of the genital branch of genitofemoral nerve, which must also be infiltrated. At this point, the surgical times are common to all techniques, and small injections of anaesthetic can be performed, if needed.

For the femoral hernias, there are no special devices, also due to the absence of important nerves in this site. An anaesthesia is practised to a plan, paying particular attention to the vessels and accurately infiltrating the hernia neck, because this represents the most sensitive spot.

Regarding the type of anaesthetic, one we find particularly useful is a rapid action anaesthetic on the surface (lidocaine) and a second one which has slightly slower but more prolonged action for deep injections (mepivacaine). The necessary dose varies widely from patient to patient, but it remains well clear of toxic quantities [10].

Because of the increasing number of hernia repairs performed in the outpatient setting, the use of a laparoscopic approach for hernia repair does not appear to provide any cost-saving benefits over existing conventional techniques [4].

25.5 Surgical Technique

Therefore, there is no difference when it comes to the surgical approach, between the elderly and the general population, concerning inguinal or femoral hernia. Thus, there is no surgical indication for direct apposition techniques, like Bassini technique (or its evolutions like Shouldice technique), except in some cases that we will discuss later.

In our experience, Bassini repair was applied until 1990 (in a lot of cases, Terranova's modification was applied) [11]. From 1992, all repairs were performed using the technique, proposed by Lichtenstein in the 1980s, which quickly spread worldwide thanks to his colleagues [12]. Basically, this theory is developed on two principles: polypropylene mesh and "tension-free" repair. Moving on from this one, many more variants have followed, based on the different personal approaches and the micro-details of each procedure. Nevertheless, what really matters are the final results and the prevention of relapses. The operation can be normally performed in local anaesthesia: preventive manual reduction, if painful, must be avoided in order to prevent any patient reaction.

After the injection of local anaesthesia (as previously explained), the incision is placed along the line between the anterior superior iliac spine and the pubic tubercle, extending 8–10 cm up. Opening the subcutaneous fat, the superficial epigastric vein is tied with laces (sometimes there could be two veins): electrocoagulation is not advisable due to the haemocoagulation problems previously mentioned.

Then the fascia of Scarpa is opened and the external oblique aponeurosis is released. Once the external inguinal ring is highlighted, the aponeurosis is incised to reveal the muscular side of the internal oblique muscle, the spermatic cord, and the ilio-hypogastric and the ilio-inguinal nerves. The spermatic cord and the inguinal ligament are divided using an instrument with a bevel edge or a swab. The inguinal ligament is now separated from the free edge of the external oblique muscle, sliding behind the pubic tubercle, and it is surrounded with a cotton band. The isolation from the other surrounding connections can be perfected with electrocoagulation. The ilio-hypogastric and ilio-inguinal nerves must be isolated and safeguarded. Doing so, the space for the following reconstructive phase is completed. Cremaster muscle can be cut longways in two halves. While the medial flap is electro-coagulated, the lateral one is cut and sutured with two laces. The lace around the inferior flap has to be sufficiently long to be found again at the end of the operation. This procedure makes the genital branch of the genitofemoral nerve and funicular vessels visible behind. Sometimes they must be sacrificed with laces in order to simplify the reconstructive time. This can cause annoying paraesthesia in the inner part of the thigh or in the region of women's great labia; however, problems like these are going to be solved spontaneously. If there is a lipoma, it must be completely isolated and then resected with a transfixed stitch.

Now, it is possible to focus on the isolation of the hernia sac. Elderly people can have such large sacs that they can reach deeply the scrotum; in order to avoid bleeding after the operation and, consequently, big hematomas, the sac must be carefully isolated from the vascular structures around, which could be numerous. On the left side, the colon could adhere to the sac: in this case, the hernia sac should not be opened, but just replaced. If the hernia sac is empty, both on the left and on the right side, it is advisable to infiltrate the neck with anaesthetic, to put a transfixed stitch, and then to resect it. Nevertheless, even if resecting the sac is not necessary, it must always be isolated backside from epigastric vessels and upside and on the medial side from the internal oblique muscle. Lastly, the sac can be replaced inside.

All the procedures described so far regard the treatment for the external oblique hernia, with or without slipping.

In the case of direct hernia, which is likely to be larger in elderly people, the isolation time can be easier than in the previously described one, but it must be done carefully. After sectioning the connections with the pubic tubercle and the external oblique muscle and seeing epigastric inferior vessels, the sac is ready to be invaginated.

Internal oblique hernias are less frequent: the treatment is the same as for the direct one, but it is not fundamental to visualise the epigastric vessels.

We are not used to opening the transversalis fascia to look for a concomitant femoral hernia, because we believe that a proper palpation from above is sufficient to exclude its presence. In our experience the link between these two hernias is as rare as the discovery of a femoral hernia during the follow-up.

The surgical technique is the same for women. Isolating the sac of an external oblique or direct hernia is not so difficult. Sometimes it can be useful to resect the round ligament in the exact place where it passes through the internal inguinal ring: in this case, its proximal edge is fixed to the internal oblique muscle with a stitch.

As already mentioned, polypropylene meshes are used during the reconstructive phase. There are many prostheses available on the market. At present, we use a preshaped model (Fig. 25.1). If necessary, a strip is fashioned from a propylene mesh 15 × 15 cm. Even though this is not treated with chemical solutions, we protect the operating field, being sure to change our gloves before applying the mesh.

Before positioning it, a 2/0 polypropylene continuous suture closes the posterior wall of the inguinal canal: this passage makes it possible to replace a sliding or direct sac. In order to clearly see the posterior wall, the spermatic cord is retracted out of the operating field with two grippers. The suture starts from the pubic tubercle: care should be taken not to pass the needle through the periosteum, which causes annoying and long-lasting pains after the operation in this area. 2–3 mm are enough to prepare a valid and secure reinforcement. The suture stops at the internal inguinal ring, without entrapping the spermatic cord. The last step includes the proximal end of cremaster muscle to protect the lower edge of the spermatic cord itself.

Now the mesh can be placed. Firstly, the medial most corner of the mesh, previously trimmed, is fixed medially to the pubic tubercle (as previously explained). Finally, the same suture is used as a polypropylene continuous one to attach the lower border of the mesh with the inguinal ligament. Wrinkles must be avoided. Alternatively, interrupted stitches can be used as well. Once the internal inguinal ring is reached, the spermatic cord is placed between the two tails of the mesh. At this stage, the nerves must be correctly positioned. The suture is continued for two centimetres and completed. The two tails are overlapped and sutured together with a stich around the spermatic cord. The mesh should lay lax on the oblique muscle; an interrupted suture in the middle can be useful to softly fix the mesh to the muscle (Fig. 25.2).

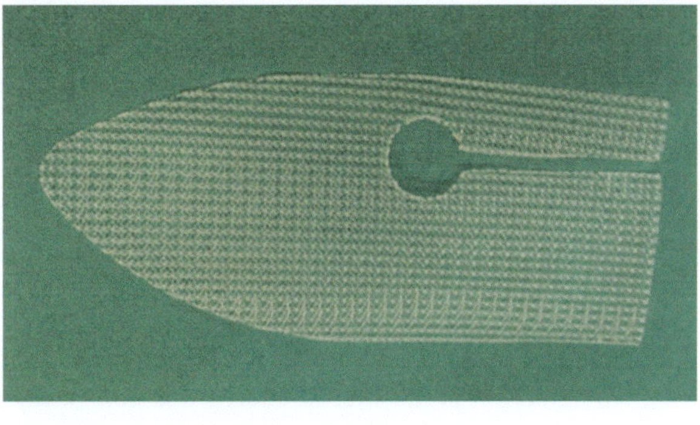

Fig. 25.1 Preshaped mesh

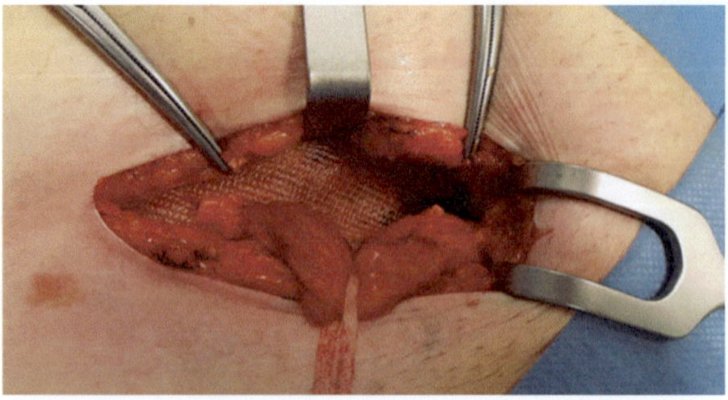

Fig. 25.2 Final aspect after mesh positioning

The reconstruction of the oblique external fascia is now possible with a continuous resorbable suture: the suture includes the distal flap of the cremaster muscle. This can avoid the slipping down of the omolateral testis as the patient sits down.

The reconstruction is the same for women. If the round ligament has been tied, a knot-shaped mesh is used: it is fixed laterally at the inguinal ligament and laid down on the oblique with one or two stiches.

The subcutaneous tissue is rebuilt with continuous or interrupted suture, to obliterate any dead space. The skin is sutured with interrupted stitches or metallic agraphes. Sometimes a continuous suture with a resorbable material is used; thus, it is not necessary to remove it.

Once the medication is done and vital parameters are checked, the patient goes to the waiting area and can walk to their bed: nowadays hygiene rules do not allow the patient to go out of the operating room on foot (this would surely be welcomed by both relatives and patients, as was commonly done in the past). The immediate postoperative period does not require particular attention: immediately after the patient can drink something warm and walk on their own feet. If the diuresis is checked and is normal, the patient can be dismissed. It is also mandatory to ensure the presence of someone able to take care of them.

The technical approach, described above, regards elective surgery. There are no contraindications for this approach in emergency cases as long as appropriate precautions are adopted. In our experience, local anaesthesia was applied in 35% of cases. In 65% of cases, general anaesthesia was required in order to perform laparotomy; in these cases, a bowel resection was performed, almost always for simultaneous intestinal necrosis. Sometimes general anaesthesia is needed for vigorous resuscitation in very serious cases. As in emergency femoral hernia operations, in a limited number of cases, bowel resection was performed through the inguinal approach. In these cases, the original or modified Bassini technique was applied without prosthetic material.

25.6 Femoral Hernia Repair

Femoral hernia is relatively uncommon and represents 3–4% of all abdominal hernias [13]. However, it is very important as more than one-third occur in surgical emergencies: strangulation is the most frequent one and results in increased morbidity and mortality [14, 15]. Scheduled surgery is performed by classical Bassini operation or Lichtenstein plug repair. In our experience, Lichtenstein technique under local anaesthesia is the primary choice in elderly patients scheduled for operation.

Otherwise, we recommend Bassini repair in an emergency situation due to the high risk of postoperative infection under these circumstances. The technical aspects do not differ in elderly patients compared to young adults. Literature reports other techniques, e.g. Lockwood's, Lotheissen's, and McEvedy's approaches, in emergency surgery [16]. In our experience a significant number of little bowel resections were performed widening the femoral orifice by means of the vertical inguinal ligament opening, so avoiding concomitant laparotomy. Results are very encouraging in terms of morbidity and rapid recovery, in the absence of postoperative mortality.

Conclusions

Hernia repair in the elderly patient, also with an asymptomatic inguinal or femoral hernia, may reduce serious morbidity and improve general health. Elderly patients with a short history of herniation should be referred urgently to hospital and receive priority on the waiting list, given that the cumulative probability of strangulation increases in the first 3 months after the onset of symptoms. Femoral hernias should be operated on with high priority to avoid incarceration. Elective surgery is safe, less traumatic, and well accepted by older patients, especially if local anaesthesia is preferred over general anaesthesia, and the procedure is performed in an outpatient setting.

References

1. Fitzgibbons RJ, Giobbie-Hurder A, Gibbs JO, Dunlop DD, Reda DJ, McCarthy M Jr. Watchful waiting vs repair of inguinal hernia in minimally symptomatic men: a randomised clinical trial. JAMA. 2006;295:285–92.
2. O'Dwyer PJ, Norrie J, Alani A, Walker A, Duffy F, Horgan P. Observation or operation for patients with an asymptomatic inguinal hernia. Ann Surg. 2006;244:167–73.
3. Compagna R, Rossi R, Fappiano F, Bianco T, Acccurso A, Danzi M, Massa S, Aprea G, Amato B. Emergency groin hernia repair: implications in elderly. BMC Surg. 2013;13(Suppl 2):S29.
4. Rutkow IM, Robbins AW. Demographic, classificatory, and socioeconomic aspects of hernia repair in the United States. Surg Clin North Am. 1993;73(3):413–26.
5. Jenkins JT, O'Dwyer PJ. Inguinal hernias. BMJ. 2008;336:269–72.
6. McGugan E, Burton H, Nixon SJ, Thompson AM. Deaths following hernia surgery: room for improvement. J R Coll Surg Edinb. 2000;45(3):183–6.
7. Spirch S, Bruttocao A, Militello C, Martella B, Nistri R, Barbon B, Lupia F, Dalla Vecchia D, Sarri C, Verdoglia S, Vecchiato V, Donà B, Terranova O. Nostra esperienza in 15 anni di chirurgia dell'ernia inguinale e crurale nel grande vecchio. In: La chirurgia dell'anziano. Napoli: De Nicola; 2000. p. 363–8.
8. Canonico S, Sciaudone G, Pacifico F, Santoriello A. Inguinal hernia repair in patients with coagulation problems: prevention of postoperative bleeding with human fibrin glue. Surgery. 1999;125(3):315–7.
9. Amato B, Compagna R, Della Corte GA, Martino G, Bianco T, Coretti T, Rossi R, Fappiano F, Aprea G, Puzziello A. Feasibility of inguinal hernioplasty under local anaesthesia in elderly patients. BMC Surg. 2012;12(Suppl 1):S2.

10. Battocchio F. Anestesia locale. In: Battocchio F, editor. Testo atlante di chirurgia delle ernie. Milano: UTET; 1994. p. 13–20.
11. Terranova O, Battocchio F, Nistri R, Martella B, Celi D. Proposte di modifica alla tecnica di Bassini per il trattamento dell'ernia inguinale. Acta Chir Ital. 1989;45:810–2.
12. Lichtenstein IL, Shulman AG. Ambulatory outpatient hernia surgery. Including a new concept, introducing tension-free repair. Int Surg. 1986;71(1):1–4.
13. Powell BS, Lytle N, Stoikes N, Webb D, Voeller G. Primary prevascular and retropsoas hernias: incidence of rare abdominal wall hernias. Hernia. 2015;19:513–6.
14. Gallegos NC, Dawson J, Jarvis M, Hobsley M. Risk of strangulation in groin hernias. Br J Surg. 1991;78(10):1171–3.
15. Dahlstrand U, Wollert S, Nordin P, Sandblom G, Gunnarsson U. Emergency femoral hernia repair: a study based on a national register. Ann Surg. 2009;249(4):672–6.
16. Chia C, Chan W, Yau K, Chan C. Emergency femoral hernia repair: 13-year retrospective comparison to the three classical open surgical approaches. Hernia. 2016;21:89–93.

Incisional Hernias

26

Carmelo Militello and Franco Mazzalai

26.1 Introduction

Incisional hernia is one of the most frequent complications of laparotomy (and one that occurs not only to general surgeons but also to vascular surgeons, gynaecologists, and urologists), with a high variable average incidence between 2 and 50%, probably depending on the heterogeneity of the cohort of patients included and the follow up duration.

In fact, this complication occurs more frequently in the first 3 years after surgery, even though it is possible that it can occur after more than 10 years [1].

The elderly population (i.e. people over 70 years old as worldwide definition) is an increasing phenomenon everywhere, especially in industrialized countries; the frequency of many diseases increases with advanced age; and consequently the number of surgical interventions for this age group is also increasing.

Incisional hernias are burdened with morbidity and mortality, especially in patients requiring more than one corrective surgery.

Elderly people often suffer from medical comorbidities that can facilitate the onset of incisional hernia [2]:

- Hypertension
- Diabetes
- Obesity
- Chronic obstructive pulmonary disease
- Use of steroids, smoking

C. Militello, MD (✉)
Geriatric Surgery Unit, University of Padua, Padua, Italy
e-mail: carmelo.militello@unipd.it

F. Mazzalai, MD
General Surgery, Treviso Hospital, Treviso, Italy

A. Crucitti (ed.), *Surgical Management of Elderly Patients*,
https://doi.org/10.1007/978-3-319-60861-7_26

- Coronary or vascular diseases
- Renal disease requiring dialysis
- Malnutrition
- Immunosuppression
- Connective tissue disorders

Constipation or ascites are conditions that increase abdominal pressure; suture technique (transverse versus midline incision, small bites versus large bites for closure, and slowly resorbable sutures such as PDS versus other resorbable stitches), emergency surgery, surgical site infections, and multiple laparotomy are other possible contributing factors [3, 4].

26.2 Surgical Approach

The Rives–Stoppa technique is the gold standard in the open treatment of incisional hernias, because it allows repairing both the anatomy and the aesthetic of the wall defect.

The main technical phases are the restoration of the deep fascial layer, retro muscular and perifascial placement of prosthetic mesh, and finally the reconstruction of the wall defect.

The first step is to perform a skin incision with excision of the previous scar, isolating the hernia sac from the subcutaneous tissue reaching the rectus muscles fascia and freeing all around the wall defect. The hernia sac should not be opened, to avoid the risk of adhesion formation (except when the peritoneal cavity must be explored, e.g. in case of occlusion of suspected ischaemia).

Then the rectus muscle must be detached from its lateral margin, exposing the retro muscular and perifascial area, where the prosthesis will be placed, using a continuous suture to close the posterior rectus sheath. This ensures that a fascial layer separates the abdominal contents from the prosthesis (if the suture leads to excessive tension and there is residual defect in the closure, we can use part of resected hernia sac or a prosthesis in resorbable material to close it).

The prosthesis is then fixed by stitches to the abdominal wall over the prepared fascial plan (in the original description, stitches were transcutaneous), and the anterior fascial layer is sutured over the prosthesis to separate it from subcutaneous tissue.

One of the main problems of this procedure is the seroma, due to the inflammatory reaction induced by the prosthesis itself (usually drains must be placed for the first day after surgery); there is lively ongoing research for materials causing less inflammatory reaction [5].

Many studies have demonstrated the feasibility of laparoscopy in the elderly [6, 7], so this technique is expanding its application fields (with a decreasing number of laparotomies), and incisional hernias of the trocars sites are less frequent [8].

The advantages of laparoscopic repair of incisional hernias are multiple:

- Allows the diagnosis of other, preoperatively unrecognized, defects
- Decreases intraoperative risk of contamination, also because no viscera are manipulated

– Allows better cosmetic results, early mobilization and refeeding of the patient, and earlier discharge from hospital

After creating the pneumoperitoneum (pressure 10–12 mmHg), the trocars are positioned as laterally as possible and far from the hernia defect to have the best possible view of the operative site. Thereafter the adhesiolysis starts freeing the contents of the hernia sac (Fig. 26.1); this is certainly the most delicate phase, and sometimes it requires a long operative time, but it is essential to avoid bowel injury (or repair immediately if created).

We must measure the diameter of the hernia defect (also with transcutaneous introduction of fine needles), to ensure an overlap of 5 cm per side [9]. The prosthesis (necessarily, with a surface ensuring the lowest bowel adhesions) is fixed to the abdominal wall by tacks (Fig. 26.2), which can have various forms (spirals, anchors) and be resorbable or not [10], creating a "double crown" around the defect, taking

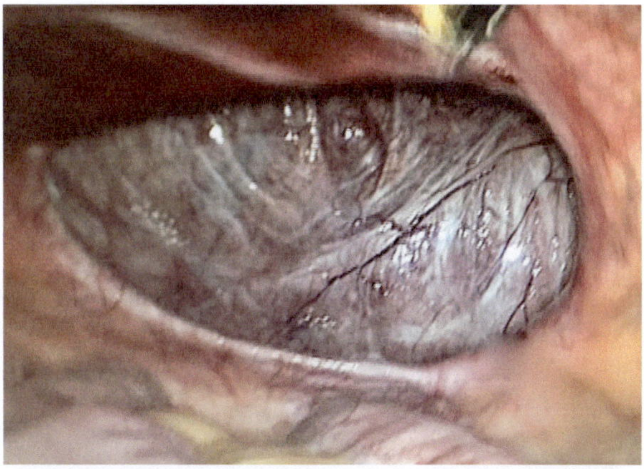

Fig. 26.1 Parietal defect at the end of the hernia contents removal

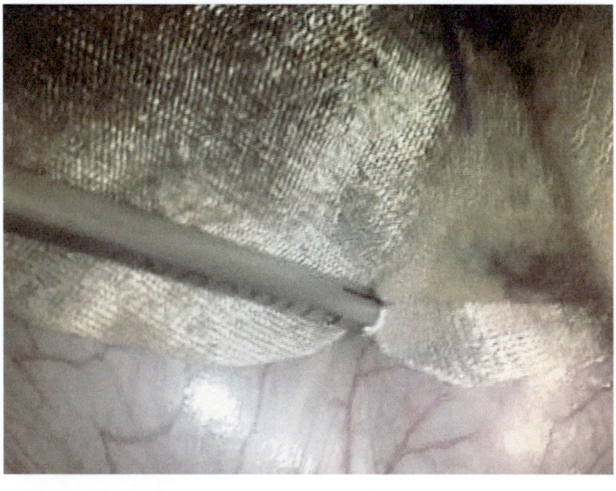

Fig. 26.2 Prosthesis fixation by tacks applicator to the abdominal wall

care not to pierce the epigastric vessels. The more tacks that are used, the higher the risk of pain (nerves entrapment).

The minimum size defect allowing laparoscopy is 3 cm, while there is no agreement on the maximum size.

Not every patient is eligible for laparoscopy: heart and severe pulmonary diseases are anaesthetic contraindications, history of previous surgery with peritonitis or multiple interventions predicts a more difficult (if not impossibility) adequate adhesiolysis, and the giant size of the defect (over 20 cm) makes it difficult to correctly place the prosthesis, as well as the border incisional hernias [11, 12].

26.3 Prosthetic Mesh

The gold standard for the repair of incisional hernias is a technique that involves the placement of a prosthesis.

The materials can vary and differ a lot, also depending on the chosen laparotomy or laparoscopic technique. In case of intraperitoneal placement of the prosthesis, this must ensure the lowest possible adhesions risk.

The main materials used are:

Polypropylene: Minimal risk of bacterial infection, it can be shaped and it is stable in time. The polypropylene microstructure promotes the structural integration with tissues and cell regrowth within its fibres. The fundamental problem of polypropylene is the visceral adhesions.

Polypropylene combined: Polypropylene mesh can be associated with a bioresorbable layer (polydioxanone—PDS) in contact with the bowel, one side coated with oxidized regenerated cellulose layer, which minimizes the formation of adhesions and is completely resorbed within 4 weeks.

This prosthesis is suitable for intraperitoneal use.

ePTFE (polytetrafluoroethylene): One of the oldest prostheses was obtained by combining a PTFE layer with polypropylene, modified subsequently to reduce the thickness and increase the porosity to encourage the colonization of fibroblasts. This prosthesis can be used in contact with the bowel.

Another one combines two layers with different porosity (the inner layer has micropores that minimize adhesion formation; the outer layer has macropores that promote tissue incorporation). It is also suitable for intraperitoneal use.

In the last few years, the use of biological prostheses, derived from animal tissue and appropriately modified, has been increasing; also, this device can be used in contaminated fields. The costs are still high, though.

Many other materials are currently being studied: the main goal is to reduce seroma, bacterial colonization, and adhesion formation, promoting the colonization of fibroblasts for the incorporation of the prosthesis [13].

26.4 Large Incisional Hernias

The width of the hernia is the most significant parameter to distinguish between easy to treat lesions and difficult or impossible ones [14]. This difference is even more evident in elderly patients.

Large incisional hernias (LIH) are those that are a 10 cm or larger in diameter at the rim, such as multiple incisional hernias [15]. In our experience their incidence was about 33% among 616 patients aged over 70 years.

Many advances in the treatment of this serious illness have been registered in the last 30 years.

They can be summarized as follows:

(1) The first advance in care is related to a "better understanding of the pathophysiological bases of the surgical treatment".

The surgeon must understand that LIH takes into account pathological ground, loco-regional lesions of the wall, distant troubles of the respiratory mechanism, and other functions. Thus, it is impossible to treat only the mechanical aspect of the LIH without considering the associated major disorders.

(a) The "pathophysiological ground" of LIH is a sort of prerequisite compound. The patients often suffer from hypertension, diabetes, respiratory disease, and obesity [16]. Most of these systemic impairments, which are both etiological and risk-increasing factors, are difficult to control and make the careful preoperative management of the patient a mandatory step. In practice weight loss and general risks corrections are desired before patient selection for surgery occurs.

(b) "Loco-regional abdominal wall impairments" concern muscles and teguments [17, 18].

Atrophy and sclero-adiposis are elementary lesions of the wall muscles responsible for their poor functional ability in LIH. This is evidenced by histological and electromyographic disorders, which are found in four out of five LIH. These lesions represent the factors inducing LIH enlargement caused by abdominal pressure and medial disinsertion of the fibres of the lateral belt muscles, which pass around the rectus abdominis to reach the midline. Muscular lesions depend on the LIH site. Since their peripheral extremities degenerate, lateral lesions are more severe once muscular fibres have been cut. In peripheral lesions with a chondrocostal, iliac, or pubis edge, fibres are destroyed and contractility cannot be preserved.

Trophic changes of the skin must be given particular attention. They culminate when a dystrophic ulceration appears at the top of the bulge (Fig. 26.3). Histologic findings confirm the trophic mechanism of the lesion by capillary thrombosis. Since the risk of infection of the ulcer is high, the surgeon must

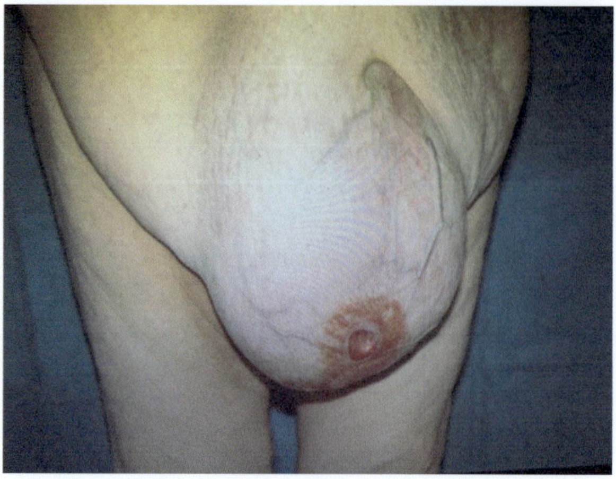

Fig. 26.3 Dystrophic ulceration at the top of the bulge of a giant hernia

treat the skin lesion before undertaking the hernia repair. Obesity often causes an apronlike cutaneous fold that is subjected to dermatosis; it must be treated and preferably resected at the time of repair.

(c) *Distant troubles* related to LIH are the following:

Respiratory troubles: They are dangerous, mostly in obese patients and in patients suffering chronic respiratory diseases, as many aged patients do. The large defect and the visceral protrusion lead to a decrease in abdominal pressure, causing respiratory and regional disorders, which are likely to influence the general status of the patient [19]. The respiratory consequences of LIH require the attention of both the surgeon and the anaesthetist. We should distinguish between two types of LIH. In the first one the visceral contents are movable through the large defect, whereas in the second one the contents of the sac are fixed in place by adhesions and cannot reintegrate into the abdomen. In the first scenario, the reduction of the viscera exposes the patient to little postoperative respiratory risk. In the second LIH type, where the herniated organs have lost their right of domain in the abdomen, the respiratory danger occurs during the reduction of the herniated viscera, when the increase of abdominal pressure impedes normal diaphragmatic action. In such a case the operative repair may be very dangerous.

Other consequences of LIH affect diverse organs. The splanchnic venous system and inferior vena cava are subjected to stasis caused by low abdominal pressure [20]. Hollow viscera are atonic and hypokinetic for the same reason. LIH may cause lumbar lordosis due to inefficient muscular support of the rectus abdominal. All of these disorders have practical consequences, which must be evaluated by the anaesthetist and the surgeon while preparing the patient for the surgical trauma.

(d) Finally, *preoperative preparation and postoperative observation* are as important as the operation itself.

Indeed, the treatment of LIH must solve two distinct problems: (1) Closure of the defect and loss of the parietal substance (mechanical problem); (2) recovery of normal respiratory function by surgical reinsertion of the lateral muscular belt of the abdomen (pathophysiologic problem).

1. Skin preparation includes decontamination and treatment of trophic ulcers and sinuses related to nonabsorbable sutures. Sometimes the operation should be delayed until 6 months after complete skin healing.
2. General and respiratory preparation may be long and complex. In older patients, the association of weight loss, cardiac disorders, diabetes, and renal failure may be the most relevant complicating problem. In the case of "very large" incisional hernias, we used progressive preoperative pneumoperitoneum, which has an interesting triple action. It enlarges the abdominal cavity and decreases the likelihood of respiratory distress due to the reduction of the contents of voluminous hernias, it facilitates the intraoperative dissection of intrasaccular and intra-abdominal adhesions, and it supports diaphragmatic functional rehabilitation producing a higher abdominal pressure [21].

Respiratory preparation is mandatory because of common pre-existing problems. It consists of respiratory physiotherapy, cough training, ceasing use of tobacco, and eventually postural drainage.

(2) The second type of advances in the care of the LIH is that the "surgeon" *understands completely the goals of the difficult treatment and correctly uses the appropriate means for reaching them.*

(a) The first goal is, of course, *closing the wall defect.* A simple repair cannot be used to treat LIH, especially in the elder patients, for whom the control of the abdominal pressure represents the main issue. Prosthetic repairs are the major improvement in the surgical technique of LIH repair, which were previously considered as inoperable. Abdominal pressure may be decreased enlarging the abdominal cavity. This can be achieved in two ways. In the first way, the defective peritoneum is replaced by suturing to its margins a non-adhesive prosthesis in direct contact with the viscera. This is followed by a prosthetic Rives repair with a polypropylene mesh [22]. In the second way, an intra-peritoneal prosthetic repair can be obtained using a double-layered composite prosthesis in direct contact with the viscera. The two surgical ways to repair LIH offer advantages in the control of abdominal pressure and in the correct tailoring of the abdominal wall. The disadvantages are the complexity of the technique and the extended operating time.

A very interesting suggestion to simplify the technique is the use of a modified Bard Composix E/X mesh as proposed by Munegato e coll. [23] (Fig. 26.4). In this composite mesh two free different flaps were created. The upper one,

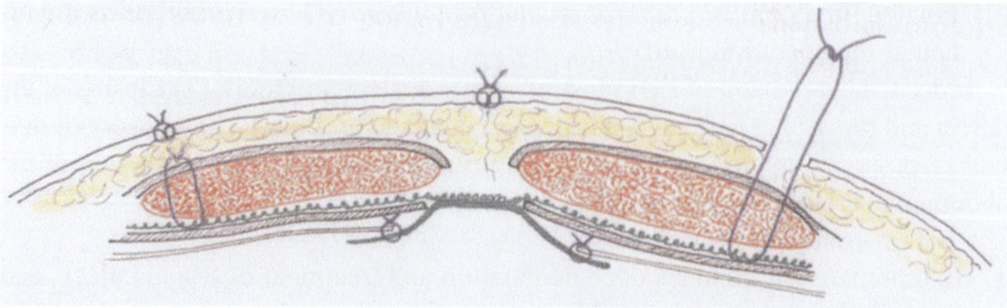

Fig. 26.4 The application of a Composix mesh is schematized. The upper polypropylene flap is placed in the retro muscular area, while the lower ePTFE one is fixed to the peritoneum

made in polypropylene, is placed in the retromuscular area according to Rives technique, while the lower one, made in ePTFE, is fixed to the peritoneum. This technique combines the advantages of Rives repair and endo-abdominal repair allowing enlargement of the abdominal cavity.

(b) The second goal is the *restoration of a correct abdominal pressure*. We think that the Goni Moreno preoperative pneumoperitoneum is a valuable choice, mostly when the contents are irreducible [24, 25]. As previously described, the choice of a large and suitable prosthesis is the main way to restore the lateral muscle belts function and carefully reach a normal internal pressure. During the operation, it is very important to avoid an increase of abdominal pressure and a reduced respiratory compliance, which may cause postoperative respiratory complications, mainly in obese and elder patients. During surgery is mandatory to measure variations of respiratory mechanics in real time. Moreover, it may be useful to measure bladder pressure at the beginning and during the surgery, as this may be sufficient to evaluate variations in abdominal pressure [26].

(c) A third important and *conclusive* consideration about the surgery of LIH is that the surgeons must know that *contraindications of surgery do exist*! Thus, patients with higher risk must be carefully prepared, and sometimes, if necessary, the operation must be deferred or cancelled.

References

1. Caglià P, et al. Incisional hernia in the elderly: risk factors and clinical considerations. Int J Surg. 2014;12(Suppl 2):S164–9.
2. Langer C, et al. Prognosis factors in incisional hernia surgery: 25 years of experience. Hernia. 2005;9:16–21.
3. Deerenberg EB, et al. Small bites versus large bites for closure of abdominal midline incisions (STITCH): a double-blind, multicenter, randomised controlled trial. Lancet. 2015;26:1254–60.
4. Ohira G, et al. Synthetic polyglycomer short-term absorbable sutures vs. polydioxanone long-term absorbable sutures for preventing incisional hernia and wound dehiscence after abdominal wall closure: a comparative randomized study of patients treated for gastric or colon cancer. Surg Today. 2015;45:841.e–5.e.

5. Tandon A, et al. Parietex™ composite mesh versus DynaMesh®-IPOM for laparoscopic incisional and ventral hernia repair: a retrospective cohort study. Ann R Coll Surg Engl. 2016;98:568–73.
6. Zhang Y, et al. Laparoscopic versus open incisional and ventral hernia repair: a systematic review and meta-analysis. World J Surg. 2014;38:2233–40.
7. Al Chalabi H, et al. A systematic review of laparoscopic versus open abdominal incisional hernia repair, with meta-analysis of randomized controlled trials. Int J Surg. 2015;20:65–74.
8. Kössler-Ebs JB, et al. Incisional hernia rates after laparoscopic or open abdominal surgery. A systematic review and meta-analysis. World J Surg. 2016;40:2319–30.
9. Le Blanc K. Proper mesh overlap is a key determinant in hernia recurrence following laparoscopic ventral and incisional hernia repair. Hernia. 2016;20:85–99.
10. Pawlak M, et al. Comparison of two different concepts of mesh and fixation technique in laparoscopic ventral hernia repair: a randomized controlled trial. Surg Endosc. 2016;30:1188–97.
11. Abet E, et al. Laparoscopic incisional hernia repair: long term results. J Visc Surg. 2014;151:103–6.
12. Ahonen-Siirtola M, et al. Complications in laparoscopic versus open incisional ventral hernia repair. A retrospective comparative study. World J Surg. 2016;39:2872–7.
13. Bondre IL, et al. Suture, synthetic, or biologic in contaminated ventral hernia repair. J Surg Res. 2016;200:488–94.
14. Wantz GE. Atlas of hernia surgery. New York: Raven Press; 1991.
15. Chevrel JP. Classification of the incisional hernia of the abdominal wall. Hernia. 2000;4:7–11.
16. Romano G, et al. Fixation-free incisional hernia repair in the elderly: our experience with a tentacle-shaped implant. Aging Clin Exp Res. 2016;29(Suppl 1):173–7.
17. Klinge U, et al. Development and pathophysiology of abdominal wall defects. Chirurg. 1997;68:304–9.
18. Franz MG. The biology of hernias and the abdominal wall. Hernia. 2006;10:462–71.
19. Trivellini G, et al. Traitement chirurgical des grandes eventrations. Etude d'une technique adaptée aux troubles de la compliance respiratoire. Chirurgie. 1984;110:116–22.
20. Jensen KK, et al. Abdominal wall reconstruction for large incisional hernia restores expiratory lung function. Surgery. 2017;161:517–24.
21. Goni Moreno I. Les pneumopéritoines dans la reparation pré-opératoire des grandes éventrations. Chirurgie. 1970;9:581–5.
22. Rives J, et al. Major incisional hernias. New York: Springer; 1987. p. 116–44.
23. Munegato G, et al. Respiratory physiopathology in surgical repair of large abdominal hernias. In: Crovella F, et al., editors. Incisional hernia. New York: Springer; 2008. p. 57–70.
24. Renard Y, et al. Management of large incisional hernias with loss of domain: a prospective series of patients prepared by progressive preoperative pneumoperitoneum. Surgery. 2016;160:426–35.
25. Elstner KE, et al. Preoperative progressive pneumoperitoneum complementing chemical component relaxation in complex ventral hernia repair. Surg Endosc. 2016;31(4):1914–22.
26. Angelici AM, et al. Measurement of intra-abdominal pressure in large incisional hernia repair to prevent abdominal compartmental syndrome. G Chir. 2016;37:31–6.

The Management of Soft Tissue Sarcoma in the Elderly

27

Sergio Sandrucci

27.1 Introduction

Soft tissue sarcomas (STSs) are a diverse group of malignant tumors that originate from mesenchymal tissue. 13,100 new cases of STS are diagnosed annually in the European Union and approximately 8500 annually in the USA [1].

Approximately one-half arise in the extremities, and one-third arise in the abdomen, pelvis, and retroperitoneum. They account for just 1% of all cancers, and despite presenting in a bimodal distribution, they are still considerably more common in the elderly (85%). There are more than 70 different subtypes of STS subcategorized by their histological appearance, although overall the group remains relatively rare compared to their benign soft tissue tumor counterparts (100:1). The most common histologic subtypes in elderly people are liposarcomas, leiomyosarcomas, and synovial sarcomas [2] (Tables 27.1 and 27.2).

STSs classically present as a slowly growing lump or swelling which may be painful. In rare cases a patient may complain of symptoms resulting from mass effect or local neurovascular invasion, especially in retroperitoneal locations. There is often a significant time delay between the initial presentation of many STSs in primary care and subsequent referral to an appropriate tertiary center, as symptoms or clinical presentation are underevaluated [3].

Ultrasonography (US), although characterized by a low accuracy, is often the first-line modality used to investigate soft tissue lesions due to its widespread availability and relatively low cost [4, 5]. Magnetic resonance imaging (MRI) is the preferred investigation; all potential STS cases should undergo an MRI prior to definitive management decisions, as it is able to characterize the tumor's boundaries and surrounding inflammatory zone, and quantify any local soft tissue or

S. Sandrucci (✉)
Sarcoma Unit, Città Della Salute e della Scienza, S. Giovanni Battista Hospital, University of Turin, Turin, Italy
e-mail: sergio.sandrucci@unito.it

A. Crucitti (ed.), *Surgical Management of Elderly Patients*,
https://doi.org/10.1007/978-3-319-60861-7_27

Table 27.1 The National Cancer Institute grading for soft tissue sarcomas

Grade 1	Grade 2	Grade 3
Well-diff liposarcoma	Pleomorphic liposarcoma	Alveolar rhabdomyosarcoma
Myxoid liposarcoma	Fibrosarcoma	Soft tissue osteosarcoma
Dermatofibrosarcoma protuberans	Malignant fibrous histiocytoma	Primitive neuroectodermal tumor
Some leiomyosarcomas	Malignant hemangiopericytoma	Alveolar soft part sarcoma
Epithelioid hemangioendothelioma	Synovial sarcoma	Mesenchymal chondrosarcoma
Spindle cell hemangioendothelioma	Leiomyosarcoma	>15% necrosis
Infantile fibrosarcoma	Neurofibrosarcoma	
Subcutaneous myxofibrosarcoma	0–15% necrosis	

The grading and staging of soft tissue sarcomas. In: Fletcher C, editor. Pathology of soft tissue sarcomas. Edinburgh, Scotland: Churchill-Livingstone; (1990). pp. 221–238

Table 27.2 Frequent histotypes in retroperitoneal sarcomas in the elderly

DD liposarcoma	43%
WD liposarcoma	20%
Leiomyosarcoma	17%
Solitary fibrous tumor	6%
Pleomorphic sarcoma	6%
Other	8%

Smith HG, Thomas JM, Smith MJ et al. Multivisceral resection of retroperitoneal sarcomas in the elderly. Eur J Cancer. (2016) Dec; 69: 119–126

neurovascular infiltration. Computed tomography (CT) is less accurate and can be used when claustrophobia prohibits a patient's willingness to undergo MRI or when this latter is contraindicated [6].

All forms of imaging should be considered an adjunct to a diagnostic biopsy, which is mandatory in most cases (and in any case of radiological features that are of concern) in order to grant a proper evaluation of a multidisciplinary team (MDT) or a tumor board prior to definitive treatment [5].

Several techniques can be used to biopsy soft tissue lesions including core needle biopsy (CNB), fine needle aspiration (FNA), and incisional (open) biopsy [6].

Regardless of biopsy technique, multiple (usually three or more) specimens should be taken, ideally from the periphery of the lesion to avoid any central necrotic tissue. An additional sample should also be taken for microbiological assessment to exclude infection. Compartmental barriers should not be breached unless absolutely unavoidable, and if curative resections are subsequently performed, biopsy tracts should be removed en bloc with the specimen [4, 6].

Surgery is the only potentially curative therapy in the management of STSs in elderly patients. The standard of care is the en bloc removal of the tumor with a cuff of healthy tissue all around, to avoid cell spillage from its surface (if no real capsule is present but a pseudocapsule of compressed cells) and allow removal of microimplants which may be present around the pseudocapsule itself [2]. The extent of resection (and the subsequent prognostic adequacy of margins) depends on a variety of factors, including histology and the presence of an intact biologic barrier (muscular fascia, vascular adventitia, periosteum, or epineurium) [4, 5].

The elderly frail patient who undergoes surgery is more likely than a fit patient to experience postoperative complications, prolonged hospital stay, discharge to nursing homes or long-term care facilities, and high mortality rates. Extended surgery may be challenging due to the high frequency of coexisting multiple or complex medical problems and geriatric syndromes (such as dementia, falls, malnutrition, sensory impairments), impaired physiologic and functional reserves, and restrictions in personal and social resources [7]. For this reason, such patients deserve a personalized treatment after an accurate multidisciplinary evaluation by a surgical, medical, and radiation oncologist jointly with other specialists (plastic surgeon, orthopedist, physiotherapist, pathologist, palliative care specialist), in order to select the best therapeutic strategy in cases in which a decreased ability to tolerate proper treatments may result [8].

27.2 Surgical Principles for Primary Operable Elderly Patients

The main concern in sarcoma surgery in the elderly is to preserve function and quality of life and to personalize treatment according to histotype, rehabilitation attitudes, and possibilities.

27.2.1 Extremities Sarcomas

STS of the extremities must represent a clinical dilemma in terms of function preservation in the elderly, as autonomy can be impaired and long rehabilitation tracks can be required. Age alone should not determine prosthetic rehabilitation: comorbidities and performance status are important determinants [8].

Surgical resection should be carefully planned based on preoperative imaging and patient's characteristics; the goal must be function sparing while achieving appropriate oncologic margins. Postoperatively, early mobilization is crucial to avoid the deleterious effects of immobility in the older person.

Soft tissue limb sarcomas often invade or are adjacent to key neurovascular structures; in this situation, the first decision to be made is whether to adopt a limb-sparing surgical approach or to perform an amputation [9]. Amputation does not increase survival when compared to limb salvage surgery: however, it can provide improved local control and symptomatic treatment in cases in which limb salvage might not be performed, such as tumors that involve the underlying bone and/or a critical neurovascular bundle (in particular, nerve rather than vessels), or in large lesions whose resection is not compatible with a functional limb [2]. The more proximal the amputation, the more energy is demanded from the cardiovascular and pulmonary systems for prosthetic gait: however, the shortened longevity emphasizes the need for timely rehabilitation to enhance the quality of the remaining years. Presurgical care and the preprosthetic phase of rehabilitation must be given attention and added to the problems common to the older patient (comorbidities, polypharmacy, immobility, and depression) [10].

Disease-free survival and time to relapse are strictly dependent from quality of margins and tumor biology. Margins are described as radical, wide, marginal, or intralesional depending on the plane of the resection's relationship to the tumor, the tumor's pseudocapsule and reactive zone, and the anatomical compartment in which the tumor is found. A reliable characteristic of STSs is their relative inability to invade the fascia or bone; Enneking [11] described a radical resection as the removal of the entire anatomical (fascial) compartment containing the STS, where tumor boundaries are respected. This principle means that a radical resection which can ensure removal of all STS tissue (microscopic and macroscopic) implies obvious functional consequences.

A wide resection includes the tumor (with an intact pseudocapsule) and the tumor's reactive zone. Although a cuff of surrounding normal tissue is excised in a wide resection, it should be recognized that in high-grade STSs, microscopic skip lesions may still be missed. In practical terms, a wide resection would normally include the involved muscle and adjacent fascia or periosteum, but not any uninvolved neurovascular structures or muscles within the anatomical compartment [12].

A marginal resection includes the tumor (with an intact pseudocapsule) but not its entire reactive zone.

A marginal excision is usually performed when a tumor's reactive zone includes adjacent or nearby neurovascular structures, whose resection may leave a significant functional impairment. Marginal excisions imply a significant risk of residual microscopic disease for high-grade tumors or infiltrative low-grade tumors. Despite this, for certain low-grade tumors (such as well-differentiated liposarcomas), marginal resections may ensure local control [13] and offer, over a wide resection, the advantage of maintaining function.

An intralesional resection leaves macroscopic remnants of tumor. This can be either planned (e.g., curettage) or unplanned as an inadvertent excision (the so-called "whoops" procedure). This latter should be avoided due to its negative impact on long-term prognosis; unplanned excisions with residual tumor have significantly lower survival probabilities and a higher amputation rate than unplanned excisions without residual disease.

If a limb-conserving procedure is chosen, a decision must then be made whether to perform a resection that will have a planned marginal or positive margin (to protect the involved neurovascular structures) or a more radical excision (accepting that the involved structures must be sacrificed).

In most low-grade lesions, microscopic infiltration of the reactive zone is unlikely, with the exception of myxofibrosarcomas (which are recognized by their high local recurrence rates [14]). As a result, long-term local control may follow a planned marginal excision combined with adjuvant radiotherapy, making this approach wholly appropriate and amputation unnecessary for these lesions.

For higher-grade lesions, the "limb-sparing versus amputation" decision is less clear-cut. Good outcomes in terms of disease-free and overall survival have been reported following less extensive, planned, limb-sparing surgeries combined with adjuvant radiotherapy. Limb salvage surgery offers better gait efficiency and return to normal living compared with amputation, but does not improve the patient's perception of quality of life and implies an intense rehabilitation track. If limb-sparing surgery is felt appropriate but significant neurovascular structures are found adjacent to a STS, a decision of whether to sacrifice these structures to gain wider histological margins must also be made. Although local recurrence rates of just 3.6% have been reported following planned, marginal STS excisions in this scenario in soft tissue tumor units [30], it should also be recognized that a major lower limb nerve resection does not necessarily lead to a nonfunctional outcome [15]. In reality, either approach can often be justified, and this decision must be made in close conjunction with patients, with frank discussions held over the implications of any neurovascular structure's sacrifice.

The current absolute indications for a primary amputation for a STS are becoming relatively rare and continue to fall as the armory of techniques available to reconstruct vascular and soft tissue defects continues to grow. Currently, only around 9% of STS patients undergo an amputation with curative intent, and a higher rate is observed in elderly patients [16].

Decisions regarding the appropriate level for amputation should be decided preoperatively in an MDT setting with input from sarcoma radiologists, specialist sarcoma surgeons, and reconstructive plastic surgeons. The role of the physiotherapist is crucial to preview the rehabilitation opportunities, and the treatment must be personalized for each patient. As a matter of fact, regardless of the chosen intervention, detailed preoperative counseling and postoperative access to limb prostheses and rehabilitation are essential.

27.2.2 Trunk Soft Tissue Sarcomas

In order to obtain wide margins in extensive superficial or fungating soft tissue sarcomas, skin removal en bloc with muscles and the tumor are necessary. Although primary wound closure is possible without reconstructive surgery in the majority of STS resection surgeries, up to 38% of patients may require some form of soft tissue reconstruction [17]. Even after re-resections following unplanned incomplete resections, soft tissue reconstruction is only required in around 17% of cases [18].

Surgical planning for potentially problematic (large) STSs should be done preoperatively with a reconstructive plastic surgeon.

Reconstruction of the abdominal wall can be achieved relatively simply using Prolene mesh, while reconstruction of the chest wall may be more complex and will require the input of a specialist thoracic surgeon.

27.2.3 Retroperitoneal Sarcomas

Elderly people account for a significant number of patients presenting with retroperitoneal sarcomas, with 60% of them occurring in patients aged over 60 years [19, 20]. Patients with retroperitoneal soft tissue sarcomas (RPS) are often asymptomatic until the mass reaches a large size (often 15 cm or greater). Symptoms include a palpable mass, early satiety, abdominal discomfort, or occasionally a new varicocele in men. Others may be incidental findings during abdominal imaging for other reasons.

Retroperitoneal sarcomas are distinct from other soft tissue sarcomas, in that local recurrence, rather than distant metastasis, is the most common cause of disease-specific mortality, accounting for 75% of deaths [21]. Extended surgical resections, encompassing adjacent uninvolved organs, have been adopted by several sarcoma centers with the aim of improving local control and patient outcomes [21, 22]. Compared to limited resections, extended resections have been shown to improve oncological outcomes (60% of patients surviving 5 years) with an acceptable perioperative morbidity.

Proper resection of RPS requires appreciation of the anatomic boundaries of the tumor [23]. CT imaging should be reviewed to identify landmarks defining the extent of the mass to determine which structures may be safely resected and which ones cannot. The *anterior* margin of a RPS is generally the ipsilateral colon and mesocolon, pancreas, liver, or stomach. The *posterior* margin is generally the psoas and iliacus muscles inferiorly, the ipsilateral kidney and diaphragm superiorly, and the ipsilateral ureter and gonadal vessels medially. However, this may vary from tumor to tumor, and some or all of these structures could be anterior to the mass, in which case they would constitute a portion of the anterior margin. The *medial* margin usually includes the spine and paraspinous muscles, the inferior vena cava (for right-sided tumors), and the aorta (for left-sided tumors). The *lateral* margin is constituted by the lateral or flank musculoskeletal sidewall, although depending on the size and location of the tumor, the kidney and/or colon could also border the lateral portion of the mass. The *superior* margin is similarly dependent on the size and location of the mass and may include the diaphragm on either side; the right lobe of the liver, the duodenum, and the head/uncinate process of the pancreas for right-sided tumors; and pancreatic tail, spleen, and splenic vessels for left-sided tumors. The *inferior* margin may include the iliopsoas muscle; the femoral nerve; the common, internal, and external iliac vessels; and the pelvic sidewall [21]. Clearly, the size and specific location of the mass determine which of the many structures mentioned above constitute which specific margin.

In general, the ipsilateral kidney, colon and mesocolon, and at least a portion of the psoas can be safely and relatively easily resected without much difficulty. Resection of the pancreatic tail and spleen can usually be performed with relatively low short-term morbidity. Resection of other structures, including but not limited to the aorta, inferior vena cava, iliac vessels, femoral nerve, diaphragm, duodenum, pancreatic head or uncinate process, and liver, entails more significant resections, with ensuing greater morbidity [24].

The proportion of elderly patients that are fit for extended resections at presentation and the outcomes of surgery in this age group is unknown. A surgical approach is still potentially beneficial in the elderly, as life expectancy is over 10 years in people of 75 years of age of either sex and does not fall below 5 years until beyond the age of 85 years [19].

However, extended resections for retroperitoneal sarcoma are a substantial undertaking. The proportion of patients treated nonoperatively is significantly higher in those aged over 65 years, with no difference in the proportion of patients presenting with unresectable disease between older and younger patients, due to unsuitability to major surgical intervention for comorbidities or surgery refusal. Perioperative morbidity has a threefold increase in patients over 65 years, but perioperative mortality does not increase compared to younger patients, and no evidence exists in identifying age as a prognostic factor [20, 25].

The location, rather than the absolute size, of retroperitoneal sarcomas is most pertinent in determining resectability, with the median tumor size in patients unsuitable for surgery being on average smaller than those proceeding to operation. In case of established renal insufficiency, the tumor must be deemed to be inoperable, as resection would necessitate a nephrectomy, which would likely render the patient dialysis dependent. Renal replacement therapy has not been shown to improve survival in the elderly when comorbidities are taken into account, and the median survival of elderly patients on dialysis is approximately 3 years [19, 24]. As such, it becomes difficult to justify an extended resection that is likely to result in end-stage renal failure, although these decisions should be made on a case-by-case basis.

The outcomes for patients managed nonoperatively are poor. The use of radiotherapy or chemotherapy is significantly less common in patients older than 65 years, likely reflecting the proportion of patients unfit for operative management. Due to the lack of effective treatment options in this situation, the patient's quality of life should be paramount in treatment planning.

27.3 Adjuvant/Neoadjuvant Radiation Therapy and Chemotherapy

Postoperative chemo-/radiotherapy has no proven efficacy in retroperitoneal sarcomas [26].

Limb-sparing surgery generally relies on adjuvant/neoadjuvant radiation therapy to minimize risk of local recurrence. The goal of radiation is to treat the margin to minimize the risk of recurrence, not necessarily to reduce the size of the tumor per se. Radiation therapy reduces the risk of local recurrence from greater than 30% to less than 10% in most series, but does not impact distant failure or overall survival [27].

Radiation therapy may be delivered as external beam radiation therapy (EBRT) or brachytherapy. EBRT may be delivered preoperatively or postoperatively. Preoperative EBRT is associated with a doubling in the rate of wound complications (35% vs. 17%) but importantly with a lower rate of late complications and tissue fibrosis and better functional outcomes. Postoperative EBRT generally has higher dose than preoperative EBRT. Brachytherapy may be delivered through afterloading catheters placed across the tumor bed at the end of surgery. The goal of brachytherapy is to deliver additional radiation to a close margin (including neurovascular structures) with minimal treatment to surrounding tissue, particularly when further EBRT is no longer feasible. This can be a desirable option for older patients.

Approximately 25–50% of patients with extremity STS develop distant metastatic disease [28]. Those with large (>10 cm), deep, high-grade STS may be considered for preoperative or postoperative chemotherapy, usually with active agents such as doxorubicin and ifosfamide (response rates of 20–40% in patients with metastatic disease). However, there are no consistently convincing data that such an approach improves overall survival for most STS histologies, and cardiac and kidney toxicities make the majority of older patients unfit for treatment.

Hyperthermic isolated limb perfusion (ILP) and infusion (ILI) have been investigated in several institutions as treatment for patients with locally advanced STS in whom limb-sparing, function-sparing surgery may not be possible, but the associated high morbidity makes this treatment not advisable for geriatric patients [29].

27.4 Histology-Specific Treatments

27.4.1 Atypical Lipomatous Tumor (ALT)/ Well-Differentiated Liposarcoma

This low-grade tumor, when arising in the extremity, has a relatively low rate of recurrence, may not recur for quite some time, and has no risk of distant metastatic spread and death, unless dedifferentiation occurs over its natural history. Dedifferentiation, if it occurs, in fact entails a risk of metastatic spread as high as 20%. In contrast, low-grade locally recurrent ALT may grow slowly for years. Therefore, such tumors arising in the extremity can be resected with a limited negative or even a positive margin especially when preserving limb function is an issue. Radiographically, ALT may be difficult to distinguish from an intramuscular lipoma, a benign entity which can also arise in deep muscle tissue. ALT/well-differentiated liposarcoma is a more threatening neoplasm when located in the retroperitoneum even in the absence of areas of dedifferentiation. In fact, local control is an issue at this site, and patients often die of locoregional failure, without developing distant metastases [2, 21].

27.4.2 Dermatofibrosarcoma Protuberans (DFSP)

DFSP is a superficial tumor which infiltrates soft tissue for centimeters beyond the obvious margins of the lesion and can recur locally following an inadequate resection. However, the more common variety of DFSP does not display metastatic behavior. Therefore, the goal of surgery should be negative margins, often necessitating reconstruction by plastic surgery. When cosmesis or function preservation is an issue, limited positive margins may be accepted, and a wider resection postponed until DFSP locally recurs.

Since DFSP is usually a relatively superficial tumor, resection of muscle deep to the tumor is not often necessary. Intraoperative frozen section margin analysis is not generally helpful, as the surrounding fat rarely freezes well for analysis. Radiation therapy is not usually recommended. Approximately 5–10% of patients with DFSP have a more aggressive fibrosarcomatous variant which may recur locally and potentially spread. Those individuals should be treated as a "conventional" sarcoma with more aggressive local therapy (including radiation) and followed with systematic imaging.

27.4.3 Myxofibrosarcoma

Myxofibrosarcoma most commonly arises in the extremities of elderly individuals. It demonstrates a 30% rate of local recurrence and 16% rate of distant recurrence [14]. Multiple local recurrences have been associated with eventual amputation. Therefore, it is critical to pursue aggressive local therapy. Wide surgical margins (2–4 cm radial margins beyond the clinical boundaries of the palpable mass, especially in more superficial tumors) should be the goal of surgery, which often requires complex wound closure or flap reconstruction by a plastic and reconstructive surgeon, as well as resection and reconstruction of vessels and/or nerves. Radiation therapy, either preoperatively or postoperatively (described below), may be considered, though the direct impact on this specific histology remains unknown.

27.4.4 Angiosarcoma

Scalp angiosarcomas are commonly multifocal, by both clinical examination and CT or MRI imaging. As radical surgery (often requiring complex flap reconstructions) is possible but rarely curative even if margins are widely negative, it may be reserved for patients who are experiencing problems with local control (bleeding from a fungating tumor) or who only appear to have a solitary site of disease by both clinical examination and imaging while undergoing systemic therapy. Angiosarcoma is sensitive to systemic chemotherapy and to radiation therapy [2].

27.4.5 Radiation-Induced Sarcomas

Radiation-induced sarcomas are rare and include a variety of histological subtypes, the most common of which are unclassified pleomorphic sarcoma, angiosarcoma, malignant peripheral nerve sheath tumors, and leiomyosarcoma. Besides the intrinsic characteristics of each histological subtype, they are all characterized by a high propensity to locally recur, given the difficulty of obtaining clear margins. This is due in part to the difficulty in distinguishing tumor infiltration of healthy tissues from radiation-induced soft tissue changes around the tumor site and in part to the discontiguous and multifocal involvement of tissue within the radiation field. The tumor should be excised with as much tissue around it as possible. This often if not always requires reconstruction and coverage by a plastic surgeon and potentially a more liberal policy of neurovascular resection and reconstruction. Systemic chemotherapy and re-irradiation are often considered, given the overall dismal prognosis, though the use of the latter must be weighed with caution [2].

References

1. Stiller CA, Trama A, Serraino D, Rossi S, Navarro C, Chirlaque MD, RARECARE Working Group, et al. Descriptive epidemiology of sarcomas in Europe: report from the RARECARE project. Eur J Cancer. 2013;49(3):684–95.
2. Samuel LC. Bone and soft tissue sarcomas. In: Yarbro CH, Wujcik D, Gobel BH, editors. Cancer nursing: principles and practice. 8th ed. Burlington: Jones &Bartlett Learning; 2018. (chapter 46).
3. Ray-Coquard I, Thiesse P, Ranchère-Vince D, Chauvin F, Bobin JY, Sunyach MP, et al. Conformity to clinical practice guidelines, multidisciplinary management and outcome of treatment for soft tissue sarcomas. Ann Oncol. 2004;15(2):307–15.
4. The ESMO/European Sarcoma Network Working Group. Soft tissue and visceral sarcomas: ESMO clinical practice guidelines for diagnosis, treatment and follow-up. Ann Oncol. 2014;25(Suppl 3):iii102–12.
5. von Mehren M, Randal RL, Benjamin RS, Boles S, Bui MM, Conrad EU, et al. Soft tissue sarcoma, version 2.2016, NCCN clinical practice guidelines in oncology. J Natl Compr Cancer Netw. 2016;14(6):758–86.
6. Noebauer-Huhmann IM, Weber MA, Lalam RK, Trattnig S, Bohndorf K, Vanhoenacker F, et al. Soft tissue tumors in adults: ESSR-approved guidelines for diagnostic imaging. Semin Musculoskelet Radiol. 2015;19(5):475–82.
7. Preston SD, Southall AR, Nel M, Das SK. Geriatric surgery is about disease, not age. J R Soc Med. 2008;101:409–15.
8. Canter RJ. Surgical approach for soft tissue sarcoma: standard of care and future approaches. Curr Opin Oncol. 2015;27(4):343–8.
9. Honoré C, Méeus P, Stoeckle E, Bonvalot S. Soft tissue sarcoma in France in 2015: epidemiology, classification and organization of clinical care. J ViscSurg. 2015;152(4):223–30.
10. Paredes T, Pereira M, Simões MR. A longitudinal study on emotional adjustment of sarcoma patients: the determinant role of demographic, clinical and coping variables. Eur J Cancer Care. 2012;21(1):41–51.
11. Enneking WF, Spanier SS, Goodman MA. A system for the surgical staging of musculoskeletal sarcoma. Clin Orthop Relat Res. 1980;153:106–20.
12. Stoeckle E, Italiano A, Stock N, Kind M, Kantor G, Coindre JM, Bui BN. Surgical margins in soft tissue sarcoma. Bull Cancer. 2008;95(12):1199–204.
13. Gerrand CH, Wunder JS, Kandel RA, et al. Classification of positive margins after resection of soft tissue sarcoma of the limb predict the risk of local recurrence. J Bone Joint Surg Br. 2001;83:1149–55.
14. Haglund KE, Raut CP, Nascimento AF, Wang Q, George S, Baldini EH. Recurrence patterns and survival for patients with intermediate- and high-grade myxofibrosarcoma. Int J Radiat Oncol Biol Phys. 2012;82(1):361–7.
15. Brooks A, Gold J, Graham D, et al. Resection of the sciatic, peroneal or tibial nerves: assessment of functional status. Ann Surg Oncol. 2002;9(1):41–7.
16. Rosemberg SA, Tepper J, Glatsein E, et al. The treatment of soft tissue sarcomas of the extremities; prospective evaluations of limb sparing surgery plus radiation therapy compared with amputation and the role of adjuvant chemotherapy. Ann Surg. 1982;196:305–15.
17. Hassan S, Gale J, Perks A, et al. Reconstruction and financial remuneration following soft tissue sarcoma surgery. Bull R Coll Surg Engl. 2013;95(5):160–2.
18. Venkasetan M, Richards CJ, McCullack TA, et al. Inadvertent surgical resection of soft tissue sarcomas. Eur J Surg Oncol. 2012;38:346–51.

19. Smith HG, Thomas JM, Smith MJ, et al. Multivisceral resection of retroperitoneal sarcomas in the elderly. Eur J Cancer. 2016;69:119–26.
20. Porter GA, Baxter NN, Pisters PW. Retroperitoneal sarcoma: a population-based analysis of epidemiology, surgery, and radiotherapy. Cancer. 2006;106:1610–6.
21. Gronchi A, Miceli R, Allard MA, Callegaro D, Le Péchoux C, Fiore M, et al. Personalizing the approach to retroperitoneal soft tissue sarcoma: histology-specific patterns of failure and post relapse outcome after primary extended resection. Ann Surg Oncol. 2015;22(5):1447–54.
22. Bonvalot S, Raut CP, Pollock RE, et al. Technical considerations in surgery for retroperitoneal sarcomas: position paper from E-surge, a master class in sarcoma surgery, and EORTC-STBSG. Ann Surg Oncol. 2012;19(9):2981–91.
23. Anaya DA, Lev DC, Pollock RE. The role of surgical margin status in retroperitoneal sarcoma. J Surg Oncol. 2008;98:607–10.
24. Smith HG, Panchalingam D, Hannay JA, Smith MJ, Thomas JM, Hayes AJ, et al. Outcome following resection of retroperitoneal sarcoma. Br J Surg. 2015;102:1698–709.
25. Berger NA, Savvides P, Koroukian SM, Kahana EF, Deimling GT, Rose JH, et al. Cancer in the elderly. Trans Am Clin Climatol Assoc. 2006;117:147–55.
26. Casali PG. Adjuvant chemotherapy for soft tissue sarcoma. Am Soc Clin Oncol Educ Book. 2015;35:e629–33.
27. Haas RL, Delaney TF, O'sullivan B, Keus RB, Le Pechoux C, Olmi P, et al. Radiotherapy for management of extremity soft tissue sarcomas: why, when, and where? Int J Radiat Oncol Biol Phys. 2012;84(3):572–80.
28. Coindre JM, Terrier P, Guillou L, Le Doussal V, Collin F, Ranchère D, et al. Predictive value of grade for metastasis development in the main histologic types of adult soft tissue sarcomas: a study of 1240 patients from the French Federation of Cancer Centers Sarcoma Group. Cancer. 2001;91(10):1914–26.
29. Jakob J, Hohenberger P. Role of isolated limb perfusion with recombinant human tumor necrosis factor α and melphalan in locally advanced extremity soft tissue sarcoma. Cancer. 2016;122(17):2624–32.
30. Sanfilippo R, Miceli R, Grosso F, et al. Myxofibrosarcoma: prognostic factors and survival in a series of patients treated at a single institution. Ann Surg Oncol. 2011;18(3):720–5.

Part VII

Trauma and Non Traumatic Emergencies

Trauma in Geriatric Age

28

Emanuele Rausa, Federico Coccolini, Giulia Montori, Maria Agnese Kelly, Baggi Paolo, Dario Piazzalunga, Cecilia Merli, and Luca Ansaloni

28.1 Introduction

The definition of the word "elderly" is not one that has been universally agreed though it is generally accepted that it pertains to a subset of population between 45 and 75 years old [1]. People are living much longer worldwide. Currently, the population over 60 years of age accounts for over 40 million persons in the United States. Over the next 20 years, the population over 65 years of age is projected to double in size, reaching 82.3 million (approximately 22% of the total population) by 2040 [2].

It is thought that the population over 65 years of age will be the fastest growing subset of population. As this population grows, so too will the need for healthcare services and their costs. In 2008, despite the fact that the elderly constituted only 13% of the US population, they represented 40% of all hospitalized adults. The total expenditure on health care reflects these data; in fact, the elderly costs twice as much as their younger counterparts (13.2% vs 6.6%, respectively) [3].

The Western lifestyle encourages old people to maintain their independence for as long as possible. In 2014, there were 5709 people over 65 killed and an estimated 221,000 injured in motor vehicle traffic crashes. Older people made up 17 percent of all traffic fatalities and 9% of all people injured in traffic crashes during the year [4].

However, physiological changes are natural and uncontrolled events that affect compensatory mechanisms and cause them to become insufficient to adequately

E. Rausa • F. Coccolini • G. Montori • B. Paolo • D. Piazzalunga • L. Ansaloni (✉)
Unit of General and Emergency Surgery, Papa Giovanni XXIII Hospital, P.zza OMS 1, 24128 Bergamo, Italy
e-mail: lansaloni@asst-pg23.it

M.A. Kelly
Department of Colorectal Diseases, St. Vincent's University Hospital, Elm Park, Dublin, Ireland

C. Merli
Unit of Emergency Medicine, Papa Giovanni XXIII Hospital, Bergamo, Italy

A. Crucitti (ed.), *Surgical Management of Elderly Patients*,
https://doi.org/10.1007/978-3-319-60861-7_28

react to injuries, illnesses, or surgery [5]. This physiological decline renders the elderly prone to traumatic injuries in the course of their daily activities. Furthermore, the higher comorbidities rate (66%) and preexisting home therapy may exacerbate and complicate the trauma and the underlying physiological mechanism [6].

The trauma mechanism in the elderly is dissimilar to that in their younger counterparts. In young patients, road trauma is most prevalent (58.4%). Other predominant trauma mechanisms are recreation (15.4%) and violence (15.3%) [7].

Blunt trauma is the dominant mechanism in elderly patients (EPs) and makes up more than 80% of all geriatric trauma [8]. Falls, which consist of a low-energy blunt trauma, account for 70% of blunt trauma cases. EPs may be more inclined to fall because of physiological change with aging and comorbidities affecting the musculoskeletal system and the brain causing tremor, rigidity, and dementia. Further blunt trauma events are motor vehicle accidents (the second most common trauma mechanism), pedestrian struck, and burn injuries [9]. Finally, there are penetrating trauma and suicide attempts. EPs account for 18% of all suicide deaths. Of note, domestic abuse and assaults represent an underrated cause of trauma, with an estimated 25,886 elderly people treated in emergency departments for lacerations, contusions, or fractures secondary to nonfatal assaults. It is estimated that roughly 85% of abuse incidents involving the elderly are not reported [10].

Despite the steady increase in geriatric trauma admissions, specific guidelines addressed toward the management of the geriatric have not been defined, and the treatment remains challenging. Demetriades et al. showed a deficiency in the proper triaging of these trauma cases [11]. EPs, even if severely injured, were underrated in 25% of cases. This bias results in a significant delay in treatment. Statistics show that 43% of patients who were considered hemodynamically stable were found to have experienced cardiogenic shock, and 54% of these cases resulted in death [12]. Mortality among those patients was substantially reduced by employing "age over 70" as an activation code for the trauma team [11].

Given the well-established relationship between age, Injury Severity Score (ISS), and mortality, a clear trauma classification at the presentation is essential as invasive procedures in EPs are widely accepted in ISS > 18, whereas in ISS < 18, the indications need to be cautiously evaluated according to the risks and benefits [13].

Due to a reduced physiological reserve, body reaction to a traumatic event is poor in both the short and the long term. EPs who are hospitalized are likely to develop a limitation in their daily abilities and functional status and need long-term care. A poor pre-injury functional status is a strong predictor of an undesirable outcome [14]. It has been evaluated as even more relevant than the admitting diagnosis in the short term (complications and in-hospital mortality) and the long term (post-hospitalization mortality) [15].

Poor functional status at the baseline, an advanced age, and a high ISS result in a longer hospital stay and increase the risk of developing nosocomial infections. As shown by Labib et al., among all the nosocomial complications, respiratory complications are those that most increase the risk for in-hospital mortality [16]. Pracht et al. showed that in patient groups aged between 65 and 74 years of age, the risk of mortality increases according to the number of comorbidities [17].

Fleischman et al. show that age is a relevant predictor of long-term prognosis. In fact, the risk of post-hospitalization mortality continues to go up until 6 months post-trauma in EPs [18]. Additionally, Davidson et al. stated that the risk of post-hospitalization mortality remains high over a 3-year post-trauma period (16%) [19]. EPs outcomes are related to multiple significant factors such as trauma mechanism, age, ISS, comorbidities (especially cardiovascular comorbidities), functional status at the baseline, and home therapy [20]. In this context, as EPs are extremely frail and feeble, it would be better to evaluate them more as individuals than as a cohort of patients.

28.2 The Physiology of Aging

Substantial physiological changes occur in aging and may affect the body's response to trauma.

In a trauma, the first body reaction is the release of catecholamine hormones, in order to raise blood pressure and provide more blood to muscles and brain. In EPs, the cardiovascular system responds to this stimulation with a consistent delay [21].

Additionally, medications such as beta-blockers or diuretic medications may mitigate the hormones' effect and exacerbate a forced status of hypotension and hypoperfusion in cases of blood loss. Figures which define the "normal blood pressure" in adults should be reconsidered in EPs. Heffernan et al. found that mortality increased in EPs with a systolic blood pressure <110 mmHg, whereas the same results were obtained when the blood pressure was <95 mmHg in younger counterparts [22].

The heart and vessels are stiff and thickened, causing a decreased compliance. Body fluid compartments are extremely narrow, and small changes among them coincide with a massive change between hypovolemia and edema because cardiac reserve is limited; atherosclerosis leads to poor vessel constriction, and the neurological system is slow in arousing the "fight or flight" response [23].

In a trauma, EPs may decompensate quickly because the respiratory reserve is decreased as well. The loss in elasticity and arthritic process makes the rib cage stiff, causing a reduction in the articular range of motion. Lungs, which are enclosed in an inflexible space, lose compliance, and the vital capacity decreases, while the dead space increases. Additionally, the pulmonary tissue changes its pattern because of fibrosis and the loss of collagen and because of chemicals and pollution in the atmosphere. Hence, early intubation is recommended in patients with borderline respiratory function [24].

The kidneys are less efficient in concentrating urine. Even temporary hypotension and hypoperfusion, radiological contrast, or nephrotoxic drugs represent a trigger for an acute kidney injury [25]. Aging acts on the musculoskeletal system, decreasing the muscle mass and strength because fat or fibrous tissue replaces muscles. In addition, osteoporosis and arthritis decrease bone density and make EPs susceptible to fracture, even in low-energy trauma [26].

Finally, another substantial physiological change is the loss of adequate thermoregulation. Even a modest trauma may easily make EPs hypothermic, resulting in a worsening of coagulopathy, which then dramatically raises the risk of mortality [27].

28.3 Neurotrauma

Physiology in traumatic brain injury (TBI) is determined by two phases. The first phase consists in a cellular disruption or death leading to a neurological impairment. The second phase results in microenviromental changes, edema, and inflammation. In EPs, these phases are exacerbated by the age-related physiological changes because aging decreases the brain's plasticity and its ability to repair the damage. Additionally, TBI conduces to further cellular loss and may boost any disease progression [28].

Medical treatment should evaluate several factors in EPs. Considering the high rate of EPs with hypertension, maintaining an appropriate blood pressure and, consequently, a correct cerebral oxygenation may be challenging [29]. In EPs, the heart ejection should be precisely calculated to determine all the further fluid management. Currently, the mainstays in TBI treatment are as follows: (1) balance hypoxia and hypotension; (2) carefully avoid hypoperfusion from hyperventilation; (3) administer anticonvulsants over the first 7 days after the trauma; and (4) do not administer steroids [30].

As the brain volume in EPs is reduced and the dead space between the brain and the head bone is enlarged, the likelihood of a substantial brain swelling with a consequent increased intracranial pressure needing surgical intervention is rare. Mannitol remains the most efficient drug in the control of increased intracranial pressure in these patients, even though a decreased function of the astrocytic gap junctions may result in a mannitol hyperfunction worsening the cerebral edema. More recently, several studies have shown that statins reduce the risk of both in-hospital mortality and 12-month adverse outcome [31, 32].

From the surgical perspective, guidelines currently recommend evacuating an acute subdural hematoma when it is >10 mm and/or midline shift is >5 mm on CT scan, regardless of the patient's Glasgow Coma Scale (GCS) [30]. While this recommendation is well established for young patients, it is vague and controversial with regard to EPs. However, EPs who underwent craniotomy for hematoma evacuation showed acceptable outcomes (in-hospital mortality 5–16%) and a similar ability to return to the baseline when compared to younger counterparts. EPs may require more scrupulous care over the period of hospitalization and a longer hospital stay and rehabilitation. Historically, the vast majority of subdural hematoma cases were treated conservatively and resulted in a chronic event. Patients have occasionally reported headache and/or minor mental changes; less than 10% have reported substantial neurological symptoms [29].

Recent studies, however, pointed out that chronic subdural hematoma (CSDH) is not a disease free of long-term complications. Miranda et al. found that the CSDH effect in the long term in EPs leads to a mortality rate of 26.3% at 6 months and 32% at 12 months [33]; similar results are reported in patients after hip fractures [34]. It might be postulated that CSDH after TBI exacerbates preexisting comorbidities and affects the brain functions, resulting in an increased rate of mortality [33].

Further studies looking at specific TBI cohorts of EPs indicated "male gender" as a predictive factor for a worse outcome. Women reported better outcomes, and it is likely to be due to estrogen and progesterone, which act in the reparation process [35].

It is well established that falls represent the most common mechanism for TBI. In this context, more efforts should be addressed toward the prevention of such injuries. Several studies listed a number of strategies to decrease the probability of these traumatic events happen. Incentivization has been suggested as an encouragement to compliance in elderly to medications, as the careful choice of the more appropriate antihypertensive (thiazide-type diuretic therapy reduces hip and pelvic fracture risk compared with other antihypertensive medications), and as the promotion of physical exercise to strengthen their musculoskeletal systems [36, 37].

Of note, the vast majority of EPs are on anticoagulation therapy, which deeply affects outcomes. Anticoagulants make treatment much more demanding and challenging [38]. Howard et al. found a relationship between an increased risk of mortality in EPs and those on warfarin who fall [39]. However, this relationship has been debated in the literature, and the data are still contradictory.

Over the last decade, new oral anticoagulants (NOACs) are available worldwide. NOACs are as efficient as warfarin but relatively safer. The action mechanism consists in the direct inhibition of the coagulation cascade. NOACs have a shorter half-life compared to warfarin (8–16 h vs 1 week, respectively) and are, thus, easier to manage. The major limitation of NOACs is the lack of a specific antidote [40]. The RE-LY trial documented that low doses of NOACs decrease the risk of intracranial hemorrhage as compared with warfarin; conversely, high doses result in a similar risk [41].

28.4 Pelvic Fracture

The pelvis is the strongest bone unit in the body and its fracture is considered to be secondary to high-energy injury (13–18%). However, comorbidities (osteoporosis, arthritis, and osteopenia), preexisting conditions (previous surgery, metastases), and age may weaken the bone pattern and make it prone to fracture even in cases of low-energy trauma [42].

Comparing EPs to their younger counterparts, differences in the mechanism, hospitalization, and outcomes are evident. While younger patients typically sustain such fractures from high-energy traumas, such as motor vehicle collisions, in EPs, low-energy trauma—usually falls from standing—is the most common cause [43]. Therefore, prevention of falls should be taken into consideration when striving to decrease the risk factors. In addition, pelvic fractures are more prevalent among males in younger patients and among females in EPs. The difference in prevalence between sexes is presumably attributable to the hormonal changes in females (estrogen and progesterone decline) which unleash subsequent osteoporosis [44]. In 64% of pelvis fractures, preexisting osteoporosis is present and this rises to 94% in <60-year-old patients [45].

Mortality in EPs (7.6%) is mostly related to hemorrhage; this is four times higher than in younger patients, where morbidity is due to incomplete healing and/or nerve damage [46]. Pelvic fracture management is standardized in two groups, whether or not the patient is hemodynamically stable [47].

Due to the anatomy, pelvic trauma may involve different organs and systems (bones, genitourinary viscera, rectum, small intestine, major vessels, and pudendal nerves); thus, the management of such trauma may be demanding and require a polyspecialistic treatment. Moreover, in EPs, bones are weaker and ligaments and the skin are less flexible; thus, the incidence of more complex fractures such as Morel-Lavallee, Malgaigne, or open-book fracture increases. Nonetheless, concomitant drugs, such as anticoagulants, which EPs are often on, may contribute to persistent bleeding and increase of the hemodynamic instability risk [48].

Primary classification is based on the fracture stability. Stable fractures are defined as fractures of the pelvic ring, acetabular fractures, and pubic branch. Unstable fractures are characterized by pelvic fractures in more sites (Malgaigne fracture or open-book fracture). The Young and Burgess system is the most accepted worldwide (Fig. 28.1) [49]. According to this classification, angiographic embolization is predominantly required in anterior posterior compression, in vertical shear, or in combined fracture patterns (Fig. 28.1) [50].

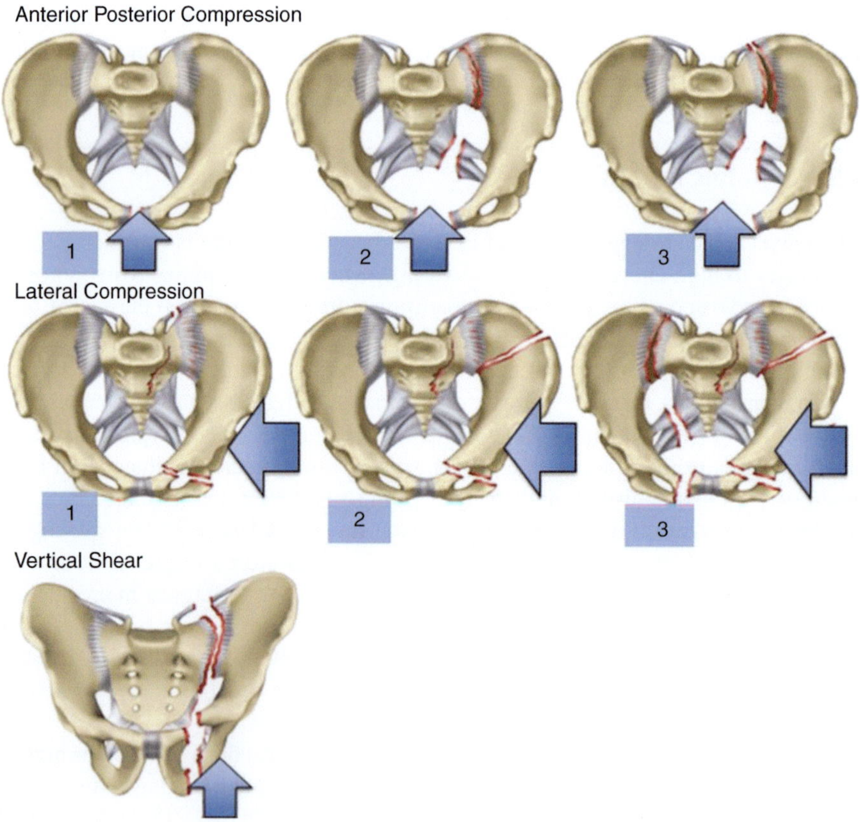

Fig. 28.1 Young and Burgess pelvic fracture classification

According to ATLS, the first assessment is based on clinical findings and pain site. Physical examination is essential to determine the anatomical site entailed in the trauma, which requires further investigations. Bimanual compression of the iliac wings can rule out either vertical or rotational instability [51]. Pelvic X-ray represents the first radiological investigation. Inlet, outlet, or judet views may offer additional data. CT scan may be useful in suspected active bleeding in order to define the site of a subsequent angiographic embolization if necessary [52]. When underlying osteoporosis is suspected, an extensive investigation, including of levels of calcium, thyroid function, and sexual hormones in the serum, should be carried out [48].

As previously mentioned, management is primarily based on the clinical presentation. In EPs who have a poor physiological reserve to get through a trauma, a comprehensive assessment of the patient should be carried out. Comorbidities should be taken into consideration, especially for potential medication interactions. It is likely that home therapy might interact with drugs administered over the course of hospitalization, causing confusion and obnubilation. A prompt correction of coagulopathy in patients on anticoagulants is essential (Table 28.1), while desmopressin may help to treat patients with chronic kidney disease [53].

The clinical examination and the radiological investigations looking at potential bleeding define the diagnostic phase. Once the site of bleeding is identified, and even supposing there is active bleeding but the patient is hemodynamically stable, conservative treatment (bed rest, minimally invasive interventions, and pain control) is preferred. Occasionally, the sites of hemorrhage are multiple, and in one third of pelvic fractures, sources of bleeding are outside of the pelvic borders [54].

Table 28.1 Commonly antiplatelet/anticoagulants agents

Antiplatelet/ anticoagulant agents (brand name)	Half-life	Duration of action	Mechanism of action	Reversal agents
Warfarin (Coumadin)	20–60 h	2–5 days	Vitamin K antagonist (inhibits factors II, VII, IX, and X)	Fresh frozen plasma, vitamin K, prothrombin complex concentrate
Aspirin	20 min	Life of the platelet (7–10 days)	Antiplatelet: thromboxane inhibitor	Desmopressin; platelets may give temporary reversal
Clopidogrel (Plavix) Prasugrel (Effient) Ticlopidine (Ticlid)	6–7 h 6–7 h 12 h	7–10 days	Antiplatelet: ADP receptor/P2Y12 inhibitors	Desmopressin; platelets may give temporary reversal
Abciximab (ReoPro) Eptifibatide (Integrilin) Tirofiban (Aggrastat)	10–30 min 2.5 h 2 h	48 h 96 h 48 h	Antiplatelet: glycoprotein IIb/IIIa inhibitors	Desmopressin; platelets may give temporary reversal
Fondaparinux (Arixtra) Enoxaparin (Lovenox)	17–21 h 4.5–7 h	2–4 days 12 h	Bind antithrombin	Protamine sulfate (more effective with heparin)
Dabigatran (Pradaxa)	12–17 h	2–4 days	Direct thrombin (II) inhibitor	Unknown

Usually, any small amount of bleeding in hemodynamically stable patients is controlled by putting in place a pelvic binder, which stabilizes the fracture. Although arterial bleeding is unusual, its presence should be investigated with radiological investigations when suspected. Such bleeding is unlikely to be controlled with immobilization, and more invasive treatment (i.e., angioembolization and/or surgery) is required [55].

A mobilization as early as possible is recommended to prevent the bone resorption and to decrease the risk of pulmonary infection and vascular or gastrointestinal complications. The average hospital stay for EPs who sustain a pelvic fracture is around 21 days. Subsequently, a long rehabilitation is frequently required; however, a complete return to the motility at the baseline is rare, and EPs may need a cane to resume daily activities [56].

28.5 Penetrating Trauma

Trauma is the fifth leading cause of death in EPs. Blunt trauma (falls, motor vehicle injuries, or pedestrian collision) is the most common, but outcomes are favorable [57]. The same cannot be said for penetrating trauma, which is relatively rare but with an extremely poor prognosis. This poor prognosis is due to the scarce physiological reserve in association with several comorbidities; of note is preexisting cardiovascular disease, which requires the administration of anticoagulants.

Penetrating trauma is most commonly due to a suicide attempt. Social context (urban setting) and comorbidities (depression and chronic pain) may deeply affect EP quality of life. Self-inflicted injury rates increase with aging (46.2% between 65 and 74 years of age and 51.5% over 75 years of age). This type of injury represents a clear public issue [58].

In 80% of suicide attempts, firearms are predominantly employed, and the head is the site most commonly involved (54.2%), with an extremely high mortality (over 90%). Additional anatomical sites of penetrating trauma are the thorax (13.5%) and abdomen (8.2%). In assaulted patients, the thorax and abdomen are the most commonly involved area (43%), followed by the extremities (16.9%). Higher mortality is recorded in suicide attempts (60%) as compared to assault-related patients (25%) or unintentional penetrating injuries (9%) [58].

Given the complex history and home therapy often present in EPs, these patients should be closely assessed and monitored. It has been demonstrated that the classic hemodynamic criteria (systolic BP <90 mmHg or heart rate >120/min), which are typically applied in trauma team activation, are inadequate in EPs. Heffernan et al. compared the blood pressure and the heart rate in geriatric and younger patients and found that vital signs are unreliable in geriatric patients. In fact, this study showed that mortality in geriatric patients increases when the blood pressure and the heart rate are <110 mmHg and >130 beats/min, respectively. Conversely, in their younger counterparts, vital sign limits are <95 mmHg and >90 beats/min, respectively [22].

This difference is presumably attributable to a substantial physiological change in EPs causing a poor reserve, in addition to medications (such as beta-blockers, anticoagulants, and diuretics) which may affect the vital signs and lead to a misleading trauma classification. In these patients, a sudden deterioration has always to be expected, even though hemodynamically stable on presentation; thus, prompt and aggressive treatment should be preferred [59].

Demetriades et al. found that assigning a specific activation code for severely injured patients over 70 years of age reduced the risk of misleading trauma classification and is helpful in enabling the prompt treatment of the patient. Applying these criteria, this study reported a consistent reduction in mortality ($p = 0.003$) [11].

A recent study reported better outcomes for severely injured patients transported to trauma hospital rather than a non-trauma center [60]. As soon as the patient is admitted, a detailed history should be gathered and any home therapy scrupulously evaluated. As bleeding in EPs may be a challenge to control, the anticoagulants need to be promptly interrupted and the coagulopathy corrected if the ISS is high [59]. Multiple hemoglobin tests may help in assessing EPs whose vital signs are affected by anticoagulants and beta-blockers. In these patients, vital signs "wrongly" considered stable may conceal potentially life-threating bleeding. ATLS guidelines should be adopted. Radiological investigations need to be completed while monitoring vital signs continuously, and angioembolization or aggressive interventions should be considered in the first phase of the evaluation [61].

Fluid administration needs to be managed carefully because the physiological response between hypovolemia and edema in EPs is extremely thin. However, a regulated hydration and bicarbonate administration reduce nephropathy. In trauma patients, thermoregulatory response may be dysregulated, causing hypothermia, acidosis, and coagulopathy. Therefore, hypothermia prevention through the administration of warm fluids represents a mainstay in the management of trauma [62].

Surgical management is related to the injured area and whether or not vital signs are stable. If vital signs are stable, further investigations (such as CT scan, endoscopy, and bronchoscopy) should be considered and a conservative treatment evaluated. Patients with penetrating trauma to the neck need an emergency operation if the vascular or aerodigestive system is involved and vital signs are unstable. Historically, less than 15–20% of penetrating neck injuries need surgery [63, 64].

In cases of chest trauma with hemodynamic instability, the surgical approach preferred is an emergency thoracotomy or median sternotomy, depending on the site involved. In cases of penetrating trauma to the lower part of the left thorax, a diagnostic laparoscopy might be considered to evaluate the diaphragm. The vast majority of cases of penetrating trauma to the chest (nearly 80%) may be managed with a chest drain [65].

Penetrating trauma to the abdomen which results in peritonitis or in hemodynamic instability requires an emergency laparotomy [66]. An emergency laparoscopy should be taken into consideration in left thoracoabdominal trauma in order to rule out lacerations to the diaphragm [61].

References

1. Adams SD, Cotton BA, McGuire MF, Dipasupil E, Podbielski JM, Zaharia A, et al. Unique pattern of complications in elderly trauma patients at a Level I trauma center. J Trauma Acute Care Surg. 2012;72(1):112–8.
2. Projections of future growth of the older. population. 2016. Available at: http://www.aoa.gov/aoaroot/aging_statistics/future_growth/future_growth.aspx#age. Accessed 24 Feb 2017.

3. Wier LM, Levit K, Stranges E, et al. HCUP facts and figures: statistics on hospital-based care in the United States, 2012. Rockville: Agency for Healthcare Research and Quality; 2014. Available at: http://www.hcup-us.ahrq.gov/reports.jsp.
4. NHTSA Traffic Safety Facts. 2014. Older population. Available at: https://crashstats.nhtsa.dot.gov/Api/Public/ViewPublication/812273.
5. Carpenter CR, Shelton E, Fowler S, Suffoletto B, Platts-Mills TF, Rothman RE, et al. Risk factors and screening instruments to predict adverse outcomes for undifferentiated older emergency department patients: a systematic review and meta-analysis. Acad Emerg Med. 2015;22(1):1–21.
6. Bergeron E, Lavoie A, Clas D, Moore L, Ratte S, Tetreault S, et al. Elderly trauma patients with rib fractures are at greater risk of death and pneumonia. J Trauma. 2003;54(3):478–85.
7. Ogilvie R, Curtis K, Lam M, McCloughen A, Foster K. The burden of youth: major traumatic injury in adolescents and young adults managed in the Australian Capital Territory. J Trauma Nurs. 2014;21(5):218–27.
8. Vieira ER, Palmer RC, Chaves PH. Prevention of falls in older people living in the community. BMJ. 2016;353:i1419.
9. Brown CV, Rix K, Klein AL, Ford B, Teixeira PG, Aydelotte J, et al. A comprehensive investigation of comorbidities, mechanisms, injury patterns, and outcomes in geriatric blunt trauma patients. Am Surg. 2016;82(11):1055–62.
10. Centers for Disease Control and Prevention, National Center for Injury Prevention and Control. WISQARS fatal injuries: mortality reports. Available at: https://webappa.cdc.gov/sasweb/ncipc/mortrate.html.
11. Demetriades D, Sava J, Alo K, Newton E, Velmahos GC, Murray JA, et al. Old age as a criterion for trauma team activation. J Trauma. 2001;51(4):754–6. discussion 6-7.
12. Martin JT, Alkhoury F, O'Connor JA, Kyriakides TC, Bonadies JA. 'Normal' vital signs belie occult hypoperfusion in geriatric trauma patients. Am Surg. 2010;76(1):65–9.
13. Tornetta P, Mostafavi H, Riina J, Turen C, Reimer B, Levine R, et al. Morbidity and mortality in elderly trauma patients. J Trauma. 1999;46(4):702–6.
14. Hashmi A, Ibrahim-Zada I, Rhee P, Aziz H, Fain MJ, Friese RS, et al. Predictors of mortality in geriatric trauma patients: a systematic review and meta-analysis. J Trauma Acute Care Surg. 2014;76(3):894–901.
15. Maxwell CA, Mion LC, Mukherjee K, Dietrich MS, Minnick A, May A, et al. Preinjury physical frailty and cognitive impairment among geriatric trauma patients determine postinjury functional recovery and survival. J Trauma Acute Care Surg. 2016;80(2):195–203.
16. Labib N, Nouh T, Winocour S, Deckelbaum D, Banici L, Fata P, et al. Severely injured geriatric population: morbidity, mortality, and risk factors. J Trauma. 2011;71(6):1908–14.
17. Pracht EE, Langland-Orban B, Flint L. Survival advantage for elderly trauma patients treated in a designated trauma center. J Trauma. 2011;71(1):69–77.
18. Fleischman RJ, Adams AL, Hedges JR, Ma OJ, Mullins RJ, Newgard CD. The optimum follow-up period for assessing mortality outcomes in injured older adults. J Am Geriatr Soc. 2010;58(10):1843–9.
19. Davidson GH, Hamlat CA, Rivara FP, Koepsell TD, Jurkovich GJ, Arbabi S. Long-term survival of adult trauma patients. JAMA. 2011;305(10):1001–7.
20. Sammy I, Lecky F, Sutton A, Leaviss J, O'Cathain A. Factors affecting mortality in older trauma patients-A systematic review and meta-analysis. Injury. 2016;47(6):1170–83.
21. Haddad F, Hunt SA, Rosenthal DN, Murphy DJ. Right ventricular function in cardiovascular disease, part I: anatomy, physiology, aging, and functional assessment of the right ventricle. Circulation. 2008;117(11):1436–48.
22. Heffernan DS, Thakkar RK, Monaghan SF, Ravindran R, Adams CA Jr, Kozloff MS, et al. Normal presenting vital signs are unreliable in geriatric blunt trauma victims. J Trauma. 2010;69(4):813–20.
23. Greenwald SE. Ageing of the conduit arteries. J Pathol. 2007;211(2):157–72.
24. Bonomo L, Larici AR, Maggi F, Schiavon F, Berletti R. Aging and the respiratory system. Radiol Clin N Am. 2008;46(4):685–702, v–vi.

25. Candela-Toha AM, Recio-Vazquez M, Delgado-Montero A, del Rey JM, Muriel A, Liano F, et al. The calculation of baseline serum creatinine overestimates the diagnosis of acute kidney injury in patients undergoing cardiac surgery. Nefrologia. 2012;32(1):53–8.
26. Lach HW, Lorenz RA, L'Ecuyer KM. Aging muscles and joints: mobilization. Crit Care Nurs Clin North Am. 2014;26(1):105–13.
27. Vaughan MS, Vaughan RW, Cork RC. Postoperative hypothermia in adults: relationship of age, anesthesia, and shivering to rewarming. Anesth Analg. 1981;60(10):746–51.
28. Powers R. Neurobiology of aging. In: Cummings J, Coffey CE, editors. Textbook of geriatric neuropsychiatry. Washington: American Psychiatric Press; 2000. p. 33–79.
29. McIntyre A, Mehta S, Aubut J, Dijkers M, Teasell RW. Mortality among older adults after a traumatic brain injury: a meta-analysis. Brain Inj. 2013;27(1):31–40.
30. Bratton SL, Chestnut RM, Ghajar J, McConnell Hammond FF, Harris OA, Hartl R, et al. Guidelines for the management of severe traumatic brain injury. I. Blood pressure and oxygenation. J Neurotrauma. 2007;24(Suppl 1):S7–13.
31. Schneider EB, Efron DT, MacKenzie EJ, Rivara FP, Nathens AB, Jurkovich GJ. Premorbid statin use is associated with improved survival and functional outcomes in older head-injured individuals. J Trauma. 2011;71(4):815–9.
32. Wible EF, Laskowitz DT. Statins in traumatic brain injury. Neurotherapeutics. 2010;7(1):62–73.
33. Miranda LB, Braxton E, Hobbs J, Quigley MR. Chronic subdural hematoma in the elderly: not a benign disease. J Neurosurg. 2011;114(1):72–6.
34. Shoda N, Yasunaga H, Horiguchi H, Matsuda S, Ohe K, Kadono Y, et al. Risk factors affecting inhospital mortality after hip fracture: retrospective analysis using the Japanese diagnosis procedure combination database. BMJ Open. 2012;2(3):e000416.
35. Gibson CL, Gray LJ, Bath PM, Murphy SP. Progesterone for the treatment of experimental brain injury; a systematic review. Brain. 2008;131(Pt 2):318–28.
36. Kendrick D, Kumar A, Carpenter H, Zijlstra GA, Skelton DA, Cook JR, et al. Exercise for reducing fear of falling in older people living in the community. Cochrane Database Syst Rev. 2014;28(11):Cd009848.
37. Puttnam R, Davis BR, Pressel SL, Whelton PK, Cushman WC, Louis GT, et al. Association of 3 different antihypertensive medications with hip and pelvic fracture risk in older adults: secondary analysis of a randomized clinical trial. JAMA Intern Med. 2017;177(1):67–76.
38. De Bonis P, Trevisi G, de Waure C, Sferrazza A, Volpe M, Pompucci A, et al. Antiplatelet/anticoagulant agents and chronic subdural hematoma in the elderly. PLoS One. 2013;8(7):e68732.
39. Howard JL, Cipolle MD, Horvat SA, Sabella VM, Reed JF, Fulda G, et al. Preinjury warfarin worsens outcome in elderly patients who fall from standing. J Trauma. 2009;66(6):1518–22. discussion 23-4.
40. Kundu A, Sardar P, Chatterjee S, Aronow WS, Owan T, Ryan JJ. Minimizing the risk of bleeding with NOACs in the elderly. Drugs Aging. 2016;33(7):491–500.
41. Eikelboom JW, Wallentin L, Connolly SJ, Ezekowitz M, Healey JS, Oldgren J, et al. Risk of bleeding with 2 doses of dabigatran compared with warfarin in older and younger patients with atrial fibrillation: an analysis of the randomized evaluation of long-term anticoagulant therapy (RE-LY) trial. Circulation. 2011;123(21):2363–72.
42. Lorich D, Gardener M, Helfet D. Trauma to the pelvis and extremities. In: Norton J, Barie P, Bollinger R, Chang A, Lowry S, Mulvihill S, et al., editors. Surgery basic science and clinical evidence. New York: Springer; 2008. p. 505–20.
43. Stahel PF, Hammerberg EM. History of pelvic fracture management: a review. World J Emerg Surg. 2016;11:18.
44. Morris RO, Sonibare A, Green DJ, Masud T. Closed pelvic fractures: characteristics and outcomes in older patients admitted to medical and geriatric wards. Postgrad Med J. 2000;76(900):646–50.
45. Krappinger D, Kammerlander C, Hak DJ, Blauth M. Low-energy osteoporotic pelvic fractures. Arch Orthop Trauma Surg. 2010;130(9):1167–75.
46. Balogh Z, King KL, Mackay P, McDougall D, Mackenzie S, Evans JA, et al. The epidemiology of pelvic ring fractures: a population-based study. J Trauma. 2007;63(5):1066–73. discussion 72-3.

47. Dechert TA, Duane TM, Frykberg BP, Aboutanos MB, Malhotra AK, Ivatury RR. Elderly patients with pelvic fracture: interventions and outcomes. Am Surg. 2009;75(4):291–5.
48. Bazylewicz D, Konda S. A Review of the definitive treatment of pelvic fractures. Bull Hosp Jt Dis. 2016;74(1):6–11.
49. McCormack R, Strauss EJ, Alwattar BJ, Tejwani NC. Diagnosis and management of pelvic fractures. Bull NYU Hosp Jt Dis. 2010;68(4):281–91.
50. Rommens PM, Ossendorf C, Pairon P, Dietz SO, Wagner D, Hofmann A. Clinical pathways for fragility fractures of the pelvic ring: personal experience and review of the literature. J Orthop Sci. 2015;20(1):1–11.
51. Coccolini F, Stahel PF, Montori G, Biffl W, Horer TM, Catena F, et al. Pelvic trauma: WSES classification and guidelines. World J Emerg Surg. 2017;12:5.
52. Schicho A, Schmidt SA, Seeber K, Olivier A, Richter PH, Gebhard F. Pelvic X-ray misses out on detecting sacral fractures in the elderly – Importance of CT imaging in blunt pelvic trauma. Injury. 2016;47(3):707–10.
53. Kaufmann JE, Vischer UM. Cellular mechanisms of the hemostatic effects of desmopressin (DDAVP). J Thromb Haemost. 2003;1(4):682–9.
54. White CE, Hsu JR, Holcomb JB. Haemodynamically unstable pelvic fractures. Injury. 2009;40(10):1023–30.
55. Wagner D, Ossendorf C, Gruszka D, Hofmann A, Rommens PM. Fragility fractures of the sacrum: how to identify and when to treat surgically? Eur J Trauma Emerg Surg. 2015;41(4):349–62.
56. Ojodu I, Pohlemann T, Hopp S, Rollmann MF, Holstein JH, Herath SC. Predictors of mortality for complex fractures of the pelvic ring in the elderly: a twelve-year review from a German level I trauma center. Injury. 2015;46(10):1996–8.
57. Nagy KK, Smith RF, Roberts RR, Joseph KT, An GC, Bokhari F, et al. Prognosis of penetrating trauma in elderly patients: a comparison with younger patients. J Trauma. 2000;49(2):190–3. discussion 3-4.
58. Lustenberger T, Inaba K, Schnuriger B, Barmparas G, Eberle BM, Lam L, et al. Gunshot injuries in the elderly: patterns and outcomes. A national trauma databank analysis. World J Surg. 2011;35(3):528–34.
59. Talving P, Benfield R, Hadjizacharia P, Inaba K, Chan LS, Demetriades D. Coagulopathy in severe traumatic brain injury: a prospective study. J Trauma. 2009;66(1):55–61. discussion -2.
60. Sugerman DE, Xu L, Pearson WS, Faul M. Patients with severe traumatic brain injury transferred to a Level I or II trauma center: United States, 2007 to 2009. J Trauma Acute Care Surg. 2012;73(6):1491–9.
61. Biffl WL, Leppaniemi A. Management guidelines for penetrating abdominal trauma. World J Surg. 2015;39(6):1373–80.
62. Brown CV, Shoemaker WC, Wo CC, Chan L, Demetriades D. Is noninvasive hemodynamic monitoring appropriate for the elderly critically injured patient? J Trauma. 2005;58(1):102–7.
63. Montorfano MA, Pla F, Vera L, Cardillo O, Nigra SG, Montorfano LM. Point-of-care ultrasound and Doppler ultrasound evaluation of vascular injuries in penetrating and blunt trauma. Crit Ultrasound J. 2017;9(1):5.
64. Colip CG, Gorantla V, LeBedis CA, Soto JA, Anderson SW. Extremity CTA for penetrating trauma: 10-year experience using a 64-detector row CT scanner. Emerg Radiol. 2016;24(3):223–32.
65. Kuhajda I, Zarogoulidis K, Kougioumtzi I, Huang H, Li Q, Dryllis G, et al. Penetrating trauma. J Thorac Dis. 2014;6(Suppl 4):S461–5.
66. Hajibandeh S, Gumber AO, Wong CS. Laparoscopy versus laparotomy for the management of penetrating abdominal trauma: a systematic review and meta-analysis. Int J Surg. 2016;34:127–36.

Bowel Obstructions

29

Gennaro Perrone, Luca Ansaloni, Federico Coccolini,
Salomone Di Saverio, Massimo Sartelli, and Fausto Catena

In elderly patients, bowel obstruction (BO) accounts for 10–12% of the PS access for abdominal pain and are intestinal obstructions [1]. Obstruction is three times more common in older adults than in younger patients [2]. After biliary disease, BO is the second most common reason for emergency surgical interventions in this group [3].

The ileum is the most common site of obstruction (most mobile tube, smoother, thinner, therefore more exposed to adhesions and hernias compared to the large bowel). The three most common causes of all small bowel occlusions (SBO) are adhesions (50–75%), hernias (15%), and neoplasms (15%). Gallstone ileum is a rare disease that accounts for 1–4% of mechanical obstructions.

Intra-abdominal adhesions following abdominal surgery represent a major unsolved problem. They are the first cause of SBO (Fig. 29.1). Diagnosis is based on clinical evaluation, water-soluble contrast follow-through, and computed tomography scan. Adhesive SBO requires appropriate management with a proper diagnostic and therapeutic pathway. Indication and length of nonoperative management (NOM) and appropriate timing for surgery may represent an insidious issue. Single therapeutic strategies are typically unsuccessful in preventing peritoneal adhesions due to the

G. Perrone • F. Catena (✉)
Department of Emergency Surgery, Maggiore Hospital, Parma, Italy

L. Ansaloni • F. Coccolini
General Surgery Department, Papa Giovanni XXIII Hospital, Bergamo, Italy

S. Di Saverio
Department of Surgery, Maggiore Hospital, Bologna, Italy

M. Sartelli
Department of Surgery, Macerata Hospital, Macerata, Italy

A. Crucitti (ed.), *Surgical Management of Elderly Patients*,
https://doi.org/10.1007/978-3-319-60861-7_29

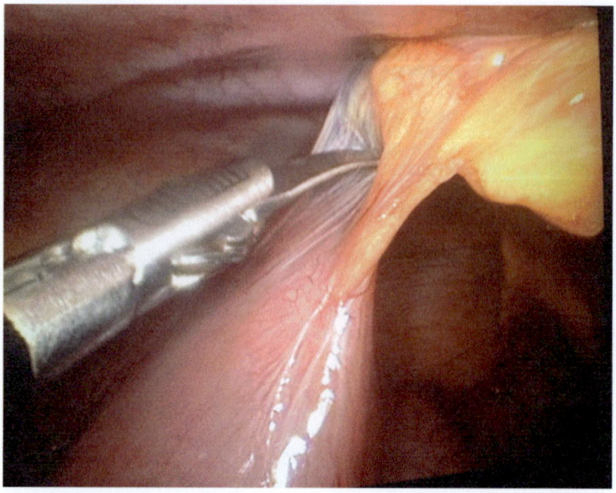

Fig. 29.1 Small bowel obstruction from adhesions

multifactorial nature of adhesion pathogenesis. Extensive literature on the subject demonstrates both the complexity of the issue and the myriad resources allocated to this condition, yet few interdisciplinary studies have been conducted involving experts from different fields. Currently the medical community only recognizes the "tip of the iceberg" and will continue treating the condition inadequately until it is more comprehensively explored [4]. In the case of suspected strangulation or after failed conservative management, open surgery is the preferred method for the surgical treatment of adhesive SBO, but laparoscopy (Fig. 29.2) is gaining widespread acceptance especially in a selected group of patients. "Good" surgical technique and anti-adhesive barriers are the main current concepts of adhesion prevention. The World Society of Emergency Surgery 2013 guidelines stated that in the absence of signs of strangulation or peritonitis, NOM can be prolonged up to 72 h. After 72 h of NOM without resolution, surgery is recommended. The risk of adhesions is greater in patients of less than 40 years of age undergoing abdominal surgery. The increase in life expectancy has resulted in an increase of the "old youngs who underwent multiple surgeries" that in life have had several occlusive episodes. A Van Goor's study underlines that patient age and three or more previous laparotomies appeared to be independent parameters predicting inadvertent enterotomy. Patients with inadvertent enterotomy had significantly more postoperative complications and urgent re-laparotomies, a higher rate of admission to the intensive care unit and parenteral nutrition usage, and a longer postoperative hospital stay [5].

In an unselected patient series of intestinal obstruction, a history of previous gynecologic pathology is a significant factor contributing to the total number of instances of intestinal obstruction in females. Surgical peritoneal closure may also result in an increase in the incidence of intestinal obstruction [6].

There are no guidelines for surgical management of malignant BO caused by peritoneal carcinomatosis, mainly when it involves the elderly; so, its treatment is still debated. In outlining indications and benefits of palliative surgery for

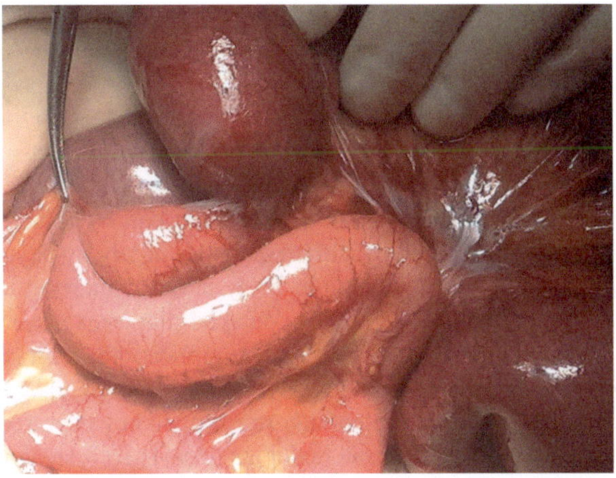

Fig. 29.2 Laparoscopic lysis of small bowel adhesions

obstructive carcinomatosis and in determining what prognostic factors, including age, have independent and significant association with outcome, surgical palliation can provide relief of obstructive symptoms as well as improved survival in well-selected patients, even if elderly.

Despite advances in diagnostic modalities, small bowel tumors are notoriously difficult to diagnose and are often advanced at the time of definitive treatment. Small intestinal neoplasms are uncommon cancers. They may occur sporadically, in association with genetic diseases (e.g., familial adenomatous polyposis coli or Peutz-Jeghers syndrome) or in association with chronic intestinal inflammatory disorders (e.g., Crohn's disease or celiac sprue). Benign small intestinal tumors (e.g., leiomyoma, lipoma, hamartoma, or desmoid tumor) usually are asymptomatic but may present with complications. Primary malignancies of the small intestine, including adenocarcinoma, leiomyosarcoma, carcinoid, and lymphoma, are often symptomatic and may present with intestinal obstruction [7].

Since the small intestine is relatively inaccessible to routine endoscopy, diagnosis of small intestinal neoplasms is often delayed for months after the onset of symptoms. Recently the increase of small bowel endoscopy and other diagnostic tools allows earlier nonoperative diagnosis. Even though radical resection of small bowel cancer plays an important role, 5-year overall survival remains low [8].

SBO in an oncology patient is a common and serious medical problem which is associated with diagnostic as well as therapeutic dilemmas. While the condition is most commonly caused by postoperative adhesions and peritoneal carcinomatosis, other causes have been reported—linitis plastica caused by metastatic lobular carcinoma of the breast, patterns of malignant melanoma's metastasis to the small bowel, intussusception in a patient treated for osteosarcoma with history of multiple metastases, a case of jejunal intussusception with gastrointestinal bleeding caused by metastatic testicular germ cell cancer.

While adhesions are the most common cause of SBO, hernias remain the most frequent cause of strangulation in patients presenting with this condition [9]. In the physical examination of an elderly patient with SBO, care should be taken to examine the hernial sites; an irreducible mass or tenderness calls for immediate operation. Obstruction by widespread intraperitoneal malignancy is the result of fixation and puckering of the bowel, often in several places. After the bowel has been decompressed, there is usually no call for any surgical procedure other than lateral anastomosis to relieve the obstruction. Abdominal hernias may be classified as groin hernias (femoral and inguinal) and ventral hernias (umbilical, epigastric, spigelian, and incisional). Strangulated hernias remain a significant challenge, as they are sometimes difficult to diagnose purely by physical examination yet require urgent surgical intervention. Early surgical intervention of a strangulated hernia with obstruction is crucial as delayed diagnosis can lead to bowel resection with longer recovery and its attendant complications. Strangulated hernias can have serious deleterious effects such as bowel obstruction, bacterial translocation, and intestinal wall necrosis (potentially resulting in bowel perforation). It poses a significant risk to emergency hernia repair, as there is an increased incidence of surgical field contamination, leading to high rates of postoperative infection and probably recurrence. Patients should undergo emergency hernia repair immediately when intestinal strangulation is suspected (grade 1C recommendation). Unfortunately, morbidity and mortality rates remain high for patients who undergo emergency repair of abdominal hernias. Early diagnosis of strangulated obstruction maybe difficult, and delayed diagnosis can lead to septic complications. However, in the case of suspected bowel strangulation, the benefits outweigh the risks of surgery, and patients should undergo immediate surgical intervention [10].

Lumbar hernias are rare conditions, and about 300 cases have been reported since the first description by Barbette in 1672. Therefore, strangulation or incarceration is also exceptionally encountered. Lumbar hernia is seen mostly in association with other abdominal wall hernias in elderly patients. They can also be bilateral as seen in this case. It was reported that the coexistence of lumbar hernia and other abdominal wall hernia is observed in 13% of patients. These reports suggest that a patient presenting with a lumbar hernia should be explored for the presence of a coexisting hernia, such as inguinal, femoral, or obturator hernia. In our case, except for the contralateral lumbar hernia, no other type of abdominal wall hernia was seen [11].

Obturator hernia was first described by Ronsil in 1724 [12]. The incidence is nearly 1% of all hernias [13]. With the nickname "little old lady's hernia," it usually occurs in multiparous and elderly emaciated women due to a wider pelvis and enlarged obturator canal. The other risk factors include chronic obstructive pulmonary disease, chronic constipation, and ascites. The cardinal clinical symptom is acute intestinal obstruction. The patient can have a positive Howship-Romberg sign, which is caused by the intermittent irritation of the obturator nerve. It was reported that 15–50% patients of obturator hernia may have positive Howship-Romberg. To examine the thigh, adductor reflex might be valuable for differentiating osteoarthritis from obturator hernia. The loss of the adductor reflex, named as the Hannington-Kiff sign, sometimes is observed on the affected side, while the patellar tendon reflex was intact on the same side [14].

Paraduodenal hernia is an unusual form of internal hernia that results from a congenital midgut malrotation. It is classified as either right or left, depending on anatomic features and embryologic origin. Left hernias are three times more common than right. Clinical symptoms may be intermittent and nonspecific, such as nausea, distention and abdominal pain, or sometimes acute SBO or ischemia. The average age at diagnosis is usually 38 years. The paraduodenal hernia is an uncommon disorder characterized by extremely variable clinical manifestations, from absolute asymptomatic to occlusion with ischemia or intestinal infarction. The importance of putting in the differential diagnosis of this disease in the case of occlusive pictures without an obvious cause is not to be underestimated. The instrumental images, and in particular the TACs, show quite a characteristic picture and are difficult to interpret by the radiologist or the experienced surgeon when not aware of this pathological condition. In a review of the literature, we found the disease in only six elderly patients (73–95 years), most of them carrying a left paraduodenal hernia. This is indicative of the rarity of the disease and thus the likelihood of a correct diagnosis [15].

Nutritional status is very important, especially in older adults because of its effects on quality of life. Phytobezoar, for instance, that can lead to SBO has risk factors such as excessive consumption of foods with high-fiber content and inadequate chewing. These factors are related to dietary habits. Furthermore, the aging process and some related physiologic changes can predispose older adults to phytobezoar formation [16].

Internal abdominal hernias present an infrequent surgical diagnosis and are usually encountered accidentally during surgery. They are generally considered as an extremely rare cause of ileus.

The incidence of the diverticulum of the SB varies from 0.2 to 1.3% in autopsy studies to 2.3% when assessed on enteroclysis. It occurs mostly in patients in the sixth decade of their life. Of all small bowel diverticula, jejunal diverticulum is the most common type. This rare entity is usually asymptomatic. However, they may cause chronic nonspecific symptoms for a long period of time like dyspepsia, chronic postprandial pain, nausea, vomiting, borborygmi, alternating diarrhea and constipation, weight loss, anemia, and steatorrhea or rarely lead to complications like hemorrhage, obstruction, and perforation. Obstruction can be due to enterolith, adhesions, intussusception, and volvulus. The condition is difficult to diagnose because patients generally present with symptoms that mimic other diseases. Only 27 cases of SBO by enterolith expelled from small bowel diverticula have been reported in the literature. Jejunal diverticular disease should be considered in the differential diagnosis of mechanical small bowel obstruction without an obvious cause, especially in the elderly population.

The prevalence of inflammatory bowel disease (IBD) increases in the elderly population. There is no increased risk for developing intestinal cancer among patients with elderly onset IBD in this population-based cohort. There are increased risks of developing lymphoproliferative and myeloproliferative disorders in all IBD. Thiopurine exposure was not found as associated with an increased risk to lymphoproliferative disorders. These data reinforce the difference between elderly onset IBD as compared with patients with a younger age at IBD onset [17].

Among elderly patients, the incidence of ulcerative colitis (UC) is higher than that of Crohn's disease (CD). Elderly patients with a new diagnosis of UC are more likely to be male and have left-sided colitis. Elderly patients with a new diagnosis of CD are more likely to be female and have colonic disease. Conversely, increasing age at diagnosis has been associated with a lower likelihood of having any family history of IBD, perianal disease in CD, and extraintestinal manifestations. This increase in inflammatory diseases in the elderly has meant that it is increasingly common to find older people with bowel obstruction from Crohn's disease [18].

The large bowel obstructions (LBO) are caused by carcinomas of the colon which slowly progress to give complete obstruction, inflammatory disease, fecal impaction, sigmoid volvulus, and cecal volvulus. Malignancy accounts for 80% of LBO. Acute obstruction of the colon rectum is a more serious emergency than occlusion of SBO because of the risk of cecal distention, necrosis, and perforation. The onset of peritonitis due to cecal perforation in the elderly patient is insidious, and the seriousness of the situation may not be apparent until the patient goes into shock. Among patients with malignant large bowel tumors, obstruction in the left colon is more common than in the right colon.

Colorectal cancer (CRC) is a major source of morbidity and mortality in the elderly population, and surgery is often the only definitive management option. Emergency surgery for acute colonic obstruction is associated with a significant risk of mortality and morbidity and with a high percentage of stoma creation (either temporary or permanent). Right-sided colonic obstructions are usually treated by one-stage resection with primary anastomosis for all but the frailest patients, whereas controversy continues to revolve around emergency management of obstructed left colon cancer (OLCC). The WSES's consensus conference of 2010 aimed to analyze the available scientific evidence on treatment modalities for OLCC and how this is implemented in clinical practice. The goal of the authors was to offer practical and scientifically supported suggestions to manage OLCC. The committee made every effort to collect and classify the best available scientific evidence on treatment of OLCC [19].

Age itself is not a risk factor for the development of complications in patients undergoing surgery for colorectal cancer. Age alone should not be a reason to avoid therapeutic or palliative surgery in these patients; instead patient selection should focus on clinical condition and ASA levels.

One-stage surgery appears to be superior to two- or three-stage procedures. Stenting is a promising option, allowing the resection to be carried out in an elective setting. Stenting appears to be a safe and effective addition to the armamentarium of treatment options for colorectal obstructions [20].

Volvulus of the intestine is a surgical emergency. Volvulus of the small bowel is more common in children and is most often secondary to malrotation. Colonic volvulus is a rare cause of large bowel obstruction but more common than small bowel volvulus in the elderly. Cecal volvulus (Fig. 29.3) is most commonly due to lack of fixation. Colonic volvulus has a specific radiographic appearance; however, small bowel volvulus is difficult to distinguish from other causes of small bowel obstruction by radiographic means. New surgical techniques with minimally invasive surgery are increasingly being applied to this old problem with good results in selected cases. The incidence of small bowel volvulus in adults varies widely with

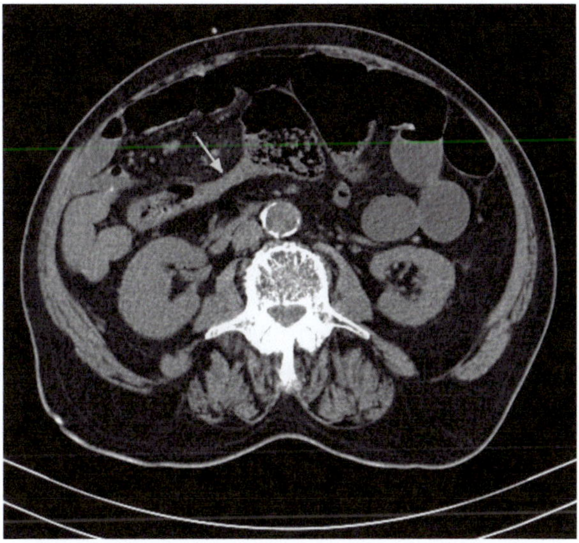

Fig. 29.3 Cecum volvulus

geographic location. In the Western world, it is rare and accounts for 1.7–6.2% of all SBO. Obstructions can be viewed as either primary (in a normal abdominal cavity) or, more commonly, secondary (due to anatomic malformations, malrotation, adhesions, tumors, or diverticula). Presentation is that of an acute small bowel obstruction, with abdominal pain, nausea, and vomiting. Peritoneal signs, palpable mass, fever, and leukocytosis are indicators of gangrenous bowel. Plain abdominal radiographs usually show a nonspecific pattern of SBO. Treatment is laparotomy with either detorsion or resection if the bowel involved is compromised, with correction of the underlying cause as appropriate. Volvulus of the colon accounts for 10–13% of all large bowel obstruction in the United States. It can involve any segment but most frequently occurs in the sigmoid or cecum. Volvulus of the sigmoid colon is the most common large bowel volvulus; it occurs in 70–80% of cases. It is usually secondary to a redundant colon, which may be associated with several illnesses. It is more common in the elderly, institutionalized patient. Typical radiographic findings are the “bent inner tube” with the point usually directed to the right upper quadrant. The preferred approach in the stable patient who can undergo a bowel preparation would be elective sigmoid resection. Other options range from cecostomy, transverse colostomy, sigmoid colostomy, operative detorsion, and emergent resection [Hartmann procedure, obstructive resection (Paul-Mikulicz), primary anastomosis] to elective resection with primary anastomosis. Other less frequently used options would include tube sigmoidostomy, mesocoloplasty, sigmoidopexy to the transverse colon, sigmoidopexy to the parietes, and fixations of the sigmoid mesentery. In patients with peritoneal signs where compromised bowel is suspected, definitive treatment with laparotomy and bowel resection is indicated. Ten to twenty percent of colonic volvulus is cecal volvulus. It is associated with lack of fixation of the right colon to the peritoneum and is more prevalent in a younger patient population. It manifests in two main forms: axial rotation of the cecum and the ileum around the mesentery (true volvulus) and the less common cecal bascule, where the bowel folds up on itself. Radiographic findings are those of large bowel obstruction with a "coffee bean" deformity directed toward the left upper quadrant. Patients with cecal volvulus are more likely to need initial surgical treatment, with cecopexy, cecostomy, or resection. Detorsion alone is not recommended due to the high recurrence rate. Volvulus of the transverse colon is rare (2–4%), and splenic flexure volvulus is the least common site. Diagnosis is usually intraoperative, and resection is the preferred treatment. A minimally invasive approach is feasible both in the acute and especially the elective settings but depends on the surgeon's experience [21].

The incidence of diverticulitis increases with age. Although left-sided colonic diverticulosis is more common among elderly patients, the most common acute mode of presentation is intestinal obstruction due to an exacerbation of the peridiverticular inflammation or to the adhesion of a loop of small bowel to the inflamed colon. The obstruction may be complete and require a defunctioning proximal colostomy for its relief. The decision regarding surgical treatment must be based on the severity of the underling diverticulitis, the degree of intestinal obstruction, and also the clarified presence of malignant colorectal disease [22].

The fecal impactions ("fecaloma") are dehydrated fecal masses that form in the bulb rectal, especially in bedridden elderly patients, who, sometimes, for reasons of central vascular disease and/or dementia, have no cognizance of reflection of defecation. So, the incomplete evacuation of stool may lead to the formation of a large mass of hard and unmovable stool in the rectum, in fact, "fecal impaction." The rectosigma becomes distended, and the hard irregular mass (stercoroma) is not sufficiently plastic to be expelled through the disproportionately small anal canal by the patient, who tries a generally weak defecation. The RX direct abdomen is an examination which is usually performed to assess whether there are "air-fluid levels" or worse "free air in the abdomen," radiological signs of acute surgical abdomen, or more simply "signs of fecal impaction," e.g., U-bends, vision of feces in the rectal ampoule, etc., or even bowel obstruction.

The frequency of fecal impaction is higher in geriatric patients admitted and treated in psychiatric hospitals. Patients who are immobilized for a long period (e.g., those with myocardial infarction or orthopedic problems) tend to develop a fecal impaction if not administered with mild laxatives for constipation. A careful rectal examination is not harmful in these patients and should be done routinely for early detection of impaction or occult intestinal bleeding.

Interesting complications but with rare conditions that accompany fecal packing are hernia, volvulus applicant megacolon, ileus, adynamic and leveling with gaseous distention, rectal prolapse, dystocia, and intestinal obstruction [23]. A fecaloma in the small intestine is extremely rare. However, this should be considered in differential diagnosis when symptoms of acute mechanical SBO develop in a child with constipation. Diagnosis is usually made from radiographic findings of a mobile intraluminal mass with a smooth outline and no mucosal attachment. Most fecalomas are successfully treated by conservative methods such as laxatives, enemas, and rectal evacuation. When conservative treatments have failed, a surgical intervention may be needed.

Laparoscopic techniques are gradually replacing many common surgical procedures that are performed in an increasingly aging population. Laparoscopy places different physiologic demands on the body to open surgery. PubMed was searched for evidence related to the use of laparoscopy in the elderly population to treat common surgical pathologies. Randomized trials, systematic reviews, and meta-analyses were preferred. Currently, over 40% of all surgeries performed in the United States are on patients older than 65 years. By the end of the twenty-first century, Americans are expected to live 20 years longer than the current average. However, elderly patients clearly show higher rates of surgical morbidity and mortality overall. Laparoscopic techniques show decreased wound complications, postoperative ileum, intraoperative blood loss, and reduced need for postoperative rehabilitation. In conclusion, laparoscopic surgery is safe in the elderly population and affords multiple advantages including decreased pain and convalescence. However, the physiology of laparoscopy places demands on elderly patients that typically present with more medical comorbidities. Elderly patients represent a large cohort of surgical patients and are therefore profoundly affected by this shift in care. Where feasible, laparoscopic surgery is becoming the gold standard in the treatment of many common pathologies that disproportionately affect elderly patients. The benefits of laparoscopy have been well documented, including decreased postoperative pain, decreased length of hospital stay, improved cosmesis, and a quicker return to normal activity. On the contrary, laparoscopy may be more technically challenging, owing to a significant learning curve among surgeons, and carries with it a distinct milieu of physiologic demands on the elderly patient. The surgical requirements for laparoscopic surgery place unique physiological demands on the patient and present a distinct challenge in the elderly patient. The insufflation of carbon dioxide gas can create acid-base disturbances, changes in blood gas balance, and alterations of cardiovascular and pulmonary physiology. While most of these changes do not result in clinical significance, they can become more of a factor in patients with comorbidity conditions, especially those that result in decreased cardiopulmonary reserve, as is common in elderly patients [24].

Utilization of abdominopelvic computed tomography (CT) in geriatric patients presenting to the emergency department (ED) with acute abdominal symptoms strongly influences clinical management and significantly affects disposition. As the US population ages, the clinical impact of emergent CT in the elderly will intensify [25].

Intussusception is defined as a segment of the gastrointestinal tract and mesentery within the lumen of an adjacent segment. It is a rare condition that in adults can occur anywhere in the gastrointestinal tract from the stomach to the rectum. Only 5% of all intussusceptions are presented in adults and in 1–5% of all cases of intestinal obstruction.

Conclusions

Most operations on elderly subjects are performed to correct or avert serious lesions. Once a decision is made that surgical treatment is indicated, the advanced age of the patient is a good reason for operating without delay. The improved outlook in recent years can be attributed to a more hopeful attitude on the part of the surgeon, better anesthesia, and an increase in our knowledge. It is in the care of the sick, elderly, surgical patient that the value of a medical team drawn from several specialties is most evident.

References

1. Kizer KW, Vassar MJ. Emergency department diagnosis of abdominal disorders in the elderly. Am J Emerg Med. 1998;16:357–62.
2. Telfer S, Fenyo G, Holt PR, et al. Acute abdominal pain in patients over 50 years of age. Scand J Gastroenterol Suppl. 1998;144:47–50.
3. Hendrickson MH, Naparst TR. Abdominal surgical emergencies in the elderly. Emerg Med Clin North Am. 2003;21:937–69.
4. Coccolini F, Ansaloni L, Manfredi R, Campanati L, Poiasina E, Bertoli P, Capponi MG, Sartelli M, Di Saverio S, Cucchi M, Lazzareschi D, Pisano M, Catena F. Peritoneal adhesion index (PAI): proposal of a score for the "ignored iceberg" of medicine and surgery. World J Emerg Surg. 2013;8:6.
5. Van Der Krabben AA, Dijkstra FR, Nieuwenhuijzen M, Reijnen MM, Schaapveld M, Van Goor H. Morbidity and mortality of inadvertent enterotomy during adhesiotomy. Br J Surg. 2000;87:467–71.
6. Stricker B, Blanco J, Fox HE. The gynecologic contribution to intestinal obstruction in females. J Am Coll Surg. 1994;178:617–20.
7. Catena F, Ansaloni L, Gazzotti F, Gagliardi S, Di Saverio S, De Cataldis A, Taffurelli M. Small bowel tumours in emergency surgery: specificity of clinical presentation. ANZ J Surg. 2005;75:997–9.
8. Coco C, Rizzo G, Manno A, Mattana C, Verbo A. Surgical treatment of small bowel neoplasms. Eur Rev Med Pharmacol Sci. 2010;14:327–33.
9. Ihedioha U, Alani A, Modak P, Chong P, O'Dwyer PJ. Hernias are the most common cause of strangulation in patients presenting with small bowel obstruction. Hernia. 2006;10:338–40.
10. Sartelli M, Coccolini F, van Ramshorst GH, Campanelli G, Mandalà V, Ansaloni L, Moore EE, Peitzman A, Velmahos G, Moore FA, Leppaniemi A, Burlew CC, Biffl W, Koike K, Kluger Y, Fraga GP, Ordonez CA, Di Saverio S, Agresta F, Sakakushev B, Gerych I, Wani I, Kelly MD, Gomes CA, Faro MP Jr, Taviloglu K, Demetrashvili Z, Lee JG, Vettoretto N, Guercioni G, Tranà C, Cui Y, Kok KYY, Ghnnam WM, Abbas AE-S, Sato N, Marwah S, Rangarajan M, Ben-Ishay O, Adesunkanmi ARK, Lohse HAS, Kenig J, Mandalà S, Patrizi A, Scibé R, Catena F. WSES guidelines for emergency repair of complicated abdominal wall hernias. World J Emerg Surg. 2013;8:50.
11. Fokou M, Fotso P, Ngowe MN, Essomba A, Sosso M. Strangulated or incarcerated spontaneous lumbar hernia as exceptional cause of intestinal obstruction: case report and review of the literature. World J Emerg Surg. 2014;9:44.
12. Ziegler DW, Rhoads JE Jr. Obturator hernia needs a laparotomy, not a diagnosis. Am J Surg. 1995;170:67–8.
13. Lo CY, Lorentz TG, Lau PW. Obturator hernia presenting as small bowel obstruction. Am J Surg. 1994;167:396–8.
14. Hannington-Kiff JG. Absent thigh adductor reflex in obturator hernia. Lancet. 1980;1:180.
15. Andreani S, Cimbanassi S, Pugliese R, Chiara O. An unusual cause of small bowel obstruction in the elderly. Ann Ital Chir. 2006;77:513–6.
16. Akrami M, Sasani MR. Dietary habits affect quality of life: bowel obstruction caused by phytobezoar. Iran J Public Health. 2016;45:1080–2.

17. Cheddani H, Dauchet L, Fumery M, Charpentier C, Marie Bouvier A, Dupas JL, Pariente B, Peyrin-Biroulet L, Savoye G, Gower-Rousseau C. Cancer in elderly onset inflammatory bowel disease: a population-based study. Am J Gastroenterol. 2016;111:1428–36.
18. Stepaniuk P, Bernstein CN, Targownik LE, Singh H. Characterization of inflammatory bowel disease in elderly patients: a review of epidemiology, current practices and outcomes of current management strategies. Can J Gastroenterol Hepatol. 2015;29:327–33.
19. Ansaloni L, Andersson RE, Bazzoli F, Catena F, Cennamo V, Di Saverio S, Fuccio L, Jeekel H, Leppäniemi A, Moore E, Pinna AD, Pisano M, Repici A, Sugarbaker PH, Tuech J-J. Guidelines in the management of obstructing cancer of the left colon: consensus conference of the world society of emergency surgery (WSES) and peritoneum and surgery (PnS) society. World J Emerg Surg. 2010;5:29.
20. Tan CJ, Dasari BV, Gardiner K. Systematic review and meta-analysis of randomized clinical trials of self-expanding metallic stents as a bridge to surgery versus emergency surgery for malignant left-sided large bowel obstruction. Br J Surg. 2012;99:469–76.
21. Valsdottir E, Marks JH. Volvulus: small bowel and colon. Clin Colon Rectal Surg. 2008;21:91–3.
22. Sartelli M, Catena F, Ansaloni L, Coccolini F, Griffiths EA, Abu-Zidan FM, Di Saverio S, Ulrych J, Kluger Y, Ben-Ishay O, Moore FA, Ivatury RR, Coimbra R, Peitzman AB, Leppaniemi A, Fraga GP, Maier RV, Chiara O, Kashuk J, Sakakushev B, Weber DG, Latifi R, Biffl W, Bala M, Karamarkovic A, Inaba K, Ordonez CA, Hecker A, Augustin G, Demetrashvili Z, Melo RB, Marwah S, Zachariah SK, Shelat VG, McFarlane M, Rems M, Gomes CA, Faro MP, Pereira GA Jr, Negoi I, Cui Y, Sato N, Vereczkei A, Bellanova G, Birindelli A, Di Carlo I, Kok KY, Gachabayov M, Gkiokas G, Bouliaris K, Çolak E, Isik A, Rios-Cruz D, Soto R, Moore EE. WSES guidelines for the management of acute left sided colonic diverticulitis in the emergency setting. World J Emerg Surg. 2016;11:37.
23. Falcón BS, López MB, Muñoz BM, Sánchez AÁ, Rey E. Fecal impaction: a systematic review of its medical complications. BMC Geriatr. 2016;16:4.
24. Bates AT, Divino C. Laparoscopic surgery in the elderly: a review of the literature. Aging Dis. 2015;6:149–55.
25. Gardner CS, Jaffe TA, Nelson RC. Impact of CT in elderly patients presenting to the emergency department with acute abdominal pain. Abdom Imaging. 2015;40:2877–82.

Acute Peritonitis

30

Massimo Sartelli, Federico Coccolini, Fausto Catena, and Luca Ansaloni

30.1 Introduction

Compared with elective surgery, emergency abdominal surgery is associated with increased morbidity and mortality, especially in elderly patients [1, 2].

Emergency laparotomies for acute peritonitis in elder patients are high-risk procedures with associated high mortality.

The improvement in living conditions and the achievement of high standards of care in the past two decades resulted in an increase in life expectancy and in an increase in the age of patients admitted with acute peritonitis. With this continuous ageing of the population, the number of elderly patients requiring emergency surgery for acute peritonitis is rising.

Elderly people express an epidemiologically different disease pattern, such as those demonstrated for perforated gastroduodenal ulcers [3].

30.2 Outcome of Elderly Patients with Acute Peritonitis

Short- and long-term outcomes of elderly patients having an acute peritonitis are often associated with higher mortality, increased morbidity, consequently higher utility of intensive care resources and longer hospital stay and even limitations on the ability to live an independent life after the septic insult.

M. Sartelli (✉)
Department of Surgery, Macerata Hospital, Macerata, Italy

F. Coccolini • L. Ansaloni
General Surgery Department, Papa Giovanni XXIII Hospital, Bergamo, Italy

F. Catena
Emergency Surgery Department, Maggiore Hospital, Parma, Italy

A. Crucitti (ed.), *Surgical Management of Elderly Patients*,
https://doi.org/10.1007/978-3-319-60861-7_30

In 2014, the World Society of Emergency Surgery (WSES) designed a global prospective observational study (CIAOW study) [4, 5].

The complicated intra-abdominal infections worldwide observational (CIAOW) study is a multicenter observational study undergone in 68 medical institutions worldwide during a 6-month study period (October 2012 to March 2013). The study included 1898 patients older than 18 years undergoing surgery or interventional drainage to address complicated intra-abdominal infections (IAIs). All the risk factors for occurrence of death during hospitalization were evaluated. According to stepwise multivariate analysis (PR = 0.005 and PE = 0.001), several criteria were found to be independent variables predictive of mortality, including patient age (OR = 1.1; 95%CI = 1.0–1.1; $p < 0.0001$).

30.3 Risk Factors of Elderly Patients with Acute Peritonitis

Elderly patients with acute peritonitis are usually in poor clinical condition due to poor physiological reserve and the additional stress caused by sepsis response. Moreover octa- and nonagenarians with acute peritonitis present with fewer signs of peritonitis and have the risk of long delays to definitive treatment and increased risk of mortality [6].

Ageing is an inexorable intrinsic process that affects all individuals; due to a diminished homeostasis and increased organism frailty, it causes a reduction in the response to environmental stimuli and, in general, is associated with an increased predisposition to illness and death.

Several studies investigating ageing physiopathology report that old age is followed by a low-grade inflammatory process, which may be upregulated during sepsis and surgical procedures [7].

Frailty is an important potential risk factor in treating elderly patients.

Frailty is defined as a decline in the physiological reserves that may make the person vulnerable to even the most minor of stressful events, and appears to be a valid indicator and predictor of risk and poor outcome, but is difficult to monitor or manage in the emergency setting.

Risk scores are not generally available universally [8, 9] for elderly population.

A new Sepsis Severity Score for patients with complicated intra-abdominal infections, validated on a global level by a prospective study, was published in 2015 [10]. The score included the clinical conditions at the admission (severe sepsis/septic shock), the origin of the cIAIs, the delay in source control, the setting of acquisition and any risk factors such as immunosuppression and age (Table 30.1).

The statistical analysis showed that the Sepsis Severity Score has a very good ability to distinguish those who survived from those who died. The overall mortality was 0.63% for those who had a score of 0–3, 6.3% for those who had a score of 4–6 and 41.7% for those who had a score of ≥7. In patients who had a score of ≥9, the mortality rate was 55.5%; those who had a score of ≥11, the mortality rate was 68.2%; and those who had a score of ≥13, the mortality rate was 80.9%.

Table 30.1 WSES Sepsis Severity Score for patients with complicated intra-abdominal infections (range, 0–18)

Clinical condition at admission	
• Severe sepsis (acute organ dysfunction) at the admission	3 score
• Septic shock (acute circulatory failure characterized by persistent arterial hypotension. It always requires vasopressor agents) at admission	5 score
Setting of acquisition	
• Healthcare-associated infection	2 score
Origin of the IAIs	
• Colonic non-diverticular perforation peritonitis	2 score
• Small bowel perforation peritonitis	3 score
• Diverticular diffuse peritonitis	2 score
• Post-operative diffuse peritonitis	2 score
Delay in source control	
• Delayed initial intervention (preoperative duration of peritonitis (localized or diffuse) > 24 h))	3 score
Risk factors	
• Age > 70	2 score
• Immunosuppression (chronic glucocorticoids, immunosuppressant agents, chemotherapy, lymphatic diseases, virus)	3 score

Comorbidities are very common in elderly patients.

Several studies have shown that the incidence of comorbidity in the elderly with acute abdominal disease requiring emergency operation was more than 50% [11–13].

Moreover, unlike elective surgery, many risk factors are not amenable to modification at the time a patient requires emergency surgery; Wu et al. [14] recently confirmed this by demonstrating how hypoalbuminemia was associated with higher rate of morbidity and mortality after emergent abdominal surgery in geriatric critically ill patients.

30.4 Healthcare System Implications

A crucial issue in managing elderly patients with acute peritonitis is post-operative care: elderly patients frequently demand intensive care, rehabilitation and longer recovery times even after minor surgery, and solid social support is necessary for a full recovery. Therefore, management of elderly patients with acute peritonitis has great clinical and healthcare system implications, and an adequate organization of emergency care is mandatory to better treat elderly patients.

Conclusions

Faced with the admission of an elderly patient, surgeons must decide whether surgical treatment is justified balancing eventual benefits and surgical risks markedly increased in the older population because of pre-existing illness and frailty.

Improving outcomes in emergency surgery for the geriatric population is a multifaceted task.

Management of elderly patients with acute peritonitis has great clinical and healthcare system implications, and an adequate organization of emergency care is important to better treat elderly patients.

References

1. Arenal JJ, Bengoechea-Beeby M. Mortality associated with emergency abdominal surgery in the elderly. Can J Surg. 2003;46(2):111–6.
2. Zerbib PH, Kuick JF, Lebuffe G, Khoury-Helou A, Pleiner I, Chamnbon JP. Emergency major abdominal surgery in patients over 85 years of age. World J Surg. 2005;29(7):820–5.
3. Thorsen K, Soreide JA, Kvaloy JT, Glomsaker T, Soreide K. Epidemiology of perforated peptic ulcer: age and gender-adjusted analysis of incidence and mortality. World J Gastroenterol. 2013;19(3):347–54.
4. Sartelli M, Catena F, Ansaloni L, Leppaniemi A, Taviloglu K, van Goor H, et al. Complicated intra-abdominal infections in Europe: a comprehensive review of the CIAO study. World J Emerg Surg. 2012;7(1):36. https://doi.org/10.1186/1749-7922-7-36.
5. Sartelli M, Catena F, Ansaloni L, Coccolini F, Corbella D, Moore EE, et al. Complicated intra-abdominal infections worldwide: the definitive data of the CIAOW study. World J Emerg Surg. 2014;9:37.
6. Søreide K, Desserud KF. Emergency surgery in the elderly: the balance between function, frailty, fatality and futility. Scand J Trauma Resusc Emerg Med. 2015;23:10.
7. Candore G, Caruso C, Jirillo E, Magrone T, Vasto S. Low grade inflammation as a common pathogenetic denominator in age-related diseases: novel drug targets for anti-ageing strategies and successful ageing achievement. Curr Pharm Des. 2010;16(6):584–96.
8. Desserud KF, Veen T, Søreide K. Emergency general surgery in the geriatric patient. Br J Surg. 2016;103(2):e52–61.
9. Søreide K, Desserud KF. Emergency surgery in the elderly: the balance between function, frailty, fatality and futility. Scand J Trauma Resusc Emerg Med. 2015;23:10.
10. Sartelli M, Abu-Zidan FM, Catena F, Griffiths EA, Di Saverio S, Coimbra R, et al. Global validation of the WSES sepsis severity score for patients with complicated intra-abdominal infections: a prospective multicentre study (WISS study). World J Emerg Surg. 2015;10:61.
11. Feny G. Acute abdominal disease in the elderly. Am J Surg. 1982;143:751–4. https://doi.org/10.1016/0002-9610(82)90052-6.
12. Mcintyre R, Reinbach D, Cuschieri RJ. Emergency abdominal surgery in the elderly. J R Coll Surg Edinb. 1997;42:173–8.
13. Ozkan E, Fersahoğlu MM, Dulundu E, Ozel Y, Yıldız MK, Topaloğlu U. Factors affecting mortality and morbidity in emergency abdominal surgery in geriatric patients. Ulus Travma Acil Cerrahi Derg. 2010;16:439–44.
14. Wu S-C, Fu C-Y, Hsieh C-H, et al. Early predictors for tissue healing deficit and leakage in geriatric critically ill patients receiving emergent abdominal surgery: a case control study. Int J Surg. 2014;12:315–9.

31 Upper and Lower Gastrointestinal Bleeding

Paola Fugazzola, Giulia Montori, Camilla Bing, Fausto Catena, Massimo Sartelli, Luca Ansaloni, and Federico Coccolini

31.1 Epidemiology

More than 1% of people aged 80 years and older are hospitalized each year because of gastrointestinal bleeding [1], and rates of both upper and lower GI hemorrhages increase significantly with aging. The incidence of hospitalization in patients older than 75 years old for upper GI bleeding and lower GI bleeding is 425.2/100.000 and 380.1/100.000, respectively [2]. The mortality rate also increases with aging, and it is 3% in patients ages 65–84 and 5.2% in patients over 85 years old [2].

GI bleeding in such elderly people can originate from lesions common to all age groups or from lesions associated specifically with aging [3]. Gastrointestinal bleeding can be classified as acute (presenting as hematemesis, melena, or hematochezia) or chronic, presenting as occult GI blood loss or anemia.

In elderly people, morbidity and mortality from GI bleeding are determined by both the nature and the entity of bleeding and the presence of comorbid medical conditions.

P. Fugazzola • G. Montori • L. Ansaloni • F. Coccolini (✉)
General, Emergency and Trauma Surgery Department, Papa Giovanni XXIII Hospital, Bergamo, Italy

C. Bing
General Surgery Department, San Giuseppe Hospital, Empoli, Italy

F. Catena
Emergency Surgery Department, Parma University Hospital, Parma, Italy

M. Sartelli
General and Emergency Surgery Department, Macerata Hospital, Macerata, Italy

A. Crucitti (ed.), *Surgical Management of Elderly Patients*,
https://doi.org/10.1007/978-3-319-60861-7_31

31.2 Clinical Features of GI Bleeding in Elderly vs Younger Patients

Although the approach to the diagnosis and management of gastrointestinal bleeding is not specific to elderly people, they differ from younger people for several aspects of clinical presentation and outcomes [4]:

- Elderly people usually have important comorbid conditions influencing outcomes, including cardiovascular and pulmonary disease.
- They are commonly prescribed numerous medications which may compromise mucosal integrity and predispose bleeding (aspirin, NSAID, anticoagulant, and antiplatelet medications).
- They have fewer antecedent symptoms (abdominal pain, dyspepsia, heartburn).
- They present higher rates of hospitalization.
- They present higher rates of rebleeding.
- They have higher mortality rate.

The widespread use of aspirin for the primary prevention of coronary events caused an increase in major GI events [5]. Furthermore, in the population older than 80 years who are prescribed with anticoagulant and antiplatelet medications, major hemorrhagic events have an incidence of 13.1% patients during the first year of anticoagulation (compared to an incidence of major hemorrhage of 4.7%/years in individuals younger than 80) [6].

Therefore, although the basic principles of managing GI bleeding are the same in elderly and younger patients, in several studies, mortality remains high in the elderly, despite strict adherence to modern algorithms [7]. Thus, elderly patients need particular attention, and the standard management might not be adequate for these patients.

31.3 Upper GI Bleeding (UGIB) in Elderly Patients

UGIB is characterized by bleeding that originates proximal to the ligament of Treitz, including the stomach, duodenum, and esophagus. The 70% of acute UGID episodes occur in patients older than 60 years old, and the incidence of UGID increases with aging [8, 9]. Furthermore, older age was identified as a risk factor for mortality among patients with UGIB [8].

31.3.1 Clinical Presentation

Patients with UGIB may present with symptoms such as hematemesis (vomiting of fresh, bright red blood), coffee ground emesis, or melena (passage of black, tarry, foul-smelling stools as a result of degradation of blood to hematin). Melena is suggestive for bleeding proximal to the ligament of Treitz but can be due to bleeding from a more distal GI source, as far as the cecum. Furthermore, rapid and high-volume UGIB can result in hematochezia (passage of bright red blood per rectum, with or without stool). However, UGIB may be chronic, presenting with hemoccult-positive stools or with microcytic anemia. Symptoms may include light-headedness, orthostatic hypotension, and syncope, related to blood loss and hypovolemia, even in the absence of overt bleeding [2, 3]. Nasogastric intubation that returns bloody aspirate can confirm UGIB. A clear or bilious nasogastric lavage, however, does not exclude UGIB [3].

The presentation of UGI disease, particularly of peptic ulcer, in elderly patients, can be subtle, and late presentation is not uncommon. It is reported that 26% of elderly patients with peptic ulcers may not have pain [10]. In a comparative study by Kemppainen et al. [11] (age >65 vs age <65 years, $n = 125$), typical epigastric pain in the older age group was rare (35 vs 91%, $p < 0.001$). In addition ulcer bleeding was more common in the older age group (50 vs 14%, $p < 0.001$). As late diagnosis can cause bad outcomes and complications, especially in these patients, a diagnostic tool in the form of a questionnaire has been developed, to reduce misleading and unrecognized diagnoses in these patients. The UEGISQUE [12] is a 15-item questionnaire evaluating five symptom clusters: abdominal pain syndrome, reflux syndrome, indigestion syndrome, bleeding, and no-specific symptoms. The predictive value of this test was reported as good (area under ROC curve 0.78, CI 0.73–0.83).

UGIB is estimated to be five times more common than lower GI bleeding (LGIB) [13]. Furthermore, it is important to remember that one of the most important sources of blood per rectum is actually the upper GI tract, and therefore UGIB should always be considered first [2].

31.3.2 Risk Factors

Despite the decreased frequency of admissions and mortality from peptic ulcer disease among young patients, admission and mortality rates for gastric and duodenal ulcer hemorrhage have increased among the older population. This can be explained by the different etiology of peptic ulcer between the young and older population [14, 15]. There are two reasons for the higher incidence of peptic ulcer in elderly patients: the increasing use of NSAIDs including aspirin and the high prevalence of *H. pylori* infections [15]. Furthermore, several studies showed that in the elderly, there is an imbalance in the equilibrium between aggressive factors on gastrointestinal mucosa (gastric acid and pepsin) and the mucosal protective mechanisms (mucus, bicarbonate, prostaglandins) [16–20]. In addition gastrointestinal transit time and gastric emptying is slower in the elderly, increasing exposure of the gastric mucosa to the ingested medications [21].

However, because many elderly patients require analgesic or antithrombotic medications, it is important to find an optimal strategy to minimize their gastrointestinal adverse effects [15]. There is significant evidence to support the concomitant treatment with PPI in the prevention of NSAID-induced and aspirin-induced ulcers both in short-term and long-term NSAID users [22, 23]. Moreover, current evidence supports the advance of PPI over H2RAs for NSAID- and aspirin-related ulcer prevention [24]. In elderly patients, if treatment with NSAIDs cannot be avoided, a combination of a COX-2 inhibitor with a PPI may offer the best gastrointestinal protection [15].

Nevertheless, there are also some concerns about PPI use in elderly patients. First, some studies have suggested that aging may reduce the efficacy of antisecretory drugs, due to a defect in the negative feedback mechanism between intragastric pH and gastrin secretion [25]. Furthermore, there are concerns over the risks associated with long-term PPI use in the elderly populations. A retrospective study by Maggio et al. [26] showed that the use of PPIs is associated with an increased risk of all-cause death in older patients discharged from intensive care hospitals. The main risks associated with PPI use are:

- Significant higher risk of *C. difficile* infection (OR 2.15, 95% CI 1.81–2.55) [27].
- Higher risk of community-acquired pneumonia (OR 1.36, 95% CI 1.12–1.65 [28]) due to the alteration in gastric pH that allows the colonization of certain bacteria species, leading to microaspiration and colonization of the lung. Furthermore, PPIs may alter the pH of seromucinous secretion of the respiratory tract, promoting bacterial growth [15].
- Higher risk of fracture (OR 1.44, 95% CI 1.21–1.70 [29]); the mechanism is still unknown, possible theories include an inhibition of osteoclastic H-K adenosine triphosphatase and a reduction in intestinal calcium absorption [15].
- Higher risk of nutritional deficiencies such as hypomagnesemia, iron and vitamin B12 deficiency.

It is important to ensure the appropriate use of PPIs, to identify what patients can gain maximum benefit from PPI therapy and what patients need alternative therapies such as H2RAs, which is associated with less adverse effects, even if they are less effective in some cases [15].

A separate discussion should be made about critically ill patients. They are at increased risk for development of stress gastritis, and the major risk factors identified are mechanical ventilation, traumatic brain injuries, major burn wounds and trauma injuries.

31.3.3 Etiology

In Table 31.1 the main causes of UGIB in the elderly are reported.

The most common sources of UGIB in the elderly are peptic ulcer disease and gastropathy which together account for between 55 and 80% of patients presenting to emergency department with UGIB [3]. Esophagitis and esophageal/gastric varices account for the remaining sources of bleeding.

Peptic ulcer disease is the most common cause of UGIB, also in elderly people [2, 3, 30]. UGIB related to portal hypertension is mostly seen in patients younger than

60 years old. The mortality of patients who present with *esophageal varices* hemorrhage historically exceeded 30%, but there are data to suggest that has recently declined. Available data suggest that mortality after variceal hemorrhage correlates with the Child-Turcotte-Pugh score and not with advanced age [31].

Although overt hemorrhage is an uncommon manifestation of *esophagitis or gastropathy*, these lesions are implicated as bleeding sources more frequently in elderly than in younger people [3].

The risk of *UGI malignancy* increases with age, and GI bleeding is often the first presentation of malignancy [30].

Although the prevalence of *gastric antral vascular ectasia* does not increase with age, it is associated with certain medical comorbidities, such as end-stage renal disease and cirrhosis. It typically causes occult or subacute blood loss and transfusion-dependent anemia [3].

Aortoenteric fistula (*AEF*) develops in 0.5% of patients who have undergone aortoiliac bypass surgery [32] and can also develop after endovascular aortic repair, a procedure increasingly performed in the elderly [30]. AEF is also described in patients with native anatomy and after enteral stent placement. The classic presentation is with a herald (sentinel) bleed followed by exsanguinating hemorrhage. Because of the delay in its diagnosis (the median time to diagnosis of an AEF after presentation is approximately 10 days), short-term mortality exceeds 30% even after accurate diagnosis and repair [33].

Dieulafoy's lesion is a dilated submucosal artery that can rupture and result in overt gastrointestinal hemorrhage. These lesions can occur in elderly people, but are not specific to this range of population.

Less common etiologies are reported in Table 31.1.

31.3.4 Risk Assessment for Outcome

Several risk assessment scores have been developed to predict outcomes, such as the need for an intervention, and the risk of rebleeding or death. Using these scores, a

Table 31.1 Etiology of UGIB in the elderly [2, 3, 30]

Common etiology
Peptic ulcer (gastric or duodenal)
Gastroduodenal erosions and gastropathy
Esophagitis
Esophageal and gastric varices
Mallory-Weiss tear
Esophageal and gastric cancer
Less common etiology
Portal hypertensive gastropathy
Dieulafoy's lesion and Boerhaave's syndrome
Gastric antral vascular ectasia
Hemobilia
Hemosuccus pancreaticus
Aortoenteric fistula

subgroup of patients who are at very low risk of adverse outcomes can be identified, and they could be candidates for early discharge or even for nonadmission with a planned early outpatient endoscopy. Furthermore, these scores allow early identification of high-risk patients who need appropriate inpatient intervention [30].

The Glasgow-Blatchford Score (GBS) and the abbreviated "admission" (pre-endoscopic) Rockall score use only clinical and laboratory data to assess the risk and therefore can be used shortly after presentation to hospital [34, 35].

Before endoscopy, the Rockall risk scoring system is recommended, and it's the most widely used scoring system, being validated by several studies. It can predict patient's outcome, death, and estimated rebleeding risk. Patient's age, systolic blood pressure, pulse rate, and presence of comorbidities are included in the score. Patients with a score of 0 could be considered for nonadmission or early discharge; if the score is above 0, there is a significant risk of mortality and endoscopy is recommended [36].

The GBS is based on blood urea level, hemoglobin level, systolic blood pressure, pulse rate, the presence of melena or syncope, and the history of liver disease or cardiac failure. It can predict the need of intervention and mortality [30].

Conversely, the full Rockall score requires endoscopy to predict outcome and includes age, pulse rate, systolic blood pressure, comorbidity, endoscopic diagnosis (Mallory-Weiss tear or no lesions vs malignant lesions vs all other diagnoses), and the presence of stigmata of hemorrhage (no stigmata or dark spot on ulcer vs presence of blood, adherent clot, visible/spurting vessel) [36].

In literature, there is not a consensus about which score system is better. In a recent study including 335 elderly patients with UGIB, authors found the Rockall score to be clinically the most useful for predicting mortality (for complete Rockall score: area under ROC curve 0.788, 95% CI 0.726–0.849, $p = 0.001$ [36]) and rebleeding (for complete Rockall score: area under ROC curve 0.787, 95% CI 0.716–0.859, $p = 0.001$ [36]) and the GBS to be superior in predicting lenght of stay and need for blood transfusion.

31.4 Lower GI Bleeding (LGIB) in Elderly Patients

A LGIB is an Intestinal bleeding from a source distal to the ligament of Treitz. While LGIB is less common than UGIB in the general population, the incidence of LGIB is higher in the elderly [2], and it is more common in men than in women [37]. One retrospective study estimated a greater than 200-fold increase in the incidence of LGIB from the third to the ninth decade of life [13]. This trend is given by the age-associated increase in incidence of diverticular hemorrhage, which is the most common cause of LGIB in elderly people. Nearly 80% of patients presenting with LGIB will stop bleeding without intervention: however, the recurrence rate can be as high as 25% [38].

31.4.1 Clinical Presentation

LGIB can be acute, occult, or obscure. Acute LGIB presents as melena or hematochezia. The source of melena is most often from the UGI tract, but it may also be from the small intestine or right colon. Occult bleeding, usually detected with stool guaiac testing, is the most common presentation of LGIB in the elderly, occurring in 10% of adult population. Patients can lose up to 100 mL of blood per day and still have a grossly normal appearing stool [37]. Obscure bleeding is a bleeding in which the source is difficult to detect on routine endoscopic and radiologic examination.

The onset and pace of LGIB can provide additional clues to the etiology. The abrupt onset of painless, hemodynamically significant hematochezia is characteristic of diverticular hemorrhage. Cramping abdominal pain or abdominal tenderness suggests colitis. However, common presenting symptoms of LGIB may not be evident in the elderly. For example, in elderly patients who are taking NSAIDs, abdominal pain may not be present [37].

Anoscopy and digital rectal examination are recommended as a standard component of the initial physical examination. Nasogastric intubation and lavage can be useful, not only to evaluate for UGIB presenting as rectal hemorrhage but also to rapidly purge the bowel in preparation for urgent colonoscopy.

31.4.2 Risk Factors

The increase in incidence of LGIB in the elderly is due to three factors:

- The increased incidence of GI disease specific to elderly patients such as *diverticulosis coli*, vascular ectasia, ischemic colitis, and colonic neoplasm.
- The presence of comorbidity that are associated with an increased incidence and severity of LGIB such as cardiovascular disease, cirrhosis, renal disease, diabetes mellitus, and malignancy [39]. Atherosclerotic cardiovascular disease affecting the splanchnic circulation is a cause of ischemic disease; atrial fibrillation is associated with embolic events leading to ischemic bowel disease, and aortic valvular disease is associated with vascular ectasia of the colon. Furthermore, after hemorrhage, the presence of serious concurrent illness is the second most important factor in predicting mortality among patients with LGIB [39].
- Polypharmacy. The use of anticoagulants and NSAIDs increases LGIB risk because can cause ulcerations of the small intestine and colon [4].

31.4.3 Etiology

In Western Europe and in the United States, the most common causes of LGIB are diverticular disease and vascular ectasia. Less common causes are inflammatory disease of the colon, neoplasms, post-polypectomy hemorrhage and hemorrhoids [40, 41] (Table 31.2). In Asia, however, the most common causes of LGIB are hemorrhoids, anal fissures, and malignant colorectal neoplasms, while *diverticulosis coli* is a remarkably rare cause [42].

In Western Europe and in the United States, the incidence of *diverticulosis coli* increases with age from approximately 5% at the age of 40 to 65% at the age of 85 [43]. LGIB occurs in approximately 3–5% of patients with diverticular disease, usually in the form of hematochezia [38]. Diverticular hemorrhage can be severe with a morbidity and mortality rate of 10–20%. Fifty to ninety percent of diverticular LGIB occurs from right-sided colonic diverticula [44], but diverticula may also arise in the small intestine, where they may be a source of obscure bleeding. Diverticular LGIB presents as painless acute hematochezia and usually ceases spontaneously, with less than 1% of patients requiring greater than four units of blood [43]. However, bleeding can become more hemodynamically significant in elderly patients, due to comorbid conditions or to the use of anticoagulants or NSAIDs [4].

Vascular ectasia, also termed angiodysplasia, can occur in the colon (especially in the cecum) or in the small intestine. It is a degenerative lesion of previously normal blood vessels, due to repeated episodes of colonic distension associated with transient increases in both luminal pressure and size. This results in multiple episodes of increased wall tension and obstruction of submucosal venous outflow. This process leads to dilatation of venules and capillaries with the development of vascular ectasia [45]. Colonic vascular ectasia is noted in over 25% of asymptomatic individuals over the age of 60, and it causes LGIB in 12–40% of patients. The LGIB due to vascular ectasia is usually subacute but can be chronic and recurrent or can be massive in up to 15% of patients [46, 47].

Inflammatory bowel disease (*IBD*) has a bimodality distribution, with a second peak occurring between the age of 60 and 70. Approximately 15% of all patients with IBD develop symptoms after the age of 65. Severe hematochezia is infrequent [48–50].

Ischemic colitis accounts for 3–9% of all cases of LGIB in the elderly [51]. Colonic atherosclerosis is almost universal in the elderly and predisposes to ischemic colitis (nonocclusive mesenteric ischemia). This is due to a reduced blood supply to the colon because of a variety of factors, such as hypotension and vascular embolic events. Additional risk factors include vasculitis, dehydration, and the use of diuretics and vasoactive agents. Patients often present with lower abdominal cramping pain, followed by hematochezia. LGIB is rarely severe. It is often unresponsive to standard colitis treatment and may be complicated by perforation or stricture formation that requires surgical intervention [37]. Ischemic colitis is

Table 31.2 Etiology of LGIB in the elderly [3, 37, 40, 41]

Common etiology
Diverticular hemorrhage
Vascular ectasia (telangiectasia)
Inflammatory bowel disease
Neoplasms
Hemorrhoids
Ischemic colitis
Infectious colitis
Drug-associated colitis
Less common etiology
Post-polypectomy bleeding
Stercoral ulcers
Solitary rectal ulcer
Radiation proctitis
Dieulafoy's lesion
Colorectal varices

different from both chronic mesenteric ischemia (intestinal angina) and acute mesenteric ischemia caused by mesenteric arterial or venous occlusion.

The mortality due to *infectious colitis* increases with age. LGIB is rarely massive in these patients. Hematochezia is noted in less than 10% of cases. The most common causes in the elderly are *Campylobacter*, *Salmonella*, *Shigella*, *E. coli* 0157:h7, and *Clostridium difficile* [52–54].

Malignant and benign neoplasm of the colon and rectum are the cause of 10–20% of LGIB. LGIB is the initial presenting symptom in up to 26% of patients with colorectal neoplasm [55, 56]. Although LGIB from colorectal neoplasms is usually occult, it can be massive if there is erosion into a large vessel or if patients take anticoagulants or NSAIDs.

LGIB is a complication of *colonoscopic polypectomy* in 0.7–2.5% of cases, and post-polypectomy hemorrhage is the source of LGIB in approximately 3% of patients [57–59].

Stercoral ulcers are the result of mucosal damage by hard impacted stool in the rectum or by foreign body injury, such as from a rectal tube. Solitary rectal ulcer syndrome is due to rectal prolapse and mucosal damage because of constipation and straining. These diseases can be a source of massive LGIB in the elderly [60].

Radiation proctitis occurs in people who have undergone radiation therapy for prostate, genitourinary, or gynecologic malignancies. It can develop years after treatment and can result in either overt rectal hemorrhage or chronic transfusion-dependent blood loss [3].

31.5 Obscure GI Bleeding (OGIB) in Elderly Patients

In 5% of GIB, the source of hemorrhage is not identified by either colonoscopy or esophagogastroduodenoscopy (EGDS), and it is defined as obscure GI bleeding. In this situation, the source of the bleeding may be the small intestine, or it may be a source in the UGI tract or colon that was not visualized in previous diagnostic attempts.

31.6 Diagnosis

31.6.1 Endoscopy

Endoscopy, including EGDS and colonoscopy, is the diagnostic test of choice for GI bleeding and may also allow therapeutic intervention. Both EGDS and colonoscopy are safe and effective in elderly populations. EGDS allows a diagnosis in over 90% of patients [61], while colonoscopy in the setting of acute LGIB has an accuracy that ranges from 72 to 86% with a cecal intubation achieved in 95% of patients [62–64]. Both the exams require conscious sedation that is generally well tolerated in elderly patients. According to recent studies, midazolam is successfully tolerated but can cause desaturation in geriatric patients [65]. Furthermore, elderly patients may also be at increased risk of aspiration and of perforation during endoscopy. The presence of certain anatomic lesions such as Zenker's diverticulum or cervical spine osteophytes can increase the risk of perforation. Then it is necessary to pay particular attention when performing endoscopic exams in these kinds of patients. It is necessary to continuously monitor the vital signs because older patients may experience an unexpected respiratory arrest that may necessitate emergent endotracheal intubation. Current guidelines from the American Society for Gastrointestinal Endoscopy recommend heightened attention to the dose and to the effects of standard sedatives used during endoscopic procedures on the elderly. They also emphasize the importance of lower initial dose of sedatives with more gradual titration [2].

Regarding colon preparation, polyethylene sulfate purge causes less associated water and electrolyte abnormalities and may be preferable to saline purge in elderly patients with comorbid renal or cardiovascular disease. If the patient is unable to take the purgative by mouth, the placement of a nasogastric tube is necessary.

31.6.2 Angiography

Angiography allows the localization of the bleeding source when the rate is as low as 0.5–1 mL/min. The accuracy of this test is 27–77% for bleeding localization, depending on the series [37]. This procedure is safe and well tolerated in elderly patients. Adverse events can be correlated to complications in the puncture site, such as bleeding, hematomas, and pseudoaneurysms, especially in patients who take anticoagulant or antiplatelet medications. Another adverse event is acute kidney injury (AKI) associated with the administration of iodinated intravenous contrast, especially in patients with comorbid renal diseases and diabetes mellitus and in patients with dehydration prior to the procedure. Interventions to reduce this adverse event include administration of acetylcysteine and bicarbonate fluid hydration. In recent studies, acetylcysteine was shown to provide minimal protection from AKI, while bolus infusion of sodium bicarbonate, in addition to standard hydration, may decrease AKI [2]. Angiography possesses the added benefit of potential therapeutic intervention, with angioembolization and vasopressin injection.

31.6.3 Computed Tomographic Scanning

Contrast-enhanced multidetector-row helical computed tomography (MDCT) scanning has been reported to detect bleeding rates as low as 0.4 mL/min [66]. It has the advantage of being noninvasive and widely available and avoids the risks associated with arterial puncture. However, MDCT has the disadvantage of complications related to the use of intravenous contrast and radiation exposure. Furthermore, it doesn't allow for a therapeutic intervention.

31.6.4 Nuclear Medicine

Nuclear scintigraphy involves Tc-99m-labeled red blood cells or Tc-99m sulfur colloid and has the ability to detect bleeding rates as low as 0.1–0.5 mL/min, although the sensitivity of the test may vary among institutions. The accuracy of this test is 24–78%, depending upon the series [37]. Its advantages are the noninvasiveness and its sensitivity for very slow bleeding, but, like MDCT, it doesn't allow a therapeutic intervention. The often-intermittent nature of some kinds of hemorrhagic lesions means that scintigraphy, MDCT, and angiography can fail to detect the culprit lesion in some patients. Up to 25% of patients with LGIB and a negative scintigraphy result, will experience recurrent bleeding [67, 68].

31.6.5 CT Enterography

CT enterography utilizes orally delivered, neutral contrast material which improves the visualization of pathology within the lumen of the intestine. With this method, active hemorrhage can be visualized more easily than with traditional CT. In addition to the adverse effects related to CT, the large volume of oral contrast liquids necessary for the procedure exposes elderly patients to the risk of aspiration.

31.6.6 Capsule Endoscopy

Capsule endoscopy is useful in small bowel exploration and in identifying the source of small bowel blood loss [69]. This test is safe and well tolerated in the elderly. Inability to swallow the capsule, battery failure before capsule reaches the cecum, and capsule retention are some of the important problems associated with this procedure in elderly as well as in younger patients [70]. Unfortunately, this exam is purely diagnostic, and it doesn't allow for any kind of intervention.

31.7 Management

The primary goals in treating elderly patients with gastrointestinal bleedings are adequate resuscitation, localization of the cause of hemorrhage, and control of the bleeding source.

31.7.1 Adequate Resuscitation

The initial assessment should include evaluation of the airway, breathing, and circulation. With significant hemorrhage, the monitoring of vital signs and the presence of two large venous accesses are necessary. The physical examination should begin with an assessment of hemodynamics (arterial pressure, heart rate, capillary refilling, peripheral vasoconstriction signs), including postural changes. ABG (with pH, pO2, pCO2, lactates, and BE assessment) should be obtained. Particular attention should be made in the evaluation of the hemodynamic status of patients who take beta-blocker medications or have pacemaker, which can be misleading. Adequate fluid resuscitation is necessary, and this should be undertaken prior to endoscopy, to minimize complication. Hypotension at presentation is associated with high mortality among elderly people who present with peptic ulcer hemorrhage, and early aggressive resuscitation decreases mortality [71, 72]. International consensus guidelines for the management of non-variceal UGIB suggest a threshold of 90 or 100 g/L for transfusion in elderly patients with underlying cardiac disease [30]. A nasogastric tube may be placed and saline lavage performed. It is important to consider that approximately 10–15% of patients presenting with hematochezia may have an upper GI source of bleeding. Therefore, it is important to rule out an upper GI bleeding source also in patients presenting apparent LGIB. A nasogastric lavage should be performed, also in elderly patients presenting with a hematochezia, and if the lavage is positive for blood or if there is a suspicion of UGIB, an upper GI endoscopy should be performed as the first endoscopic exam. A Foley catheter should be placed to monitor urine output, and, in the suspicion of UGIB, high-dose IPP should be infused. Airway protection is of primary importance in elderly people during resuscitation, then all patients should be administered with supplementary oxygen, the head of the bed should remain elevated, and prophylactic intubation should be considered in selected cases.

Medical history collected should include prior GI bleeding, previous abdominal surgery, medications taken (aspirin, antiplatelet and anticoagulant medications, NSAID), and comorbid conditions (particularly cardiovascular or pulmonary disease). Then physical findings of chronic liver disease, portal hypertension, and altered coagulation should be sought.

Laboratory evaluation should include complete blood count, serum electrolytes, coagulation parameters, and liver biochemical tests. Thromboelastography (TEG) and thromboelastometry (TEM) can be useful in providing detailed and rapidly available information about coagulation abnormalities of the patient, especially in patients in therapy with newer antithrombotic medications. It is necessary to rapidly correct the coagulopathy and prevent large-volume infusions that may be problematic in patients with cardiopulmonary comorbid conditions. Consensus guidelines on UGIB recommend correction of abnormal coagulation as soon as possible, although endoscopy should not be delayed unless INR is above the therapeutic range [30].

Resuscitation efforts are a cornerstone in the successful management of patients with acute GI bleeding. In the majority of cases, LGIB stops spontaneously with appropriate resuscitation and supportive care [37].

An important aspect to remember is that age is clearly associated with higher mortality largely because of comorbidities. A recent population-based study showed that most UGIB-related deaths are due to non-bleeding causes (79.9%) as opposed to bleeding causes (18.4%) [30]. Therefore, it is important to manage these patients focusing on both controlling hemorrhage and providing general supportive care from the outset.

31.7.2 Localization and Control of the Bleeding Source

31.7.2.1 Endoscopy

In contrast to UGIB, in which EGDS is typically the diagnostic and therapeutic modality of choice, the range of diagnostic modalities more frequently used in patients with LGIB includes endoscopic, radiologic, and angiographic options. However, endoscopy is the primary diagnostic and therapeutic modality for both UGIB and LGIB in hemodynamically stable patients or in patients that have been hemodynamically resuscitated. Timing of upper GI endoscopy for non-variceal bleeding was studied. Evidences suggested that EGDS should be performed in an urgent, but not emergent, fashion. Endoscopy within the first 24 h from admission is safe, and more urgent endoscopy doesn't offer additional benefits [73, 74]. EGDS can identify the stigmata connoting a high risk of rebleeding or continued hemorrhage: presence of spurting vessel, adherent clot, visible vessel, and ulcer greater than 2 cm [3]. In these patients, endoscopic therapy can reduce risk of rebleeding and mortality [3]. If rebleeding occurs, most guidelines for non-variceal UGIB recommend a repeat endoscopy in the first instance, with treatment of bleeding lesions.

Concerning LGIB there is no consensus for the optimal timing for colonoscopy. Adequate visualization during colonoscopy requires bowel preparation which was shown to be safe and effective during acute GI bleeding [75, 76]. However, colonoscopy performed within the first 24 h from admission may offer benefits by providing a definitive diagnosis in up to 96% of patients [77]. If the source of bleeding cannot be controlled during colonoscopy, the bleeding site should be marked with ink tattooing in order to allow the surgeon to identify the portion of colon for resection during surgery.

Endoscopy allows treating the source of bleeding using mechanical clipping, electrical coagulation, or injection of epinephrine. A combined therapy with epinephrine injection followed by mechanical methods of hemostasis is superior in preventing rebleeding than either of these methods alone [30].

31.7.2.2 Angiographic Embolization

Another therapeutic option in hemodynamically stable patients is angiographic embolization, which is highly effective with bleeding controlled in 80–90% of patients [78, 79]. Adverse effects include contrast-induced nephropathy and bowel ischemia that has an incidence of 5% and can result in necrosis and perforation [80]. Catheter-directed infusion of vasopressin may be used to treat bleeding where arterial embolization is not an ideal choice. However, this procedure has a rebleeding rate of 50% [81], and it is not recommended in elderly patients with severe coronary artery disease or cardiac arrhythmias and may also cause bowel ischemia [2]. Rebleeding after arterial embolization is infrequent, and it can be treated with further embolization. Arterial embolization should be considered as an alternative to surgery, especially in patients with high risk of poor surgical outcomes because of advanced age or significant comorbidities. However, a recent meta-analysis showed that there were no significant differences in rebleeding or mortality between surgery and embolization, despite increased age and comorbidities in the embolization group [30].

In a randomized trial, 100 patients with LGIB were randomly allocated to urgent colonoscopy or to technetium-labeled red blood cell scintigraphy followed by angiography. Colonoscopic therapy was delivered to 17 patients, whereas angiographic therapy was performed in 10 patients. There were no differences between the groups for rebleeding rates, transfusion requirements, or the need for emergency surgery [68].

31.7.2.3 Surgery

Indications to surgery in patients with gastrointestinal bleeding are:

- hemodynamic instability
- failure of endoscopy and angiography in controlling bleeding
- transfusion of 4-6 units of blood in 24 hours for LGIB.

Emergent surgery for UGIB has a high rate of morbidity in the elderly [82]. If bleeding is suspected to be caused by a gastric source, an anterior gastrotomy should be performed with ligation of the bleeding source. In case of unlocalized UGIB, gastric devascularization (ligation of the blood supply to the stomach with the exception of the short gastric vessel) can be performed. If the bleeding source is the duodenum, a gastroduodenostomy with oversewing of the bleeding vessel is recommended. In LGIB, segment resection of colon marked by previous endoscopy or identified by a previous angiography is the treatment of choice. Subtotal colectomy may be required if the specific location of the bleeding source cannot be localized, like in patients who have pancolonic diverticular disease. Mortality rates for patients undergoing subtotal colectomy remain high, ranging from 20 to 35% [83, 84], and it's higher in elderly people (37% in patients >70 years old vs 21% in patients <70 years old [85]). Every efforts should be made to identify the bleeding source prior to referral for surgery. Blind segmental resection is associated with very high rebleeding and mortality rates of 47% and 57%, respectively [37].

31.7.2.4 Concomitant Medical Therapy

Endoscopic therapy combined with *PPI* administration results in lower rebleeding rates, shorter hospital stay, lower need of transfusion, and mortality than with endoscopic therapy alone [3, 30]. For patients with proven high-risk endoscopic stigmata, the recommended regimen for intravenous PPIs is omeprazole (or pantoprazole) 80 mg bolus, followed by 8 mg/h for 72 h. Lower doses of PPIs reduce rebleeding but do not affect mortality [30]. If there is no bleeding after 72 h, PPI intravenous therapy can be switched to oral [30].

It is usually recommended that aspirin and clopidogrel are discontinued after UGIB; however, prolonged discontinuation can increase cardiovascular and cerebrovascular risk. One randomized trial [86] suggested that immediate reintroduction of aspirin is associated with a twofold increase in the risk of recurrent bleeding but discontinuation was associated with increased 8-week cardiovascular mortality. Therefore, the decision to discontinue or reintroduce aspirin should be individualized.

The prevalence of *H pylori* infection in patients with peptic ulcer aged over 65 years has been reported to be in the range of 58–78% [87]. In a prospective study, eradication of *H. pylori* infection significantly improved long-term clinical outcomes of peptic ulcer disease in the elderly [88].

References

1. Kaplan RC, et al. Risk factors for hospitalized gastrointestinal bleeding among older persons. J Am Geriatr Soc. 2001;49:126–33.
2. Constantini TW, Kobayashi LM, Coimbra R. Intestinal hemorrhage in elderly. In: Yelon JA, Luchette FA, editors. Geriatric trauma e critical care. New York: Springer Science+Business Media; 2014. p. 145–54.
3. Yachimski PS, Friedman LS. Gastrointestinal bleeding in the elderly. Nat Clin Pract Gastroenterol Hepatol. 2008;5(2):80–93. https://doi.org/10.1038/ncpgasthep1034.
4. Farrell JJ, Friedman LS. Gastrointestinal bleeding in older people. Gastroenterol Clin N Am. 2000;29:1–36.
5. Nikolsky E, Mehran R, Stone GW. Gastrointestinal bleeding in percutaneous coronary intervention and acute coronary syndromes. Am J Cardiol. 2009;104(5 Suppl):22C–9.
6. Hylek EM, Evans-Molina C, Shea C, Henault LE, Regan S. Major hemorrhage and tolerability of warfarin in the first year of therapy among elderly patients with atrial fibrillation. Circulation. 2007;115(21):2689–96.
7. Wierzchowski P. Urgent endoscopy in elderly patients with non-variceal upper gastrointestinal bleeding. Videosurg Other Miniinvasive Tech. 2012;7(4):246–50. https://doi.org/10.5114/wiitm.2011.28907.
8. Rockall TA, et al. Incidence of and mortality from acute upper gastrointestinal haemorrhage in the United Kingdom. Steering Committee and members of the national audit of acute upper gastrointestinal hemorrhage. BMJ. 1995;311:222–6.
9. Longstreth GF. Epidemiology of hospitalization for acute upper gastrointestinal hemorrhage: a population-based study. Am J Gastroenterol. 1995;90:206–10.
10. Seinela L, Ahvenainen J. Peptic ulcer in the very old patients. Gerontology. 2000;46:271–5.
11. Kemppainen H, Raiha I, Sourander L. Clinical presentation of peptic ulcer in the elderly. Gerontology. 1997;43:283–8.
12. Pilotto A, Maggi S, Noale M, et al. Development and validation of a new questionnaire for the evaluation of upper gastrointestinal symptoms in the elderly population: a multicenter study. J Gerontol A Biol Sci Med Sci. 2010;65:174–8.
13. Longstreth GF. Epidemiology and outcome of patients hospitalized with acute lower gastrointestinal hemorrhage: a population-based study. Am J Gastroenterol. 1997;92(3):419–24.
14. Higham J, Kang JY, Majeed A. Recent trends in admissions and mortality due to peptic ulcer in England: increasing frequency of haemorrhage among older subjects. Gut. 2002;50:460–4.
15. Kyaw MH, Chan FK. Pharmacologic options in the management of upper gastrointestinal bleeding: focus on the elderly. Drugs Aging. 2014;31(5):349–61.
16. Newton JL. Improving the gastrointestinal tolerability of aspirin in older people. Clin Interv Aging. 2006;1:33–9.
17. Cryer B, Lee E, Feldman M. Factors influencing gastroduodenal mucosal prostaglandin concentrations: roles of smoking and aging. Ann Intern Med. 1992;116:636–40.
18. Goto H, Sugiyama S, Ohara A, et al. Age-associated decreases in prostaglandin contents in human gastric mucosa. Biochem Biophys Res Commun. 1992;186:1443–8.
19. Guslandi M, Pellegrini A, Sorghi M. Gastric mucosal defences in the elderly. Gerontology. 1999;45:206–8.
20. Kim SW, Parekh D, Townsend CM Jr, et al. Effects of aging on duodenal bicarbonate secretion. Ann Surg. 1990;212:332–7; discussion 337–8
21. Brogna A, Ferrara R, Bucceri AM, et al. Influence of aging on gastrointestinal transit time: an ultrasonographic and radiologic study. Investig Radiol. 1999;34:357–9.
22. Scheiman JM, Yeomans ND, Talley NJ, et al. Prevention of ulcers by esomeprazole in at-risk patients using non-selective NSAIDs and COX-2 inhibitors. Am J Gastroenterol. 2006;101:701–10.
23. Rostom A, Dube C, Wells G, et al. Prevention of NSAID-induced gastroduodenal ulcers. Cochrane Database Syst Rev. 2002;4:CD002296.

24. Yeomans ND, Tulassay Z, Juhasz L, et al. A comparison of omeprazole with ranitidine for ulcers associated with nonsteroidal antiinflammatory drugs: acid suppression trial: ranitidine versus omeprazole for NSAID-associated ulcer treatment (ASTRONAUT) study group. N Engl J Med. 1998;338:719–26.
25. Ishihara M, Ito M. Influence of aging on gastric ulcer healing activities of cimetidine and omeprazole. Eur J Pharmacol. 2002;444:209–15.
26. Maggio M, Corsonello A, Ceda GP, et al. Proton pump inhibitors and risk of 1-year mortality and rehospitalization in older patients discharged from acute care hospitals. JAMA Intern Med. 2013;173:518–23.
27. Deshpande A, Pant C, Pasupuleti V, et al. Association between proton pump inhibitor therapy and *Clostridium difficile* infection in a meta-analysis. Clin Gastroenterol Hepatol. 2012;10:225–33.
28. Johnstone J, Nerenberg K, Loeb M. Meta-analysis: proton pump inhibitor use and the risk of community-acquired pneumonia. Aliment Pharmacol Ther. 2010;31:1165–77.
29. Ngamruengphong S, Leontiadis GI, Radhi S, et al. Proton pump inhibitors and risk of fracture: a systematic review and metaanalysis of observational studies. Am J Gastroenterol. 2011;106:1209–18; quiz 1219
30. Ahmed A, Stanley AJ. Acute upper gastrointestinal bleeding in the elderly: aetiology, diagnosis and treatment. Drugs Aging. 2012;29(12):933–40. https://doi.org/10.1007/s40266-012-0020-5.
31. Hosking SW, et al. Management of bleeding varices in the elderly. BMJ. 1989;298:152–3.
32. Bergqvist D, et al. Secondary aortoenteric fistulate—changes from 1973 to 1993. Eur J Endovasc Surg. 1996;11:425–8.
33. Cendan JC, et al. Twenty-one cases of aortoenteric fistula: lessons for the general surgeon. Am Surg. 2004;70:583–7.
34. Rockall TA, Logan RFA, Devlin HB, et al. Risk assessment after acute upper gastrointestinal haemorrhage. Gut. 1996;38:316–21.
35. Blatchford O, Murray WR, Blatchford M. A risk score to predict need for treatment of upper gastrointestinal haemorrhage. Lancet. 2000;356:1318–21.
36. Wang CY, Qin J, Wang J, Sun CY, Cao T, Zhu DD. Rockall score in predicting outcomes of elderly patients with acute upper gastrointestinal bleeding. World J Gastrointest Endosc. 2010;2(5):147–54. https://doi.org/10.4253/wjge.v2.i5.147.38.
37. Chait MM. Lower gastrointestinal bleeding in the elderly. World J Gastrointest Endosc. 2010;2(5):147–54. https://doi.org/10.4253/wjge.v2.i5.147.
38. McGuire HH Jr. Bleeding colonic diverticula. A reappraisal of natural history and management. Ann Surg. 1994;220(5):653–6.
39. Comay D, Marshall JK. Resource utilization for acute lower gastrointestinal hemorrhage: the Ontario GI bleed study. Can J Gastroenterol. 2002;16:677–82.
40. Ríos A, Montoya MJ, Rodríguez JM, Serrano A, Molina J, Parrilla P. Acute lower gastrointestinal hemorrhages in geriatric patients. Dig Dis Sci. 2005;50:898–904.
41. Rockey DC. Lower gastrointestinal bleeding. Gastroenterology. 2006;130:165–71.
42. Rhee JC, Lee KT. The causes and management of lower GI bleeding: a study based on clinical observations at Hanyang University Hospital. Gastroenterol Jpn. 1991;26(Suppl 3):101–6.
43. Bokhari M, Vernava AM, Ure T, Longo WE. Diverticular hemorrhage in the elderly—is it well tolerated? Dis Colon Rectum. 1996;39:191–5.
44. Stollman N, Raskin JB. Diverticular disease of the colon. Lancet. 2004;363:631–9.
45. Reinus JF, Brandt LJ. Vascular ectasias and diverticulosis. Common causes of lower intestinal bleeding. Gastroenterol Clin N Am. 1994;23:1–20.
46. Boley SJ, Sammartano R, Adams A, DiBiase A, Kleinhaus S, Sprayregen S. On the nature and etiology of vascular ectasias of the colon. Degenerative lesions of aging. Gastroenterology. 1977;72:650–60.
47. Imperiale TF, Ransohoff DF. Aortic stenosis, idiopathic gastrointestinal bleeding, and angiodysplasia: is there an association? A methodologic critique of the literature. Gastroenterology. 1988;95:1670–6.
48. Lindner AE. Inflammatory bowel disease in the elderly. Clin Geriatr Med. 1999;15:487–97.

49. Robertson DJ, Grimm IS. Inflammatory bowel disease in the elderly. Gastroenterol Clin N Am. 2001;30:409–26.
50. Robert JH, Sachar DB, Aufses AH Jr, Greenstein AJ. Management of severe hemorrhage in ulcerative colitis. Am J Surg. 1990;159:550–5.
51. Medina C, Vilaseca J, Videla S, Fabra R, Armengol-Miro JR, Malagelada JR. Outcome of patients with ischemic colitis: review of fifty-three cases. Dis Colon Rectum. 2004;47:180–4.
52. Lew JF, Glass RI, Gangarosa RE, Cohen IP, Bern C, Moe CL. Diarrheal deaths in the United States, 1979 through 1987. A special problem for the elderly. JAMA. 1991;265:3280–4.
53. Guerrant RL, Van Gilder T, Steiner TS, Thielman NM, Slutsker L, Tauxe RV, Hennessy T, Griffin PM, DuPont H, Sack RB, Tarr P, Neill M, Nachamkin I, Reller LB, Osterholm MT, Bennish ML, Pickering LK. Practice guidelines for the management of infectious diarrhea. Clin Infect Dis. 2001;32:331–51.
54. Slotwiner-Nie PK, Brandt LJ. Infectious diarrhea in the elderly. Gastroenterol Clin N Am. 2001;30:625–35.
55. Peura DA, Lanza FL, Gostout CJ, Foutch PG. The American College of Gastroenterology bleeding registry: preliminary findings. Am J Gastroenterol. 1997;92:924–8.
56. Richter JM, Christensen MR, Kaplan LM, Nishioka NS. Effectiveness of current technology in the diagnosis and management of lower gastrointestinal hemorrhage. Gastrointest Endosc. 1995;41:93–8.
57. Kim HS, Kim TI, Kim WH, Kim YH, Kim HJ, Yang SK, Myung SJ, Byeon JS, Lee MS, Chung IK, Jung SA, Jeen YT, Choi JH, Choi KY, Choi H, Han DS, Song JS. Risk factors for immediate post-polypectomy bleeding of the colon: a multicenter study. Am J Gastroenterol. 2006;101:1333–41.
58. Mühldorfer SM, Kekos G, Hahn EG, Ell C. Complications of therapeutic gastrointestinal endoscopy. Endoscopy. 1992;24:276–83.
59. Rex DK, Lewis BS, Waye JD. Colonoscopy and endoscopic therapy for delayed post-polypectomy hemorrhage. Gastrointest Endosc. 1992;38:127–9.
60. Tseng CA, Chen LT, Tsai KB, Su YC, Wu DC, Jan CM, Wang WM, Pan YS. Acute hemorrhagic rectal ulcer syndrome: a new clinical entity? Report of 19 cases and review of the literature. Dis Colon Rectum. 2004;47:895–903; discussion 903–905
61. Jafri SM, Monkemuller K, Lukens FJ. Endoscopy in the elderly: a review of the efficacy and safety of colonoscopy, esophagogastroduodenoscopy, and endoscopic retrograde cholangiopancreatography. J Clin Gastroenterol. 2010;44(3):161–6.
62. Hilton D, Iman N, Burke GJ, Moore A, O'Mara G, Signorini D, Lyons D, Banerjee AK, Clinch D. Absence of abdominal pain in older persons with endoscopic ulcers: a prospective study. Am J Gastroenterol. 2001;96:380–4.
63. Waye JD, Bashkoff E. Total colonoscopy: is it always possible? Gastrointest Endosc. 1991;37:152–4.
64. Zuckerman DA, Bocchini TP, Birnbaum EH. Massive hemorrhage in the lower gastrointestinal tract in adults: diagnostic imaging and intervention. Am J Roentgenol. 1993;161:703–11.
65. Christe C, Janssens JP, Armenian B, Herrmann F, Vogt N. Midazolam sedation for upper gastrointestinal endoscopy in older persons: a randomized, double-blind, placebo-controlled study. J Am Geriatr Soc. 2000;48(11):1398–403.
66. Katschinski B, Logan R, Davies J, Faulkner G, Pearson J, Langman M. Prognostic factors in upper gastrointestinal bleeding. Dig Dis Sci. 1994;39(4):706–12.
67. Hammond KL, et al. Implications of negative technetium 99m-labeled red blood cell scintigraphy in patients presenting with lower gastrointestinal bleeding. Am J Surg. 2007;193:404–7.
68. Green BT, et al. Urgent colonoscopy for the evaluation and management of acute lower gastrointestinal hemorrhage: a randomized controlled trial. Am J Gastroenterol. 2005;100:2395–402.
69. Laine L, Sahota A, Shah A. Does capsule endoscopy improve outcomes in obscure gastrointestinal bleeding? Randomized trial versus dedicated small bowel radiography. Gastroenterology. 2010;138(5):1673.e1–80.e1; quiz e11–2
70. Orlando G, Luppino IM, Lerose MA, Gervasi R, Amato B, Silecchia G, Puzziello A. Feasibility of capsule endoscopy in elderly patients with obscure gastrointestinal bleeding. An up-to-date report. BMC Surg. 2012;12(Suppl 1):S30. https://doi.org/10.1186/1471-2482-12-S1-S30.

71. Baradarian R, et al. Early intensive resuscitation of patients with upper gastrointestinal bleeding decreases mortality. Am J Gastroenterol. 2004;99:619–22.
72. Hasselgren G, et al. Risk factors for rebleeding and fatal outcome in elderly patients with acute peptic ulcer bleeding. Eur J Gastroenterol Hepatol. 1998;10:667–72.
73. Qureshi WA, Zuckerman MJ, Adler DG, Davila RE, Egan JV, Gan SI, et al. ASGE guideline: modifications in endoscopic practice for the elderly. Gastrointest Endosc. 2006;63(4):566–9.
74. Sarin N, Monga N, Adams PC. Time to endoscopy and outcomes in upper gastrointestinal bleeding. Can J Gastroenterol. 2009;23(7):489–93.
75. Gilbert DA, Silverstein FE, Tedesco FJ. National ASGE survey on upper gastrointestinal bleeding: complications of endoscopy. Dig Dis Sci. 1981;26(7 Suppl):55S–9.
76. Gilbert DA, Silverstein FE, Tedesco FJ, Buenger NK, Persing J. The national ASGE survey on upper gastrointestinal bleeding. III. Endoscopy in upper gastrointestinal bleeding. Gastrointest Endosc. 1981;27(2):94–102.
77. Lipof T, Sardella WV, Bartus CM, Johnson KH, Vignati PV, Cohen JL. The efficacy and durability of super-selective embolization in the treatment of lower gastrointestinal bleeding. Dis Colon Rectum. 2008;51(3):301–5.
78. Kuo WT. Transcatheter treatment for lower gastrointestinal hemorrhage. Tech Vasc Interv Radiol. 2004;7(3):143–50.
79. Bandi R, Shetty PC, Sharma RP, Burke TH, Burke MW, Kastan D. Superselective arterial embolization for the treatment of lower gastrointestinal hemorrhage. J Vasc Interv Radiol. 2001;12(12):1399–405.
80. Kuo WT, Lee DE, Saad WE, Patel N, Sahler LG, Waldman DL. Superselective microcoil embolization for the treatment of lower gastrointestinal hemorrhage. J Vasc Interv Radiol. 2003;14(12):1503–9.
81. Clark RA, Colley DP, Eggers FM. Acute arterial gastrointestinal hemorrhage: efficacy of transcatheter control. Am J Roentgenol. 1981;136(6):1185–9.
82. Clarke MG, Bunting D, Smart NJ, Lowes J, Mitchell SJ. The surgical management of acute upper gastrointestinal bleeding: a 12-year experience. Int J Surg. 2010;8(5):377–80.
83. Gianfrancisco JA, Abcarian H. Pitfalls in the treatment of massive lower gastrointestinal bleeding with "blind" subtotal colectomy. Dis Colon Rectum. 1982;25(5):441–5.
84. Setya V, Singer JA, Minken SL. Subtotal colectomy as a last resort for unrelenting, unlocalized, lower gastrointestinal hemorrhage: experience with 12 cases. Am Surg. 1992;58(5):295–9.
85. Bender JS, et al. Morbidity and mortality following total abdominal colectomy for massive lower gastrointestinal bleeding. Am Surg. 1991;57:536–40.
86. Sung J, Lau J, Ching J, et al. Early reintroduction of aspirin with proton pump inhibitor after endoscopic hemostasis for peptic ulcer bleeding. Gut. 2007;56:A27.
87. Pilotto A. *Helicobacter pylori*-associated peptic ulcer disease in older patients: current management strategies. Drugs Aging. 2001;18:487–94.
88. Pilotto A, Franceschi M, Di Mario F, et al. The long-term clinical outcome of elderly patients with *Helicobacter pylori*-associated peptic ulcer disease. Gerontology. 1998;44:153–8.

MIX
Papier aus verantwortungsvollen Quellen
Paper from responsible sources
FSC® C105338

If you have any concerns about our products,
you can contact us on
ProductSafety@springernature.com

In case Publisher is established outside the EU,
the EU authorized representative is:
Springer Nature Customer Service Center GmbH
Europaplatz 3, 69115 Heidelberg, Germany

Printed by Libri Plureos GmbH
in Hamburg, Germany